PAIN-FREE PERFORMANCE

MOVE BETTER,
TRAIN SMARTER, AND BUILD
AN **UNBREAKABLE BODY**

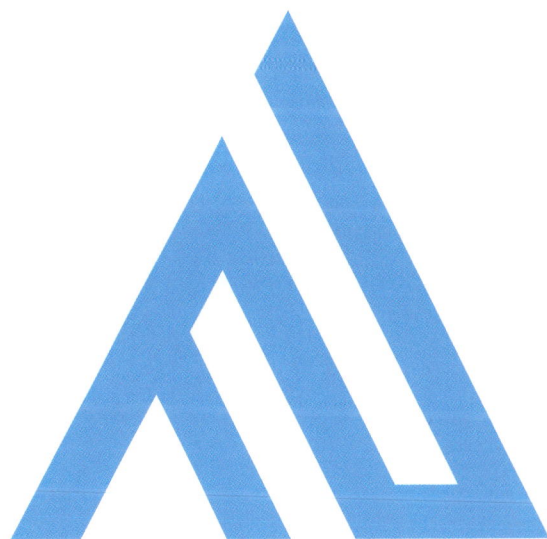

DR. JOHN RUSIN
with **GLEN CORDOZA**

VICTORY BELT PUBLISHING INC.
LAS VEGAS

First published in 2025 by Victory Belt Publishing Inc.

ISBN-13: 978-1-628605-09-9

The information included in this book is for educational purposes only. It is not intended or implied to be a substitute for professional medical advice. The reader should always consult their healthcare provider to determine the appropriateness of the information for their own situation or if they have any questions regarding a medical condition or treatment plan. Reading the information in this book does not constitute a physician-patient relationship.

The author/owner claims no responsibility to any person or entity for any liability, loss, or damage caused or alleged to be caused directly or indirectly as a result of the use, application, or interpretation of the information presented herein.

Cover design by Justin-Aaron Velasco

Interior design and illustrations by Yordan Terziev and Boryana Yordanova

Photos of John Rusin and Lalaina Duncan by Glen Cordoza

Printed in Canada

TC 0125

TO MY SON, CAM. WITH YOUR HEALTH—AND A
LOT OF HARD WORK—ANYTHING IS POSSIBLE.
CHASE YOUR DREAMS.

INTRODUCTION

"How many of you are currently in pain?"

I'm standing at the front of the room, teaching the Pain-Free Performance Specialist Certification (PPSC) to a group of elite trainers and fitness professionals.

When I ask that question, nearly half the room raises a hand.

Then I ask another:

"How many of you feel less than your best?"

Almost every hand goes up.

It always stops me for a moment. Because these aren't weekend warriors or casual gym-goers. These are some of the most skilled, experienced coaches in the industry—the top 1 percent. They know how the body works. They know what training is supposed to do.

And still, so many of them are stuck. Fighting through pain. Managing injuries. Dealing with that frustrating sense that something just isn't moving the way it should.

At first, it's hard to make sense of it. How can the people who know the most about exercise still feel broken by it?

Exercise is meant to be the fix. It's the tool we turn to for more strength, better movement, and a body that lasts. When used correctly, it recalibrates everything. It rebuilds posture, reinforces stability, restores range of motion, and reawakens the parts of us that go offline from sitting too long or moving too little. It's one of the most powerful levers we have for promoting physical health and longevity.

But only when it's done right.

Because when it's not—when training skips over the fundamentals or fails to match the needs of the individual—it stops being a solution and starts becoming a source of stress. It places more demand on a system that's already out of balance. And instead of promoting health, it pushes the body deeper into dysfunction.

Here's where most people go wrong.

They jump into training that's too advanced or too random. They chase intensity before they've earned it. They skip warm-ups, ignore pain signals, and let social media trends dictate which exercises they do—without ever asking whether those movements are right for their body.

Over time, those missteps add up. Movement quality breaks down. Injuries creep in. And training becomes another thing to work around.

At that point, it's no longer helping. It's holding them back.

That's what brought those trainers into the room with me. They were there to learn a system—one that integrates performance and pain prevention. One that would help them—and the people they coach—not only train harder but train smarter.

That's the system this book will teach you.

THIS IS WHAT YOU'RE REALLY AFTER

If you've picked up this book, chances are you're looking for a better way to train. You want to feel good in your body. You want to move with confidence and consistency. And most importantly, you want to know that your effort is building something sustainable.

That's the promise of pain-free performance. But to turn that promise into progress, it's important to understand what it means.

Pain-free means doing no harm while training. It means you are able to exercise without eliciting a pain response. It doesn't mean the absence of all discomfort. And it certainly doesn't mean you'll wake up one day and never feel pain.

After working with thousands of clients and coaches around the world, I've stopped expecting anyone to be completely pain-free. That mythical unicorn doesn't exist. Pain is part of life. But it exists on a spectrum. On one end, you've got minor aches that come and go. On the other, you've got the kind of pain that sidelines you and chips away at your confidence to move.

What matters is how you respond to it.

If you stop moving entirely—"let's take six weeks off and see how it feels"— you slide into deactivation. Muscles weaken. Posture collapses. You become a lesser version of yourself.

If you try to grind through with a "no pain, no gain" mentality, you stack wear-and-tear on top of dysfunction until something breaks—and then you're forced to stop.

Pain-free training is the middle path—one that respects your body's signals while continuing to build capacity. It's training in a way that improves how you move rather than pushing through or backing away. It means finishing workouts feeling energized, not broken down. Pain-free is about aligning your training with your individual anatomy, movement capabilities, and goals, ensuring each exercise fits you—not the other way around. Ultimately, it's about finding a sustainable approach that empowers you to move with freedom, intention, and trust in your body.

Performance is about how you feel and function in the things that matter to you. It's playing with your kids. It's excelling in your career. It's chasing a personal record in the gym, competing in sports, or completing a physical challenge you've never done before. At its core, performance is your health— how well your body supports your life, in and out of the gym.

Don't fall for the misconception that performance comes at a cost. It doesn't.

Pain-free and *performance* don't compete—they compound. You don't have to choose between feeling good and performing well. When your training stops creating pain and starts building resilience, better performance—and better health—will follow. That's pain-free performance.

PUTTING THE SYSTEM TO WORK— HOW TO NAVIGATE THIS BOOK

Safe and effective training requires structure. The better you understand how the system fits together, the more you'll get from the work you're about to do.

If you're the kind of person who likes to skip ahead or you want to start training immediately, you'll find detailed programs and training templates in Part 4. You can jump in today. But to get the most out of this process—to make your training more efficient, sustainable, and pain-free—it's worth understanding the why behind the how.

That begins with understanding what it means to move well. In Part 1, you'll learn the real meaning of *form*—not as a rigid set of rules but as a dynamic, personalized framework for safe and effective movement. You'll understand why bracing, breathing, and stabilization help you avoid injury and unlock better performance. You'll also step into the movement mastery mindset, a philosophy that places quality before quantity and intentionality at the center of every rep.

In Part 2, you'll learn the 6-phase dynamic warm-up: the go-to prep sequence that blends the best of physical therapy with the principles of performance training. More than just a warm-up, this sequence is your daily opportunity to refine your movement, alleviate pain, and create a consistent results-based practice that supports recovery and long-term progress. Each phase plays a specific role in helping you move with more control and confidence, whether you're getting ready for a workout, winding down after training, or simply restoring your body.

Part 3 is all about the core of human movement—the six foundational patterns: squat, hinge, push, pull, lunge, and carry. You'll explore how to train these patterns in the way your body was designed to move and how to select exercises that align with your anatomy and experience level. You'll learn how to screen and assess your movement to identify what your body can do well right now—and what needs to be refined, adjusted, or built upon.

You'll also discover the movement pattern pyramids—structured frameworks that clearly outline how to regress or progress exercises based on how you feel, function, and perform. These pyramids help you choose movements tailored specifically to your current capabilities, ensuring safe, effective, and continuous progress. From there, you'll dive into biomechanics, dialing in your setup and execution to ensure each movement is progressed appropriately.

In Part 4, the system comes to life. You'll get complete training programs built around everything you've learned—structured to match your movement patterns, address common pain points, and train the physical qualities that keep you strong and capable. Each program includes a dynamic warm-up, a structured workout, and a cooldown aligned with what your body needs most that day.

You'll also find linchpin blueprints—targeted mobility and stability sequences built around the 6-phase warm-up. These are designed to help you restore your most vulnerable areas, prevent and alleviate pain, and improve the way you move. Think of them as your go-to recovery and mobility plans.

Every part of this book serves a purpose. Not to overwhelm you with options, but to guide you toward clarity. To give you a starting point and process you can trust.

This is your blueprint. Your path to pain-free performance.

NEED A VISUAL? SCAN THE QR CODE.

Throughout this book, you'll find QR codes that link to demo videos for every exercise. These demos were created to help you apply the information more effectively—to give you a moving visual reference for all the exercises covered.

Scan the codes. Watch the demos. Use them as a quick reference for unfamiliar exercises or to verify that you're moving with proper form.

01

PRINCIPLES
OF PAIN-FREE
PERFORMANCE

THE FOUNDATIONS OF PAIN-FREE PERFORMANCE

Form matters.

We've all heard the adage that form matters—that to minimize risk of pain and injury and optimize performance, we must move with good form. But what exactly does "form" mean, and why does it matter?

FORM refers to the specific technique and alignment used during movement to enhance motor control and motor unit recruitment. It involves the proper sequencing, symmetry, and stability of the body to ensure movements are smooth and controlled.

And form matters because it promotes

▼
SAFETY:
Proper form acts as a safeguard against pain and injury by minimizing strain on joints, ligaments, and soft tissues. It encourages efficient biomechanics that avoid unwanted stress on vulnerable areas.

▼
EFFECTIVENESS:
Correct form targets muscles and muscle groups accurately. Dismissing exercise form based on your anatomy and functional abilities can undermine the intended focus by shifting the workload away from the targeted muscles, hindering performance and progress.

▼
PROGRESSION:
Form isn't static; it's a stepping stone to growth. It paves the way for gradual advancement and exploration of new exercises.

▼
EFFICIENCY:
Ideal form optimizes energy and effort, leading to better results in less time.

▼
CONSISTENCY:
Continual adherence to and progressive advancement of proper form amplify the exercise-enhancing, performance-boosting, and injury-protective benefits while promoting movement skills that transfer from the gym to everyday physical activities.

Knowing what form means—and why it matters—is central to pain-free performance because how you move influences your emotional and physical state, your resilience against pain and injury, and your overall performance in workouts and daily life.

But form is subjective. There is no one perfect way to move. Someone's "good form" might be less than ideal for someone else and vice versa. It's not about right and wrong or chasing perfection; it's about knowing what is optimal or suboptimal for your body and seeking continual improvements. It's about following universal principles and guidelines that unlock your movement potential and cater to your unique needs, regardless of the exercise you are performing, your experience, or your functional abilities.

This section delves into these core principles and guidelines (mindset, stabilization, and breathing strategies) that underpin safe, effective, and efficient form, marking the beginning of your journey toward pain-free performance.

MOTOR CONTROL refers to the nervous system's ability to coordinate and execute movements effectively. It encompasses the planning, execution, and regulation of movement patterns, integrating sensory input (like balance and feedback) with muscular output to ensure precise performance.

MOTOR UNIT RECRUITMENT is more specific and refers to the process by which the nervous system activates motor units (a motor neuron and the muscle fibers it innervates) to generate force. The greater the demand for force in a movement, the more motor units are recruited. It's about how many muscle fibers are activated to perform a task and how effectively they are used to produce strength or power.

In the context of form, **MOTOR CONTROL** ensures the movement is executed efficiently and safely, while **MOTOR UNIT RECRUITMENt** ensures the correct amount of muscle fibers are activated to meet the physical demands of the movement.

THE MOVEMENT MASTERY MINDSET

Moving meaningfully is a cornerstone practice for pain-free performance. Whether in structured training or unstructured physical activity, you must adopt a movement mastery mindset. That is an intention to become a master of your movement patterns—to critique, improve, and maintain the quality of your movement forever.

*I'm sitting in the bleachers closely observing my client—
an internationally ranked top ten tennis player—work with her
coach ahead of the Australian Open.*

Nearly three hours have passed, and I can't help but marvel at the level of meticulous detail they're pouring into her serving technique. They're making tiny, barely perceptible adjustments to her stance and body position to get her a fraction of a percent better. Every motion is an embodiment of finesse and precision. There is a reason she is one of the best competitors in the world. She has a deep respect for the game, and she's willing to spend countless hours refining movement skills, delving into the minutiae of form, all for the sake of optimized performance.

It's a trait that's common to every professional athlete I've had the honor of working with. They dedicate four to six hours daily to honing their intricate sport-specific skills, driven by an unwavering pursuit of movement mastery. For these athletes, movement mastery embodies a mindset characterized by purposeful intention, continuous refinement, and precise execution. It's about cultivating synergy between mind and body and embedding movements so deeply that they become second nature during competition. It's this fusion of acute mental focus and physical efficiency that defines their approach— the orchestration of technique that merges mindfulness with motion.

As the trainer to these athletes, I was brought in for a specific purpose: to help them achieve pain-free performance. With a background in sports performance and physical therapy, I designed strength and conditioning programs around the demands of their sport while addressing whatever pain or injury they had with individualized training. It was my job to keep them healthy—to build their strength and make them more resilient so they had less pain and better performance in their sport.

The tennis star, for example, was banged up from toes to crown. She had ankle and foot issues, hip and back pain, shoulder problems, and the list went on—and changed from day to day. Finding exercises that she could perform without pain was straightforward. I would simply scale the exercise and load to match her current level of performance for whichever movement pattern she was performing (an approach that you will learn how to implement in Part 3). However, getting her to perform these movements with the same level of intent and focus that she put into her tennis serve was a challenge.

On the court, she had a movement mastery mindset. She was focused on her body position, sequencing and coordinating her actions to be as effective and efficient as possible. In the gym, however, she essentially punched the clock, did the work, and went home. She did not apply the movement mastery mindset to training, which surprised me. After all, we're talking about a world-class athlete who routinely spends several hours focused on one sport-specific skill—and who often struggles performing to her true potential due to constant pain.

In our sessions, we're building foundational movement patterns that are intrinsic to human biomechanics, aiming primarily to improve the quality of her movement: enhancing muscle coordination, increasing joint stability, and ensuring pain-free motion. If she improved in these areas, she would have more capacity and less pain performing the skills in her sport. She would get stronger and more resilient everywhere—and for everything. But she hadn't connected those dots.

Interestingly, this disconnect wasn't unique to her. Many professional athletes I worked with over the years had a similar mentality. They pursued movement mastery within their sport, but rarely applied it to their exercise form in the gym. It's not that they didn't have the ability to perform exercise movements with pristine form. They have a level of movement mastery that most of us can only dream of. It's that they didn't make the connection between their exercise form and the positive impact it would have on their sport performance, longevity, and overall movement health.

We can all relate to this. We devote a ton of focus and energy to the things we enjoy (even if it hurts us) and half-ass the things we don't (even when it is good for us). What we need to do is shift our perspective and approach exercise form with the same level of intent we would have when performing the activities that we are training for. Whether you are perfecting a serve for the Australian Open, seeking an edge in the next pickleball tournament, or simply training to feel and move better, adopting a movement mastery mindset in the gym can lead to improved performance and resiliency in sport and in life. It will help you build your skills faster and prime your mind and body for better, safer movement. Because when you strive to improve the quality of your movement, you get stronger, faster, and more efficient. You will have fewer occurrences of pain and more reliable functional abilities in all areas and for every activity.

MOVE WITH PURPOSE

In the early 1990s, Anders Ericsson—a Swedish psychologist renowned for his research on human performance—published a paper along with his colleagues titled "The Role of Deliberate Practice in the Acquisition of Expert Performance." In this paper, they introduce the concept of deliberate practice, emphasizing the role of purposeful training to improve performance and expertise. Ericsson's work debunks the mere reliance on innate talent and underscores the significance of quality over quantity in practice.[1]

To achieve movement mastery, you must apply the concept of deliberate practice in your training. Deliberate practice refers to a systematic and focused regimen designed to improve certain aspects, offer feedback, and refine performance. It involves pushing beyond your comfort zone, identifying weaknesses, and making continuous, targeted improvements—every single time.

This is the exact approach that the tennis prodigy and her coach used when practicing her serve. They broke down the overarching skill into individual components (stance, body position, sequencing, etc.) with a keen understanding of each nuance, and then refined them based on her performance. She didn't mindlessly repeat the movement. Together they sought ways to make every repetition better with a specific objective: improving the efficiency and repeatability of her serve.

Mastering the modality-specific movements in the 6-phase warm-up in Part 2, as well as the foundational movement patterns in Part 3, requires a similar approach with the same goal. You need

▼ MINDFUL AWARENESS:
To engage mentally with the movement, being present and in tune with your body's feedback so you can recognize potentially problematic patterns and make the necessary adjustments.

▼ VALUE OF QUALITY:
To prioritize quality over sheer effort or speed.

▼ CONTINUOUS LEARNING:
To be open to feedback, whether from trainers, peers, or self-assessment, and adjust accordingly to refine your form.

▼ MIND-MUSCLE-MOVEMENT CONNECTION:
To develop a deeper connection between the mind, movement, and muscles being used, ensuring accurate activation, tension, and fluency.

▼ CONSISTENCY:
To engage in regular and deliberate practice, ingraining the proper movement patterns until they become second nature.

Put together, the components of deliberate practice provide a process not only for achieving a high level of skill but also for patterning efficient and automatic movement. When it comes to exercise form, intuitive execution is the ultimate goal. It's the "why" that influences the "how"—the driving force behind your purposeful practice.

THE RELIABLE AUTOPILOT

Learning a movement, like a squat or a tennis serve, requires considerable mental engagement. Initially, each motion might feel awkward as your brain and body work to internalize the correct pattern. But as you practice and refine the movement, your nervous system becomes more efficient at coordinating the muscles and joints involved. With time and deliberate practice, properly executed movements become intuitive, requiring less conscious thought and more automatic execution. When a movement becomes second nature through repetition and correct motor learning, it's like switching on a reliable autopilot for your body. You don't have to think about every little detail of the movement; the body "knows" what to do, just as an autopilot manages the nuances of flight once activated.

This is the essence of movement mastery. The foundational movement patterns are *foundational* because they are the basis for human movement, meaning they are patterns buried in the daily activities of life. Your practiced movements in the gym translate to real-life situations. When you strengthen them, and you can control them through your full ranges of motion, you encode a reliable autopilot for movement that is there to assist you when your focus is elsewhere—whether that is catching yourself from an unexpected fall or moving in a way that places less wear and tear on your body. It's a protective mechanism against injuries, much like an autopilot can ensure the plane stays on a safe and efficient course even in turbulence or challenging conditions. Stated differently, you have a level of proficiency that is automatic, so you don't need to put conscious effort into moving effectively when it matters the most.

In this way, the gym is a place where you rehearse for life's unexpected scenarios. The more repetitions of quality movement you do, the better you can fortify yourself against unforeseen challenges. When a challenge comes, you've put in enough focused reps that efficient movement is reactionary. This isn't about forecasting every challenge but about preparing your mind and body to respond with precision. Whether you're performing an exercise in the gym or just moving through life, the goal is to program an autopilot for movement that is reliable—that will fly you where you need to go, regardless of the task or activity.

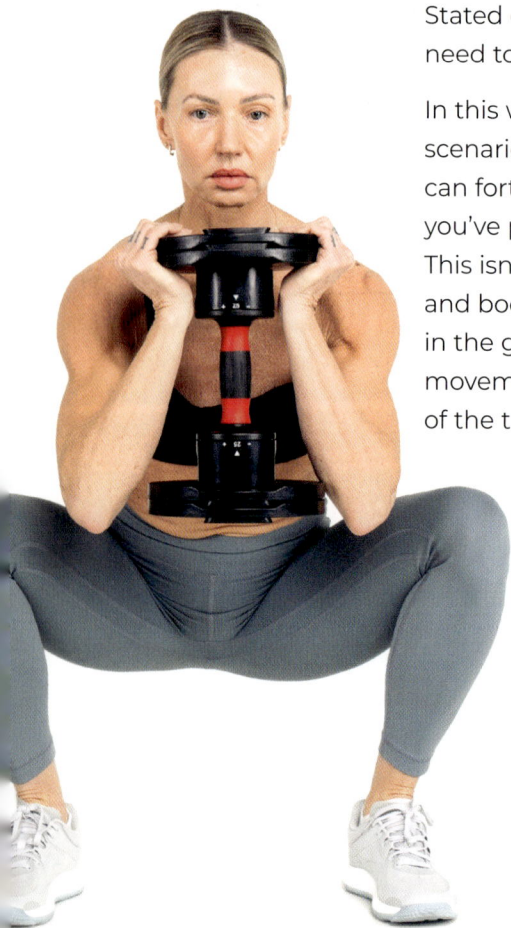

REPROGRAMMING THE INTUITIVE AUTOPILOT

What feels natural may not be optimal. Take the foundational movement patterns you perform daily: squatting, hinging, lunging, pushing, pulling, and carrying (locomotion). While these actions are intuitive and ingrained, their efficiency and reliability are not assured, especially if you haven't consciously refined these patterns or adapted them to your unique physical needs.

This is where challenge meets opportunity—to reprogram your intuitive autopilot. The goal isn't to discard what you already know about your body but to unlock your movement potential by refining and enhancing what already exists within you. This demands a comprehensive approach, transcending mere adjustments to a squat or tweaks to a lunge. It's about awakening and optimizing the skills built into the patterns, custom-fitted to your anatomy and capabilities. Through this process, you will make quality movement not just a practice but a habit, effortlessly integrated into every action, ensuring a lifetime of pain-free performance.

THE MOVEMENT MASTERY FRAMEWORK

A reliable autopilot means using the correct muscles at the right time, with the appropriate force, and in a functional manner. To sequence and control your movement without having to think about it. That's what you're after.

But how do you get to that point? I realize that simply telling you to be purposeful with your training isn't that helpful, even if the concepts are clear and actionable. So, let's map out a path to movement mastery that you can apply to the modalities and exercises in the coming chapters.

It starts with an intention to move well.

Any voluntary movement begins with an intention in the brain. This intention generates a neural blueprint or plan for the movement. An intention to move well refers to a conscious commitment to optimize the quality of your movements in all physical activities, but especially the exercises you perform in the gym. This involves a proactive mindset that does the following:

▼

Prioritizes proper form, biomechanics, and body alignment, ensuring every motion is purposeful, efficient, and safe

▼

Grounds you in the present, enhancing your awareness of body mechanics

▼

Strengthens neural connections that power pain-free movement, enriching physical engagement with every activity you undertake

▼

Deepens your respect and appreciation for your exercise form, harmonizing your attention with the universal movement principles and guidelines explored in this book

Rather than mindlessly pushing through training sessions, you will engage fully with your body, transforming your workout into a mindful practice where every movement is imbued with intentionality and control.

With an intention to move well guiding your practice, channel it toward the development of motor control proficiency.

In the realm of exercise and movement science, *motor control* refers to the process of initiating and directing voluntary movements. It involves the coordination and integration of various body parts and systems—including muscles, joints, and the neurological system—to perform a specific task or activity.

COGNITIVE STAGE

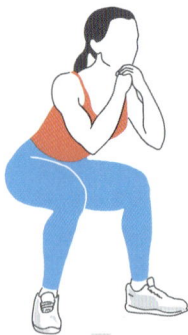

Developing proficient motor control is a step-by-step process, often illustrated in stages.[2] First, there's the **cognitive stage**, which requires a high level of conscious involvement as you work to understand the nuances of what needs to be done. The key is to remain patient, move slowly, and stay engaged. Performance is typically inconsistent in this stage, and errors are to be expected. If you're squatting, for example, you may not know where to place your feet, how to coordinate your body, or how deep to go. This is the stage where you're working out the technique with the goal of cultivating a strong mind-muscle-movement connection (thinking about and feeling the muscles that power the movement pattern you're working to develop).

ASSOCIATIVE STAGE

Second is the **associative stage**, which involves associating cues with the required motor actions. This is where you start to apply the components of deliberate practice to refine your skill, reduce errors, and become more consistent. Keeping with the squat example, you will start noticing areas of improvement. You might realize, "If I keep my knees aligned over my toes, I feel more stable," or, "When I engage my hips, shoulders, and core, I don't feel pain in my lower back." Every adjustment and refinement develops motor control proficiency. You will get stronger, enhance your mobility, and gain confidence as your movement quality improves.

AUTONOMOUS STAGE

The third stage is where you start to develop a reliable autopilot. It is the **autonomous stage** where the skill becomes automatic. You don't need to consciously think about the movement; you can perform it reliably and efficiently. For example, you will be able to squat without analyzing every detail, progress to more complex variations, and make intuitive in-the-moment corrections to maintain excellent form.

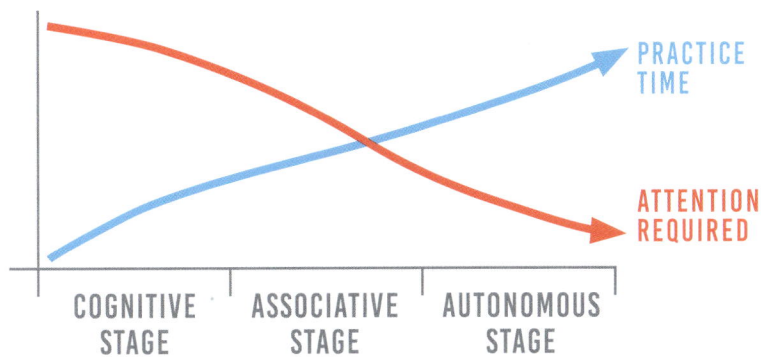

PRACTICE TIME

ATTENTION REQUIRED

COGNITIVE STAGE ASSOCIATIVE STAGE AUTONOMOUS STAGE

Once quality movement becomes automatic, direct your attention toward other aspects of performance and explore deeper levels of movement mastery.

With your mind freed up and your actions coordinated, it's time to get creative and find novel ways to challenge your body. Typically, this is achieved through progressive overload (doing more over time) by increasing the load, effort, volume, range of motion, and so on. These methods are valuable—ones that you should certainly utilize—but I want you to take it a step further by exploring variations that uniquely test your movement patterns.

The reason for this is simple. When you progress from having to think about every aspect of a movement to execution without conscious thought, you develop motor control proficiency—meaning you can control every aspect and position of the movement. If you were to pause the movement at any point, you could demonstrate control and positional mastery. This reduces your susceptibility to pain and injury by channeling strain to the muscles, which are the primary stabilizers for your joints, rather than to ligaments and tendons, which are secondary stabilizers. It also amplifies performance because your actions are coordinated and in sync with the rest of the integrated parts. You control every gap and range. This is what it means to move with good form.

But you can only control what you've trained. If you perform only one squat variation, from the same stance, using the same range of motion, with the same form, then you're only pursuing mastery within one narrow aspect of the squat movement pattern spectrum. You want to cast a wide net by hitting as many positions, angles, and depths as possible—to close the motor control gaps that leave you vulnerable to pain and injury.

As you expand your movement repertoire, you will reach higher levels of skill. You will reduce your vulnerability to injury. You will have the power to redefine your ability to move in a variety of situations, ensuring it's based on optimal, efficient, and safe movement patterns rather than limitations or inefficiencies.

HOW YOU MOVE BECOMES THE WAY YOU MOVE

There's an evergreen trend in the fitness industry to sensationalize opposite ends of the extreme when it comes to exercise form. On one end, you must move with picture-perfect, textbook form no matter what you are doing. If you fail to mirror this approach, you are destined for injury and suboptimal performance.

On the other end, form doesn't matter, even if it defies principles of movement science and biomechanics. Less pain and improved performance will come as a result of moving, not how you are performing the movements.

Like many things in life, the truth isn't in the extremes, but in the balance between them.

It's not about chasing an elusive "perfect" movement based on someone else—and it's not about moving with zero awareness or skill. It's about homing in on efficient and effective movement for your unique anatomy and functional abilities and then matching it to the demands of the activities you're engaged in. Understand this: your form doesn't cloak you in an impenetrable shield against pain and injury. However, when you tailor exercise variations, adapt your stance, and adjust your range of motion to align with your body's nuances, you become more resistant to them. Fewer injuries and less pain translate to more consistent training, refined movement patterns, and ultimately, peak performance.

This is why you must prioritize exercise form. **How you move becomes the way you move—and the way you move can make or break your longevity in fitness and in life.** You want an autopilot that is programmed for your body, not someone else's. I have anatomical variations, mobility restrictions, adaptations, and conditioned patterns that are specific to me. You have qualities that are specific to you. If I were to tell you to move exactly like me, then I would be neglecting the aspects that resonate with your unique body and objectives. What's more, if you dismiss form altogether, then your autopilot program might be setting you up for a crash. You're leaving your form to chance and surrendering to the environmental pressures and habits that can misshape your movement patterns in ways that can put your orthopedic health at risk.

Consider the modern-day desk jockey. Hours stuck in a chair, hips anchored at a right angle, and shoulders hunched in devotion to the digital world—a sedentary snapshot that we're all familiar with. The confinement to this posture shackles the hips, limiting hip mobility and driving unwanted forces into the lower back. Overstretched shoulder and upper back muscles jeopardize mobility and joint stability. Repetitive movement patterns can also cause biomechanical repercussions. Baseball and tennis players, for example, develop asymmetries from throwing and serving that can compromise their exercise form.

In Part 3, I will teach you how to screen for these asymmetries and offer strategies for improving them. For now, it's essential to understand that compensations (undesirable deviations in movement form) conditioned by your environment and activities can compromise joint stability, muscular activation, and place excessive strain on the joints, tendons, ligaments, and bones that support movement. It's a ticking time bomb: diminished stability coupled with muscular inefficiency invariably compromises movement health.

The ethos behind pain-free performance training is to counteract and preempt these widespread vulnerabilities that are both a bane to performance and a precursor to pain. Your mission? To fortify your body to withstand the challenges of daily life. To build the strongest engines with the highest capacities possible to overcome the demands that we inevitably face. But—and this is crucial—you must navigate this mission with individualization and customization in mind. While there are many universal principles and cues that apply to everyone, you still need to tailor the movement to suit your individual needs. That way, you pattern a pain-free way of moving that you can consistently replicate when it's time to perform.

In the next chapter, you'll learn how to stabilize and brace your hips, shoulders, and core (referred to as "the pillar"). Exercise form plays a huge role here. It's the basis from which all safe and effective movement stems. From there, you'll discover how to enhance and strengthen your pillar in the preparation phase or warm-up. Then you'll carry these lessons into the foundational movement patterns, where you will learn how to individualize them using targeted screens and assessments to find your optimal setup, stance, and range of motion—as well as how to select and progress exercise variations to match your abilities and goals.

Remember, the road to movement mastery doesn't have a final destination. It's a process that you must constantly undertake. Resolve to start that process now.

THE PILLAR

Movement mastery hinges on organizing your joints in optimal positions and then creating adequate tension to control those positions while moving. Your hips, shoulders, and core, including breathing and bracing strategies, synergistically work together to deliver safe and effective movement. They form the pillar that supports all your training endeavors.

I'm standing behind a mountain of a man—one of the strongest powerlifters on the planet.

"Wrap your arms around my body," he tells me. We've been deep in conversation about bracing—the act of creating tension to stabilize the body—and he is poised to demonstrate its power by giving me a hands-on lesson. Given my relatively meager strength compared to his, I comply without hesitation, awkwardly hugging my arms around his massive torso.

"Tighter," he bellows. Intimidated, I tighten my embrace, pressing my chest into his back and constricting my arms against his sides.

"You ready?" he asks.

Before I can respond, he draws an enormous breath, his chest, belly, and back swelling like they're drawing in the power of a storm. In an instant, his entire body transforms into an unyielding statue, breaking my grasp as every muscle fires to life.

Having made his point, he turns to face me and states simply, "That is how you lift a thousand pounds."

At the time, I thought I knew what it meant to brace. Every trainer has a commonsense understanding of "getting tight" when lifting heavy weight. Creating tension is necessary to maintain control during loaded movements and prevent the body from defaulting into potentially harmful positions. It's a concept I learned early in my introduction to the iron game. And I had been practicing and teaching it to clients for years. However, I didn't have a refined system when it came to applying this all-important skill. That is, until I started working with powerlifters.

When the objective is to lift the heaviest weight possible, there's a greater emphasis on creating tension and stabilizing the body because the consequences of failure are amplified by the load. If one segment is lax, force seeps from the system, causing the body to compensate into weaker, less stable positions. Because of this, powerlifters focus on getting into the most stable positions possible before a lift, maximizing muscle engagement and strength in a way that protects their body. To them, getting tight is much more than just bracing the spine by contracting core muscles. It's a deliberate and rehearsed sequence with the hips, shoulders, core, and breath working as one—a technique refined through focused repetition.

That's exactly what this strange yet illuminating demonstration taught me—not only what it means to get tight but to approach bracing with a movement mastery mindset. When he asked me to wrap my arms around his body, he knew what was going to happen because he had done it countless times. Turning his body into an unyielding statue was part of his reliable autopilot, a volitional skill that he could turn on and off and scale up and down at will, which is the goal.

Fortunately, you don't need to hug a powerlifter to get your "aha" moment and feel what it is like to truly brace. In this chapter, you will learn a systematic approach to creating tension and stability that is scalable and repeatable. That you can emulate, feel, and apply to your unique body, giving you greater control of your movement, improving your functional range of motion, and reducing the likelihood of flaring up pain or getting injured.

SHOULDERS, HIPS, AND CORE—TOGETHER

World-renowned powerlifter Dave Tate once told me, "Brace what you want to protect." In the realm of strength training, much of the focus is on protecting the spine—and for good reason. Spinal injuries can be devastating, and the lower back is among the most common sources of pain for both novice and seasoned lifters. However, if you truly aspire to shield your spine, you must treat your shoulders, hips, and core as an indivisible functional unit. Together, they comprise the central stability line—the pillar—that supports the entire body.

Let's examine this concept through a rudimentary anatomical lens. At the core, there's the spine, the epicenter of our protective efforts. Above the core lie the shoulders, the most mobile joints in the human body. Below the core are the hips, our second most mobile joints.

Now envision a scenario where you brace your spine by contracting your core muscles but fail to create tension in your hips and shoulders. As you introduce a load and initiate movement, the shoulders and hips seek stability—often defaulting into positions with much less muscular control—and force bleeds into your spine. Even with a firmly braced core, the spine is ill equipped to withstand the additional force, leading to potentially harmful compensatory patterns that wear on the vertebrae (individual spinal segments).

When it comes to bracing, your aim is not isolated tension, but rather the harmonious integration of tension across all three segments of the pillar. To achieve such synergy, you first must examine the anatomical positions that facilitate maximal strength and stability for the shoulders and hips. Only then can you successfully brace the spine by creating tension through the core.

HARMONIOUS TENSION VS. ISOLATED TENSION

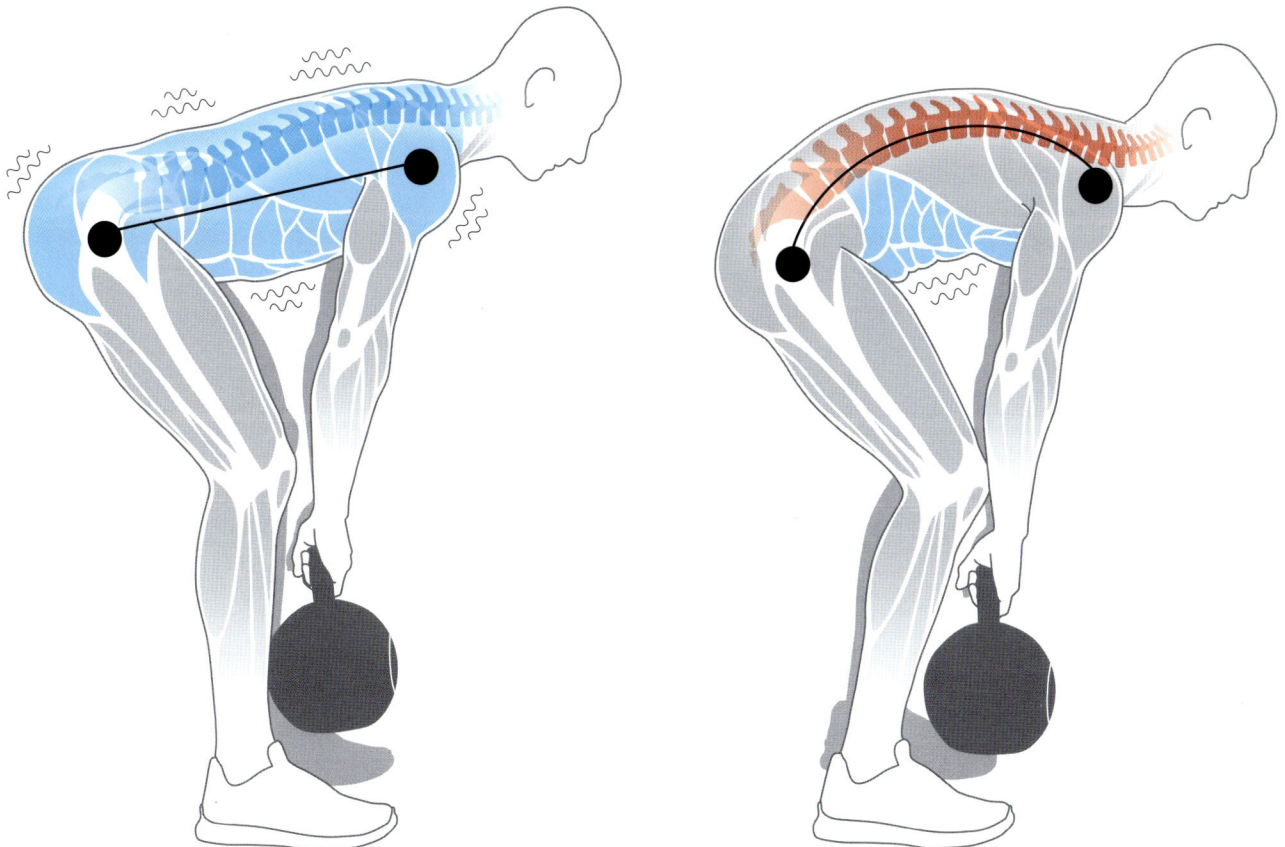

SETTING THE PILLAR
(THE NEUTRAL AND CENTRATION ZONE)

Your strongest position is your safest position. And your safest position is the one from which you can generate the most muscular activation and proximal stability to produce pillar-wide tension and control. You achieve it by aligning your shoulders, hips, and spine into a neutral position so that your muscles can effectively stabilize your joints.

Interestingly, discovering your neutral alignment involves creating tension through muscular contractions. In other words, it's not about getting into the correct neutral alignment and then contracting your muscles to stabilize the position; it's about using muscular contractions to set your neutral alignment, which enables strong and safe positions.

JOINT CENTRATION

The hips and shoulders are ball-and-socket joints. The closer you get to aligning the head of the ball in the center of the joint socket, the more muscle activation you can generate and the stronger the position becomes. This is called joint centration, meaning you have maximal bony surface area contact in the joint.

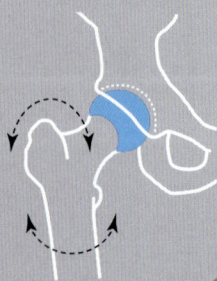

HIP JOINT

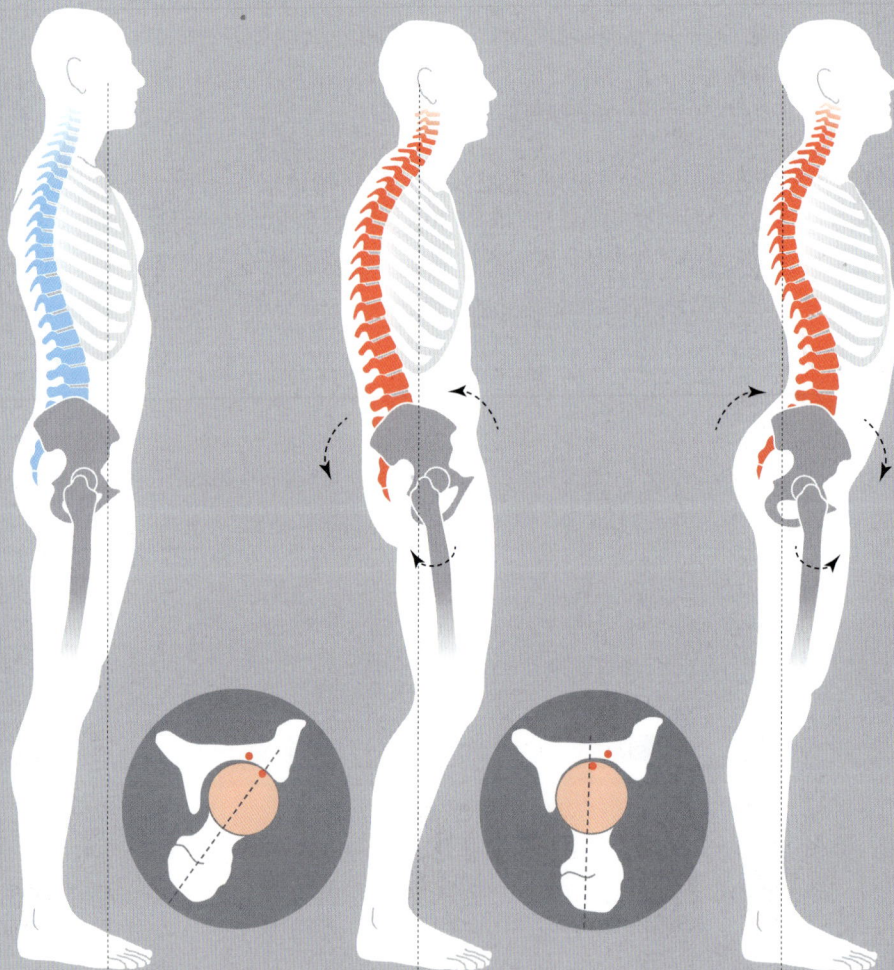

It just so happens that the neutral alignment that facilitates the highest levels of muscular engagement and joint stability is determined by the structural bony alignment of your hips and shoulders.

It's crucial to realize that neutral position varies slightly from person to person due to anatomical variations and postural adaptations. So don't worry if your neutral position doesn't precisely align with the illustrations or resemble someone else's seemingly perfect posture. **There is no universal neutral position that looks exactly the same on everyone. There is only your neutral position.**

With this understanding, let's explore how to stabilize the pillar—and how to achieve joint centration and your ideal neutral position by creating tension.

When your shoulders and hips are in a neutral position, the natural curvature of your spine automatically aligns within your neutral zone.

SHOULDER JOINT

UNDERSTANDING YOUR NEUTRAL ZONE

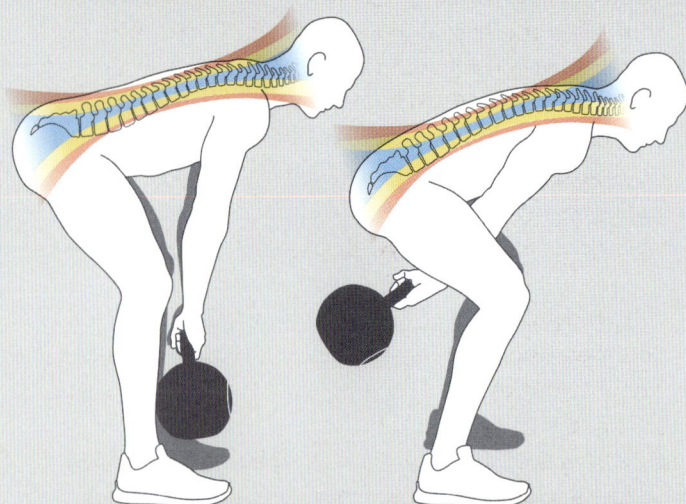

■ NEUTRAL ZONE ■ BUFFER ZONE ■ DANGER ZONE

While the directive is to seek neutral hip, shoulder, and spinal positioning, it's nearly impossible to stay perfectly neutral during dynamic and loaded movements. Take, for instance, a flawlessly executed kettlebell swing where the back appears to be perfectly neutral, meaning the spine stays rigid and there is minimal forward or backward (flexion or extension) motion. Studies show that, even with a neutral spine, there is up to 37 degrees of flexion at the L4-L5 segments.[1] This deviation from a perfectly straight line doesn't mean the movement is incorrect or harmful. In fact, our spine has a "buffering" zone, which allows for some degree of flexion and extension without compromising safety or performance. The same could be said for the hips and shoulders.

The reason you're putting tension in your hips, shoulders, and core is to create and maintain stability. Typically, the less movement that occurs from the pillar, the more stability and control you have over your body and the movement you're performing. But—and this is important to remember—there will be some movement. Your aim: to contain this movement within your neutral zone.

I'm saying "your" neutral zone, not "the" neutral zone, because just as neutral positioning looks different on everyone, your neutral zone is entirely specific to you. It might be a narrow zone or a wider zone based on several interconnected factors:

EXPERIENCE: Those with more movement and exercise experience tend to have better body awareness and greater capacities, which often translates to a wider neutral zone. Take powerlifters,

for example; many deadlift with kyphotic curves (forward rounding) in their upper back but can lift massive weights without pain or injury. They've expanded their neutral zone through gradual adaptation. However, it's a calculated risk. Some operate at the edge of their neutral zone to lift more weight, reducing their safety buffer.

Novices generally have less awareness of their bodies and should operate within a narrower zone until they've learned and patterned proper technique and execution. If you are learning a new movement, experimenting with a different way of performing a movement, or progressing to a more advanced variation, keep your zone narrow before testing your boundaries. Just because a powerlifter deadlifts with a rounded back, doesn't mean you should too. The more you train a movement, and the better you get at maintaining pillar stability during the movement, the wider your zone becomes. It's all about progressing based on your capacity, goals, and abilities.

PRESENCE OF PAIN: When pain is a factor, it can decrease muscle function, leading to reduced stability. This necessitates a more conservative approach to movement, maintaining a range that avoids flaring up the pain. If pain is present, it's prudent to restrict movement within a smaller, more controlled zone, even if you're typically capable of a broader range.

SENSITIVITIES: Like pain, specific sensitivities can alter your neutral zone. For instance, sensitivity to lumbar hyperextension (arching through the lower back) might mean that you have to reduce the range of motion for certain movements and maintain a rigid zone for exercises that stress the area, such as hinge movement patterns.

MOVEMENT PATTERN: The complexity and challenge of a particular movement pattern can vary greatly depending on individual factors such as past injuries, inherent mobility, and your level of experience with the movement. These factors can either expand or restrict your neutral zone. For instance, if you have a history of lower back pain, movements that place a high demand on the lumbar region may require a narrower neutral zone to avoid discomfort. Conversely, if you're highly skilled and conditioned for a specific pattern, you can safely access a wider range of motion within your neutral zone for that movement.

ANATOMY: The unique structural makeup of each person's body, including the degree of spinal curvature or the depth of the hip sockets, directly affects the range of motion that is safe and sustainable. Those with greater flexibility or hypermobility may need to be more vigilant and exert extra control to ensure stability.

INJURY HISTORY: A history of injuries often leads to the body's development of protective mechanisms, resulting in a tightened neutral zone to safeguard against re-injury. For instance, if you've previously strained your back during a kettlebell swing, deadlift, or by squatting too deeply, heightened pillar vigilance is crucial. Tailoring the movement to fit your body's current condition is key, and the assessments outlined in Part 3 will serve as a guide. These adjustments help not only in avoiding further injury but also in accommodating any sensitivities that have arisen as a result of that injury.

LOAD: The weight you're lifting has a substantial impact on your neutral zone. When managing heavier loads, your neutral zone usually narrows, demanding a more precise and controlled range to ensure stability and safety. Conversely, lighter loads can afford a more generous neutral zone, allowing a broader safe range for movement. However, this isn't a one-size-fits-all rule. The specifics—such as the type of movement, your personal lifting experience, and the interplay of other elements like your anatomy and injury history— all contribute to determining the appropriate breadth of your neutral zone under different loads.

SPEED: The pace at which a movement is executed has a direct effect on your neutral zone. For dynamic, unweighted actions such as throwing, the body naturally employs a wider range of motion, allowing for significant rotation and spinal flexion and extension. This means a broader neutral zone is acceptable and often necessary. In contrast, when speed is combined with load—as seen in exercises like kettlebell swings—precision and control become paramount. A tighter rein on the neutral zone is crucial here to maintain stability and to safeguard against the risks associated with the increased momentum and force.

FATIGUE: Fatigue dramatically affects the size and manageability of your neutral zone. As fatigue sets in, muscle endurance wanes, and the ability to maintain optimal form diminishes. This reduction in muscular support demands a narrower zone, as the body is less capable of safely handling deviations from ideal alignment. The risk of straying outside this zone and encountering injury escalates with fatigue, emphasizing the need for increased pillar tension and careful monitoring of physical exhaustion levels during workouts. In the presence of fatigue, it's crucial to adjust the intensity, load, and complexity of movements to preserve stability and ensure safe practice within a temporarily constricted neutral zone.

By recognizing these factors, you can work on your stability within your specific neutral zone, which can be different each day, for each movement, and across various conditions.

Given the variability, there's no need to obsess over precise angles or textbook positions when it comes to your neutral zone. Instead, shift your focus toward internal bracing, breathing, and how your body responds to a movement or range.

When you feel stable, controlled, and pain-free, you're likely operating within your neutral zone, regardless of how it might look.

As a general rule, start with a narrow zone, especially when introducing new movements or loads. As you gain proficiency with the cueing sequence (page 34), test boundaries with caution, and only expand your neutral zone through strategic and incremental progressions.

Ultimately, injuries frequently occur due to sudden, uncontrolled deviations beyond your neutral zone, particularly during the eccentric or lowering phase of movements. For example, dropping into a squat, lowering the weight in a deadlift, or reaching the bottom of a kettlebell swing, are critical moments where the risk of moving outside of your neutral zone increases. With the combined pressures of the load as muscles are lengthening under tension and the need to manage movement against gravity, maintaining heightened awareness during eccentric motions is crucial.

Recognizing and respecting your unique neutral zone—and the factors that shape it—can lead to greater stability, control, and pain-free performance across all your movements. This awareness leads to a more informed approach to your workouts, allowing you to adjust your technique, load, and speed in a way that respects your body's current capabilities and limits. By leveraging the full extent of your movement potential within a safe range, you can minimize the occurrences of pain and injury, ensuring that each exercise contributes positively to your overall health and performance.

STABILIZING THE PILLAR

STABILIZING YOUR SHOULDERS

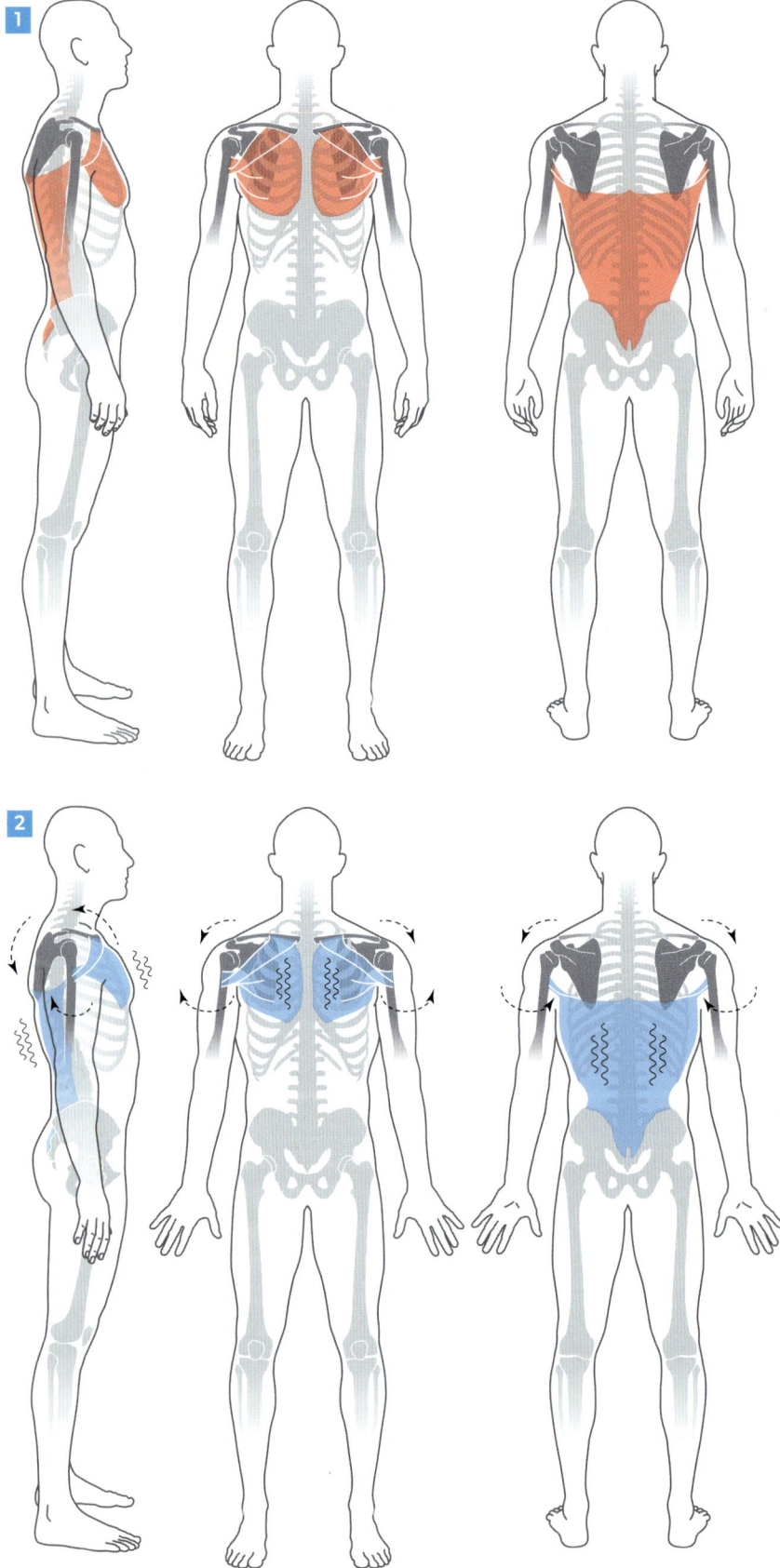

When the goal is to be strong, you want as much musculature involved as possible because—again—what is strong is stable; what is stable is safe; and what is safe is pain-free performance.

Finding your neutral and joint centration zone primes the biggest, broadest, and strongest muscles of the human body. Muscles provide stability, but to create that stability, you need to add tension to the system and let your body, with its unique structure, dictate your neutral position. There are two synergizing steps to this process.

1. Create tension from the inside out. This is achieved by simply co-contracting the muscles that connect and control movement for the shoulders and hips. The position that allows for maximal co-contraction is your neutral and joint centration zone. But don't just take my word for it; feel it for yourself with this simple test.

Stand with your feet straight or slightly turned out, positioned roughly shoulder width apart, and your arms relaxed at your sides. To stabilize your shoulders, create tension by co-contracting your pecs and lats. This is a simultaneous action. In other words, you're not contracting your pecs and then lats, but rather engaging both at the same time.

STABILIZING YOUR HIPS

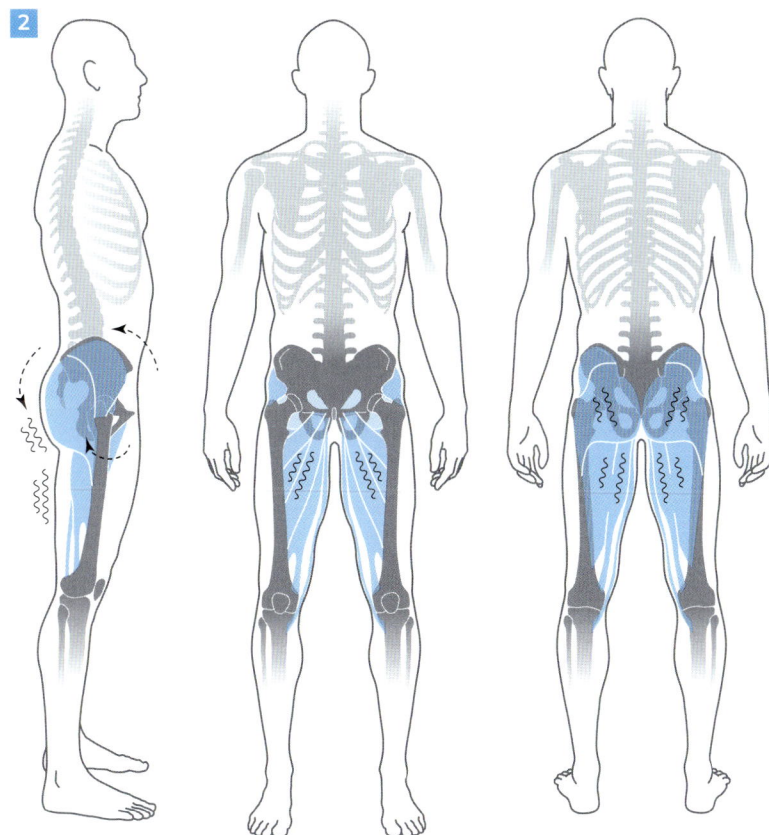

To stabilize your hips, create tension by co-contracting your glutes and adductors. Again, this is a concurrent action. It's difficult to engage your adductors without also contracting your quadriceps. However, maximally contracting your glutes also fires your adductors, so place your focus there—and notice that as you squeeze your glutes, the muscles of your adductors turn on.

Perform each in isolation—shoulders and then hips or hips and then shoulders—and test the level of activation you can achieve based on your position. For example, roll your shoulders forward and then contract your pecs and lats. Do the same thing by pulling your shoulders back. Notice that you can't generate equal levels of activation across both muscles when you venture outside of your centration or neutral zone.

The same is true for your hips and spine. When you dump your pelvis forward or backward (anterior or posterior pelvic tilt) and hyperextend or flex your spine, you can't maximally contract your glutes and adductors or the abdominal and back muscles to the same degree.

STABILIZING YOUR SHOULDERS

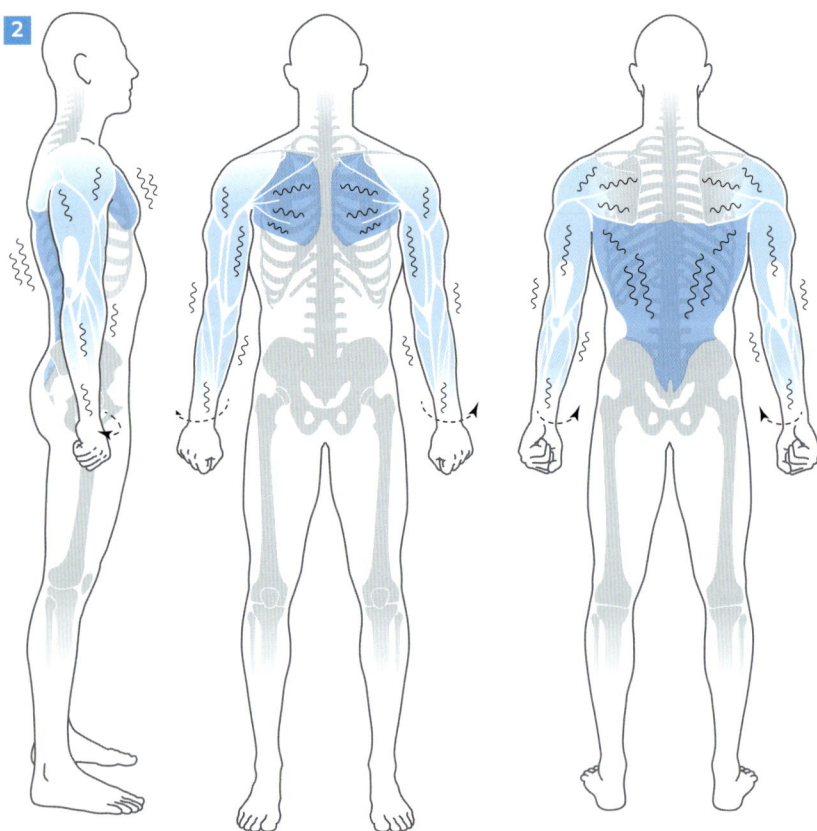

2. Create tension from the outside in. This is achieved through torque and irradiation. Torque and irradiation work in tandem to enhance muscular engagement and joint stability by harnessing rotational forces and the spread of tension across connected muscle groups. Torque involves creating rotational force, which aligns joints and bones for optimal power and safety. Irradiation amplifies this effect by spreading tension from the engaged muscle to neighboring muscles, increasing overall stability and force production. Together, they ensure that movements are performed in the strongest, safest positions, optimizing the body's mechanical advantage and protective mechanisms against injury.

To test this concept, perform the previous test, starting with your shoulders. Co-contract your pecs and lats, and then clench both fists as hard as you can by engaging every muscle in your arms and shoulders to maximize grip strength. Notice the subtle, natural rotation that occurs through the wrist, elbow, and shoulder (torque), as well as the increased isometric contraction in your pecs and lats (irradiation).

In practical terms, when you apply torque and irradiation—by gripping a barbell or dumbbell tightly, or even clenching the fist of your non-working hand during unilateral (single arm) exercises—you not only enhance the muscle activation in your primary movers like pecs and lats but also ensure greater strength and stability across your shoulders.

STABILIZING YOUR HIPS

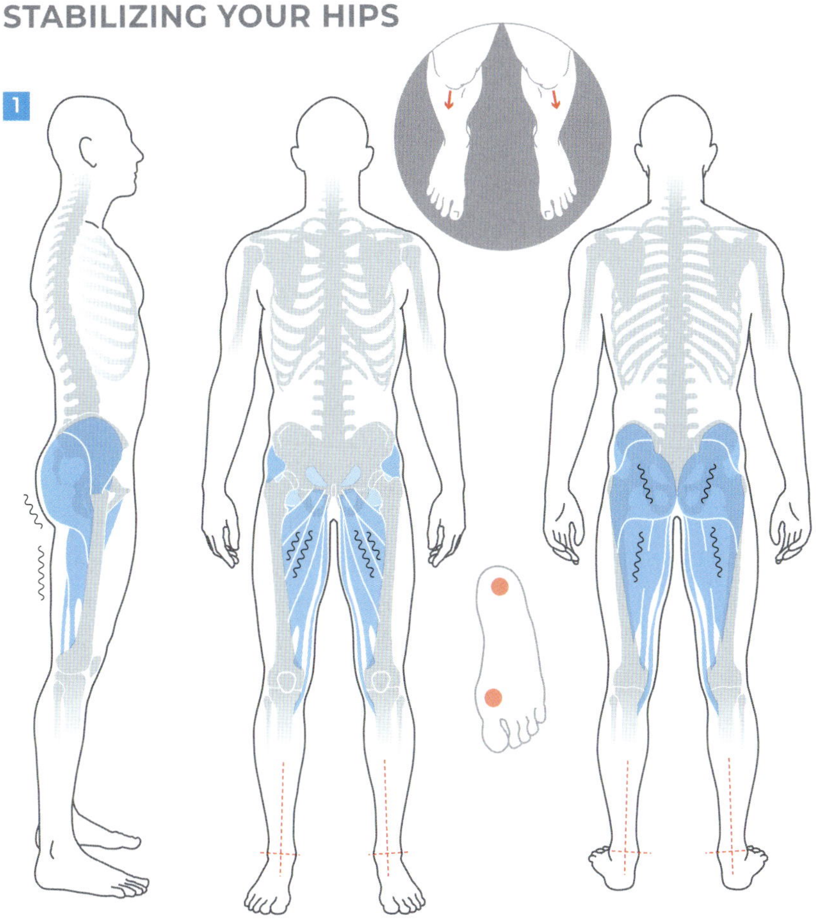

1

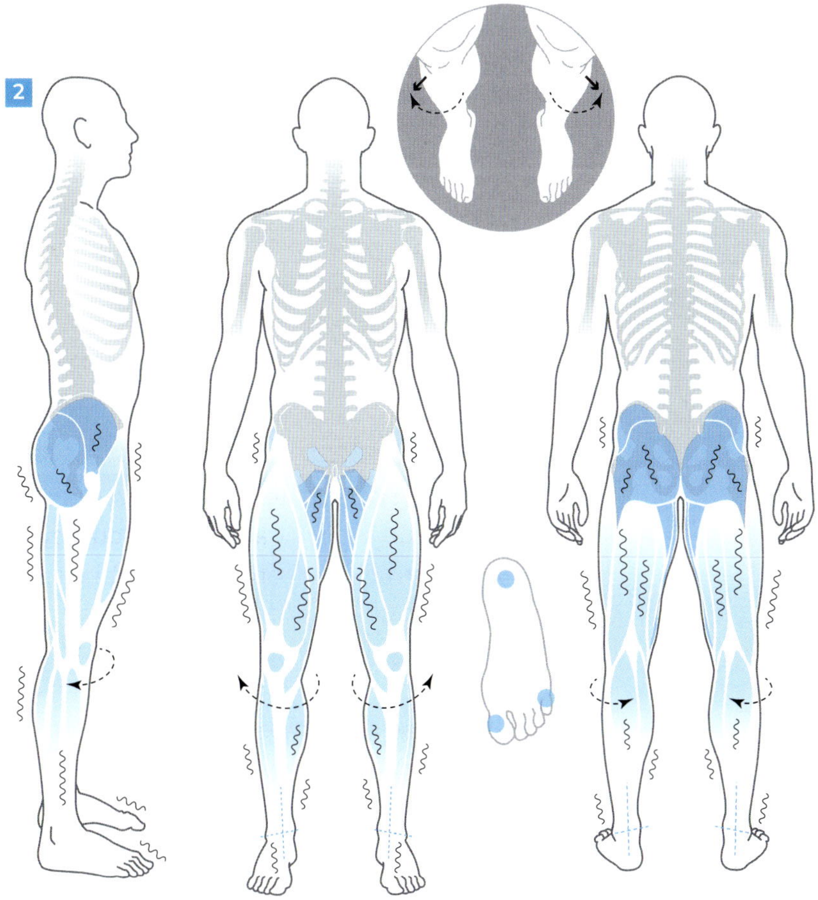

2

Now let's apply this concept to the hips. Again, co-contract your glutes and adductors. Then "screw" your feet into the floor by pressing your big toes down and outwardly rotating your legs without moving your feet. Your big toes are a key driver of irradiation up the chain into your glutes, while the rotational aspect (torque) activates your adductors. Just as you experienced with your shoulders, screwing your feet into the ground creates a chain reaction that bolsters tension in your glutes and adductors, solidifying the stability of your hips.

Whether you are in a bilateral or unilateral (single-leg or lunge) stance, the process is the same. Think grip and rip. You're gripping the ground with your big toe and ripping the floor to stabilize the position.

Don't overcomplicate this step. You're simply creating torque in a way that amplifies the co-contraction. If you increase the engagement and feel more stable, then you're doing it correctly. If you lose tension and stability, then you might be overexaggerating the rotational aspect or rotating in the wrong direction.

Now that you understand how to create tension to find your neutral position—and how to amplify that tension through torque and irradiation—let's tie in the core and put it all together into one sequence.

THE CUEING SEQUENCE
(PUTTING IT ALL TOGETHER)

The cueing sequence is a step-by-step process for establishing a stable pillar. It is the rooting mechanism for controlled and efficient movement upon which you can build a reliable autopilot—a trusted system that safeguards your body and optimizes performance for all loaded movements. Each step is marked by specific cues that initiate targeted actions. Approach this sequence with intent, adopting a mindset geared toward movement mastery.

STEP 1:
SHOULDERS

Stand with your feet under your hips and your arms at your sides. Co-contract your pecs and lats maximally. Holding this contraction, clench your fists, digging your fingertips into your palms and engaging all the muscles in your arms and shoulders.

STEP 2:
HIPS

Co-contract your glutes and adductors maximally. Keeping your glutes and adductors engaged, screw your feet into the ground by pressing your big toes into the floor, creating an arch in your foot, and turning your knees outward without moving your feet.

STEP 3:
BREATHE

Inhale fully through the nose, with a 360-degree expansion through your diaphragm.

STEP 4:
BRACE

As you reach maximal tidal volume (the maximum amount of air you can voluntarily inhale), hold your breath and engage the muscles of your core. Think about creating tension through 360 degrees around your torso by "crunching" down the distance between the bottom portion of your sternum and top of your pubic bone. Keep everything stable and maximally tensioned for a few seconds. Then exhale and relax.

That's what it feels like to brace. The purpose of the cueing sequence is to generate maximal tension correctly—as if you were getting ready to lift a thousand pounds. I want you to experience the feeling of turning your body into an unyielding statue because bracing is how you stabilize and protect your body. But it's not enough to simply create tension while standing upright in a static position. You must be able to apply this sequence in different positions with movement, which you will practice in the 6-phase dynamic warm-up and when training the six foundational movement patterns. Equally important, you need to be able to scale your level of tension to match the stability demands of the task or activity.

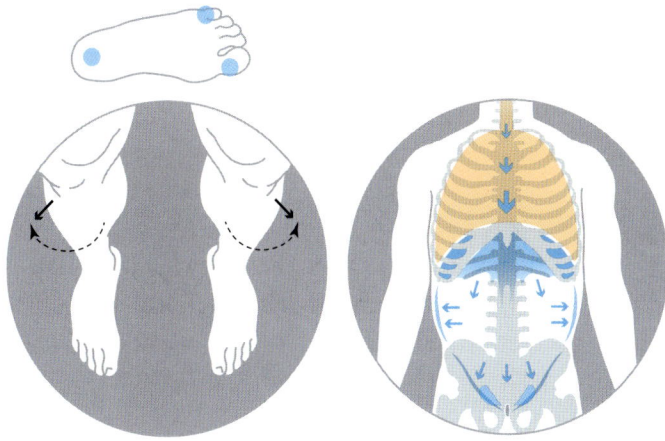

START POSITION	SHOULDERS	HIPS	BREATHE	BRACE

THE PREPLANNED AND REACTIVE BRACING STRATEGIES

Not all bracing strategies are created equal—what works in a controlled gym setting may not directly translate to the unpredictable nature of sport and play. When it comes to bracing, you must adapt to the context of the movement and activity: whether it's the steady precision required for a heavy squat or the instant reactivity needed for a sprint. Navigating the spectrum from the meticulous control of a loaded barbell to the agility demanded on the field hinges on mastering both preplanned and reactive bracing. Let's explore how these distinct strategies underpin your movement and performance, ensuring you're braced for success, no matter the challenge.

THE PREPLANNED BRACING STRATEGY: FOR SLOW AND PREDICTABLE MOVEMENTS

In the gym, most exercises are performed in a single plane of motion, where movements follow a predictable path such as up and down, side to side, or forward and back.

Consider the squat: You begin standing, descend, and then rise again, moving in a defined up-and-down motion. The movement is predictable, with minimal directional variability, and is usually performed under load, requiring slow, careful execution. During a squat, maintaining the integrity of your hips, shoulders, and core—your pillar stability—is crucial. A loss of stability can lead to force being misdirected into weaker areas, making it difficult to regain a proper, stable posture under the constant weight.

Knowing this, it's essential to brace your body at the start, establishing a rigid, tension-filled base through a neutral pillar. This conscious preparation ensures that you can uphold that stability throughout the movement, preserving the effectiveness and safety of the pillar while in motion.

THE REACTIVE BRACING STRATEGY: FOR FAST AND LESS PREDICTABLE MOVEMENTS

In sports and daily life, movements typically involve multiple planes, engaging your body in complex, multi-directional patterns.

Imagine the dynamic actions in field sports—sudden cuts, jumps, and quick changes in direction. In such fast-paced situations, your movements are less predictable and more varied, often requiring rapid responses to changing scenarios. Here, bracing isn't about setting up a rigid, premeditated brace; it's about responding to stabilization demands on the fly. Whether it's channeling force from your limbs to the ground or vice versa, this form of bracing is less about muscular tension and more about force transference—it's a synergistic, reflexive response rather than a deliberate creation of tension.

Understanding the distinction between the two bracing strategies is vital: **With single-direction loaded movements, bracing is a conscious, deliberate act of creating tension, whereas with multi-directional high-speed movements, it shifts to a more instinctive, reactive brace (often out of non-neutral postures) to maximize speed and adaptability while moving.**

In this chapter and throughout the book, we emphasize the cueing sequence (the preplanned bracing strategy) because that is what you will utilize most in your training. However, it's important to realize that by mastering the cueing sequence, you are also building your reactive capabilities.

In other words, enhancing your preplanned brace with single-plane movements under load builds the foundation for a more efficient reactive brace with multi-plane movements under speed. You practice the cueing sequence in a controlled environment so that you develop a reliable autopilot that intuitively responds when the challenges are unpredictable, ensuring safe, effective movement regardless of the activity.

SCALING TENSION

When training, the mandate is clear: a stable pillar is non-negotiable. This isn't about rigidly locking down with maximal tension at all times; it's about fine-tuning tension to each specific movement and load. With unloaded movements, such as a bodyweight squat, you may only need 10 to 20 percent tension to maintain pillar stability, whereas with maximal-effort movements like a one-rep-max deadlift, you need 100 percent tension. Scaling tension—the art of bracing—involves creating just enough pillar stability to stay within your neutral zone.

SCALING TENSION TO LOAD

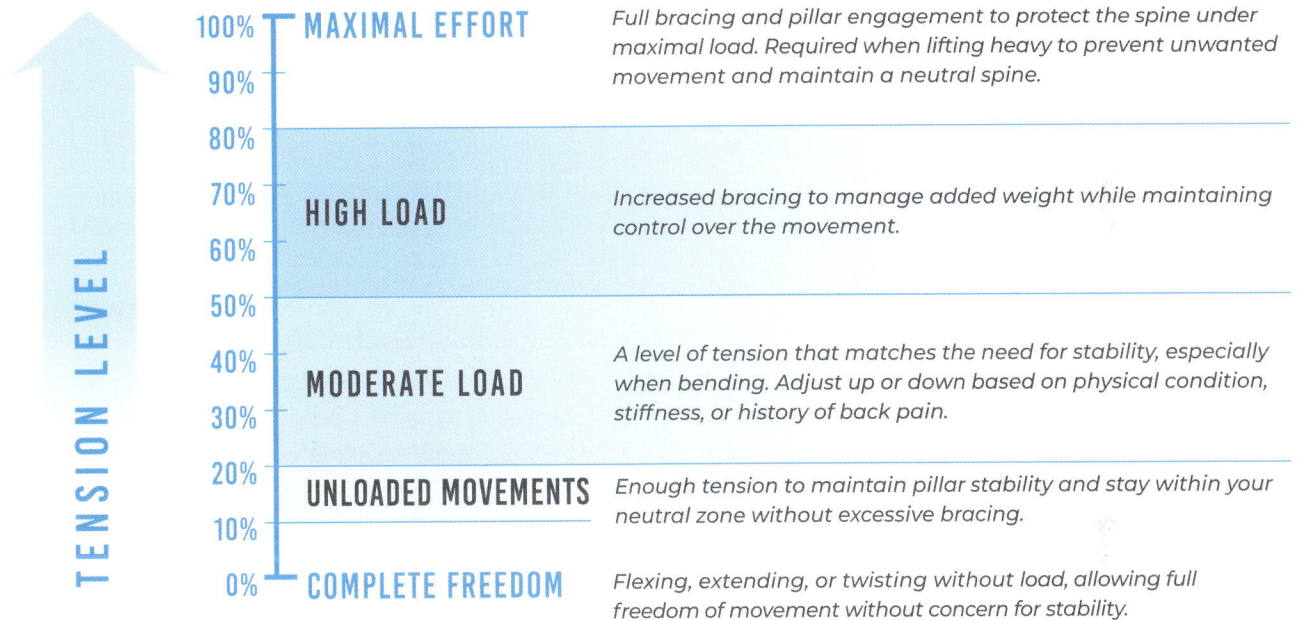

TENSION LEVEL		
100% / 90%	**MAXIMAL EFFORT**	*Full bracing and pillar engagement to protect the spine under maximal load. Required when lifting heavy to prevent unwanted movement and maintain a neutral spine.*
80% / 70% / 60%	**HIGH LOAD**	*Increased bracing to manage added weight while maintaining control over the movement.*
50% / 40% / 30%	**MODERATE LOAD**	*A level of tension that matches the need for stability, especially when bending. Adjust up or down based on physical condition, stiffness, or history of back pain.*
20% / 10%	**UNLOADED MOVEMENTS**	*Enough tension to maintain pillar stability and stay within your neutral zone without excessive bracing.*
0%	**COMPLETE FREEDOM**	*Flexing, extending, or twisting without load, allowing full freedom of movement without concern for stability.*

The only time you scale tension down to zero is when the activity demands complete freedom of movement and there is no threat to your body. Take yoga, for example. You can break the rules of tension and neutrality by flexing and extending your spine because you are not moving with load. Squatting ass-to-grass or hinging with a rounded back when there is no challenge on your body is very different from squatting or deadlifting with a heavy barbell.

Managing pillar stability through activities of daily living is another important consideration—you may need maximal tension or zero tension based on the interplay between your physical condition and the specific context of your movement.

For instance, picking up an object as light as a feather might seem trivial, yet it's often in these unsuspecting moments that minor lower back strains occur—especially when bending and twisting are involved. It's a common misconception that such injuries are reserved for moments of heavy lifting, but the reality is starkly different. The act of bending over to retrieve something from the ground, regardless of its weight, can be the very instance that sidelines you from training.

That's why adjusting tension in your pillar hinges significantly on your current physical state. If you're feeling strong, well-rested, and free from pain, minimal or zero tension might suffice for mundane tasks. However, if you're experiencing stiffness, feeling cold, or particularly run down, especially with a history of lower back issues, adopting a bracing strategy akin to preparing for a heavy deadlift might be necessary. These precautions are paramount when you're not at your best—when soreness, dehydration, or lack of sleep have taken their toll, making you vulnerable to injuries over seemingly inconsequential movements.

This variability underscores the importance of being both aware and adaptable. Being able to deadlift twice your body weight means little if bending over to pick up your laundry could cause a strain. Such paradoxes highlight the ever-evolving nature of controlling tension and managing your pillar stability. The art of scaling your brace isn't static; it requires continuous customization based on your individual state, the preparation you've undertaken, and the demands of the activity at hand. Over time, as you master the skill set to fine-tune your approach to bracing, you develop a more reliable autopilot. This refined intuition allows for seamless adjustment to your body's needs, ensuring you maintain optimal performance and protection against pain, without the constant need for conscious adjustment.

SCALING TENSION TO PAIN

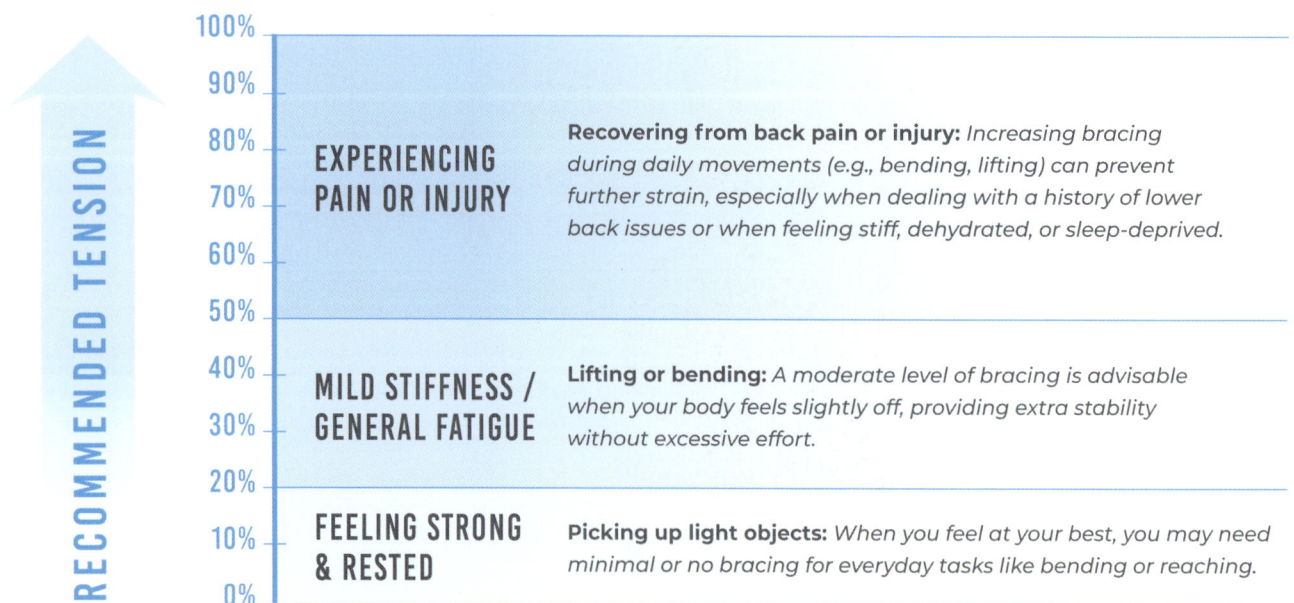

RECOMMENDED TENSION		
100%		
90%		
80%	**EXPERIENCING PAIN OR INJURY**	**Recovering from back pain or injury:** *Increasing bracing during daily movements (e.g., bending, lifting) can prevent further strain, especially when dealing with a history of lower back issues or when feeling stiff, dehydrated, or sleep-deprived.*
70%		
60%		
50%		
40%	**MILD STIFFNESS / GENERAL FATIGUE**	**Lifting or bending:** *A moderate level of bracing is advisable when your body feels slightly off, providing extra stability without excessive effort.*
30%		
20%		
10%	**FEELING STRONG & RESTED**	**Picking up light objects:** *When you feel at your best, you may need minimal or no bracing for everyday tasks like bending or reaching.*
0%		

As you start practicing these adjustments, it may feel like a concentrated effort—finding that sweet spot where you create just enough tension to maintain your neutral zone will involve some trial and error. You will overshoot it or undershoot it—and that is OK. With the right intention and practice, the process will eventually become intuitive. The 6-phase warm-up includes exercises that will help you develop it. And the movement pattern progressions will help you scale and refine your bracing strategies to match the exercise.

Remember, scaling tension is not on and off at 100 percent. It's a dimmer switch that you turn up or down based on the demands of the movement and the other factors mentioned. The controller on that dimmer switch—the mechanism that allows you to modulate tension—is regulated to a large extent by your breathing strategy, which is the focus of the next chapter.

BREATHING STRATEGIES
(FOR BETTER MOVEMENT, RECOVERY, AND PERFORMANCE)

Life demands breath. Pain-free training demands breathing strategies. To optimize your exercise form and strengthen the connection between your mind, body, and the movements you are performing, you must control your breath—and align your breathing strategies with the demands of your life and training.

"Inhale deeply through your nose, and exhale slowly through your mouth."

The words from legendary strength coach Buddy Morris float through the air, a stark contrast to his usual roaring commands. "Feel your belly rise and fall. Relax into each breath."

I'm in the football weight room at the University of Buffalo, surrounded by modern-day gladiators, lying on their backs, legs propped up on benches, being guided through a breathing exercise. As a young athlete with little experience and no expertise, I watch in silent curiosity, my teenage mind trying to make sense of what I am witnessing.

On any other day, the gym would pulse with the anthems of Metallica, reverberating with the clang of iron and the guttural shouts of exertion. The coaches, hailing from the famed powerlifting gym Westside Barbell, embody the physical supremacy they instill in their athletes. Typical training sessions are a masterclass in power and strength. Energizing. Inspiring.

But this day is different. The atmosphere is quiet, calm, and introspective. The silence of concentration fills the room, punctuated by controlled breathing. In this unexpected setting, I find myself grappling with questions. What significance does breathing hold in the realm of strength training? This practice, so far removed from the high-octane ethos I had come to associate with athletic excellence, leaves me bewildered. How could such a serene exercise contribute to sports performance? Departing with more questions than answers, I'm enveloped in a mix of astonishment and confusion, pondering the unseen connections between the calm of controlled breathing and the storm of athletic training.

Nearly a decade passes...

In the intervening years, my academic and professional journey—culminating in a degree in exercise science, followed by a doctorate in physical therapy and a transition to personal training—did little to connect me with the art and skill of breathing. It remained a background function, secondary to the more physical aspects of fitness and rehabilitation. It wasn't until I moved to San Diego, living next door to two Navy SEAL brothers, that the insights from that memorable session in the UB weight room began to take root.

"You should check out SEALFIT," the brothers told me. "That's where we train for fun."

Being new to the area, I was doing everything I could to network and attract personal training clients. I was particularly intrigued by the brothers, who trained like absolute beasts, and who—like me—were obsessed with human performance. Inspired by their training and overall badassery, I researched SEALFIT and its founder, former SEAL Mark Divine. Based on his training methods, I quickly realized this was no ordinary gym. SEALFIT embodied the training regimens of Navy SEALs, but it had been adapted for civilians and athletes keen to test their limits. It was a crucible for physical and mental transformation, blending military discipline with cutting-edge sports science. As with Buddy Morris years earlier, they embraced strategies that stretched beyond the conventional boundaries of strength and conditioning, incorporating breathwork, yoga, and mindset techniques—aspects I had yet to fully explore.

Driven by curiosity and the goal to expand my client base, I immersed myself in the SEALFIT community by participating in their challenges and experiences. This involvement gave me the opportunity to work closely with SEALs and other high-level athletes as personal training clients while also exposing me to a transformative breathing strategy pivotal to SEAL training.

One day, while observing a particularly grueling training session, I noticed some of the athletes taking deep, systematic breaths during the workout. They weren't just huffing and puffing, frantically trying to recover. They were controlling each inhale and exhale, remaining incredibly focused and calm despite the intensity. Intrigued, I asked one of the trainers about it.

"It's called box breathing," he told me. "It involves a deliberate breathing pattern in four-second intervals." He explained how it was pivotal for regulating the nervous system and sharpening attention, enabling athletes to maintain composure and precision under high-stress situations. The benefits were evident not just during the peak of their training but also during their recovery phases, demonstrating how controlled breathing could profoundly influence both mental and physical recuperation.

At the time, my personal training approach revolved around enhancing movement patterns to facilitate pain-free training. This meant concentrating on the physical aspects of movement, rehab, and training, such as prescribing specific exercises to strengthen imbalances and weak links or modifying movements to suit individual anatomy and abilities. While this physical focus was effective—it forms the foundation of this book and contributed significantly to keeping the athletes I trained healthy—I had not completely grasped the critical role of the nervous system, nor had I recognized how strategically applied breathing techniques could influence focus and recovery to create a more fruitful and injury-free workout experience.

In working with these athletes, I learned that intentional, structured breathing strategies like "box breathing" allow for a smooth transition from the high-alert state of the sympathetic nervous system to the more calming influences of the parasympathetic nervous system. Such a practice not only facilitates faster recovery but also enhances mental clarity and the precision of each movement—critical for SEALs who must perform complex tasks under life-threatening stress.

Mark Divine's insight that these strategies could significantly benefit elite operators as well as the general population resonated deeply with me. While most of us will never endure the extremes of combat or the rigors of Hell Week, we encounter our own battles with stress and anxiety daily and push our bodies to personal extremes. Recovery and nervous system regulation are just as vital to our health and performance as they are to these elite warriors and athletes.

Motivated by these revelations, I decided to integrate the SEALFIT-inspired methods into the fitness boot camps I was teaching at the time—specifically, deep breathing and yoga at the end of intense physical workouts. The impact was astounding. Everyone loved it. After pushing their heart rates to 190 with expressions of sheer exhaustion plastered on their faces, they would, just minutes later, be hugging me, sharing how life-changing the experience was. They went from peak stress to feeling rejuvenated, ready to tackle whatever challenges the day had in store. I knew right then what Buddy was doing all those years ago.

In a domain where the drive is to build capacity—to be faster, stronger, and more formidable—the imperative to recover is often overshadowed. Buddy understood that breathing is the linchpin of recuperation. He was training hardened athletes essentially preparing for war. On top of the intense physical training, the football players were under immense pressure to perform—stressors that ultimately inhibit recovery and performance.

The deep breathing exercise Buddy put his players through didn't require any specialized equipment or expertise. He was giving them an essential life skill that they could do anytime, anywhere. Most importantly, he knew that to influence and promote recovery, he needed to get his players to relax and decrease their vital metrics (heart rate, blood pressure, and stress) after training. Once in a relaxed state, the physiological and psychological processes that enhance post-exercise recuperation would take over.

Breathing strategies, such as Buddy Morris's post-exercise recovery drill and the "box breathing" method popularized by Mark Divine, stand out because they offer unique advantages that traditional gym routines lack: instant gratification and immediate results.

To put this in perspective, consider the varying timelines for training benefits: the effects of a warm-up are felt within minutes; the impact of a typical workout, within hours; and the outcomes of strength and physique goals, often over months or even years. Yet, the benefits of intentional, effective breathing are experienced instantly.

The benefits of intentional, effective breathing are experienced instantly.

Utilizing deep, controlled breathing to focus and calm the mind and body was my gateway to appreciating the true power of breathwork, elevating the act of breathing from a subconscious routine to a deliberate practice— crucial for achieving pain-free performance across all areas of training and life. But I was only scratching the surface when it came to breathing strategies and techniques that enhance function, recovery, and performance. As I evolved as a trainer and started working with professional and Olympic athletes, powerlifters, and endurance competitors, I learned that efficient movement and optimal performance are only possible when you understand how to breathe, as well as how to match the right breathing strategy to the task or goal at hand.

Now, as I share these strategies, my mission is to equip you with a breathing strategy for every facet of training, ensuring that each breath moves you closer to your peak potential, both physically and mentally.

BENEFITS OF DEEP BREATHING FOR POST-EXERCISE RECOVERY

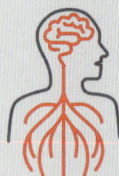

ACTIVATE THE PARASYMPATHETIC NERVOUS SYSTEM: Deep breathing can stimulate the parasympathetic nervous system (the "rest and digest" system). This is in contrast to the sympathetic nervous system, which is activated during exercise (the "fight or flight" system). You can't recover in a sympathetic state. By stimulating the parasympathetic system, the body is brought back to a state of calm, promoting faster recovery.

REDUCTION IN HEART RATE: During post-exercise, the heart rate can remain elevated. Deep breathing exercises can help lower heart rate more quickly, guiding the body toward its resting state.

DECREASED STRESS HORMONES: Exercise, especially intense exercise, can increase levels of cortisol and other stress hormones. Deep breathing can help reduce these hormone levels, thereby promoting recovery.

RELAXATION OF MUSCLES: Focused, deep breathing can help in the relaxation of muscles that might have become tense during exercise. Relaxed muscles recover more efficiently and are less prone to injury.

MENTAL RECOVERY: Deep breathing exercises, especially when combined with mindfulness or meditation techniques, can also aid in mental recovery. They can reduce feelings of anxiety or stress that might be associated with intense training sessions or competitive events.

BETTER CIRCULATION: Deep breathing helps facilitate blood flow, improving overall circulation. Efficient blood circulation is crucial during post-exercise recovery as hemoglobin carries essential nutrients and oxygen needed for healing and recuperation.

IMPROVED OXYGENATION: Intense exercise increases the demand for oxygen in muscles. Deep breathing post-exercise can help meet this demand by increasing the oxygen supply, which aids in the repair and recovery of muscle cells. The enhanced oxygen flow also helps in the removal of carbon dioxide, a by-product of metabolism.

HARNESSING THE POWER OF BREATH:
PAIN-FREE PERFORMANCE BREATHING STRATEGIES

Breathing underpins every motion, every thought, and every moment of stillness and stress in your life. It has the dual power to relax and restore, guiding you into deeper states of awareness and aiding in post-exercise recuperation, or to ignite your internal fires and ramp up your system, giving you the energy, focus, and strength required to conquer strenuous tasks. At its most fundamental level, breathing is automatic. Yet every inhale and exhale you take is more than a physiological process—it's an integral movement that can either amplify your physical and mental prowess or undermine your best efforts to perform.

To harness the transformative power of breath, you must treat breathing mechanics as a foundational motor skill and approach respiration with the same intent and rigor as you would any other movement pattern you're working to master. When you view breathing through this lens, you can move beyond thinking of it as an automated function and start to apply the principles of exercise form to each breath.

This requires a holistic approach that integrates breathing strategies tailored to the demands and scenarios you face in training and everyday life. For instance, to stabilize your body during movement, which you learned about in the previous chapter, you need to create tension in your hips, shoulders, and core (the pillar). Your breathing strategy plays a key role here. You need strategies that cover you from 0 to 100 percent tension—from a one-rep max to a 20-rep set and everything in between. You also need strategies for regulating your central nervous system (CNS)—whether it is downregulating into a parasympathetic state to relax and recover, ramping up the CNS for a max-effort lift, or managing stress after a sympathetic spike.

In this chapter, you will learn six battle-tested breathing strategies, each designed for a specific purpose:

1.
PRONE BREATH CORRECTIVE:
Establishes fundamental diaphragmatic breathing mechanics, laying the groundwork for effective respiration (page 46).

2.
DOUBLE BREATH TECHNIQUE:
Optimizes hip, shoulder, and core stability during movement (page 49).

3.
90/90 SUPINE PARASYMPATHETIC POSITIONAL BREATHING:
Expedites recovery and helps reset your central nervous system (page 54).

4.
SYMPATHETIC HUFF BREATH:
Amplifies performance for max-effort lifts and movements (page 57).

5.
RHYTHMIC BREATHING:
Improves endurance and refines mechanics in locomotion-based activities like walking, running, and biking (page 59).

6.
TACTICAL BREATH:
Aids in managing sympathetic stress responses and facilitates recovery between training sets (page 62).

Progress through them in sequence, learning the why, when, and how behind each strategy and technique. Then integrate them into your workout regimen as circumstances demand. You'll find, as I did, that pain-free training is accessible—and game-changing results are possible. It simply takes the right type of breath.

HOW TO BREATHE CORRECTLY:
THE PRONE BREATH CORRECTIVE

When it comes to breathing and bracing mechanics, it's helpful to start from a blank slate. Despite breathing since birth, most of us have never been taught or even felt what it is like to breathe diaphragmatically with a 360-degree core expansion—essential for modulating stress and managing pillar stability. Consequently, we rely on our untrained default breathing strategies that don't always match our goals and needs. For instance, most people resort to chest breathing, which activates secondary breathing muscles like the scalenes, sternocleidomastoid (SCM), upper trapezius, and pec minor. This is undesirable in most situations because it sparks a sympathetic response that limits your ability to take in full breaths and brace to create pillar-wide tension.

Remember, you need to do more than just breathe—you need to optimize each breath. That starts with learning how to breathe correctly and then applying the principles of movement mastery to make it second nature. However, considering that the average person takes over 20,000 breaths per day, fixing suboptimal breathing mechanics can be hugely challenging. In most cases, verbal cues and corrections are ineffective. Enter the Prone Breath Corrective. Using the ground as a tactile cue from the prone position, this strategy will help you "feel" what it is like to properly expand your diaphragm through 360 degrees. With each proper inhale and exhale, you are effectively re-engineering faulty patterns, allowing for correct motor learning and skill transference to occur.

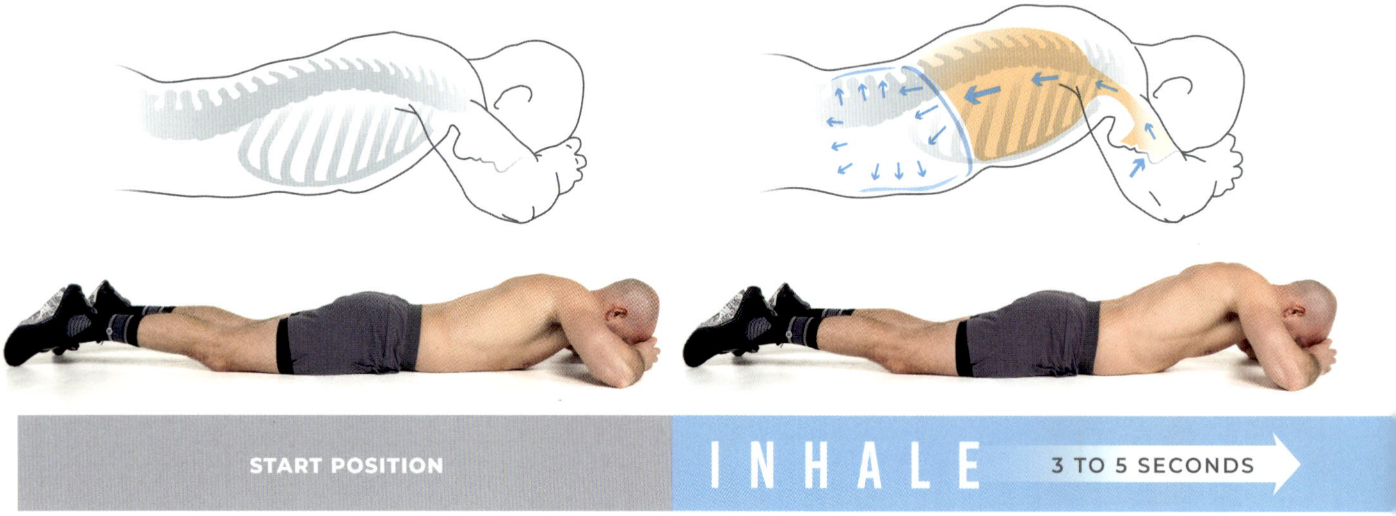

START POSITION

INHALE 3 TO 5 SECONDS →

WHEN TO USE THIS TECHNIQUE

This technique is used primarily in the early stages of breath repatterning, especially for those having difficulty distinguishing compensatory chest breathing from authentic deep diaphragmatic (belly) breathing. Just 1 to 3 minutes of Prone Breath Corrective daily—ideally as the first component of a dynamic warm-up sequence—can help you break old habits and establish new ones.

Once you've corrected the pattern and you can repeat it during daily activities and training, it's not necessary to keep it in your program.

HOW TO EXECUTE THE PRONE BREATH CORRECTIVE

In any movement correction strategy, the emphasis must be on quality, not quantity or intensity. This principle dictates that each breath should be executed with precision, aiming for habitual, flawless execution.

Here is the setup for the Prone Breath Corrective:

1. Start in a prone position (lying face down on your stomach) on the floor.

2. Bring your fists together and let your forehead rest gently on them.

3. Extend your legs and point your toes straight back.

4. Allow your body to relax fully into this position.

Propping your head on your fists will feel a bit unnatural at first, but it serves two important purposes. First, it places your head and neck in a neutral position (avoiding rotation), opening up your airway. Second, elevating your hands and arms relaxes the secondary respiratory muscles, allowing for more authentic diaphragmatic breaths.

Once you are positioned correctly, you can focus on the execution and quality of the breath by

▶ Inhaling slowly through your nose

▶ Breathing into your belly against the floor, expanding through the sides of your torso and lower back

▶ Exhale slowly through your nose

HOLD 2 TO 4 SECONDS → **EXHALE** 4 TO 6 SECONDS →

For tactile feedback on this expansion, have a partner place hands on your sides or put a yoga block or balance pad on your lower back to press against as you breathe.

INHALE
3 to 5 seconds

HOLD
2 to 4 seconds

EXHALE
4 to 6 seconds

Once you've grasped the proper expansion pattern, shift your focus to the tempo of your breaths. Make sure your exhale is longer than your inhale and allow for a short pause after you inhale fully. This approach is key for enhancing gas exchange and experiencing the full 360-degree expansion that is the aim of this corrective exercise.

After getting a feel for the Prone Breath Corrective with proper tempo while lying down, repeat the 360-degree belly breathing pattern in different developmental positions—go from lying down to kneeling, then to standing, for example. The goal is to habituate proper breathing across all postures through gradual progressions. As this breathing pattern becomes second nature, you'll be better equipped to master the more advanced breathing strategies covered in this chapter, which utilize similar base breathing mechanics.

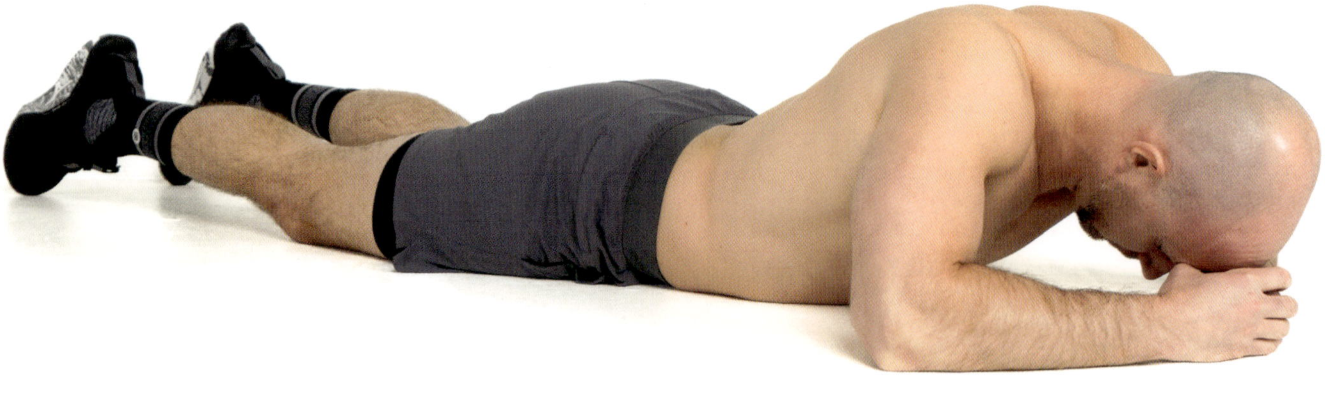

HOW TO OPTIMIZE PILLAR STABILITY:
THE DOUBLE BREATH TECHNIQUE

One of the most troubling misconceptions in strength training is the common recommendation to inhale and exhale fully during reps under load. While it's of course necessary to breathe during extended sets with high rep counts, there is an optimal way to do it and a suboptimal way that places the body—and more specifically, the spine—in destabilized positions due to a lack of core stiffness and control. Bracing effectively during any loaded movement creates the base of pain-free training. And with full breaths in and out, it's physiologically impossible to maximize, maintain, or scale the brace and breath cycle to meet the demands of the movement. There is a better way—one that not only protects the body against pain and injury but also improves top-end performance under load.

The Double Breath Technique is essential to this process. Once you understand how to maximize pillar tension during your setup with the Double Breath Technique, the next step is to scale your breath cycle to control tension during movement. I adopted this technique while working with powerlifting legend Dave Tate at the Elite FTS S5 Compound many years ago, and it instantly upgraded the quality of my brace. Since then, I've taught it to all my clients, and they have experienced the same benefits. I'm confident it will do the same for you.

WHEN TO USE THIS TECHNIQUE

Every time you approach the bar or attempt to move a weight, you must treat the setup, execution, and dismount of load with the utmost respect. That means utilizing the Double Breath Technique as a preplanned bracing strategy for each and every loaded movement, regardless of the weight.

In other words, don't neglect your bracing strategy when the load is light. You still need to control your hips, shoulders, and core with a solid brace to protect your body, no matter how much weight you are lifting. Consider the contrast between executing a deadlift with a robust brace and a neutral spine and lifting light dumbbells with zero brace and a flexed spine. Even though the weight is minimal, you are more likely to harm your body with the lighter load. Say you are cold, sore, and more vulnerable due to prior back injuries. In this scenario, a single lapse with a poor bracing strategy could result in immediate pain. For those less vulnerable, pain and injury may not be a concern, and the chances of getting hurt when lifting loosely without a brace might be extremely low. But, over time, the unwanted compensatory stress on the spine can catch up with you. It's not a problem until it is—and you shouldn't wait for pain to do something about it.

The best defense is to treat every lift, whether it is heavy or light, with a fine-tuned setup and a quality brace. In addition to safeguarding your body, you'll likely experience improvements in your overall lifting mechanics and performance.

HOW TO EXECUTE THE DOUBLE BREATH TECHNIQUE

To effectively brace, you must first organize your shoulders, hips, and spine into a neutral position. Only then can you tap into the potential of the diaphragm and create tension in your shoulders, hips, and core musculature with an active brace. The cueing sequence on page 34 took you step-by-step through this process. Let's revisit this sequence by examining the Double Breath Technique in more detail—and take a deeper dive into the nuances of each breath and brace step.

To begin, stand with your feet underneath your hips and your arms at your sides. Co-contract your pecs and lats, making a tight fist with both hands. Then co-contract your glutes and adductors, engaging your feet into the ground through external rotation. Now, maintaining this tension, go through this four-step breathing process:

1. **INITIAL DEEP BREATH:** Start by inhaling deeply through your nose.

2. **HOLD AND BRACE:** As you reach full lung capacity, hold your breath for a split second.

3. **SECOND GULP BREATH:** Still holding the air from your first breath, take a second, shallower breath by gulping in air through your mouth. This second breath tops off your lung capacity with a 360-degree expansion of your core.

4. **BRACE:** Maximally contract the core musculature around your entire trunk (front, back, and sides) while holding your breath.

THE DOUBLE BREATH TECHNIQUE

START POSITION	INHALE 3 SECONDS	HOLD	MOUTH GULP 1 SECOND	BRACE	MOVE

The initial nose breath takes around 3 seconds. It's imperative to inhale slowly and expand through your belly. The goal with this first breath is to emphasize diaphragmatic belly breathing, similar to what you experienced with the Prone Breath Corrective on page 46. If you feel your chest rise, shoulders elevate, and upper back expand, start over. Again, the diaphragm, not the chest, is the primary mover in this step. This begins to pressurize the abdomen and thoracic cavity for an optimal brace and primes your diaphragm for the second breath.

To maintain intra-abdominal pressure, you must hold your breath through your nose for a split second while taking your second breath through your mouth. This gulping inhale through your mouth tops off the lungs and expands the diaphragm by an additional 5 to 15 percent. With the increased intra-abdominal pressure from the Double Breath Technique, you enhance the quality of your brace and the degree of tension you can create through the pillar. Stated differently, the more air you're holding in your diaphragm, the more tension and pillar stability you can create by bracing. Conversely, the less air you're holding in your diaphragm, the less tension you can create by bracing.

After both the full nose inhalation and mouth gulp, the last step is to lock in the position by actively engaging your abdominals through a 360-degree contraction. From this maximal brace, the next step is to scale tension to meet the demands of the movement (load and rep range)—and scale your breath cycle to meet the demands of your brace. In other words, bracing and breathing just enough to maintain pillar stability through the duration of the set (see "How to Brace and Breathe" to learn how this is done).

TEMPO:

NOSE INHALE
3 seconds

MOUTH GULP
1 second

BRACE and BREATHE

As covered above, maximizing the brace starts with a calm and controlled breath through the nose, which is typically about 3 seconds. But by no means should you feel restricted to that time frame. Take as long as you need during the initial inhale to expand your diaphragm fully; that might be 3 seconds or 5, depending on your lung capacity. The secondary gulp should take no more than a second. From here, scale your tension and breathing to the demand of the movement—and, more specifically, the rep counts associated with the desired training effects. When in doubt, breathe more slowly and under control, and look to bracing quality as the indicator of what breathing tempo works best for you.

HOW TO BRACE AND BREATHE

When learning to properly scale and match your brace and breath cycle, always start with a maximal preplanned brace, as guided by the cueing sequence and Double Breath Technique. Starting strong is crucial because you can't reclaim a good position under load once it's lost, despite any increase in tension. For instance, imagine you're performing a set of goblet squats. If you start with insufficient tension—meaning you aren't braced enough to support the weight—you'll likely compensate into positions with less muscular control, placing unwanted stress on your joints. Once the weight is in motion, increasing tension does little to safeguard your body because you're already moving with suboptimal form. Conversely, if you initially brace with more tension than necessary, your body is protected from the start, allowing you to fine-tune the tension downward without compromising pillar neutrality and stability. Think of it like overinflating a balloon and then slowly letting out just enough air to achieve the perfect size; it requires less effort than trying to blow more air into a balloon that's already pressurized.

While it's recommended to brace maximally and then scale down accordingly, there comes a point when it's not always necessary to apply the Double Breath Technique to every setup. Once you've developed an intuitive sense of how to synchronize the required tension to perform movements safely and effectively—essentially, your reliable autopilot—you can reserve the Double Breath Technique for max-effort lifts. For most other movements, particularly movements with light to moderate loads, you will follow the cueing sequence to brace, but rather than bracing maximally and scaling down, you will simply brace and breathe to perfectly meet the demands of the movement and set. This tailored approach to bracing and breathing is an art, as it varies depending not only on how you feel and the specific movement performed but also on the load and number of repetitions in the set.

For rep counts of 1 to 3 in a pure power scheme (max-effort lift), complete all reps with a single breath hold. One common mistake in this range is performing what are essentially three back-to-back single lifts—that is, breaking at the top of the movement and re-bracing with the Double Breath Technique. As you've learned, you can't re-brace effectively under load. Resting at the top, as many do with hard sets of 3 to 5 repetitions, contradicts the principles of effective bracing. It's a practice typically seen among those who have not mastered proper bracing and breathing techniques from the start. So, for maximal lifts, execute all reps consecutively without pausing to inhale. If necessary, you may exhale slightly with pursed lips—this creates resistance so that you don't let out too much air and lose the brace—during the concentric or lifting phase. Be aware of symptoms like dizziness, blurred vision, or sudden weakness, which could indicate you're pushing too hard without adequate oxygen. Passing out during a max-effort lift does not fall into the category of pain-free performance.

For sets ranging from 3 to 8 reps, it's essential to manage your breathing to maintain optimal muscle function and brace integrity. The key is not to take full breaths between reps, which can disrupt your form and reduce the effectiveness of your brace. Instead, sip air at the top of the movement as if through a straw and exhale slowly against resistance (pursed lips) as you lift the weight (concentric phase). This method helps maintain the brace during critical points of exertion, often resulting in the natural occurrence of grunting during loaded reps.

Further emphasizing this technique, it's crucial to avoid "resetting" or attempting to rebrace between reps. Doing so can cause you to lose your established pillar position, the synergistic tension among muscle groups, the beneficial effect of diaphragmatic expansion, and the constant muscular tension that is crucial for achieving the desired training effect. In this method, you allow for only about 10 percent air exchange with each rep, ensuring that your pillar is engaged and protected throughout the set.

For sets of more than 8 repetitions, focus on synchronizing your breath cycle with the tension of your brace. As a general rule, the less tension required to maintain pillar stability, the more air you can exchange, and vice versa. So, for a hard set of 8 to 20 reps, you may only exchange 20 to 30 percent of your total lung capacity every other rep. For lower load sets extending beyond 20 reps—say 20 to 50 reps—you may take a half breath every other rep, or every 3 reps. This breath cycle largely depends on your lung capacity, the load, and your effort (how fast you are performing the movement). For example, someone who is 6 feet and 200 pounds might take one half breath in and out over 3 reps, whereas someone who is 5 feet and 120 pounds might take two half breaths over 3 reps for the same exercise and rep count. However, this breath cycle or tempo might increase if the weight is heavier or the movement is performed at a faster rhythm, or decrease if the weight is lighter or the movement is performed slower. Given these variabilities, the best strategy is to concentrate on matching your breath cycle—breathing just enough—to maintain pillar stability through the duration of the set, whether it is for 8 or 50 reps. In other words, don't worry so much about the tempo of your breath cycle, trying to time your inhale and exhale with a specific number of reps during the set. As you fatigue, your tempo may change, meaning you may require more breaths to keep optimal blood oxygenation as the set progresses. In short, allow your breath cycle to occur naturally based on the precise level of tension required to preserve pillar stability.

To reiterate, you will never complete a full breath cycle during loaded movements—you would lose the initial brace and tension through the pillar and be unable to regain a quality brace during the set. Even with higher rep counts, you should never exchange more than half of your air during a single breath cycle, otherwise you will not be able to maintain the integrity of your brace.

Take these guidelines into consideration every single time you set up for a lift. Your preplanned bracing strategy should not only encompass the degree of tension required to maintain pillar stability, but also how much you are breathing to maintain that stability. A common mistake is to treat an 8-rep set like a 1-rep set, or a 20-rep set like an 8-rep set, accelerating fatigue. As fatigue sets in—because you are bracing too much and breathing too little to match the time under tension—you will default to taking bigger, faster breaths. It's a reflexive impulse when there is not enough air exchange to fuel the effort. The more you fatigue, the more air you have to take in. And the more air you take in, the harder it is to maintain a quality brace. As a result, you either can't hit the desired rep count (not ideal), or you will compensate and finish the set with suboptimal form (don't do this).

Remember, there is a skill and art to breathing and bracing. The better you get at synchronizing your brace and breath cycle, the more intuitive the process will become. You will be able to adjust based on how you are feeling and moving—this is your reliable autopilot. Put another way, the more intent you place behind your preplanned bracing and breathing strategy—that is, knowing how much you will need to brace and breathe to complete the set—the more efficient your movement and the less likely you are to compensate into potentially harmful positions.

SINGLE BREATH HOLD — 1-3 REPS

HEAVILY LOADED BARBELL BACK SQUAT

STRAW SIP BREATHS — 3-8 REPS

Sip air at the top of the movement as if through a straw.

Exhale slowly against resistance (pursed lips) as you lift the weight.

AIR EXCHANGE: *10% of total lung capacity*

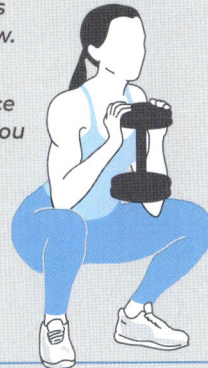

GOBLET SQUAT

HALF BREATHS — 8+ REPS

Take a half breath every other rep, or every 3 reps.

AIR EXCHANGE: *20% to 50% of total lung capacity*

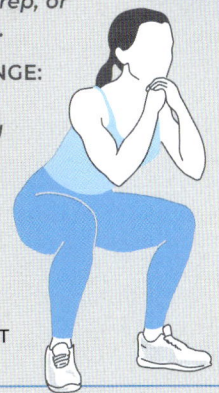

BODYWEIGHT SQUAT

HOW TO EXPEDITE RECOVERY:
90/90 SUPINE PARASYMPATHETIC POSITIONAL BREATHING

Achieving gains in muscle, strength, and athletic performance hinges not only on the intensity and quality of your training but also on effective recovery management between sessions. Despite its importance, the recovery phase often takes a backseat to training, overlooking its crucial role in allowing the body to heal from training-induced stress.

What strategies, then, can speed up recovery and make training sessions more productive, ensuring steady progress? Key factors like proper nutrition, adequate hydration, and stress management significantly contribute to both enhanced performance and faster recovery. Yet an often-overlooked recovery aspect is the shift from a sympathetic response to a parasympathetic state, which kick-starts the recovery process.

Minimizing the central nervous system's transition time from post-workout arousal to a recovery-friendly state is vital. Incorporating recovery breathing techniques as the concluding "exercise" of your workout can effectively ease this shift, serving as a critical link between rigorous training and the body's inherent healing mechanisms that support sustained, pain-free performance.

WHEN TO USE THIS TECHNIQUE

When I was younger, I thought I could get away with skipping warm-ups and cool-downs, and as a result, my fitness routines focused solely on the workout: get in, train hard, and get out. This pattern led to a predictable crash a couple of hours later, marked by a racing heart, trembling body, dizziness, and profuse sweating. It was as if my body was hitting the brakes for me, signaling the urgent need to slow down and recuperate.

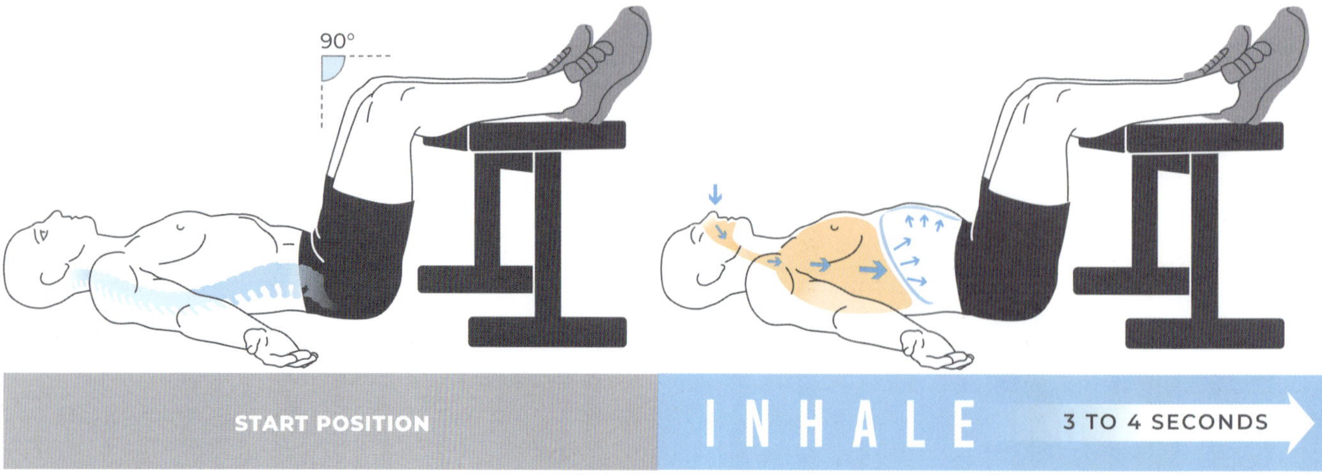

90°

START POSITION

I N H A L E — 3 TO 4 SECONDS →

This pattern isn't unique to me; many who train hard, particularly in the mornings, experience similar overtraining symptoms. The training ignites a sympathetic response, and then they remain in that elevated state throughout the day, which not only hampers recovery but can also create a barrier to strength, muscle growth, and performance due to the neurological and systemic strain it places on the mind and body.

The 90/90 Supine Parasympathetic Positional Breathing drill is one viable strategy to effectively break that cycle. When I began implementing this breathing strategy into my post-training routine, my symptoms of overtraining vanished. I recovered faster and felt a noticeable improvement in my physical state—I didn't get as sore and was able to transition more quickly from training to work. What astonished me most, however, was the mental clarity it brought. At the time, I was taking every continued education course and certification that I could, literally studying every minute of my free time. It was as if my brain had been supercharged. I honestly believe had I not added breathwork, I would have crashed and burned.

Initially, when I observed Buddy Morris leading his team through this simple breathing exercise, I didn't grasp its significance. Today, it's a staple in all my programs. Don't underestimate the power of this simple yet profound breathing practice. It's not a supplement to your workout—it's as essential as the exercises themselves, ensuring you exit your workout feeling better than when you started.

NOTE: *This breathing exercise can also be done before training to promote a parasympathetic response—see phase 0 of the warm-up on page 77. It's not exceedingly common and is often implemented when someone enters the gym already in sympathetic overdrive, too stressed to begin the first phase of the warm-up.*

HOW TO EXECUTE RECOVERY BREATHING

While it's important to take slow, rhythmic deep breaths with this exercise, the emphasis centers more around the setup and position of your body than on the actual breath tempo. To spark the recovery process, it's important to

▶ Elevate your limbs in a way that aids in the centralized drainage of lymphatic fluid—that is, built-up metabolites (waste products such as lactic acid accumulated in the muscles)—to reduce soreness and improve circulation

▶ Maintain a neutral spine to minimize any potential stress response from your body

▶ Find the most comfortable position possible to help shift your CNS away from its post-training state

HOLD	2 TO 3 SECONDS	EXHALE	6 TO 8 SECONDS

Find a quiet area in the gym, or put on your headphones with serene music to block out ambient noise, and follow these steps:

1. Lie down with the back of your head resting on the floor.

2. Elevate your legs above heart level with your hips and knees bent to about 90 degrees.

3. Position your arms out to your side, keeping them relaxed.

4. Close your eyes and consciously release any tension in your body.

5. Breathe in and out through your nose.

From this position, try to relax every muscle while breathing in and out through your nose in a slow, steady rhythm. You can exhale through your mouth if that feels better, especially if you are still out of breath from your workout, but just make sure to control the exhalation with a 6 to 8 second exhale. This is done by pursing your lips, which creates resistance to slow the exhale. Remember, rapid breathing, particularly mouth breathing, heightens the CNS response—the opposite effect of what you're trying to achieve here.

TEMPO:

INHALE
3 to 4 seconds

HOLD
2 to 3 seconds

EXHALE
6 to 8 seconds

Given that many athletes and lifters have trouble slowing down, particularly in the gym, using a specific tempo can be very useful with this breathing strategy.

The main focus is a deliberate, unhurried inhalation followed by a long, controlled exhalation. Inhale deeply over 3 to 4 seconds, pause for a moment, and then emphasize an extended exhalation lasting for about 6 to 8 seconds. The aim is to settle into a slow rhythm. Try not to fuss over the precise timing of your breaths—the tempo is merely a guide for you to habituate a natural breath cycle that promotes recovery.

Keep in mind that this period is meant to turn off the sympathetic switch before you leave the gym. Sidestep thoughts about upcoming tasks or anything else that's likely to induce stress. And steer clear of watching the clock. Instead, set a timer for 1 to 2 minutes, engage in positive visualization, and revel in your rest, celebrating the effort you just put into your workout.

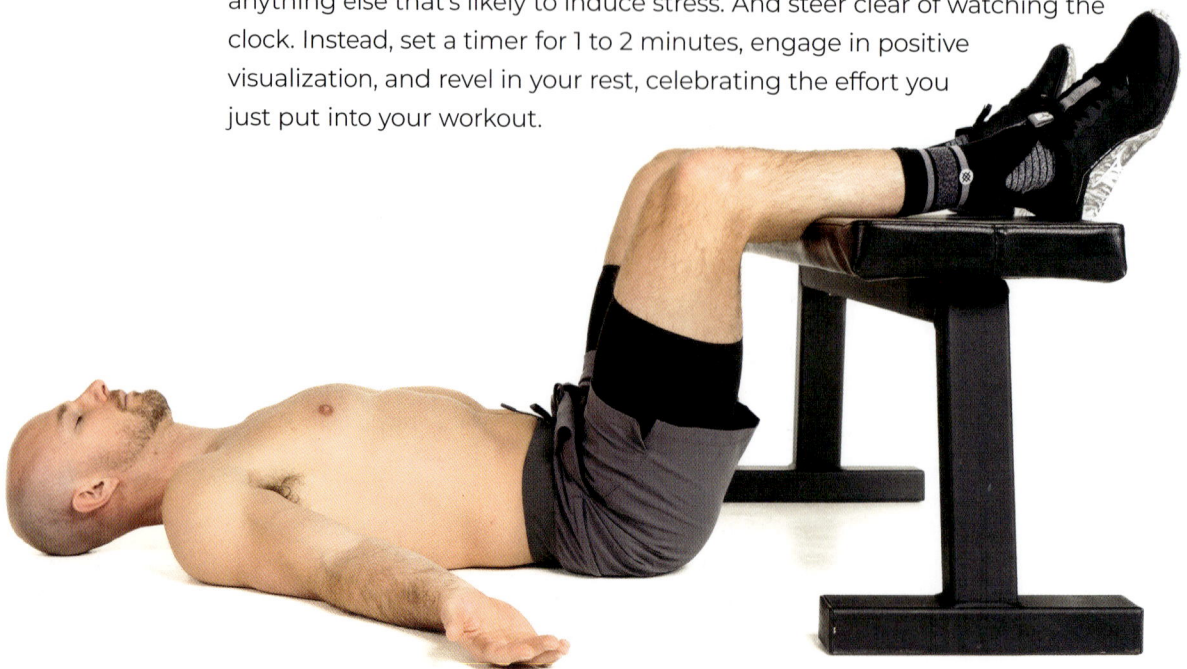

HOW TO RAMP UP FOR A BIG LIFT AND AMPLIFY PERFORMANCE:
THE SYMPATHETIC HUFF BREATH

Most breathing strategies in this chapter center around downregulating the central nervous system with a parasympathetic emphasis—and rightfully so, given that many of us live in a state of chronic stress. However, when a lift demands a surge of strength and power, such as a one-rep-max back squat, you want the opposite effect. In this situation, you don't want to calm down; you want to ramp up. This is where the Sympathetic Huff Breath comes in. It's a breathing strategy that upregulates the CNS, priming the mind and body for peak exertion.

WHEN TO USE THIS TECHNIQUE

Regardless of your training objective or how you orchestrate your program, each training session should revolve around a primary performance goal or key performance indicator (KPI). This KPI is the heart of your workout, denoting the most demanding exercise or skill you're aiming to conquer and improve. It is during these critical moments, particularly in your heaviest or fastest set, that you should utilize the Sympathetic Huff Breath.

When applied strategically and with precision, the sympathetic spark can provide a powerful performance boost. However, indiscriminate usage—say during lighter, dynamic warm-up or accessory exercise sets—can overtax the system, leading to diminished power and increased fatigue. Imagine being in a gunfight with limited ammunition; you need to make each shot count.

For an effective and balanced approach, incorporate 1 to 3 sets of Sympathetic Huff Breaths each session, carefully selecting the right moment to employ this powerful breathing technique. To optimize performance and prevent fatigue, limit the total weekly usage to no more than 8 sets.

HOW TO EXECUTE THE SYMPATHETIC HUFF BREATH

In contrast to the full 360-degree diaphragmatic breathing strategies emphasized throughout this chapter, the Sympathetic Huff Breath intentionally diverges from this approach. This strategy involves taking quick, shallow breaths through the chest to ignite the CNS—the opposite of how you should normally breathe. Here's how to properly execute this technique:

1. Stand straight in a neutral posture, with your arms relaxed at your sides.

2. Elevate your elbows, drawing them back slightly, and shrug your shoulders. Accompany this movement with a quick inhalation through your nose, directing air into your chest.

3. Instantly follow with a powerful exhale, emitting a "huff" against resistance, by pushing air out through your mouth. This action involves forcefully compressing your chest and dropping your shoulders and arms, facilitated by pursing your lips to restrict airflow. Repeat this breathing cycle 2 to 4 times.

THE SYMPATHETIC HUFF BREATH

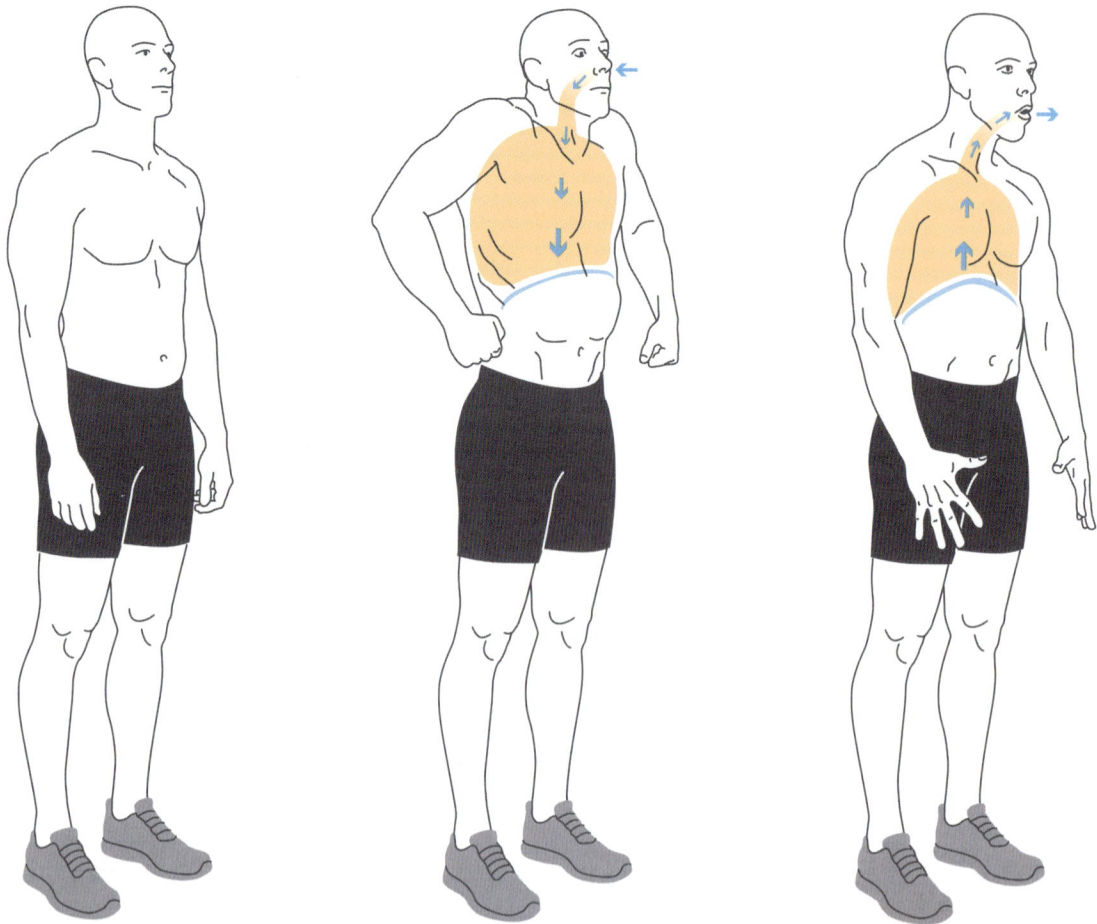

START POSITION	INHALE	EXHALE

TEMPO:

Rapid inhale followed by a forceful exhale

Tempo is crucial with this breathing strategy. When taking the 2 to 4 sympathetic huff breaths pre-set, focus on speed and precision. Each inhale and exhale should take less than one second.

After the breathing cycle, immediately employ the Double Breath Technique to create and maintain pillar stability before transitioning into your key performance indicator, or KPI—the hardest, heaviest lift of the workout session.

MAXIMIZE CARDIOVASCULAR FITNESS
AND IMPROVE BIOMECHANICAL EFFICIENCY:
RHYTHMIC BREATHING

Endurance activities like running rank among the highest for injury rates in all forms of physical exercise, a consequence of global popularity as well as the cumulative strain from repeated movement patterns. Biomechanical factors related to form and tissue preparedness certainly play a role. However, there is another contributing factor that often flies under the radar: breathing.

For those aiming to maximize cardiovascular fitness while minimizing injury risk, the Rhythmic Breathing strategy can be a game changer. Adopting a steady, rhythmic breathing cadence that alternates with each footfall can help balance mechanical stress and retrain the neuromuscular system toward enhanced efficiency.

While cardiovascular health is essential for everyone, no matter the demographic or activity of choice, it shouldn't come at the expense of your orthopedic health. Here's how to use the Rhythmic Breathing strategy to mitigate such risks.

WHEN TO USE THIS TECHNIQUE

When engaged in intense physical activities, the sympathetic side of your central nervous system spikes, priming your body for a fight-or-flight reaction. While useful in short bursts, consistently redlining your system can provoke injuries and diminish long-term performance, especially in activities extending beyond 10 to 15 seconds.

For traditional cardiovascular exercises like walking, running, biking, and cardio machine training, mitigating the sympathetic response is key to reaping training benefits. This mitigation involves aligning your breath with your movements to preserve proper exercise form and pillar stability.

In running, the moment of greatest stress occurs when the foot contacts the ground, often bearing 3 to 4 times one's body weight. Runners in a sustained sympathetic state often resort to rapid, shallow breathing from the chest, accelerating fatigue. Compounding this, they usually exhale when one foot—more frequently on one side than the other—hits the ground. With each exhale, the diaphragm rises, reducing core stability and transmitting uneven forces from the foot through the knee, hip, and spine. This results in a disproportionate impact on the favored side, which is a predictor for injuries.

Rhythmic Breathing, with a 3:2 tempo—three counts for inhalation and two for exhalation—offers a solution, particularly in activities like running and walking, where limbs move in opposition. This breathing technique is advisable for any reciprocal endurance activity of low to moderate intensity lasting over 15 seconds, helping distribute impact more evenly. Initially, Rhythmic Breathing enhances performance. Long-term, it minimizes occurrences of pain and injury.

HOW TO EXECUTE RHYTHMIC BREATHING

Like any other motor skill, rhythmic breathing must be intelligently implemented into training with a predictable step-by-step approach to mastery.

Believing you can shift from an uneven breathing pattern during a run one day to a flawless 3:2 tempo the next without a decrease in performance is a bit of a stretch. However, you can expedite the learning phase using the same stepwise approach you would employ to rebuild a movement pattern (bearing in mind that locomotion is a foundational movement pattern). Think of it like a corrective exercise: you're employing a specific exercise sequence to pattern a new motor skill. There are no set or rep recommendations, simply play with the movement until it "clicks" and then move on. For Rhythmic Breathing, you will use a three-phase progression strategy.

1. SUPINE 3:2 BREATHING WITH MARCH

Begin by lying on your back with your knees bent and feet flat on the ground. With both feet grounded, this position enables easier mental transfer to the dynamics of walking and running. To perform the movement, elevate your hips into the bridge and bring your knee toward your chest, keeping roughly a 90-degree angle in your knee and hips. Maintaining the bridge position, bring your foot down to the start position and then immediately perform the same movement with your other leg. Repeat this back-and-forth movement while coordinating your leg movements with your breathing: inhale over three-foot movements, then exhale over the next two. Once you get the rhythm down, proceed to standing.

START POSITION

INHALE ➔   EXHALE ➔

2. STANDING 3:2 BREATHING WITH MARCH

March in place, maintaining the 3:2 breathing rhythm: three footfalls on the inhale and then two on the exhale. This cadence ensures alternating steps on consecutive exhales, evenly dispersing force between both feet.

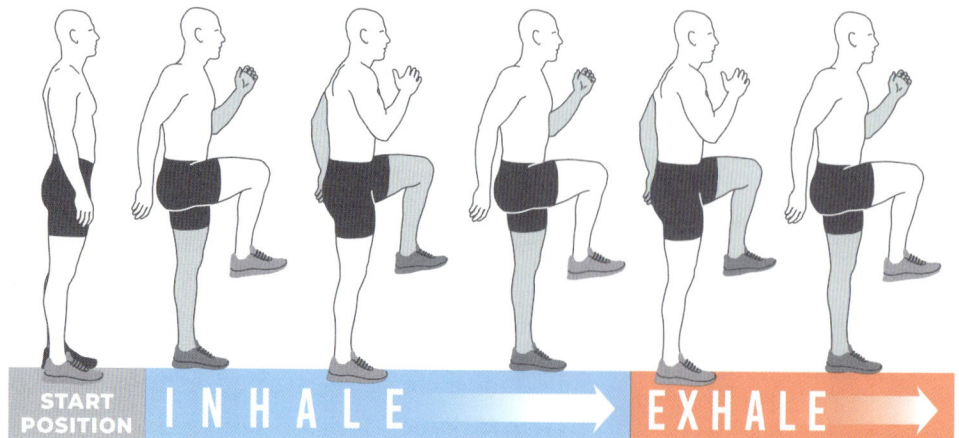

START POSITION   INHALE ➔   EXHALE ➔

3. LOCOMOTION WITH 3:2 BREATHING

The culmination of this strategy involves integrating the 3:2 breathing pattern with walking, eventually progressing to brisker paces like jogging and running. Start slow, only walking or running as fast as you can while preserving the breathing cycle—three steps on the inhale, two on the exhale. This skill will evolve with practice, with the ultimate aim of it becoming automatic.

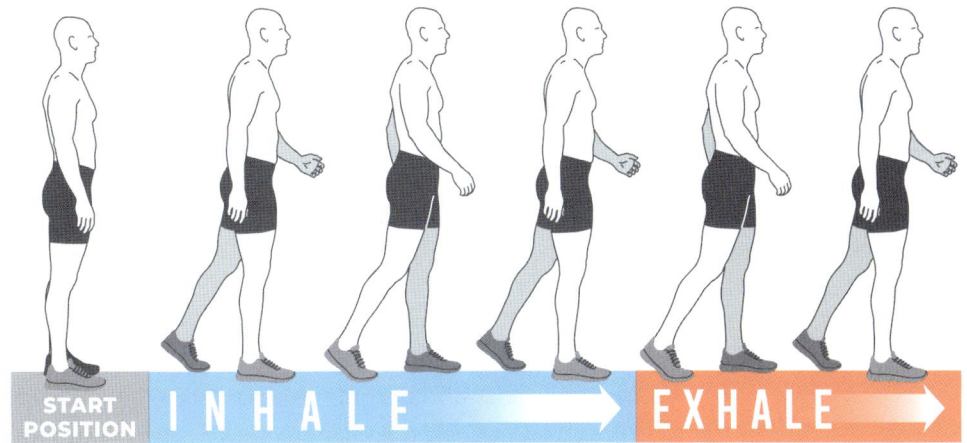

START POSITION — INHALE — EXHALE

TEMPO:

INHALE 3 counts

EXHALE 2 counts

As the name implies, Rhythmic Breathing focuses on the cadenced tempo of breath in harmony with bodily movements. Most runners and endurance athletes default to a 2:2 breathing pattern, which can be problematic. Typically, exhaling coincides with the foot strike of the same foot, leading to imbalanced forces on the body's right and left sides.

The 3:2 breathing rhythm presents a straightforward resolution. This pattern alternates the foot that hits the ground on exhalation, equalizing the load on both sides.

Alternating strike patterns might seem trivial in the short term. However, over longer durations, repetitive cycles with one side bearing the brunt of the impact during exhalation—and an unstable core affecting joint stability—stress can accumulate, potentially leading to pain and injuries. By systematizing your breathing with cardiovascular activity, you're not only performing optimally but also protecting your body.

FOOT STRIKE AT POINT OF FULL EXHALATION

FOOT STRIKE AT POINT OF FULL EXHALATION

INHALE			EXHALE		INHALE			EXHALE	
RIGHT STRIKE	LEFT STRIKE	RIGHT STRIKE	LEFT STRIKE	RIGHT STRIKE	LEFT STRIKE	RIGHT STRIKE	LEFT STRIKE	RIGHT STRIKE	LEFT STRIKE

HOW TO MITIGATE SYMPATHETIC STRESS RESPONSES AND RECOVER BETWEEN SETS:
THE TACTICAL BREATH

When we think about the highest-level physical performers, our minds typically gravitate toward professional athletes. Sure, there are some serious freaks of nature who are nothing short of astonishing, but overlooking the phenomenal capabilities of elite tactical athletes, such as Navy SEALs, would be a glaring omission.

This isn't about equating military operations with gym routines—the disparity is vast and obvious. It's about adopting the sophisticated techniques that forge such remarkable resilience in tactical athletes, especially under duress, and applying it to our training. A prime example of such a technique is the Tactical Breath.

WHEN TO USE THIS TECHNIQUE

Like many innovative methods, the Tactical Breath (also known as box breathing) was birthed from necessity. My formal introduction to the Tactical Breath was through the teachings of ex–Navy SEAL Mark Divine. There's nothing routine about a firefight, no matter how much experience you have in the field. In such high-stress moments, you're hardwired to enter fight-or-flight mode: heart racing, blood pressure soaring, pupils dilating, primed for survival.

This primal reaction, while useful, doesn't always serve us when fine motor skills and peak performance are required. Consider a highly trained sniper—if they succumb to sympathetic shakes upon spotting a target, their effectiveness would be compromised. Similarly, not all training should mimic the high stakes of competition. Often, it's more about managing the sympathetic surge during workouts to maintain control as intensity and volume ramp up.

In essence, the Tactical Breath serves as a tool to enhance the recovery phase within resting intervals, promoting both mechanical and systemic recuperation. This, in turn, enhances focus, the quality of movement patterns, and training performance. The quicker you can recover between sets, the more efficient your training becomes. And when training is efficient, energy is conserved and can be channeled more productively into the workout.

Deploy the Tactical Breath whenever you need to dampen a sympathetic surge and return to baseline, be it from a taxing exercise set or an acute stressor in life.

HOW TO EXECUTE TACTICAL BREATHING

First, it's crucial to nail down the 360-degree belly breathing technique. Review the Prone Breath Corrective on page 46 to ensure your diaphragmatic breathing is on point. Shallow, rapid chest breathing, the default for many, will only heighten the stress response you're aiming to mitigate with this strategy.

While the ultimate goal is to use the Tactical Breath to accelerate recovery during workouts, that is not the best time to learn this skill. A much better approach is to practice the breathing pattern in a calm environment with minimal movement and distractions. When starting out, sit in a comfortable position with an upright posture and then go through these steps:

1. Sit with your spine in a neutral posture and close your eyes. This encourages deep, natural breathing, reduces sensory input, and enhances relaxation.

2. Inhale over 4 seconds, drawing air in through your belly.

3. Hold this inhalation for a 4-second count.

4. Exhale through your nose over 4 seconds. If you prefer to exhale through your mouth, purse your lips to restrict air flow and slow your exhalation.

5. Briefly pause for 1 to 4 seconds before your next inhale.

TEMPO:

INHALE 4 seconds
HOLD 4 seconds
EXHALE 4 seconds
HOLD 1 to 4 seconds

Referred to as "box breathing" for the equal time given to each part of the cycle, this practice excels across a spectrum of tough scenarios. Yet, for recovery during exercise, a quicker cadence can be beneficial—because muscles need a faster oxygen refresh and you'll likely be out of breath from a hard set.

In this situation, tweak the last pause post-exhalation to 1 to 2 seconds. This change can boost recovery significantly, as it increases the frequency of breathing cycles during rest. The customary box breath cycle is 16 seconds; with the alteration, it's 13 seconds. That's precious time for a recuperating athlete.

In summary, adopt a 4:4:4:1 breathing tempo to optimize recovery between intense training sets. Outside of training, the standard 4:4:4:4 box breathing rhythm is your go-to tempo for managing stress and anxiety.

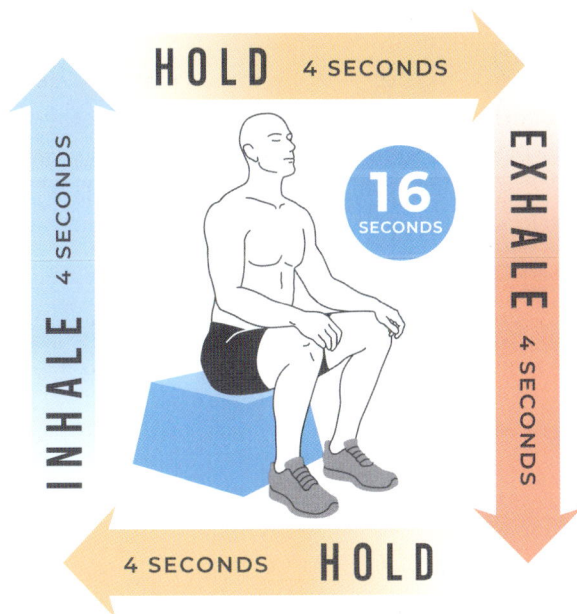

STANDARD BOX BREATHING TEMPO
(for managing stress)

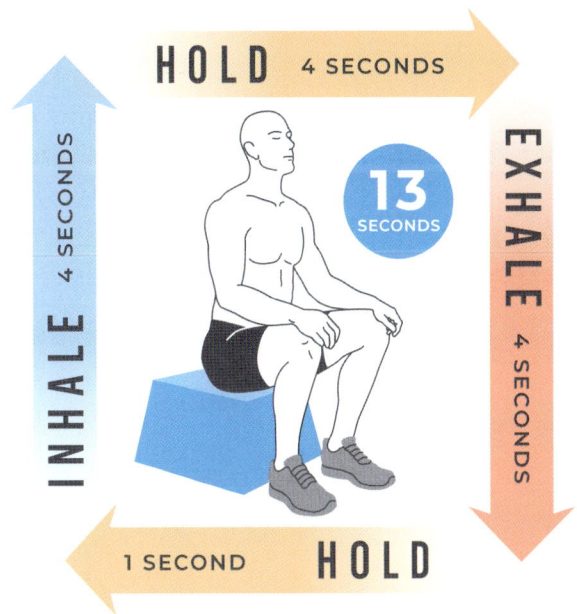

TACTICAL BREATHING TEMPO
(recovering between training sets)

02

THE 6-PHASE DYNAMIC WARM-UP

THE 6-PHASE DYNAMIC WARM-UP

Never waste another warm-up.

You're training to feel and perform at your best—and you want results.

The 6-phase dynamic warm-up sequence is the first step in that process and one of the most important pillars supporting your health and fitness efforts. It's neither an optional add-on to the beginning of a workout that you can skip nor a long, complex list of random exercises with zero benefit.

Let's get it right. The focus is training, and the 6-phase dynamic warm-up sequence is the on-ramp that prepares you to move safely and effectively—to get you feeling your best so that you're ready to crush the workout. It plays an indispensable role in pain-free performance and sets the tone for the training session by helping you

▶ Increase resilience against training-related pain and injuries

▶ Prime your mind and body for the training session

▶ Enhance performance potential for the workout

▶ Learn, practice, and refine movement skills

▶ Pinpoint and strengthen weak links that cause pain or limit functional abilities

But to get the most from the warm-up, you must follow a structured and purposeful plan—a minimum effective dose of the best therapeutic exercise modalities and performance-boosting techniques that express and amplify the short- and long-term benefits of training. The 6-phase dynamic warm-up takes all of this into account. It includes

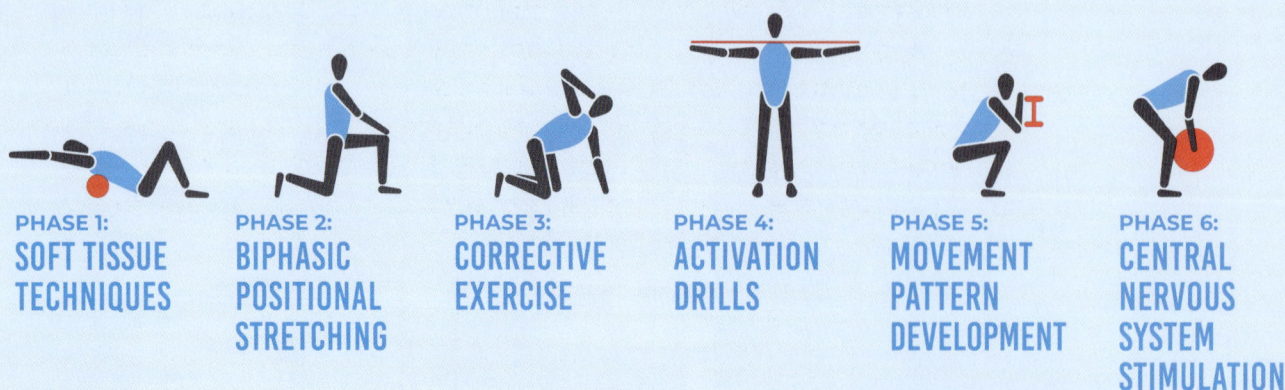

PHASE 1:
SOFT TISSUE TECHNIQUES

PHASE 2:
BIPHASIC POSITIONAL STRETCHING

PHASE 3:
CORRECTIVE EXERCISE

PHASE 4:
ACTIVATION DRILLS

PHASE 5:
MOVEMENT PATTERN DEVELOPMENT

PHASE 6:
CENTRAL NERVOUS SYSTEM STIMULATION

In this part of the book, you will learn why you need to warm up using this 6-phase sequence, the purpose of each phase, and how to program and perform the exercises. With this knowledge, you will practice a step-by-step system for warming up that is

▼
EFFECTIVE:
It will get you ready to perform by improving how you feel and move.

▼
EFFICIENT:
It is purposeful, with no time wasted.

What's more, you can apply this warm-up to any sport, fitness modality, or physical therapy practice—any setting where the goal is to reduce the risk of injury, alleviate pain, improve movement quality, and prepare the mind and body for the challenges of life and training. In this way, the warm-up is more than just an exercise preparation sequence; it is your toolkit for maintaining your body, maximizing your recovery, and enhancing your movement health. Put simply, it is

> The warm-up is more than just an exercise preparation sequence; it is your toolkit for maintaining your body, maximizing your recovery, and enhancing your movement health.

▼
SCALABLE:
It works for everyone, regardless of age, fitness level, or training activity.

▼
ADAPTABLE:
It serves as a pre-training sequence, can be manipulated to function as a post-training recovery, or acts as a standalone regenerative protocol.

▼
SUSTAINABLE:
It can be repeated no matter how you feel or how much time you have.

Don't waste another second on a warm-up that doesn't complement your training or make the best use of your time. With just a 10-minute daily investment, you can optimize movement, mobility, and recovery, all of which compound over time. The more consistently you do it, the better you get at it, leading to greater returns on your investment. Plus, this warm-up can adapt with you, meeting your evolving needs while building resilience and movement mastery. Embrace the 6-phase dynamic warm-up, commit to a daily practice, and reap the rewards in your health, function, and performance.

PREPARATION TENETS

The 6-phase dynamic warm-up is a 10- to 12-minute exercise preparation and body maintenance template to get you feeling and performing your best both in and out of the gym. But, to maximize the benefits from each phase—and the pre-training and recovery system as a whole—there are key tenets that are crucial to understand, along with some general guidelines that you must follow.

Watch any professional athlete warm up, and you'll witness a meticulously crafted symphony of preparation.

They perform dynamic movements to increase blood flow and unlock mobility, ensuring that every joint and muscle is primed and ready. They incorporate specific drills designed to sharpen their technique and coordination so that they can deploy their refined, precise skills when it matters most. Visualization and breathing exercises steady their nerves and hone their concentration, readying their minds for the challenges ahead. By the time they finish the warm-up, their bodies are finely tuned instruments, and their mental state is focused and unbreakable—prepared to tackle the grueling demands of high-intensity training and competition.

For professional athletes, the stakes are incredibly high—careers, sponsorships, and millions of dollars are on the line. That's why their preparation must be meticulous and unwavering. Warming up isn't just a preparatory step. It's a foundational practice. Never skipped. Always prioritized. Because when it comes to their performance, it's not just about winning or losing; it's about staying in the game.

Injuries are the ultimate gatekeepers. Pain is a performance inhibitor. An athlete's skill can only rise to the level of how they feel physically, mentally, and emotionally. Injury and pain not only restrict physical capabilities but also erode mental focus and emotional resilience, creating a triad of obstacles that prevent athletes from performing at their true potential. And if they can't perform to their potential, everything they've worked for is at risk. Look at the exit rates in professional sports— those exits are almost never about lack of skill but about getting injured and then being unable to perform. A well-structured warm-up keeps them in the game, acting as their shield against pain and ensuring they can perform at their best, day in and day out. It safeguards them from preventable injuries that could sideline them for weeks, months, or even permanently.

Athletes and trainers know this well, which is why they place so much emphasis on and spend so much time warming up. I can personally attest to it. When I was training professional and Olympic athletes, the warm-up was the bedrock of our training regimen, routinely spanning upward of 40 minutes. Each phase of the warm-up, consisting of a targeted set of exercises, was designed with a specific purpose: to prime the athletes' bodies and minds for pain-free performance. We performed soft tissue techniques, stretches, and corrective exercises to eliminate friction points that could impede training and movement quality. We implemented activation and mobility drills, homed in on technique, and utilized other performance-based strategies that mirrored their training and sport, creating a seamless transition into the workout or competition. In short, it was a strategically sequenced, phase-based dynamic warm-up that accounted for all aspects of physical, mental, and emotional preparation.

Given the well-established importance and effectiveness of a purposefully designed dynamic warm-up—and the resounding success my athletes experienced with the routines I crafted for them—I naturally adopted the same approach in my own training. I figured if it worked for elite athletes, it was a necessity for me as well. Considering myself an athlete, I wanted to maximize my time in the gym, especially in terms of enhancing my functional abilities and reducing my susceptibility to pain and injury. I viewed the warm-up—the same warm-up my professional athletes were doing—as a crucial piece of my performance puzzle.

For several years, I followed the same routine, warming up for nearly 40 minutes before every training session. I never got hurt, and I felt good. That is to say, I felt as good as I'd always felt—no better, no worse. However, as time went on, the extensive time and energy spent on my warm-up began to wear on me. Unlike professional athletes—who are often required and have the time to warm up for 40 minutes, and who might need drawn-out warm-ups to prepare for long games and intense workouts that push their bodies to the absolute limit—I was training to feel and look good and to be the healthiest version of myself. Without the motivational inputs that push athletes to perform at the highest level, my enthusiasm began to decline. As a result, my strength and muscle gains plateaued, my focus diminished, and my excitement for training waned. Despite these signs, I didn't question the efficacy of my lengthy warm-up. Instead, I blamed my stagnation on not training hard enough, believing that to gain more, I needed to do more.

Then everything changed. When my son Cam was born, time suddenly became my most precious resource. Running a business, training clients, balancing fatherhood, and trying to maintain my fitness routine became a juggling act. The reality hit me: I wasn't a professional athlete getting paid to exercise, and I didn't have 40 minutes to spend warming up. This forced a deep introspection and personal audit of my training time—because every minute spent in the gym was time that I wasn't spending with my son or providing for my family.

In light of this, I began to think more methodically about the purpose of the warm-up for general health and fitness, knowing that for the average person, a well-designed warm-up can make all the difference in getting results and achieving consistent, pain-free performance. What's more, I knew the phasic approach I used with my athletes worked because—again—they were getting results.

This presented a conflict I had to resolve. Most people, like me, don't have 40 minutes to warm up. But we still need to warm-up using the same phasic approach as professional athletes because the stakes are just as high—it's our health and performance that are on the line. Getting sidelined with pain, wasting time in the gym, and not making progress can have real consequences. It can lead to frustration, decreased motivation,

and even skipping the warm-up or giving up on exercise entirely. So, I asked myself: How could I make the warm-up more efficient and less overwhelming? How could I improve it to ensure consistent progress while preventing pain and injuries?

Reflecting on these questions, I concluded that an effective warm-up shouldn't be excessively long or burdensome. It should

- Be just enough to prepare anyone, regardless of age or background, for optimal performance without detracting from the main workout

- Address every aspect of movement health: prime the nervous system, enhance mental and physical readiness, fine-tune exercise form, reduce susceptibility to pain and injury, and set the stage for efficient recovery and cool-downs

- Align with common training goals and continually evolve as each milestone is reached, ensuring that engagement remains high and movement quality steadily improves

Taking an honest and objective assessment of my warm-up through this refined lens, it became clear that I was doing too much. The more I thought about it, the more I realized that my plateau wasn't due to a lack of effort or intensity in my training. Rather, it was because I was fatigued going into my most important lifts. Digging deeper, I uncovered another flaw in my approach: I was treating the warm-up as a formality, not the finely tuned prelude to the workout that it should be. I wasn't focused on improving the movements or progressing the exercises; I was simply going through the motions because it was the routine I had always followed, with decent success.

In other words, I was following a routine guided by default, and as a result, I was mentally and physically checked out. Instead of critically evaluating the efficiency of my routine with questions like, "Is this the best use of my time?" or "Is this exercise or strategy enhancing my workouts and health?" I had fallen into a ritualistic practice—a mindless routine devoid of intent and focus.

This insight not only sparked a recalibration of my pre-training routine but also made me understand why there's a tendency to overlook or even skip the warm-up. When warming up becomes a monotonous, time-consuming routine with zero perceived benefit, people burn out and give up. They may go from warming up extensively to not warming up at all. Initially, such a strategy might even prove beneficial. With more time and energy to direct into the workout, many experience gains in strength and performance, cementing the idea that a warm-up might not be necessary. But I can tell you from firsthand experience that these benefits are short-lived.

When I began the process of refining my warm-up, I decided to strip it down to nothing. Starting from a blank slate and gradually adding in phases (modalities) seemed the best way to identify which strategies and exercises were truly effective. The immediate results from this minimalist approach were eye-opening. I felt fresh going into my most important lifts and could push harder with less neural and mechanical fatigue—the precise reason why many powerlifters and bodybuilders champion not warming up.

However, it didn't take long before the lack of mobility and focused exercises started to catch up to me. After a few weeks, my progress had stalled. I felt stiff and stagnant. Not surprisingly, I encountered the same pitfalls as those who skip warm-ups for extended periods: tension, pain, and a plateau in progress. In essence, I was trading short-term gains for long-term losses, and it took my experience of briefly experimenting with no warm-up to realize this fundamental truth.

With a renewed perspective, I started reintroducing phases individually to my warm-up, but with a more concentrated and deliberate approach, adopting the minimum effective dose mentality. I evaluated each phase and technique to determine its effectiveness, adding exercises that contributed to my goals and removing those that didn't. I experimented with the order of the routine, continually assessing the benefits of each change. All of this was guided by my intention to free up more time for other important aspects of my life. The updated warm-up needed to be more efficient, accomplishing everything the old warm-up did—priming the mind and body, enhancing movement and mobility, preventing pain and injuries—without compromising time, energy, and focus for the main workout. To achieve this goal, I completely shifted my mindset. I went from a ritualistic approach that was repetitive, unfocused, and excessive to a results-driven approach that was efficient, attentive, and purposeful.

RITUALISTIC PRACTICE:	vs.	RESULTS-BASED PRACTICE:
Just going through the motions		Focused on specific outcomes
Zero intention or purpose		Clear intention and purpose
Doing the same thing every time		Tailored to individual needs and goals
Emphasis on quantity over quality		Emphasis on quality over quantity
Routine becomes monotonous		Regularly adjusted based on feedback and progress
Lack of measurable progress		Uses measurable metrics to track improvement
Overemphasis on tradition and habit		Engages variety to prevent monotony
Neglects individual needs and goals		Prioritizes efficiency and effectiveness
Resistant to change or new methods		Incorporates evidence-based techniques
Focuses on completion rather than improvement		Encourages continual learning and adaptation

I continued this process for several years, rigorously testing and fine-tuning to find the best sequence. The end result is the 6-phase dynamic warm-up covered in this section. At just 10 to 12 minutes, it retains all the pain-preventing and performance-promoting qualities of the 40-minute warm-up I used with professional athletes, but in a fraction of the time—allowing you to efficiently tackle multiple issues head-on without diminishing the effectiveness of the warm-up.

Motivation stays high, making it easier to commit to daily. The concise format prevents you from becoming overwhelmed, ensuring you start your workout energized rather than drained.

Movement and mobility improve significantly. The targeted exercises in each phase are designed to enhance joint mobility and range of motion, making every movement smoother and more controlled.

Each phase facilitates movement mastery. By incorporating specific drills that sharpen technique and coordination, you can execute exercises with precision and confidence. This attention to detail translates to better overall movement quality and effectiveness.

It strengthens weak links. Identifying and addressing imbalances or vulnerabilities in your body ensures that these areas become robust, preventing potential injuries and enhancing overall strength.

You manage training stress better. The inclusion of breathing exercises and mental preparation techniques helps regulate the nervous system, making it easier to handle the physical demands of intense training sessions.

Recovery is quicker and more efficient. By priming your body correctly, you reduce post-workout soreness and accelerate the healing process. This means you can train more consistently without the setbacks of prolonged recovery times.

Consistent muscle and strength gains become achievable. The optimized warm-up prepares your body to lift heavier and perform better, leading to steady progress and visible results over time.

In summary, the 6-phase dynamic warm-up is not just efficient—it's transformative. It addresses every aspect of physical health, performance, and longevity. If you were to do nothing else other than this, your body would feel and function well. The benefits will compound and lead to significant improvements over time. While it may not directly elicit muscular hypertrophy or a strength adaptation, it will potentiate you to take the next step, ensuring you are prepared for further physical development and performance.

And the best part? The multi-modality phasic approach also serves as a proactive post-training recovery template that facilitates improvements in mobility, movement, and pain prevention. Simply put, the 6-phase dynamic warm-up is a system designed not just for pre-training but for your cool-downs, recovery days, and long-term movement health.

To fully harness the potential of this 6-phase dynamic sequence, it's essential to grasp the underlying principles. As we transition into exploring the key tenets, remember that each one is a guideline to help you get the most from the sequence as a whole. Together, they make up the framework that ensures you don't just go through the motions but actively engage in a process that will help you achieve pain-free performance.

The 6-phase dynamic warm-up is a system designed not just for pre-training but for your cool-downs, recovery days, and long-term movement health.

NEVER SKIP THE WARM-UP—
EVEN WHEN YOU ARE SHORT ON TIME

I'll be the first to admit that the warm-up is not the sexiest of topics. Most people just want to get into the gym, work hard, and see results. They're not turned on by foam rolling, stretching, or activating key stabilizers—they would rather skip the foreplay and get straight to the workout.

But that runs counter to the goals of pain-free performance. A lot of people hold the misguided belief that foam rolling is pointless, stretching doesn't work, corrective exercises are a waste of time, and so on. They will say, "I don't do any of those things, and I still end up training pain-free."

It's true, you can get away with skipping the warm-up and exit the training session pain-free. But you potentially miss out on the performance-enhancing, injury-preventing, and movement-amplifying components of the sequential phases. And what happens when you do end up with training-related pain? Or you miss that personal record (PR)? Might it have been avoided, and could you have done better with a properly executed warm-up?

Remember, the 6-phase dynamic warm-up is about facilitating movement mastery and cleaning up functional loose ends that create pain and impede performance. Most important, it's about physical and emotional preparation for the workout—supercharging your movement system to be awesome that day.

Once you are familiar with the phases and how to progress through them, the 6-phase dynamic warm-up becomes an easy and necessary segue into training. You'll feel better, and your workouts will improve. The best part is, it only takes 10 minutes. There is no excuse to ever skip the warm-up.

PERFORM EACH PHASE IN SEQUENCE—
START SLOW TO GO FAST

The six phases are strategically programmed in a specific order, and each phase works off of the last to produce numerous benefits. Put another way, there is synergy—a binding power—between phases that makes the exercises far more valuable as a stepwise sequence than as standalone practices for training preparation.

The research on foam rolling and stretching as independent warm-up modalities isn't great. Corrective exercises by themselves aren't that effective. Activation drills have a place but are not the best in isolation. You see where I'm going with this—the six phases are stronger as a system than as individual parts.

Even so, people will sensibly question the efficacy of the phases. They will argue, "If the primary goal of the warm-up is to prepare the mind and body to move with load and speed, why should I foam roll and stretch? If I'm not in pain and don't have an obvious movement limitation, what's the point of doing corrective exercises? I just get my body temperature up, gradually introduce more load and speed, and I'm good to go."

Though reasonable, this line of thinking fails to consider how the mind and body are connected or, more specifically, the role the nervous system plays in regulating how we move, feel, and perform.

THE CNS SPECTRUM

To appreciate the logic underpinning the order of the six phases, it's important to understand the two polarizing sides of the central nervous system spectrum and how they harmonize training and performance.

On one side of the spectrum, there's the sympathetic nervous system (known as the fight or flight response), which prepares you to perform against a threat or challenge. On the other side of the spectrum, there's the parasympathetic nervous system (known as rest and digest), which helps regulate recovery and regeneration.

When it comes to training, sympathetic nervous system activity is necessary to perform at the highest level. But you want to avoid punching the gas on the CNS when the warm-up starts because, if you're like most people, you show up to the gym in a sympathetic state with alarmingly high vital metrics. Your heart rate is elevated, your blood pressure is high, and your stress tolerance is diminished.

I call this running the red line. People are literally fighting for survival the moment they walk in the gym. They drive themselves into the ground and are neurologically cooked before the workout even begins. Throw in some sympathetic training at the start of the training session, and their susceptibility to pain and injury increases, their performance suffers, and they risk burning out and giving up. Just as the engine in your car will eventually cease under sustained high-intensity stress, so will your mind and body.

It's like this: life is crazy before you show up to the gym, and it will be crazy after you leave. You must use the training session as an opportunity to better your life, not run yourself into the ground and perpetuate unnecessary stress. Equally important, you should leave feeling better and stronger, not worse and broken.

To accomplish that, you will start slow to go fast. You need to bring the system into balance before you ramp it up to perform. You only want to be in a highly sympathetic state when it's advantageous for your physical and mental performance, and the way you do that is by regulating the CNS response at the beginning of the training session with a parasympathetic emphasis and then gradually riding the sympathetic wave to its peak as you enter the workout.

You begin with parasympathetic exercises like soft tissue work and stretching because these are restorative modalities that help decrease vital metrics—they lower the heart rate, calm you down, and bring you into the moment. They help you find homeostasis where you feel grounded and centered, allowing

OPTIMIZING THE CNS SPECTRUM

The mind and body are connected via a vast network of nerves and cells that include our central nervous system (CNS) and peripheral nervous system (PNS). The autonomic nervous system—a subsystem of the PNS—regulates processes you don't think about, such as heartbeat, blood pressure, and stress tolerance. These physiological changes are driven by either the parasympathetic nervous system or the sympathetic nervous system. The goal of the early phases of the warm-up is to get you into a parasympathetic state and then gradually increase the demands on the system to prepare for performance. If you jump into a warm-up with sympathetic-driven exercises while in a sympathetic state, you can push yourself past the red line—the point at which you break down and burn out—potentially increasing your susceptibility to pain, injury, and more.

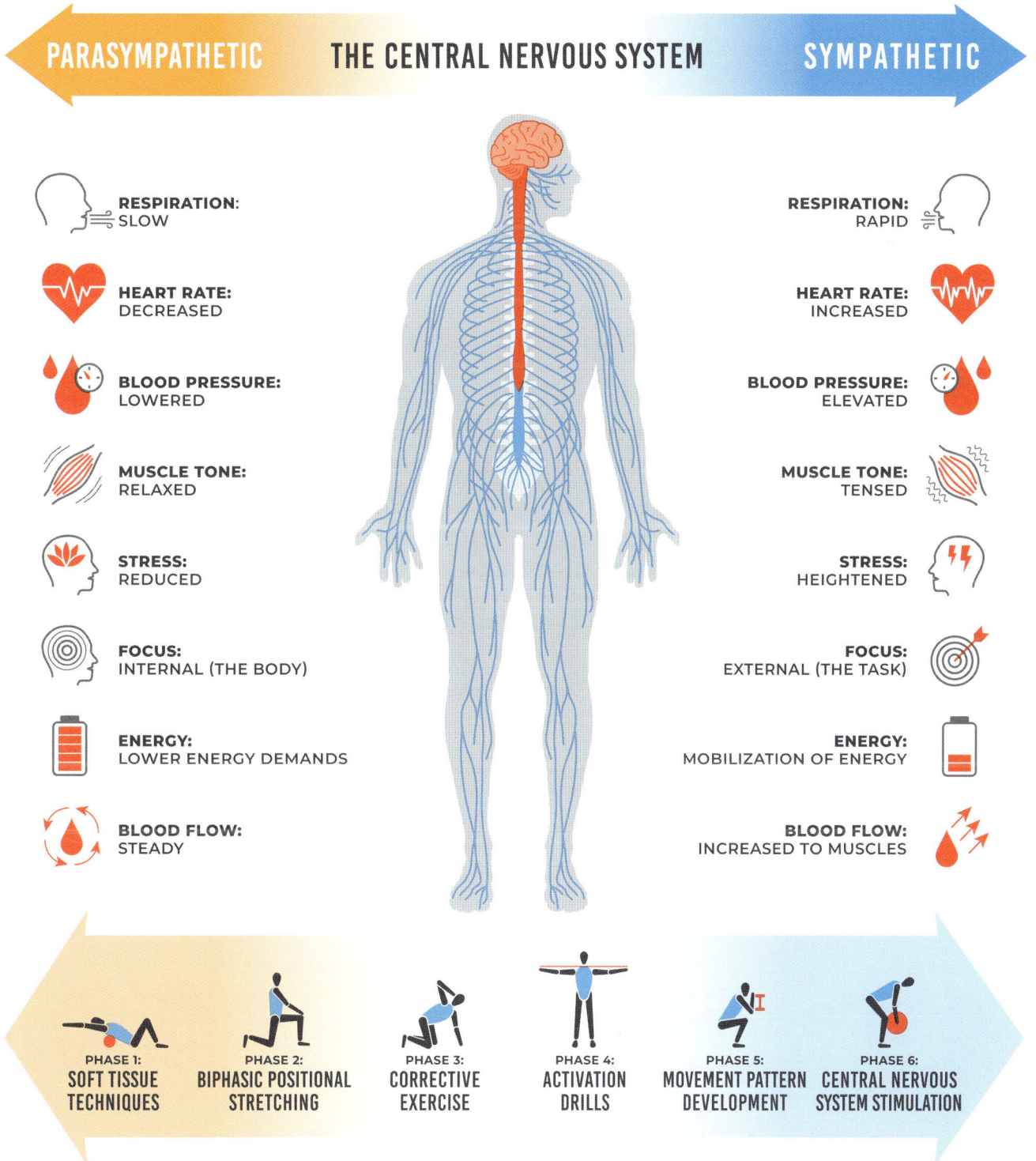

PARASYMPATHETIC — THE CENTRAL NERVOUS SYSTEM — SYMPATHETIC

PARASYMPATHETIC	SYMPATHETIC
RESPIRATION: SLOW	**RESPIRATION:** RAPID
HEART RATE: DECREASED	**HEART RATE:** INCREASED
BLOOD PRESSURE: LOWERED	**BLOOD PRESSURE:** ELEVATED
MUSCLE TONE: RELAXED	**MUSCLE TONE:** TENSED
STRESS: REDUCED	**STRESS:** HEIGHTENED
FOCUS: INTERNAL (THE BODY)	**FOCUS:** EXTERNAL (THE TASK)
ENERGY: LOWER ENERGY DEMANDS	**ENERGY:** MOBILIZATION OF ENERGY
BLOOD FLOW: STEADY	**BLOOD FLOW:** INCREASED TO MUSCLES

PHASE 1: SOFT TISSUE TECHNIQUES

PHASE 2: BIPHASIC POSITIONAL STRETCHING

PHASE 3: CORRECTIVE EXERCISE

PHASE 4: ACTIVATION DRILLS

PHASE 5: MOVEMENT PATTERN DEVELOPMENT

PHASE 6: CENTRAL NERVOUS SYSTEM STIMULATION

you to disengage from the stressors that followed you into the gym. That, in turn, opens you up for better movement in the subsequent phases and helps you manage the stress from the training session more efficiently.

This is the function of the sequential phasic approach—and why you are doing them in a specific order. Each phase makes the next phase better. They build on one another. By the time you finish the sixth phase, you are ready to perform and you're feeling your best.

The bottom line is that the orchestration of the phases is hugely beneficial to the training session and will set you up to finish better than when you started. Just as you should never skip a warm-up, never skip a phase—and perform each phase in order.

THE DYNAMIC WARM-UP SEQUENCE

BLOCK 1:
RESTORATIVE
(PARASYMPATHETIC EMPHASIS)

PHASE 1:
SOFT TISSUE TECHNIQUES

PHASE 2:
BIPHASIC POSITIONAL STRETCHING

PURPOSE:
Relaxing and opening up ranges of motion

GOOD FOR:
- Reducing stress and bodily tension
- Connecting with your body
- Improving range of motion
- Alleviating pain

FOCUS ON:
- Breathing
- Relaxing
- Smiling

BLOCK 2:
CORRECTIVE
(PARASYMPATHETIC TO SYMPATHETIC TRANSITION)

PHASE 3:
CORRECTIVE EXERCISE

PHASE 4:
ACTIVATION DRILLS

PURPOSE:
Learning and feeling

GOOD FOR:
- Improving movement quality (closing the motor control gap)
- Activating key stabilizers (hips and shoulders)
- Enhancing the mind-muscle-movement connection
- Expressing new ranges of motion

FOCUS ON:
- Sequencing, stability, smoothness, and symmetry
- Specific aspects of the movement pattern (isolated by body region)
- Feeling muscle engagement

BLOCK 3:
STIMULATION
(SYMPATHETIC EMPHASIS)

PHASE 5:
MOVEMENT PATTERN DEVELOPMENT

PHASE 6:
CENTRAL NERVOUS SYSTEM STIMULATION

PURPOSE:
Practice and performance preparation

GOOD FOR:
- Addressing movement and positional faults
- Grooving the movement pattern
- Improving motor control
- Getting primed for the workout

FOCUS ON:
- Skill acquisition
- Global aspects of the movement pattern (entire body)
- Amplifying pillar stability

PHASE 0: PARASYMPATHETIC POSITIONAL BREATHING

When you're in pain or you are passing the redline due to chronic stress, your top priority is to slam the brakes on that sympathetic drive.

Foam rolling and stretching (phases 1 and 2) are great for that. For most people, they're the first step in moving the needle toward the parasympathetic end of the spectrum. But in times of extreme stress and acute pain timed with the training session, you may need more time and strategies to bring the system back into homeostasis.

You have two options here. The first is simply to add a minute or two to phases 1 and 2—and that might be enough to downregulate the system. But that doesn't work all the time, especially if you're coming off an all-day or weeks-long sympathetic bender. If you get into phase 1 and you're hyperventilating and just going through the motions, then you may need to take a step back and begin again with phase 0, which is the second option.

Pain and stress make you apprehensive. Foam rolling and stretching without slow, rhythmic breathing is ineffective. Phase 0 strips away the external implements and puts the focus solely on your breath, which is predicated on the science and application of mindfulness meditation—it's all about observing your sensory inputs with open awareness and an intentional emphasis on deep, controlled breathing. It becomes a buffer zone between walking into the gym and getting to work.

One to 3 minutes of Positional Parasympathetic Breathing can be a game changer for downregulating your system. It will put you in the right mindset to extract the maximum benefit from the warm-up. But you don't need to do it before every warm-up (it is usually reserved as a cool-down protocol, as covered on page 83). Here are some commonsense strategies to help you determine when to employ phase 0:

- Elevated resting heart rate (120 bpm or higher)
- Acute or subacute pain
- Extreme, chronic stress
- Hyperventilating or heavy chest breathing

Go to page 54 for a step-by-step breakdown.

COACHES' CORNER

There are three signs to look for to define whether you should put a client through phase 0 or overemphasize phases 1 and 2.

- Most people can't fake pain or stress—they will grimace instead of smile, for example. Their facial expressions will say it all, and you can use them to determine whether phase 0 is necessary.

- Look at how they are moving. Are they limping? Are their movement patterns jerky or different? Check the quality and smoothness of their movement from the moment they walk into the gym and use that as your initial screen.

- If they are unable to get any benefit from phase 1 within 1 to 2 minutes—they are holding their breath and unable to relax—it might be a good time to revert to a phase 0 protocol.

If your client wears a heart rate monitor, then that is another tool you can use. Say they're foam rolling with a heart rate of 160. That is a good indication that they should start with phase 0.

10 MINUTES—
THAT'S THE MINIMUM EFFECTIVE DOSE

When it comes to pre-training preparation, people typically do too much or not enough. The 6-phase dynamic warm-up finds the sweet spot at 10 to 12 minutes. Each phase takes between 1 and 2 minutes, making it easy to complete efficiently and effectively.

In the forthcoming chapters, I provide specific programming guidelines for each phase—and explain why the sets, reps, and rest periods are set up the way they are. This tenet simply serves as a reminder to be efficient and disciplined with your time.

To be clear, there is flexibility in the program, and you can adjust the time you spend in each phase based on your specific needs. For example, I routinely spend an extra minute or two in phases 1 and 2 because it feels good, and, like most people, I spend way too much time sitting. A little bit of extra time in the early phases helps reduce stiffness and opens me up for better movement. However, I'm careful not to turn my warm-up into a glorified recovery session by expanding every phase. A little bit of added mobility work goes a long way to counter the pressures of the modern lifestyle. But you must remain judicious. Remember, you're not recovering from a workout; you're preparing to perform.

After 10 to 12 minutes, there is a diminishing return. If you add time to your warm-up, try to keep your total time under 16 minutes. To stay on track, be sure to

STICK TO A PLAN:
Design or follow a program based on what you want to improve that day (see Part 4 for guided templates). Set a timer if it's helpful and respect the programming guidelines for each phase.

MANAGE REST PERIODS:
The goal is to seamlessly flow through the warm-up with intent and focus. There is no need to rest between sets or phases. It's not a workout, and you're not going to failure on anything. It will take 10 to 15 seconds to transition from one exercise to the next, which is plenty of rest.

BE IN THE MOMENT:
Stay physically and emotionally engaged (don't rest, as if you're training, and avoid checking your phone or multitasking).

SET YOUR ENVIRONMENT:
For many, adhering to this guideline is key to completing the warm-up in under 12 minutes. Organize your station with everything you need to complete all the phases (make sure you have a foam roller, band, kettlebell, etc.) before you start.

CHOOSE ONE PRIMARY FOCUS:
The key performance indicator (KPI) and linchpin provide a framework for selecting exercises and navigating the sequence. You will pick either a movement pattern that you want to improve (KPI) or a weak link (linchpin) that you want to strengthen to guide the sequence (see the next tenet).

PRE—DYNAMIC WARM-UP ROUTINE

Many people start their workout with a few minutes on the treadmill or bike. This is especially common for folks who live in cold climates. If this is part of your routine, you don't have to stop. Just do it better and more efficiently. The goal isn't to sustain a high heart rate or break a sweat but to get your heart rate up just enough to increase tissue and body temperature.

Here's how to do it right:

▼

Duration: Spend 90 seconds to 2 minutes on a low-intensity activity like walking or biking.

▼

Heart Rate Zone: Aim to reach a higher zone 2 or a zone 3 heart rate (see page 447). As soon as you feel your heart rate start to increase or your breathing pattern change, you're done. This typically happens around 120 beats per minute (bpm).

▼

Transition: The moment you hit that heart rate zone, move on to phase 1 of the dynamic warm-up. There's no need to sustain the heart rate—this isn't about cardio conditioning.

This quick pre-warm-up helps you tap into the sensations of your body and get into the mindset for training. It ensures you're warm and ready, making your transition into the 6-phase dynamic warm-up smooth and effective.

CHOOSE ONE PRIMARY FOCUS—
EITHER A MOVEMENT PATTERN OR LINCHPIN

At a glance, the number of phases in the warm-up and the options within each phase can be a bit overwhelming. It seems like a lot to tackle in a 10-minute time frame. Without a coherent plan, many get paralysis by analysis—they don't know what areas to target or which exercises to select, and they get stuck.

There are two options that provide a framework for the six phases, both of which will streamline your approach and remove the friction points.

The first is based on pain and functional limitations. Say you have acute pain or a specific area of weakness—a linchpin that affects your ability to move with good form. In this scenario, your goal is to be pain-free, so you need to program exercises that target those weak links and help alleviate your acute pain sources. Because we're living in a world that encourages sitting, and, like it or not, we all find ourselves glued to computers and phones for a good chunk of the day, we share similar linchpins, such as tight hips, lower back pain, and a stiff thoracic spine. To make programming for these collective issues more accessible—and to prevent paralysis by analysis—I provide structured templates you can follow that address the most common linchpins (see page 467).

The second option is based on performance. If you don't have any glaring linchpins, then your goal is to get the most from the training session by choosing one primary focus. For most people, that is the biggest, most demanding exercise of the day—what we refer to as the key performance indicator (KPI). If the priority is to PR on a squat or simply to improve some aspect of the squat movement pattern (form, range of motion, etc.), then that is your KPI—and everything that you do in the warm-up should prepare you to perform in that movement.

While the goal is to progress all movement patterns, there is only so much you can do in a single training session. It's not realistic to improve them all in one day. If you don't clearly define your KPI, then you're just putting random things together and hoping they work. This is a big reason why people plateau on their strength, performance, and aesthetic goals. They have multiple priorities, their focus becomes scattered, and as a result, nothing gets prioritized and nothing improves.

That doesn't mean you're not training the other patterns—you can still place an intentional focus on advancing skills in other areas of training. But you can't PR or go balls-to-the-wall with every exercise every day. You need to choose one movement pattern and go as hard as you can. Everything else is supplemental. This is ultimately less stressful on your mind and body. You're not worried about getting in more reps or lifting more weight with the other movements because they are ancillary. Instead, you're focusing on moving with pristine form and getting in the volume necessary to maintain muscle, strength, and fluency in the pattern (more on this in the Training Tenets chapter).

In summary, the KPI provides a focal point that directs each phase of the warm-up and the workout as a whole. The exercises you choose will revolve around your KPI, giving you the best opportunity to PR or improve the movement pattern that is your central focus for that training session. Think of the KPI-directed warm-up as riding the performance wave to its peak. The warm-up sets you up for a record that day, and everything that follows will provide supplemental benefits.

In the warm-up templates offered in Part 4, you'll notice that there is overlap between the linchpin programs and the KPI programs. That's because the exercises that prepare you to perform also clean up functional limitations. They are one and the same. Knowing this, don't overcomplicate your programs by trying to fix everything. Simply find the program that matches your KPI or linchpin and go to work.

THERE ARE NO DAYS OFF—
IF YOU'RE NOT GAINING, YOU'RE MAINTAINING (THE PERFORMANCE RECOVERY SYSTEM)

If you hire me as your coach, you will do the 6-phase dynamic warm-up every day. Of course, you will need to take days off from training to recover. But that doesn't mean you do nothing. When you're training, you're using the warm-up to gain performance. On non-training days, you're using the warm-up as a regenerative and recovery protocol to maintain those gains. In this context, think of it as the 6-phase dynamic recovery sequence.

Because the intent of the 6-phase sequence differs from training to non-training days, there is flexibility in how you approach the phases—as well as some necessary modifications to the exercise intensity and volume within each phase. Here's how to adapt the 6-phase sequence to accelerate your recovery, improve your mobility, prevent pain, and feel your best every day.

BLOCK 1 (PHASES 1 AND 2): MORE TIME, MORE REGIONS

There is no time limit to foam rolling and stretching, and you are not restricted to one body region or technique. When employing these phases as a recovery protocol, you can implement a more global approach (exploring all the main regions of the body) with no time limit. Go based on feel and focus on your breathing. Stop on tight areas and connect with your body by taking slow, smooth breaths. If you have more acute soreness or pain, this is a great time to use a ball or soft tissue massage tool with more precise pressure. You are also not restricted by the individual phases. In other words, you can separate the phases by foam rolling and then stretching or combine them into a superset by rolling out a specific body region and then stretching the same area. There are no rules other than being mindful of your movement and body.

BLOCK 2 (PHASES 3 AND 4): EXPLORE NEW RANGES, ENHANCE THE PATTERN

The purpose of phase 3 is to improve range of motion with exploratory movement—keying in on symmetry, sequencing, and smoothness of the pattern. Phase 4 essentially hits the save button on that newly gained range by adding tension (muscular activation) and stability to the movement pattern. There are a couple of options here. The first is to simply choose one or two exercises from each phase and perform them just as you would when doing them in the warm-up. This is great for those who are new to the system, have a linchpin (pain or weak link they are trying to resolve), and want to focus on a specific range or skill. The second is to blend phases 3 and 4, kind of like a global mobility flow drill where you are moving, exploring, and playing with novel movements and full ranges that you don't typically do in normal life (think rotation and lateral movements). This is best for more experienced practitioners who do not have specific issues or physical limitations and want a wider grasp of mobility exercises and movements. With both options, there is no time limit or rep count. It's all about feeling good and having fun, exploring new ranges, and developing movement fluency within those ranges.

BLOCK 3 (PHASES 5 AND 6): REDUCE INTENSITY, EMPHASIZE MOBILITY AND SKILL DEVELOPMENT

These phases stimulate a training effect to prepare you for performance. But when you're implementing them outside of training, the goal is not to stimulate the sympathetic nervous system and ride that wave into the workout—you want to remain on the parasympathetic side of the spectrum. You do so by manipulating the exercises and reducing the intensity of your effort. For example, instead of doing a bilateral squat with maximal tension in phase 5, you would perform a lateral lunge and place a mobility emphasis on the movement. Think in terms of rotational and lateralized movement with a loaded stretch. In phase 6, you'll focus more on skill, stability, and deceleration as opposed to explosive acceleration-based movements. For instance, instead of a depth jump off a 2-foot box with double-leg contact into a vertical jump, you perform a single-leg catch off a 1-foot box. As with the other phases, there is no time limit. The key is to keep your heart rate and overall exertion low. So don't get crazy with your sets and reps; maintain low to moderate effort and rest as needed between exercises.

FINISH WITH LOW-INTENSITY, LOW-IMPACT, STEADY-STATE CARDIO FOR 10 TO 20 MINUTES

On non-workout days, always follow up the 6-phase dynamic recovery with some light movement, like walking or biking. I prefer walking because it's one of the foundational movement patterns (carry or locomotion); it's easy, effective, and free. To maximize the cardiovascular, regenerative, and mental benefits, be sure to walk for 10-plus minutes without stopping or changing pace (to jogging or running). Walk briskly but not so fast that you elevate your heart rate or impede your natural gait cycle. Remember, steady-state walking should not be reserved for recovery days. It is a physical practice that should take place every day, if not multiple times a day. That way, you get the most out of your body without the neural stress, physical fatigue, or risk of overtraining.

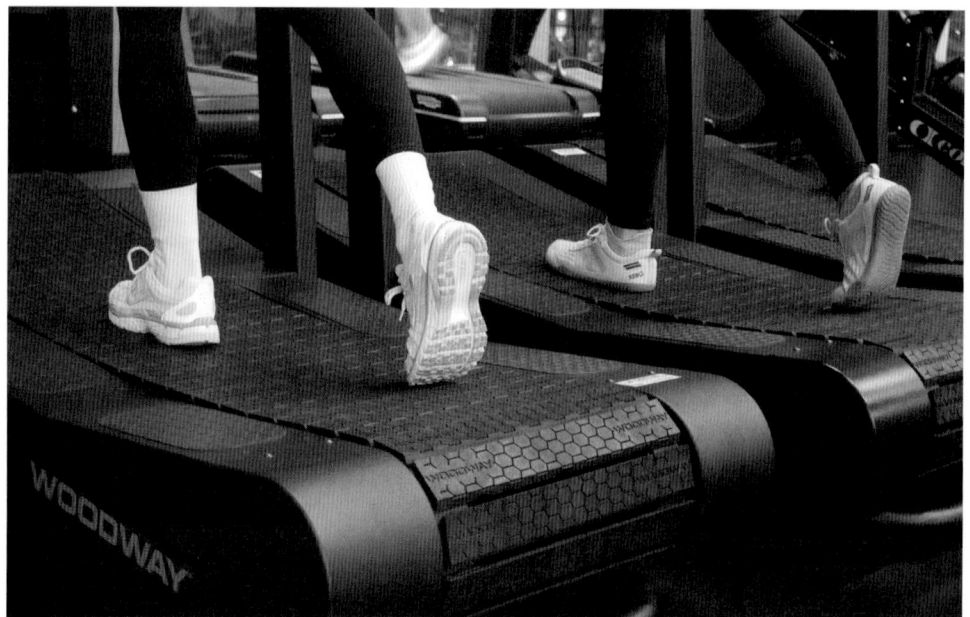

WHEN TO UTILIZE THE DYNAMIC RECOVERY PROTOCOL—
and HOW to MODIFY the PHASES

There are three main ways to program and modify the phasic warm-up sequence as a performance recovery system.

1.

POST-WORKOUT COOL-DOWN WINDOW:
parasympathetic positional breathing + soft tissue techniques + stretching

Just as it's essential to activate a parasympathetic response before training, it's equally important to calm the sympathetic storm after a workout. This transition promotes a post-training feel-good effect, reduces pain and muscle soreness, and prepares you to better handle the stressors of life outside the gym.

After the last set of the day, devote 5 to 12 minutes (depending on the time available) to programming parasympathetic-directed modalities in a strategic order. If you have only a few minutes for parasympathetic post-training recovery (cool-down), prioritize the 90/90 Supine Parasympathetic Positional Breathing technique above all other modalities. This has become non-negotiable for my clients. If you have more time, spend a few extra minutes on foam rolling and stretching, which goes a long way, especially in reducing pain and soreness. Follow the block 1 recovery guideline, focusing on the areas hit hardest by the workout. You will learn more about cool-downs on page 476. I have included guided cool-down programs and templates in Part 4.

2.

SECONDARY RECOVERY SESSIONS:
soft tissue techniques + stretching

Another way to modify the phasic sequence is to add a secondary daily recovery session— essentially a second cool-down in which you prioritize soft tissue techniques and stretching. If you train in the morning, slip an active recovery protocol into your routine later in the mid-afternoon or evening. Just make sure there's a 4- to 6-hour break after your primary training. If you train in the afternoon, you can use this protocol as a pre-bedtime routine to wind down—think of it as a perfect Netflix-and-chill moment. Again, there are no rules when it comes to techniques, timelines, and body regions. Focus on the areas that feel tight or most prone to soreness, but be gentle. Pain stimulates a sympathetic response— the opposite of what you're trying to achieve— so keep the pressure light and perform gentle stretches. When coupled with deep, rhythmic breathing, this helps bring down your CNS response and ensures better sleep quality.

3.

"OFF-DAY" ACTIVE RECOVERY TRAINING:
the 6-phase dynamic recovery sequence + walking

As I said, there should be no off days when it comes to the 6-phase sequence. Whether your goal is fat loss, hypertrophy, rehab, sports performance, or general fitness, enhancing these physical metrics is dependent on optimizing recovery and maintaining your body. That means, at a bare minimum, you should utilize the 6-phase sequence once during your off days with 10-plus minutes of low-impact-intensity steady-state cardio.

Remember, long-term, life-changing results are forged through strong daily habits and hard work—forever. If you have true aspirations to be your healthiest, you must approach each day as an opportunity to improve how you feel, function, and perform.

THE HIERARCHY OF REGENERATION AND RECOVERABILITY

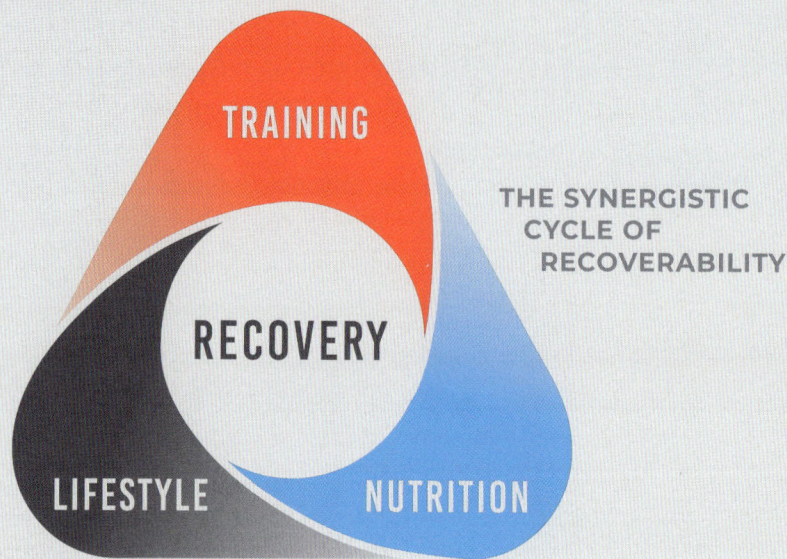

TRAINING

RECOVERY

LIFESTYLE

NUTRITION

THE SYNERGISTIC CYCLE OF RECOVERABILITY

Even if you follow the pain-free performance training system—you utilize the 6-phase dynamic warm-up and incorporate the six foundational movement patterns in your training—the modern lifestyle is replete with too much sitting, junk food, stress, and poor sleep. Left unchecked, our lifestyles can negate many of the gains we make during the training session. If you're not recovering, you're setting yourself up for pain and decreased performance. What's more, if you're not maintaining what you gained during your training sessions, you will be in a constant cycle of taking two steps forward and one step back.

While the 6-phase dynamic recovery sequence can be manipulated to suit your goals and schedule—and it certainly helps with maintaining gains and improving your movement and mobility—it will not make up for a bad night of sleep, poor food choices, and unhealthy lifestyle habits. Regeneration, recoverability, and optimizing performance require a multifactorial holistic approach that integrates training, nutrition, and lifestyle.

The graphic above is the perfect depiction of the multifactorial cycle of recoverability. Each of the three elements (training, nutrition, and lifestyle) revolve around and are dependent on each other. As a whole, they have the potential to either expedite or delay the recovery process. Train smart, eat well, manage stress, and get good sleep—that is how you optimize performance and recovery. Overlook just one element, and there is a performance-hindering, recovery-inhibiting cascade effect. For example, even if you train smart and eat well, your lifestyle (sleep quality, daily habits, relationships, stress, etc.) can undo all of it. In other words, you cannot out-train or out-eat poor sleep or the constant lifestyle stresses that strain the CNS. The same is true of the other factors. Remove one cog from the machine, and it won't run as efficiently.

While there is a synergistic relationship between your lifestyle, nutrition, and training, some factors have a bigger impact than others. That's important to realize if you want to maximize your recoverability—and avoid wasting time and money on modalities that don't give you the biggest bang for your buck.

THE HIERARCHY OF RECOVERABILITY PYRAMID

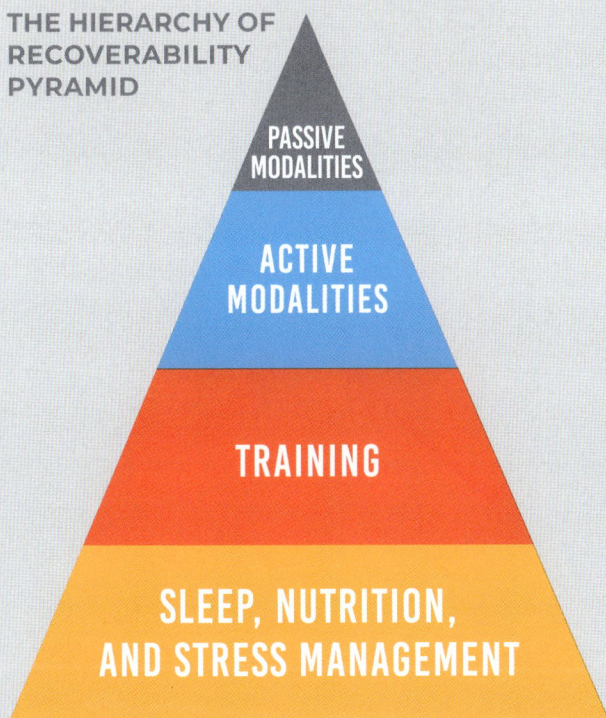

PASSIVE MODALITIES

ACTIVE MODALITIES

TRAINING

SLEEP, NUTRITION, AND STRESS MANAGEMENT

SLEEP, NUTRITION, AND STRESS MANAGEMENT

As with anything in life, you can only shake the foundations on which you stand for so long before the pillars of your health come toppling down on top of you. When it comes to your recoverability from training, your sleep, stress management, and nutrition are your foundation—and the most important factor in the hierarchy of recoverability. Only when your sleep, nutrition, and stress are managed appropriately can you take full advantage of the training and regenerative modalities to spark the recovery process. The 6-phase dynamic recovery protocol provides immense benefits—but only if you have an honest and objective intake of your stress, sleep, and nutrition.

TRAINING

The next big driver when it comes to optimizing recoverability is tied to your training. The pain-free performance training system provides a blueprint, especially for choosing the exercise variations that match your abilities. But it's up to you to adhere to a program that suits your individual needs and experience. As it's been said, you can only get better from a training stimulus that you can recover from.

ACTIVE MODALITIES

Now, we're getting at the heart of what this book can provide in terms of recoverability strategies. The 6-phase dynamic recovery sequence is your active modality. It's foam rolling, stretching, corrective exercises, activation drills, movement sequencing, and low-impact, steady-state movements—all things you can do at home without any specialized equipment. Put simply, it is exercise and movement programmed in a way that amplifies and expedites recovery and regeneration.

PASSIVE MODALITIES

Passive modalities are located at the top of the pyramid, which represents the least important of all the factors centered around the recovery process. Yet they are commonly the first modalities people use to spark recovery and regeneration. Passive modalities such as float tanks, massage, soft tissue manipulation, chiropractic, muscle activation devices, acupuncture, thermal agents (sauna), and ice baths certainly can have a place in the recovery and overall health optimization plan (I love saunas and cold plunges), but they should never take the place of an active modality. Not only will many of these passive modalities break the bank when utilized on a regular cycle or schedule, but they also create a dependency between the person and their perceived ability to recover.

Before you go spend your hard-earned dollars on passive recovery modalities—and before you become dependent on a passive-based modality to "get you feeling good" after hard training sessions—take one step down the pyramid and prioritize active self-sufficient modalities that are self-directed and free.

If you plan on unlocking longevity with your training career, don't pay someone else to do work that you aren't willing to do yourself. As physically active autonomous human beings, we need to be able to do certain things ourselves, and self-maintenance and recovery are two of those things. We are the keepers of the key that unlocks our ability to manipulate central nervous system activity and ignite the recovery process on demand, without relying solely on another powder, pill, or physio session.

The power of recovery and physical preparation is within your control. You just have to exercise it.

PHASE 1:
SOFT TISSUE TECHNIQUES

Phase 1 is all about calming the mind and body. You perform soft tissue techniques—foam rolling—to spark a parasympathetic response (relax) and reduce muscle tonicity (tightness). You're priming the mind to learn, the body to move, and the nervous system to respond. Breathe deeply and rhythmically, target one or two muscle groups, and be completely mindful for 1 to 2 minutes.

"How are you feeling today?"

is the first question I ask my clients at the start of every training session. It may seem like polite small talk, but it's much more than that. I want to know their mental state and how they are doing physically—if they have anything going on that I should be aware of.

Are they stressed?

Do they have a nagging ache or pain?

Are they sore and beat up, or do they feel good and ready to go?

The enthusiastic affirmations of "I feel great!" or "Let's get after it!" are what I hope for, yet rarely hear. Even a seemingly straightforward "I'm good" often unravels upon further probing, revealing underlying issues such as stress, tightness, or discomfort in a particular area.

The unfortunate truth is that most people do not feel their best when they enter the gym. They're working out to feel better, and it's my job to ensure that happens. Asking how they feel is an important step in achieving that objective because their answers help shape the training session ahead—what exercises we will perform, how much we should do, and how hard we can go. With intelligent programming and strategic personalization, I can get them feeling and moving better. But to achieve this outcome, I must begin the session by addressing the most common linchpins holding them back: stress, tension, and pain.

Most clients, knowingly or unknowingly, enter the gym carrying a lot of stress. They swim out into the ocean of their day, catch a sympathetic wave of anxiety, and ride it right into the training session. This stress places them in a precarious start position for the workout. With their central nervous system (CNS) locked in overdrive, fatigue sets in faster, and their mind, distracted by the demands of daily life, cannot focus with the clarity needed for safe and effective training. My task is to help them dismount the wave of stress that they rode in on so they can enter the next wave—the workout itself.

Then there's tension. Ask almost anyone, especially those over thirty, how they feel at the start of a training session, and they'll likely say something to the effect of, "I feel tight." This feeling of stiffness, often stemming from stress, sedentary habits, and insufficient self-care, compromises mobility, restricts movement, and can quickly escalate to pain. Once pain sets in, it becomes a physical barrier to performing exercises correctly and serves as a psychological hindrance, instilling a sense of limitation and apprehension.

Whether it is stress, tension, pain, or a combination of all three, you must get these symptoms under control before you do anything else—because feeling your best and getting the most from the training session is impossible under such restraints.

It's a detrimental cycle where stress begets tension, tension fosters pain, and pain circles back to stress, creating a feedback loop that undermines the very goals of fitness and health. You can break that cycle before it starts by learning how to apply soft tissue techniques—referred to as foam rolling—to downregulate the CNS and momentarily relieve muscle tension and pain. If you're like most of my clients, you'll feel your focus sharpen and the discomfort you've been carrying for most of the day quickly dissipate. This opens an opportunity window to move and feel better, which only compounds through each phase of the warm-up, leading you directly into a pain-free workout.

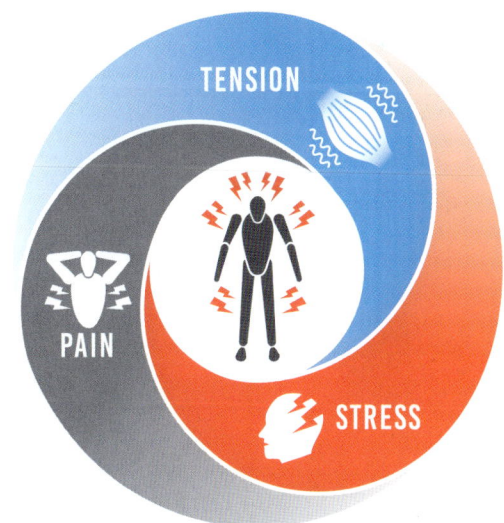

DISPELLING THE MYTHS AND MISCONCEPTIONS OF FOAM ROLLING

Many gym-goers labor under serious misconceptions about what foam rolling can and cannot do, leading to misguided practices or outright dismissal of its benefits.

For instance, the idea that foam rolling can break up adhesion or scar tissue, or can alter the anatomical length of a muscle, is a myth. The amount of poundage per square inch it takes to break up tissue adhesions is astronomical and far beyond what any foam roller can exert. And altering the length of a muscle from end-to-end? That's a job for a surgeon, not a piece of foam.

Here's the truth: foam rolling is not a magical tool that can change the mechanical structure of your muscles or eradicate scar tissue. Believing this leads to aggressive and unproductive habits. People who buy into these myths often end up just smashing their tissues, thinking more pain equals more gain. When they don't see the expected results, they double down on the intensity and adopt the "more is better" mentality. They get caught up in a ritualistic practice, expecting an outcome that soft tissue techniques can never achieve.

On the flip side are those who recognize that foam rolling doesn't achieve these mechanical changes and, as a result, dismiss it entirely. This perspective is equally flawed. It overlooks the legitimate benefits of foam rolling in favor of a black-and-white view that ignores its true purpose.

Foam rolling is fundamentally about preparing the body for movement and recovery. It's a technique that, when done correctly, can downregulate the nervous system and reduce muscle tone, setting the stage for effective training and recuperation.[1] Understanding the real capabilities of foam rolling is key to integrating it effectively into your training regimen and tapping into its true value.

THE GOALS OF SOFT TISSUE TECHNIQUES

Imagine a Ferrari F50, one of the most high-performance cars in the world. It is engineered for speed and an exhilarating driving experience. Now picture driving this Ferrari with the parking brake engaged. The car's ability to accelerate, handle corners, and reach peak performance would be drastically compromised. The parking brake creates resistance, preventing it from unleashing its full potential.

Think of your body as this Ferrari. When you carry stress, tension, and pain into a workout, it's as if you've engaged your internal parking brake. This metaphorical brake represents the internal resistance in your body, holding back your true movement potential. Just as the Ferrari wouldn't be able to showcase its full power and speed with the parking brake on, your body, when burdened with stress, tension, and pain, cannot perform optimally.

Foam rolling acts as the tool to release this internal parking brake. It primes your body—your Ferrari F50—to move with the freedom, agility, and strength it's capable of. For example, when you foam roll a region that is tight, there's a feel-good effect, the muscle momentarily relaxes, and you gain more range of motion. You're not trying to break up scar tissue, change the anatomical length of the muscle, manipulate fascial planes, or increase temperature and blood flow. You're simply trying to influence the tonicity of the tissue. When someone says, "I'm tight," that's what they're referring to—the tonicity of their tissue or the degree of tension or firmness in their muscles. Tone can increase or decrease. Through foam rolling, the aim is to decrease this tone, primarily by downregulating the sympathetic nervous system. In this way, foam rolling is as much a neurological intervention as it is a physical one—it's about influencing the mind to release tension held in the body. This relaxation fosters a mental environment conducive to motor skill development and refinement, which is one of the central goals of the warm-up.

Simply put, foam rolling serves as a critical modulator for the nervous system. It's not about the tissue, the tool, or even the specific body part—it's about the nervous system's capacity to reduce muscle tone through the entire body. This is what truly matters. The process goes something like this:

HOW FOAM ROLLING IN THE WARM-UP WORKS

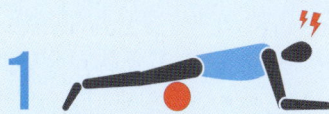

1 APPLY PHYSICAL PRESSURE WITH FOAM ROLLING

The physical pressure from foam rolling influences the nervous system by affecting mechanoreceptors, which are sensory receptors found in muscles, fascia, connective tissues, and even skin.

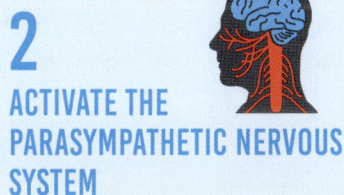

2 ACTIVATE THE PARASYMPATHETIC NERVOUS SYSTEM

By stimulating these receptors, foam rolling with appropriate intensity and deep breathing can elicit a parasympathetic response.

3 REDUCE STRESS AND MUSCLE TENSION

This stimulation promotes relaxation, which reduces stress and muscle tension.

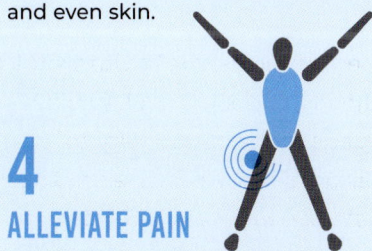

4 ALLEVIATE PAIN

Foam rolling can also produce a temporary analgesic effect, similar to massage, due to the "gate control theory" of pain where non-painful stimuli, like pressure from foam rolling, can inhibit the sensation of pain.

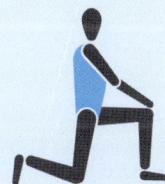

5 IMPROVE RANGE OF MOTION

Reduced pain perception further reduces tension and stress, which can improve joint and tissue range of motion, helping you get into better position when stretching in phase 2.

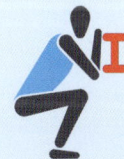

6 ENHANCE MOVEMENT

Less stress, tension, and pain leads to enhanced mobility and more fluid movement patterns through each phase of the warm-up, enhancing overall physical performance.

Remember that these effects are momentary. The key is to capitalize on that short window to facilitate longer-term results, which is the purpose of the next five phases. Once you release the internal parking brake that is constricting your mind and constraining your mobility and movement, you are more receptive to the beneficial inputs from each subsequent phase. By the time you get to the actual workout, the engine is warm, the parts are calibrated, and you're ready to perform to your potential that day.

RECOMMENDATIONS & GUIDELINES

Now that you know why you're foam rolling—and what you can expect to get from it—let's explore how to implement the soft tissue techniques in phase 1 to extract the maximum benefit.

UTILIZE TWO FUNDAMENTAL TECHNIQUES

With soft tissue techniques, you're chasing the minimal effective dose. You don't need to explore all the options and match each technique to every nuanced detail of soft tissue management. That is what recovery is for. That is what physical therapy and massage therapists are for. The goal here is to do only what is necessary to spark a parasympathetic response, which starts with the breath. Regardless of the technique, you must breathe deeply and rhythmically to get the desired effect. With that in mind, you can achieve central reduction in stress, tension, and pain by utilizing these two fundamental techniques: the oscillatory and the neurological trigger point.

OSCILLATORY TECHNIQUE

In the oscillatory technique, you're generating motion between the foam roller and your body. Think of it as a short back-and-forth movement—about 1 to 3 inches—over the length or across the muscle (referred to as the "spanning"). You'll find spots that are tighter than others. Focus your oscillation efforts over these tight pockets.

NEUROLOGICAL TRIGGER POINT TECHNIQUE

For the neurological trigger point technique, the foam roller remains stationary as you maneuver your body over it. Here, you're targeting superficial nerve bundles, those sensitive spots where nerves converge just beneath the skin and muscle surface. They are easy to find because they are more sensitive to pressure than other points. That is the "trigger point," or the area you want to target. Once you've identified the trigger point, maintain pressure while moving your limb. For example, if you are targeting the quadriceps region, you would bend your knee, curling your heel toward your glutes. This takes the "slack" out of the tissue, placing the nerve bundle in a more advantageous position to facilitate change. From there, keep the roller still and make small movements by shifting your weight over the roller. I use the term "neurological trigger point" partly because it's familiar, but also because you're trying to facilitate change "neurologically" by targeting a specific "point" that is sensitive or "triggered" when pressure is applied.

It's essential to understand, especially with the neurological trigger points, that reducing sensitivity down to zero is impossible. Nerves will always react to pressure. You could foam roll every day, all day, and they'd still be sensitive. That sensitivity is vital; it signals your brain to let go of bodily tension. However, there is diminishing return after a minute or two, so follow the guidelines and don't get caught up in trying to eliminate the sensitive points.

While both techniques are effective, and you can certainly use them in combination, don't overthink the process and try to use both equally every time you foam roll. Sometimes, one may serve you better than the other (personally, I find the oscillatory technique covers about 90 percent of what I need). Again, the true benefit lies not in the technique, but in maintaining focused, mindful breathing and a centralized approach to relaxation—not just targeting the specific area under the roller but also easing your entire body.

OSCILLATORY TECHNIQUE

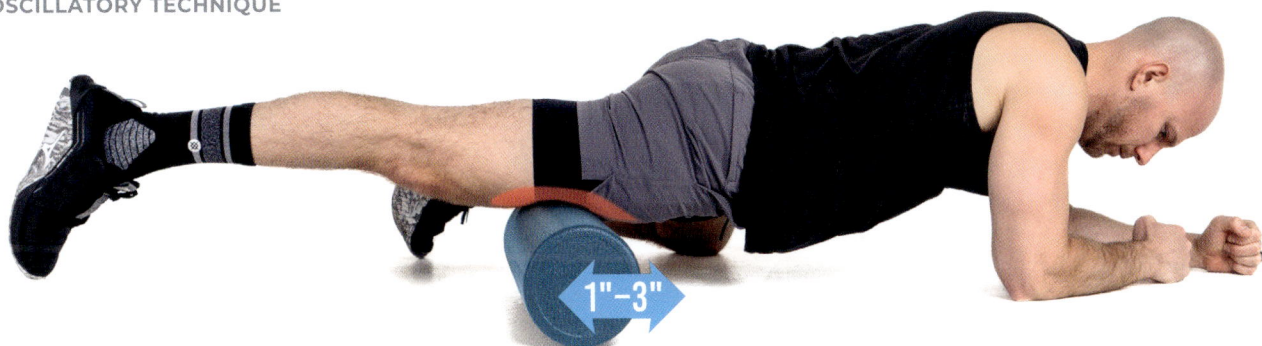

1"-3"

NEUROLOGICAL TRIGGER POINT TECHNIQUE

3 TO 4 OUT OF 10 MAX ON THE PAIN SCALE

Pain is synonymous with soft tissue techniques, or at least that is what a lot of us have been led to believe. We're often told that in order to make positive change, we must hunt for the pain sources, the most sensitive areas, and really hammer the tissue. Please don't do this. The aim is pain-free performance, not to illicit more pain to perform.

This goes back to why you are foam rolling. Remember, you can't change the mechanics of the tissue no matter how much you smash or how much pain you endure. But you can change the tonicity of the tissue by tricking the nervous system to let go of tension. That requires sensory input from the tool, so you do need to feel something. The key is to manage that input by staying below a certain pain threshold.

You can use a subjective pain scale to gauge this threshold. A 0 out of 10 means you feel nothing. A 10 out of 10 represents the worst pain you've ever felt. A 3 or 4 out of 10 is mildly uncomfortable, but you can manage it by keeping your heart rate steady and controlling your breath. This is the sweet spot where you can maintain your contact points on the ground and keep steady pressure on the roller.

To make this easier to understand, think of the "talk test." At a 3 to 4 out of 10 on the pain scale, you're able to converse freely without changes in speed, sharpness, or pattern. However, maintaining this balance requires concentration, as it's not automatic.

If you notice your breath cycle becoming erratic or your heart rate increasing, or you have to come off the roller to adjust the pressure—all signs that would change your speech pattern—you're probably going too hard and moving too far into the pain zone. It's a slippery slope because once you feel more than moderate pain, you've activated the sympathetic nervous system. Your body goes into protection mode and tightens up, which is the opposite of what you're trying to accomplish.

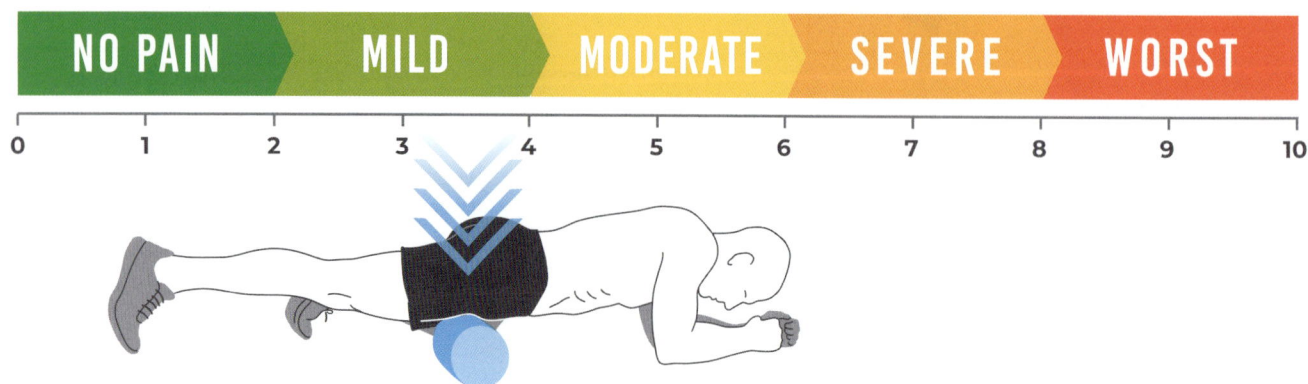

NO PAIN	MILD	MODERATE	SEVERE	WORST

0   1   2   3   4   5   6   7   8   9   10

TARGET 1 OR 2 AREAS—2 OR 3 LOCATIONS PER REGION

Knowing why you are foam rolling in phase 1 of the warm-up is super helpful because you don't need to hit every single body region that feels tight, or home in on specific muscles to achieve the central goal. However, you can still take a methodical approach by targeting the internal rotators at the front of hips and shoulders. In daily life, many of us spend long hours in forward-flexed positions—sitting, texting, or working at a computer. This constant positioning puts stress on areas that are internally rotated, causing them to become chronically tight. By targeting these areas with foam rolling, you can begin to restore postural imbalances that prepare you for better movement and stronger pillar stability in the later phases.

While the primary aim of foam rolling is to create a parasympathetic nervous system response that downregulates tension, targeting the right regions can amplify this effect. As you roll out areas like the adductors, tensor fasciae latae (TFL), or pecs, you're also stimulating nerve innervations that link back to the brain. This helps the entire system "chill out" by sending signals that reduce tension more effectively. In theory, you could roll out any muscle and achieve some relaxation, but focusing on these key areas is more strategic—you're hitting the regions that not only help reduce overall tension but also improve mobility and range of motion for your workout.

You might be thinking, "How do I choose one muscle group when everything feels tight?" Again, the goal is to reduce apprehension stored in the body and held by the mind. To that end, you just need to target one or two body regions, focusing your oscillatory and neurological trigger point efforts on two or three locations within the region to effectively reduce tension in the entire body.

UPPER BODY:

- Thoracic spine
- Pectoralis group (anterior shoulder)
- Posterior shoulder (lats)

LOWER BODY:

- Quadriceps
- Adductor group
- Lateral hip (TFL/glutes)

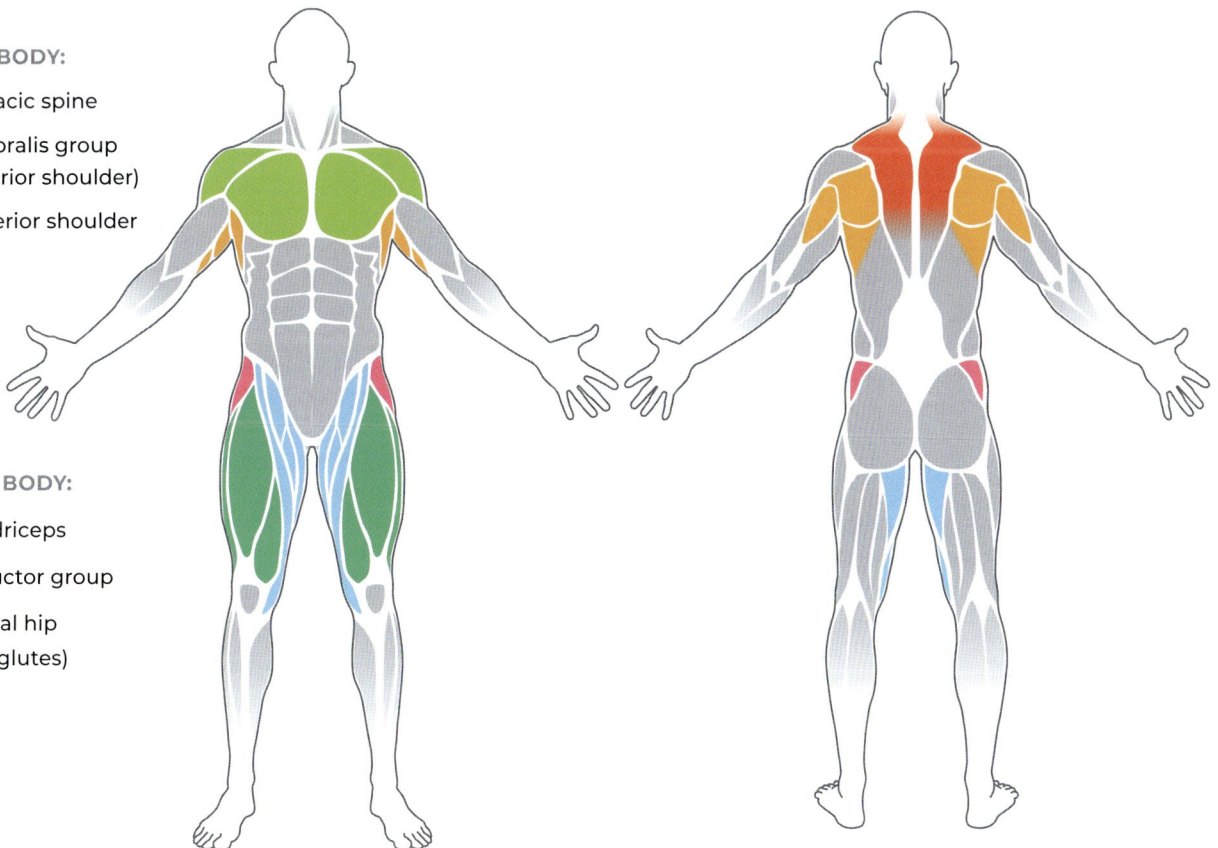

THE FOAM ROLLER: ONE TOOL TO RULE THEM ALL

In phase 1 of our warm-up routine, the primary focus is on the larger, more superficial tissues: quads, adductors, glutes, lats, pecs, and upper back (thoracic spine). You're not going after smaller areas, like aspects of the forearm, or specific muscles, like the supraspinatus. The rationale for the foam roller is simple: larger tissues require a tool with greater surface area and circumference for effective coverage.

Diving deep into the tiny structures can veer into the realm of recovery and clinical pain diagnostics, which is not the goal here. While tools tailored for specific structures can be effective, it's vital to remember what you're trying to achieve in the warm-up: downregulation of the central nervous system. Foam rollers generally don't create a lot of pain, making it easier to relax. There's also the grounding factor. When you foam roll, you're on the ground with multiple points of contact, further promoting the calming effects on the central nervous system.

The foam roller also provides the right amount of stimulus to effect change. It is versatile, combining the benefits of both broad and edged surfaces, ideal for diverse applications from the pecs to the lats. Moreover, the simplicity makes it more accessible and prevents overcomplication.

Nuanced tools and gadgets have a place, but not in the warm-up. Save the more precise tools for recovery sessions, after the workout, or during downtime. The foam roller remains an essential, affordable, and effective tool for soft tissue work. There's no need for high-end gadgets or precise tools when the foam roller can do the trick efficiently.

With that understanding, you can still be strategic when it comes to choosing which body region to target. There are two options: the most painful or restricted area (referred to as the linchpin) or the region you want to open up for that day's movement pattern (referred to as the key performance indicator, or KPI).

For the linchpin focus, ask yourself, "Where do I want to reduce pain and gain more range of motion."

For the KPI focus, ask yourself, "What region will improve the movement pattern that I want to prioritize in today's workout?"

Then target that area using one of the techniques covered in the exercise appendix at the end of this chapter.

When it comes to choosing between a linchpin or a KPI, prioritize the linchpin because that is where you are most susceptible to pain. If you don't have any pain sources, choose the KPI.

In Part 4, I offer linchpin and KPI warm-up templates that you can follow. Try not to overthink it. Just focus on the recommendations and guidelines and you will get the results you're after. Once you downregulate the CNS, which you can achieve with one soft tissue technique in one region, you've accomplished the goal. No need to keep foam rolling other areas. By all means, target more than one region if you feel a benefit. I routinely target two regions because it feels good and helps me transition mentally into the workout. But that isn't necessary for everyone. As I said, there's diminishing return, especially when it comes to time spent foam rolling in the warm-up. So limit it to two regions.

SOFT TISSUE TECHNIQUES: WARM-UP VS. RECOVERY

When it comes to soft tissue work, there's a clear distinction between what we do for pre-training preparation and what we do for post-exercise recovery. In the warm-up, the focus is triggering a parasympathetic response quickly and efficiently. Techniques like oscillatory and trigger point methods should be brief, lasting just 30 seconds to 2 minutes. You're not lingering. You're doing just enough to prime your mind and body for the workout ahead.

The goals and guidelines change when the objective is to enhance post-exercise recuperation (see the Performance Recovery System tenet on page 81). In this scenario, you want to not only ignite a parasympathetic response, but also tap into the mechanical benefits of soft tissue work—think increased blood flow for nutrient delivery and lymphatic drainage for cellular waste removal. Here, you've got more freedom, and frankly, more can be better. Instead of targeting one or two specific areas, you're covering every inch of your muscles. Rather than spending 1 to 2 minutes, there is no time limit. It's all about exploring and doing what feels beneficial and comfortable for you.

Whether it's a longer session on a foam roller or a quick go with a percussive therapy device, recovery is your time to give your body the care it needs. If it feels right, helps you relax, and doesn't cause pain, then don't hesitate to indulge in a little bit of extra soft tissue work, especially during the post-workout window, any time you feel tight, or when winding down for bed. You may find that you recover faster, feel better, and sleep deeper.

2 MINUTES TOTAL

There's only so much time to work out. Most people can only devote an hour to the training session. While the warm-up is important, it shouldn't take more than 12 minutes from the training session. With five additional warm-up phases to get through, you don't want to spend a ton of time foam rolling when you can get 90 percent of the benefit with 2 minutes of total soft tissue work (or 1 minute per side).

I know this doesn't seem like a lot of time—most people want to do more—but it's enough to elicit a parasympathetic response, especially if you focus on your breathing. Remember, when there's a finite amount of time to train, any additional time spent in the warm-up takes away from the workout. The workout provides the highest return on investment. If you spend more time foam rolling and less time training, then you are getting less benefit from the workout as a whole. More is not better when it comes to foam rolling in the warm-up.

To maximize your time in phase 1, take a moment before you plop down on the roller to synchronize your breathing and set your intention. That way, when you lie down to start foam rolling, you've already started the recalibration process to be in a more relaxed state. Spend about a minute on each side. If you're especially tight or having trouble relaxing, then add another minute or two—or implement 2 to 3 minutes of Parasympathetic Positional Breathing (phase 0). Just don't get carried away and turn it into a recovery session.

In this section, you will learn how to perform the main soft tissue techniques used during the warm-up, as well as some supplemental techniques that can be employed as a linchpin focus or during recovery sessions.

As previously mentioned, 1 minute per body region is the minimum effective dose. This means dedicating 1 minute to each side of a muscle group—such as both quadriceps or both adductors—to maintain symmetry and balance in your body.

EXERCISE APPENDIX

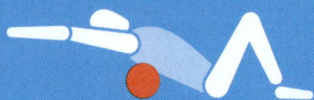

PHASE 1:
SOFT TISSUE TECHNIQUES

LOWER BODY

QUADRICEPS

TARGET ZONES: To target your lower quad (zone 1), roll from just above your knee to halfway up your quad muscle. To target your upper quad (zone 2), roll the middle of your thigh to the front of your hip. The lateral quad (zone 3) runs along the outside edge of your of your thigh—don't venture too far onto your side and target the IT band (the gap between your quad and hamstrings).

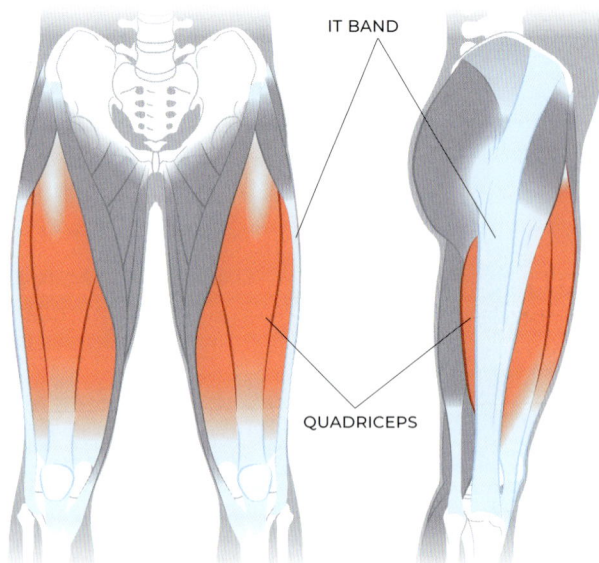

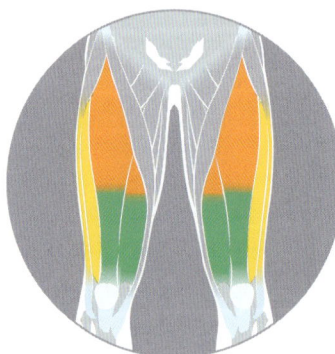

IT BAND

QUADRICEPS

- ZONE 1
- ZONE 2
- ZONE 3

Scan the QR code to access demos of each exercise.

BODY POSITION: Get into the "soldier crawl" position: elbows under shoulders, foam roller under straight leg, other leg bent to about 90 degrees. Keep your head and spine in line (neutral pillar), your shoulders below your ears, and your hips relatively level (square with the ground).

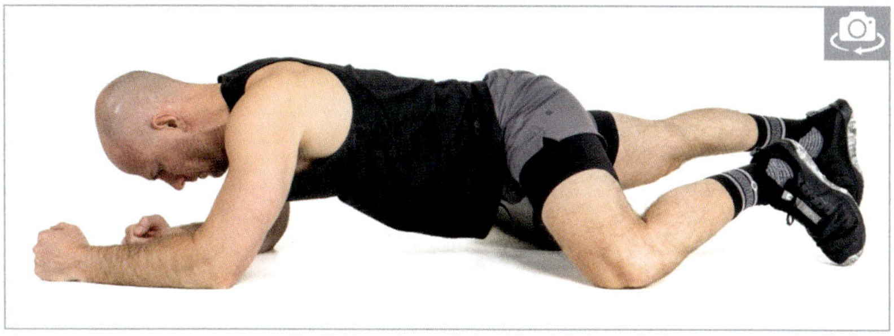

EXECUTION: Keeping your leg as straight as possible while maintaining a neutral pillar, pull and/or push your body on the roller using your arms and bent (grounded) leg. When you find a tender spot, oscillate on that area, rolling back and forth with 1 to 3 inches of movement.

Another option is to pause on the area and perform the neurological trigger point technique by bending and straightening your knee for 3 to 5 reps.

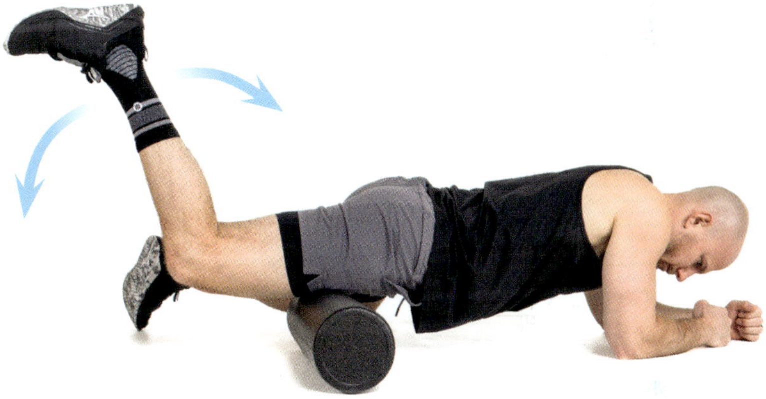

CONSIDERATIONS: If the pressure is too painful, lean more body weight onto your bent knee and/or place a towel between the roller and your thigh. If that doesn't alleviate enough pressure, you can position both quads on the roller at the same time.

OSCILLATORY

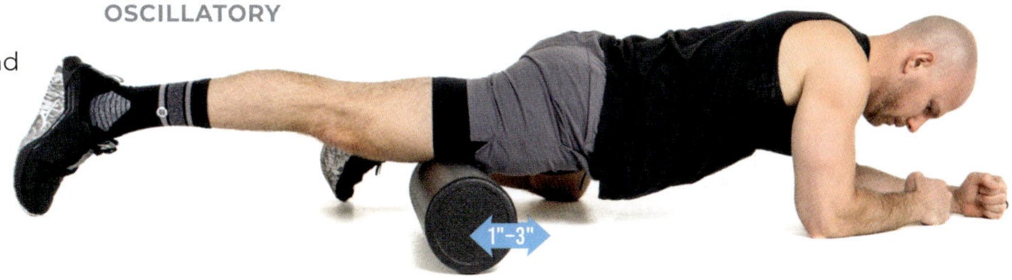

1"–3"

NEUROLOGICAL TRIGGER POINT

LATERAL HIP / TENSOR FASCIAE LATAE (TFL)

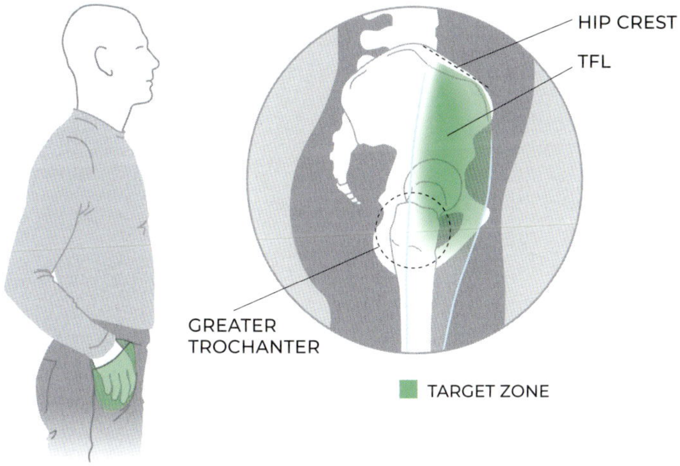

HIP CREST

TFL

GREATER TROCHANTER

TARGET ZONE

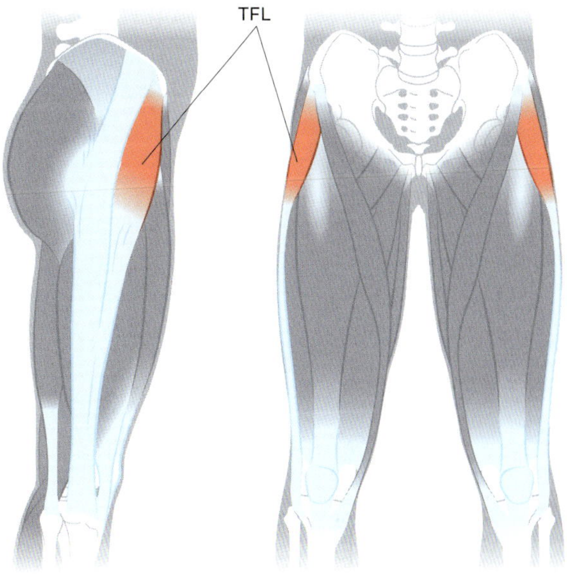

TFL

TARGET ZONES: The region between the top of the hip crest and the top of your greater trochanter—roughly where your hand would slide into a front/side pocket.

BODY POSITION: Get into a modified side plank position with your elbow under your shoulder, bent at roughly a 90-degree angle. Keep your shoulder stable (joint centration), your hips square, your spine neutral, and your bottom leg relaxed.

EXECUTION: From the start position, perform the oscillatory technique by rolling 1 to 3 inches over the target zone, using your grounded arm and top leg to guide the movement. Remaining on the tender area, you can also perform the neurological trigger point technique by lifting and lowering your bottom leg a few inches off the ground for 3 to 5 reps (not shown).

    Another option is to rotate your upper body toward your back and front side, shearing across the muscle— referred to as the spanning technique. The focus here is maintaining a neutral spine as you rotate from your hips and shoulders.

CONSIDERATIONS: To keep the intensity to a manageable to 3–4 out of 10, lean your body slightly backward (toward your glutes). This shifts pressure away from the TFL, which can be especially sensitive. If rolling up and down still feels too intense, use the spanning technique instead.

OSCILLATORY

1"–3"

NEUROLOGICAL TRIGGER POINT

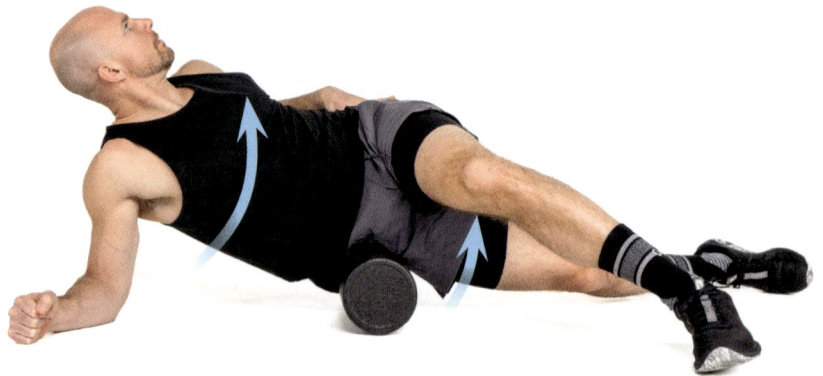

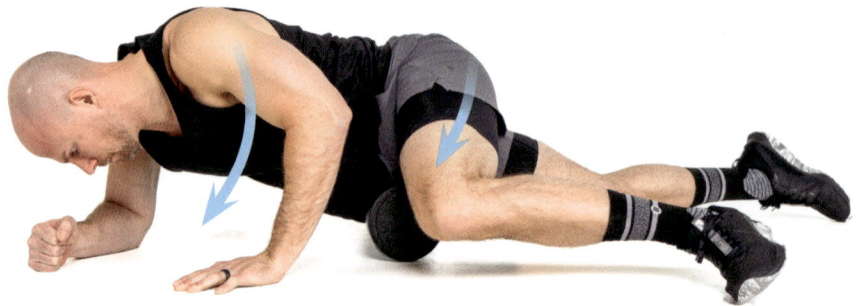

ADDUCTOR GROUP

TARGET ZONES: To target your lower adductor group (zone 1), roll from just above the inside of your knee to halfway up your adductor. To target your upper adductor group (zone 2), roll from the middle of your inner thigh to the inside of your hip.

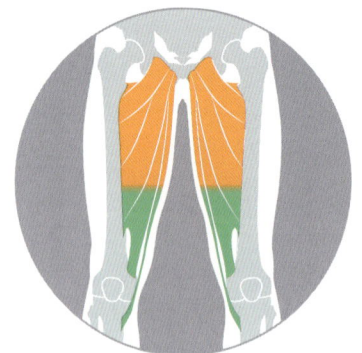

ZONE 1

ZONE 2

BODY POSITION: Get into the "soldier crawl" position: elbows aligned under your shoulders, foam roller under your leg bent at roughly 90 degrees, and your other leg straight and relaxed. Keep your shoulders below your ears and your hips relatively level (square with the ground).

If this position does not provide enough intensity, you can shift more body weight onto the roller by posting up on your toes and elevating your thigh off the ground as if you were doing a plank.

EXECUTION: Keeping your leg bent while maintaining a neutral pillar, use your arms and grounded leg to shift your weight laterally onto the roller. When you find a tender spot, oscillate on that area, rolling back and forth with 1 to 3 inches of movement. While on the tender area, you can also perform the neurological trigger point technique by straightening and bending your knee for 3 to 5 reps (think "windshield wiper" motion).

If you feel apprehensive—you're too tight or there is too much resistance to fully straighten your leg— perform shorter back-and-forth movements. Another option is to shear or span across the muscle by rotating the foot of your bent leg toward the ceiling and floor (not pictured). This technique tends to work better in zone 2.

CONSIDERATIONS: If bringing your leg up to a 90-degree hip angle in the start position is uncomfortable, open the angle of your hip by lowering your leg. This same modification applies when using a small foam roller (small diameter).

When targeting zone 1, rotating your knee toward the ground directs pressure between the quad and adductors, whereas rotating toward the ceiling shifts the emphasis to the hamstrings. Choose the position that feels more sensitive. For most people, that is on the quad side.

When targeting zone 2, you may not feel enough pressure going into your upper adductor, rolling along the length of the muscle. In this scenario, pause on the roller and shift your body back an inch or two as if you were pushing your tailbone to the wall behind you. This targets the hamstring side of the adductor, which is often the more sensitive area.

OSCILLATORY

1"-3"

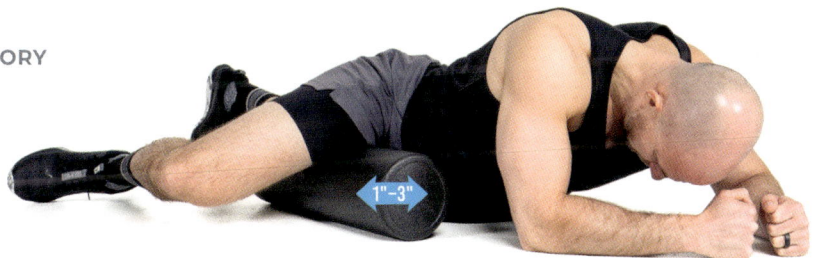

NEUROLOGICAL TRIGGER POINT

UPPER BODY

TRAPEZIUS   SCAPULAE

LATISSIMUS DORSI

■ TARGET ZONE

THORACIC SPINE

TARGET ZONES: From the bottom of your shoulder blades (scapulae) to the base of your neck.

BODY POSITION: To get set up, position the foam roller perpendicular to your spine and then lie on the roller, positioning it across your upper back at the bottom of your shoulder blades. Cross your arms—as if you were giving yourself a big hug—and tuck your chin. These actions expose the muscles you're aiming to target and reduce vertebrae contact, so that you're rolling tissue, not bone.

EXECUTION: Lift your hips a couple of inches off the ground to increase pressure, making sure to keep your hips in a stable position, and then use your legs to roll your back up and down the target zone. Focus your oscillation efforts on tight areas, rolling back and forth with 1 to 3 inches of movement.

To perform the neurological trigger point technique, flex (like doing a small ab crunch) to bring your ribs toward your hips, then extend your arms overhead. As you do this, draw your head back so your ears are between your biceps. The key here is to maintain a neutral pillar with a strong core. In other words, don't arch through your lower back or tilt your head back as you reach your arms overhead. Repeat this "flex to extend" motion for 3 to 5 reps, then move the foam roller up about 1-2 inches. Do another 3 to 5 reps from this new position. Sync your breathing with this movement by inhaling as you flex and exhaling as you extend and reach overhead.

CONSIDERATIONS: The biggest fault to avoid here is letting go of core stability, allowing your head to crane toward the ground, the ribcage to tilt up, and the pelvis to dump forward. This puts pressure and creates tension in the lower back and neck. Again, mind your pillar and keep your core engaged.

Stay within the indicated zone to prevent discomfort. In other words, avoid putting the pressure of your body weight on your lower ribs and neck muscles.

If you experience neck pain or discomfort during the thoracic spine mobilization with arms reaching overhead, keep your hands behind your head to support your neck as you flex and extend over the roller.

OSCILLATORY

1"–3"

NEUROLOGICAL TRIGGER POINT

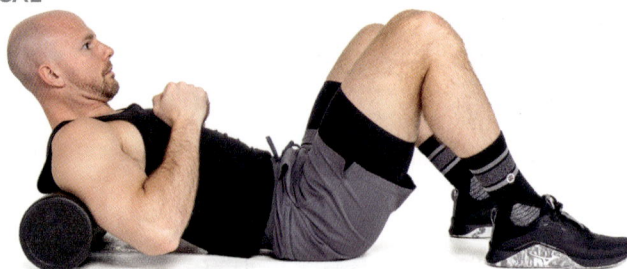

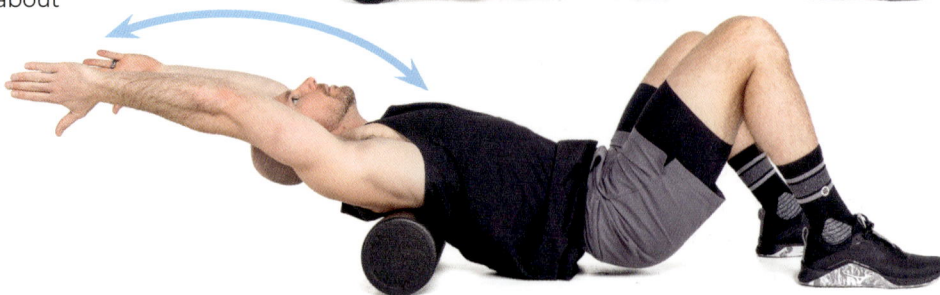

PECTORALIS GROUP

TARGET ZONES: Start where your pectoralis major (pec) attaches to your humerus, just below your clavicle and on the front of your shoulder (anterior deltoid muscle).

BODY POSITION: Lie belly down on the ground with the foam roller positioned at about a 45-degree angle relative to your head. Place the edge of the roller near the front of your deltoid and outside region of your upper pec muscle. If you are mobilizing your right arm/chest, keep your right leg straight and your left leg up at about a 90-degree angle.

Adjust the angle of your chest/arm and use your body weight to apply the appropriate amount of pressure on the foam roller while keeping your body relaxed.

EXECUTION: Say you're targeting your right pec. To execute the oscillatory technique, use your legs and grounded (left) arm to glide your shoulder and pec over the roller. Push and pull, moving back and forth 1 to 3 inches over the target zone for 30 to 60 seconds.

When you find a tender spot, which for most people is where the pec attaches to the humerus and front of the shoulder, pause on the roller and perform the neurological trigger point technique by straightening and pulling your arm back—as if you were doing a rear delt fly. You can also keep your arm extended and make a circular motion by sliding your hand in an arcing motion toward your hips.

CONSIDERATIONS: If it feels comfortable, move the roller toward the middle of your pec, positioning the end of the roller toward the edge of your armpit.

To keep pain at a 3 to 4 out of 10, you may need to lean your body weight off the roller. You should be able to maintain smooth, steady breathing even when on a tender area.

PECTORALIS MAJOR

CLAVICLE

ANTERIOR DELTOID MUSCLE

45°

HUMERUS

OSCILLATORY

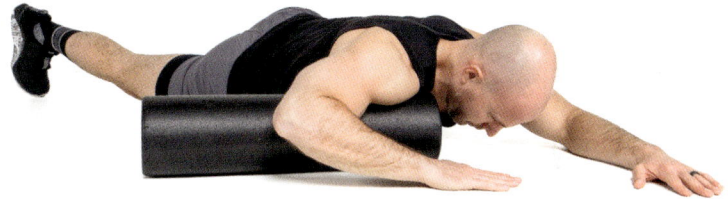

NEUROLOGICAL TRIGGER POINT

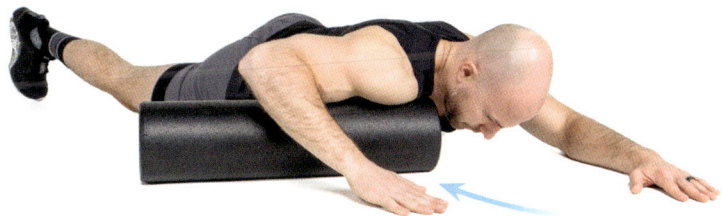

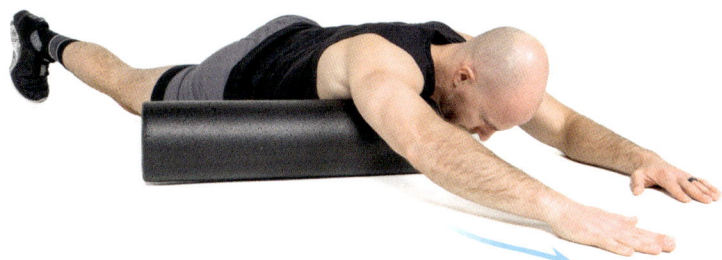

POSTERIOR SHOULDER

TARGET ZONES: For zone 1, position the roller in the crease of your armpit. This region targets the attachment points of numerous muscles: posterior deltoid, triceps, latissimus dorsi (lat), infraspinatus, teres minor, and teres major. For zone 2, position the roller just below your shoulder. You may have to lean slightly toward your backside to target your lat muscle, which wraps from the back side of your shoulder toward your lower back.

TRICEPS BRACHII

DELTOID

TERES MINOR

TERES MAJOR

INFRASPINATUS

LATISSIMUS DORSI

■ ZONE 1
■ ZONE 2

BODY POSITION: Get into the side-lying position with your legs splayed and bent at 90-degree angles. Extend your bottom arm overhead, positioning the foam roller under your armpit.

Configuring your legs in the 90/90 position, as pictured, not only provides balance and support, but also aligns with the fascial lines that cross the body, connecting the lat of the right arm across the backside of the body to the glute, lateral quad, and subpatellar tendon of the left leg. This positioning promotes good posture and functional integration, which will be the focus of future phases in the warm-up.

EXECUTION: For the posterior shoulder, the area is small, so your rolling will be minimal. Use your legs to create small oscillations, allowing your arm to rest on the ground for support and stability.

To target the lats with the oscillatory technique, use your legs to roll 1 to 2 inches up and down, being careful not to roll too low on the ribs.

When you find a tender spot, implement the neurological trigger point technique. There are three options here: 1) rotating your chest toward the ground and leaning toward your backside, 2) bending your arm at a 90-degree angle and then lowering your palm toward the ground, repeating this back-and-forth motion, or 3) raising and lowering your arm while keeping your elbow locked out.

OSCILLATORY

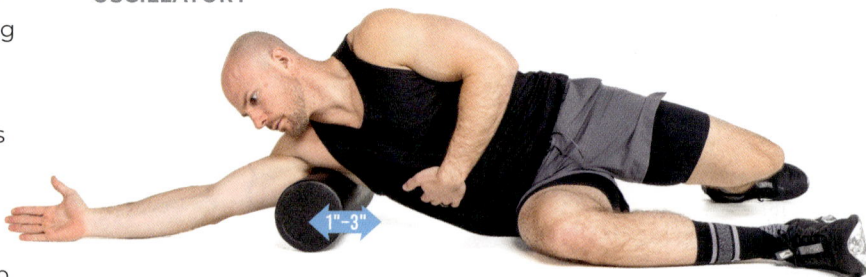

1"–3"

NEUROLOGICAL TRIGGER POINT

OPTION 1

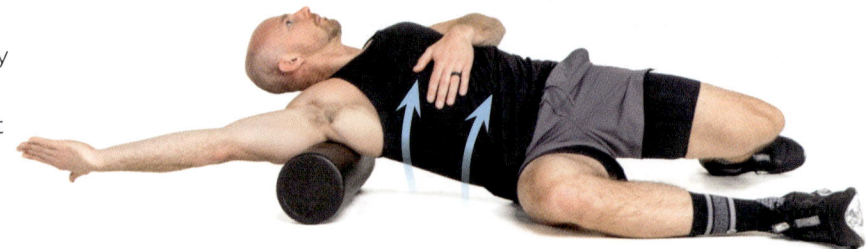

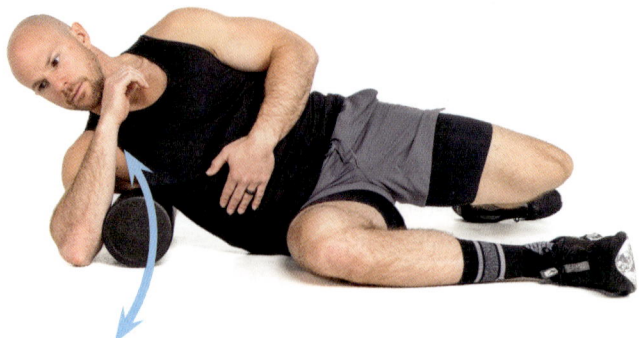

OPTION 2

CONSIDERATIONS: If your shoulder hurts when reaching overhead, reduce or change your arm angle. If you experience neck pain or discomfort, cup the hand of your bottom arm behind your head to support and alleviate tension in your neck.

OPTION 3

SUPPLEMENTAL OPTIONS

GLUTES

BODY POSITION: Sit on the foam roller, angled slightly to one side so that it targets the thickest part of your glute.

   If you're rolling your right glute, support yourself with your right hand and left foot on the ground. If this causes any wrist discomfort, you can lower yourself onto your right forearm for added support.

EXECUTION: Use your right arm and left foot to slowly roll your glute over the foam roller. Adjust your body angle by tilting forward or backward slightly to target different areas of the glute. The roller's larger surface area allows it to apply pressure to multiple hip muscles, both superficial and deep. As the surface layers begin to release, you'll be able to reach deeper layers. Spend 1 to 2 minutes on each side to facilitate this gradual release.

PROGRESSION: If comfortable, cross your right ankle over your left knee while rolling the right glute. This adds a stretch to the glute and externally rotates the femur, allowing you to access deeper layers of tissue.

   For more targeted pressure, you can progress to using a trigger point ball.

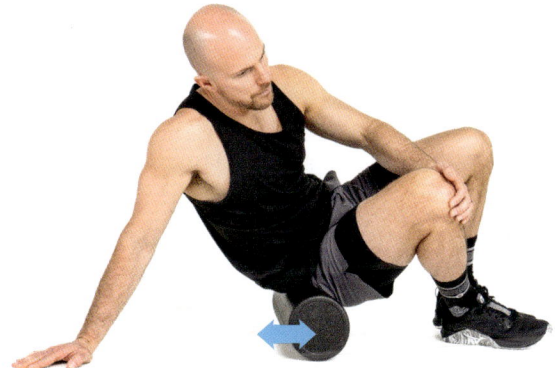

HAMSTRINGS

BODY POSITION: Sit on the foam roller at the top of your hamstring, just below your glute. Bend one leg for support and use your hands behind you to maintain stability and maximize ground contact.

   If flexibility is an issue, prop up your hands on yoga blocks or a step for added support. Alternatively, you can roll both hamstrings at the same time by leaning your torso back, making it easier to maintain balance.

EXECUTION: Focus on rolling the top half of your hamstring, working into the main belly of the muscle by pushing and pulling yourself back and forth using your bent leg. This area tends to be denser, offering more benefit than rolling all the way down to the back of your knee.

   For additional relief, try the spanning technique by turning your toes inward and outward. Think of starting with your toes pointing upright at 12 o'clock, then rotating them to 10 o'clock and 2 o'clock.

   You can also try the shearing technique: Keep a specific area of the muscle "pinned" on the foam roller while you move your body side to side. Leaning forward slightly helps apply more body weight, allowing for a deeper release.

PROGRESSION: Once you're comfortable with the foam roller's intensity, you can progress to using a trigger point ball for more targeted pressure. This allows you to access deeper areas, including the spaces where one muscle overlaps another. To do it, sit on a chair or bench and position the ball under the hamstring. In addition to rolling, you can extend and bend your knee to create more movement. The hamstring is a large muscle group, so you can target multiple spots—aim for 3 or more areas, spending 30 to 60 seconds on each with a combination of rolling and knee extensions.

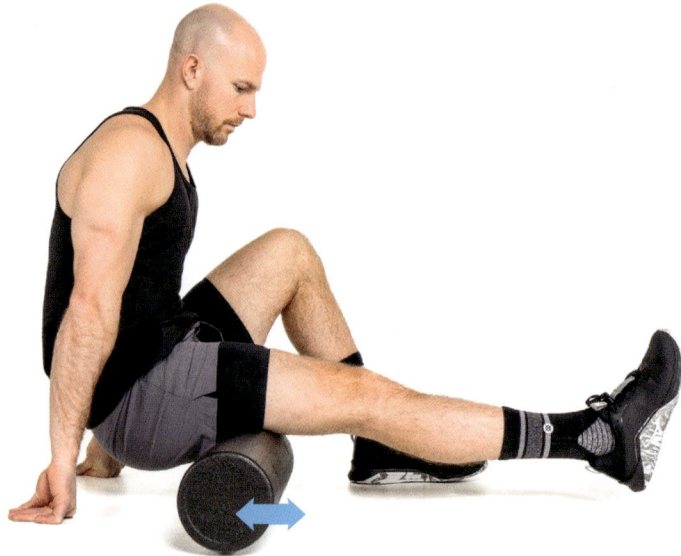

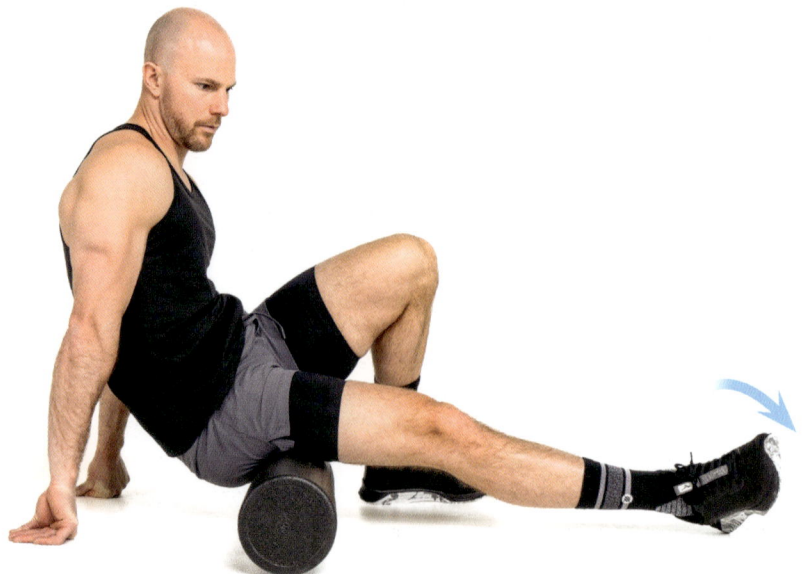

CALVES

BODY POSITION: Sit on the floor with the foam roller positioned under your straight leg, right at the base of your calf muscle, just above the Achilles tendon. Bend your other leg with your foot flat on the floor for stability, and place your hands behind you for support. (If you feel discomfort in your wrists, you can lower onto your forearms.)

EXECUTION: Use your hands and the foot on the floor to gently roll up and down through the calf. For more intensity, you can lift your hips about 1 inch off the ground to increase the pressure on the muscle. The calf can be quite sensitive, even for those who foam-roll regularly, so take your time, working through smaller sections. While holding yourself up, try to keep your shoulders back and down, encouraging a relaxed and controlled movement.

PROGRESSION: To enhance movement through the lower limb, "pin" the muscle on the roller and add toe point/flex movements or perform a few ankle circles in each direction. This can help to release deeper layers and improve range of motion in the calf and ankle.

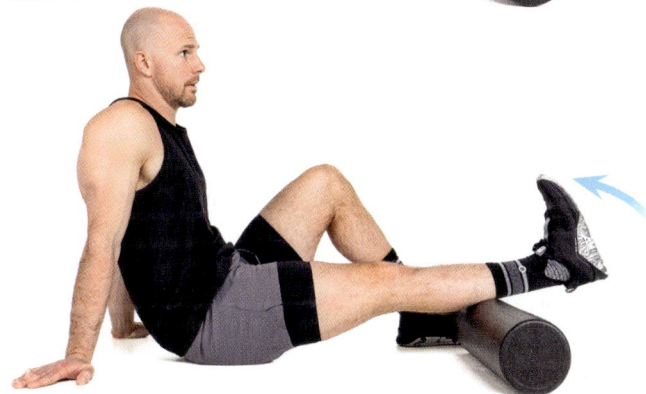

FEET

BODY POSITION: Keep your feet about hip-width apart to maintain balance while you roll the soles of your feet with a ball. This stance gives you stability and control over the pressure applied.

EXECUTION: Place the ball under the ball of your foot. Slowly work through the arch muscles by rolling from the big toe side across to the pinky toe side. A simple method is to start along a line (e.g., the big toe) and roll the ball back and forth toward your heel. Then shift to the next line (e.g., the second toe) and repeat the process, gradually working through the entire arch for about 60 seconds.

After focusing on the arch, move the ball under your heel with your toes and the ball of your foot resting on the floor—similar to the position of wearing a high-heeled shoe. Pivot your foot side-to-side, like you're putting out a cigarette, to massage the ball across the heel.

It's common for the arch area to feel tender, while the heel may not produce much sensation. However, don't skip the heel—it's still beneficial. In fact, you might notice improved range of motion or a decrease in tightness through your back-line if you test bending over to touch your toes before and after rolling your feet.

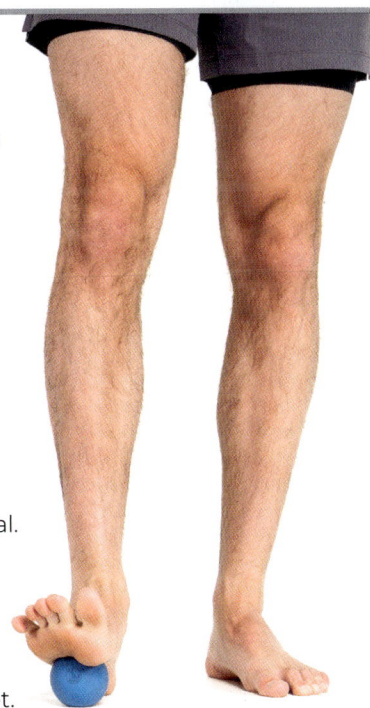

PHASE 2: BIPHASIC POSITIONAL STRETCHING

Phase 2, biphasic positional stretching, amplifies the stress-reducing, tension-relieving, pain-alleviating, and movement-enhancing benefits of phase 1, but with a more localized effect. Together, these two phases form the parasympathetic block of the warm-up sequence, sharing the same goals and general guidelines. It's not about one or the other; it's the amalgamation that holds the power.

"I'm not stretching enough."

We've all thought this before—usually right after sustaining an injury or when our movement goals hit a plateau.

"My mobility sucks. I need to stretch."

"If I take up yoga, maybe this ache would go away."

"This injury is my own doing because I neglect stretching."

This is the narrative I hear from 90 percent of clients who come to me for personal training, especially those battling pain, rehabbing an injury, or struggling with mobility. There's a deeply ingrained belief that stretching is a kind of magic bullet—the solution to all pain and performance woes. And it makes sense. Stretching is one of the oldest forms of physical self-help. When a part of our body aches, we instinctually stretch the area to find relief. When we transition from rest to activity, we intuitively stretch to warm up and prepare for movement.

Yet, despite the simplicity and age-old presence of stretching in human movement, many people still struggle to find balance with a stretching routine. People who don't stretch enough often adopt an all-or-nothing mindset, thinking all stretching is the same. They believe they need to stretch for hours every day to see any functional benefits, leading them to avoid stretching altogether, mistakenly viewing it solely as static stretching. Conversely, some individuals stretch excessively, often in compensated positions—with a rounded or arched back, for example—for long durations and at high intensity. This approach is both unsustainable and ineffective, as stretching in such positions fails to yield the desired results and can even contribute to pain and injury.

The truth I've come to understand, through both personal experience and professional practice,

is that optimal results lie in the balance, not in extremes. This book's guiding principle is the pursuit of a middle path—a results-driven approach that shuns rigid, dogmatic thinking. It's about breaking free from unproductive habits (or non-habits) and the notion that more is always better. Because anytime you venture too far toward either end of the spectrum—doing nothing or doing too much—you miss out on the benefits and risk causing more harm than good.

When it comes to stretching in the warm-up, a little can go a long way, assuming that quality (form), quantity (duration), and intensity (effort) are properly managed. Context is also important. Stretching in the warm-up is different from stretching for recovery or stretching as an independent practice. The former requires stricter guidelines, while the latter offers more flexibility. To get the most out of stretching, you need to understand why it works, how it helps, and what you are trying to accomplish, then model your approach to meet those objectives.

In other words, it's not just about the quantity of stretching but the quality and purpose behind it. Are you stretching effectively, or are you simply going through the motions without understanding how to do it correctly?

In this chapter, we'll explore the real goals of stretching within the warm-up, moving beyond the common notions that all stretching is the same and that more is better. I'll show you how stretching, when tailored to enhance pillar stability and regulate the nervous system, can significantly reduce tension, alleviate pain, and improve your overall mobility. By shifting from the mindset of "not stretching enough" to "stretching effectively," you will transform your approach to this time-tested modality, ensuring that each stretch serves a purposeful role in preparing your mind and body for pain-free performance.

THE GOALS OF STRETCHING

The primary goal of stretching in the warm-up is to downregulate the central nervous system. Remember, phase 2 is in the parasympathetic block of the warm-up sequence. As with foam rolling, the aim is to reduce stress, release tension, and modulate pain. That way, you not only feel better, but you can also improve your movement quality as you progress through the phases and ride the performance wave into the workout.

You're also stretching to improve range of motion and pillar positioning. It's a movement-based approach where you perform dynamic positional stretches that influence joint and tissue stability and mobility. It's crucial to point out that I'm not referring to the dynamic stretching movements such as leg swings and arm circles common in many sports-performance warm-ups. While such movements are indeed dynamic—and can prepare the tissues for speed-based actions like sprinting—they are limited in scope. With those types of dynamic stretches, you move through full ranges of motions and increase tissue temperature, which is useful, but you are not facilitating change in the specific positions or body regions that will have the most carryover to pillar function and resistance training.

In phase 2, you perform what resembles traditional static stretches. You get into a position and then actively stretch to gain more range of movement. The aim here is twofold: to counteract common compensatory tightness and to improve positions that will ultimately enhance movement quality. For example, the half-kneeling hip flexor stretch helps open up your hips, counteracting hours spent sitting. The 90/90 chest stretch targets your pecs and shoulders, reversing the forward hunch from constant phone use. By relieving tension and increasing range in these regions, you're able to stabilize your hips and shoulders more effectively, alleviate common pain sources linked to sedentary postures, and gain access to positions that you would otherwise struggle to get into.

To achieve these goals, however, you not only need to stretch in a good position with your hips, shoulders, and spine neutral—that is, with a stable pillar—but you also need to create enough tension in the system to maintain the position. In other words, these are not passive stretches where you completely relax and compensate (breaking the pillar) to sink deeper into the stretch. Your muscles are active, holding just enough tension to maintain hip, shoulder, and core stability. This sensation of resistance around the region you are stretching is important because it communicates to your brain that you own the position. That it is safe to be in that position and move your body into the space that you are stretching. Here's how it works:

HOW STRETCHING WORKS

1
SENSATION OF TENSION OR RESISTANCE

When you stretch a muscle, you feel a sensation of tension or resistance. This is a combination of mechanical resistance from the muscle and connective tissue as well as neural inhibition from the nervous system.

2
MUSCLE SPINDLE ACTIVATION

As the muscle is stretched, muscle spindles (sensory receptors in the muscle) send signals to the spinal cord.

3
STRETCH REFLEX (MYOTATIC REFLEX)

In response to those signals, the spinal cord sends a reflex signal back to the muscles to contract (known as the stretch reflex or myotatic reflex). It's a protective response to prevent overstretching and potential injury to the muscle.

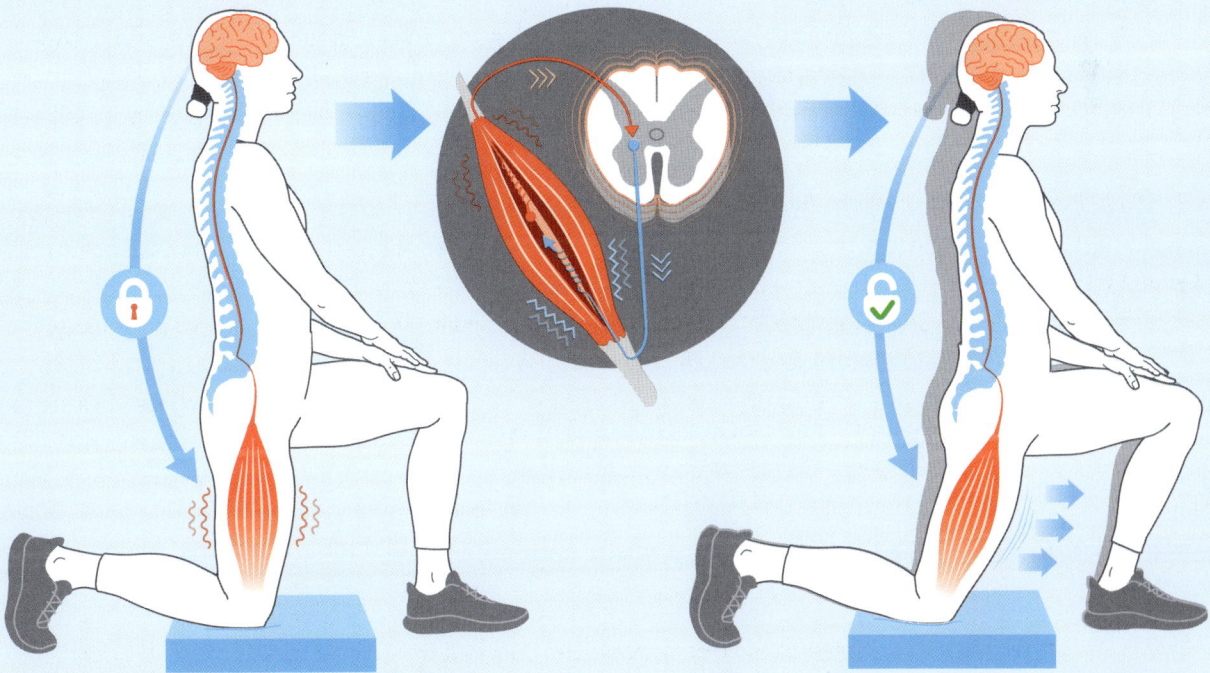

4
MUSCLE RELAXES

When you oscillate and hold the stretch in non-threatening positions at low intensity, the nervous system "lets go," releasing muscle tension. In other words, the signal telling the muscle to contract (to resist damage or further stretch) falls below the threshold that is stimulating the muscle contraction, so the muscle relaxes.

5
INCREASED RANGE OF MOTION

As the muscle relaxes, the range of motion increases, allowing for greater flexibility and movement.

6
IMPROVED STABILITY AND POSITIONING

By easing tension and expanding your range of motion, you'll more effectively reach neutral, stable positions during movement, enhancing both your exercise and overall movement form.

Like with soft tissue techniques, you are not trying to mechanically change or lengthen the muscle. Instead, you're trying to "fool" your nervous system into reducing muscle tonicity (tightness) to momentarily overcome neural inhibition (when the nervous system restricts movement to protect the body). Foam rolling has a more centralized or global effect—when you foam roll your quads, you reduce tension not just in your quads but in your entire body. Stretching has a more localized effect—when you stretch your quads, you primarily reduce tension in your quads. This is why the two are coupled. The soft tissue technique reduces tone globally so that you can increase range of motion with stretching locally, opening an opportunity window to improve specific aspects of a movement pattern as well as reduce pain in a particular region.

This is different from stretching to increase flexibility. Over time, with consistent stretching, the nervous system may "learn" to allow a greater range of motion without eliciting the stretch reflex, allowing more extensive range of motion without an automatic contraction. But just because you have access to the range of motion doesn't mean you can control the range of motion with load and speed. Therein lies the difference between flexibility and mobility.

> **FLEXIBILITY is the range of motion that you can passively access,** meaning you can access a position but with limited ability to control the position.

> **MOBILITY is the range of motion that you can actively control**, meaning you have the coordination and strength to stabilize the position during movement.

The goal in the warm-up for most people is to improve mobility and close the motor control gap—the range between your passive flexibility and active mobility—while progressing through the subsequent phases. You do that by

▼ **FOAM ROLLING**
to reduce total body tension (phase 1).

▼ **STRETCHING**
to increase range of motion and improve pillar positioning for a particular body region (phase 2).

▼ **PERFORMING STRATEGIC CORRECTIVE EXERCISES**
that express movement within that newly gained range, helping to close the motor control gap (phase 3).

▼ **STABILIZING THE RANGE WITH ACTIVATION DRILLS,**
"locking in" the newly gained or practiced range (phase 4).

▼ **APPLYING THE GAINED MOBILITY**
to functional movement patterns (phases 5 and 6)

DISPELLING THE PRE-TRAINING STRETCHING MYTHS

The debate surrounding the role of stretching in warm-ups is as old as exercise itself. Once universally accepted as crucial before any physical activity, stretching's place in pre-training routines has now come under scrutiny. Contemporary research has shifted opinions, leading many to view stretching as potentially detrimental to performance and an instigator of injury risks.

This shift is largely due to studies indicating that static stretching before certain activities can diminish muscle strength and power and disrupt neuromuscular coordination.[1] However, the broader context of these studies is frequently ignored. Many involved intense, prolonged static stretching right before engaging in high-intensity exercise. Delving deeper reveals that most of these stretches were performed on apparatuses reminiscent of medieval torture devices, with little consideration for proper form. Such extreme routines, far removed from the functional stretching positions advocated in this phase, inevitably led to decreased performance and increased injury risk, exacerbating the very motor control issues that you aim to remedy.

This is not the approach in phase 2. Your strategy should follow a moderate, results-driven stretching warm-up routine that focuses on a combination of dynamic and static stretches, each carefully chosen to prime the body for peak performance, improve biomechanical function, and build a stronger, more adaptable physique over time. To truly appreciate the value of stretching in phase 2 of the dynamic warm-up, you must discard these misguided views based on flawed premises. Because when implemented correctly, biphasic stretching plays an essential role in the warm-up, enhancing mobility, strength, and overall physical capacity.

So, as you advance through the six phases, you incrementally gain mobility and motor control around the pillar that carries over into the movement patterns you will perform in the workout.

Now, it's important to note that not everyone needs to improve mobility. For those of you who already have stellar mobility, your focus should shift to stability and motor control—because improving mobility isn't the goal when you already have it.

Hyper-mobile athletes—people with an excessive range of motion in their joints—may need to use more restrictive ranges of motion when stretching to stay within their neutral zone. In this scenario, you're not chasing the stretch sensation but rather ramping up tension through the pillar and locking in the position that maximizes stability in your hips and shoulders.

In summary, everyone can benefit from improving pillar stability and motor control. That is always the goal, no matter which phase you are in or how much mobility you possess. However, in phase 2, less flexible people should focus on improving mobility to access better, more stable positions, while more flexible people should concentrate on stabilizing neutral positions so they can carry that sensation into subsequent phases.

In both cases, it's a deliberate approach that enhances how you feel and how you move, setting you up for safe and effective movement through each phase. The key to unlocking the benefits—mobility, stability, and motor control—of stretching in phase 2 and beyond is understanding which techniques to utilize and how and when to implement them.

RECOMMENDATIONS AND GUIDELINES

When you know why you are implementing a particular strategy or technique—and how it will benefit you—the intention becomes clear. And that intention is what powers the efficient and purposeful pain-free training that you're after.

With phase 2, the intention is similar to phase 1: to heighten the parasympathetic response, reduce muscle tonicity, and improve range of motion. While the recommendations and guidelines are similar, there are nuances in the techniques and execution that will align your efforts with the intended goals.

UTILIZE TWO FUNDAMENTAL TECHNIQUES

There's a lot in the name. "Biphasic positional stretching" isn't just a fancy title to make it sound more scientific and technical—it captures the essence of the techniques and how you should approach them.

"Biphasic" refers to executing the two fundamental stretching techniques in two phases: the dynamic oscillatory stretch followed by the static end-range stretch. Say you're doing the half-kneeling hip flexor stretch (see below). Begin with the dynamic oscillatory stretch, moving in and out of end range for 30 seconds (or 6 to 8 oscillations), and then seamlessly transition into the static end-range stretch, holding the position for 15 to 30 seconds. Two distinct stretching phases (biphasic) performed in sequence as a single drill.

"Positional" relates to the mechanics of the body and the authenticity of the stretch. To effectively target the intended muscle and area, you must prioritize your position by setting and maintaining pillar stability—proper alignment and tension in the hips, shoulders, and core. Without any external load, a mild bracing tension of about 10 percent is sufficient to prevent unwanted compensations: twisting, turning, arching, bending, pelvic tilting, etc.

The effectiveness of a stretch is measured not in the range that you can gain through compensation but in the range you can authentically control.

Remember, just because you feel the stretch doesn't mean you're getting the most from it. If you compensate to increase range, the stretch is dispersed away from the targeted area, increasing sensation in the compensating regions. For example, if you arch your lower back during the half-kneeling hip flexor stretch, you'll feel it in your hips and quads (the areas you want to target) but also in your lower back (an area you don't intend to target). Additionally, sacrificing pillar positioning leads to less overall stability. A predictable response to insufficient stability is increased muscle tonicity—compensatory stability, if you will—which is the opposite of what you're trying to achieve here.

The effectiveness of a stretch is measured not in the range that you can gain through compensation but in the range you can authentically control. To display the mobility gained in this phase—and apply it to the movement patterns you want to improve—seek positional mastery with the stretching techniques.

COMPENSATION VS. AUTHENTIC POSITIONING

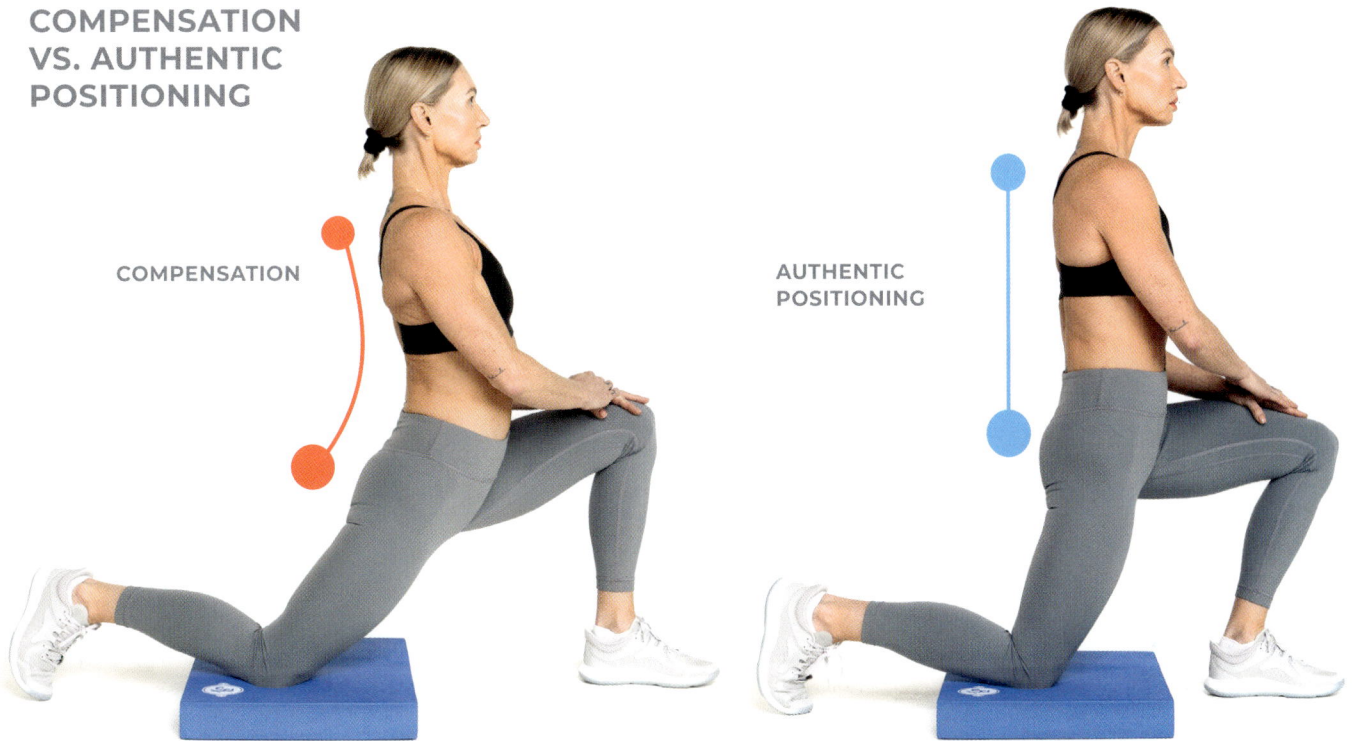

COMPENSATION

AUTHENTIC POSITIONING

DYNAMIC OSCILLATORY STRETCH

To begin, get your hips, shoulders, and core into a neutral position, and then stabilize the pillar by creating just enough tension to maintain the structural integrity of the position. Next, move into the end range of the stretch (defined as the farthest range you can achieve without compensating or breaking the pillar), and then back off by ½ inch to 1 inch, keeping tension in the stretch as you move. Repeat this oscillatory motion, trying to eke out just a little bit more range with each oscillation, for 30 seconds. For example, go forward an inch, back up three-quarters of an inch, then go forward another inch, and back up three-quarters of an inch, and repeat 6 to 8 times.

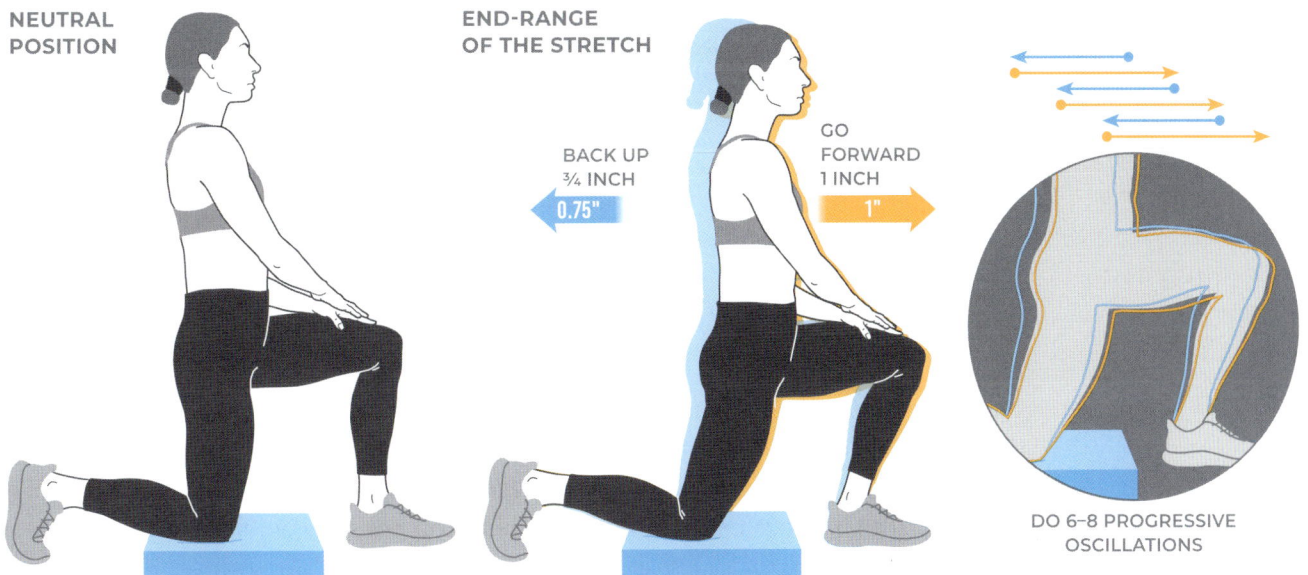

NEUTRAL POSITION

END-RANGE OF THE STRETCH

BACK UP ¾ INCH
0.75"

GO FORWARD 1 INCH
1"

DO 6–8 PROGRESSIVE OSCILLATIONS

STATIC END-RANGE STRETCH

After 30 seconds or roughly 6 to 8 progressive oscillations, seamlessly transition into your new end-range position and hold for 15 to 30 seconds.

Slow and smooth cadence of motion coupled with deep rhythmical diaphragmatic breaths is crucial. Move too fast and your body will go into protection mode, limiting the authentic range of motion you're trying to accentuate. Heavy chest-breathing patterns will drag you toward the sympathetic side of the spectrum, which is the opposite of what you're trying to accomplish.

If the oscillation motion feels clunky or restricted, you may be overbracing with too much tension. Back off just enough to maintain pillar stability and stay focused on your breath cycle.

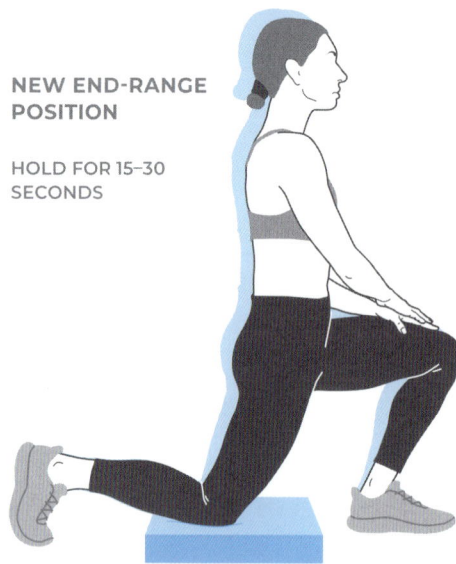

NEW END-RANGE POSITION

HOLD FOR 15–30 SECONDS

3 TO 4 OUT OF 10 ON THE PAIN SCALE

Similar to soft tissue techniques, you're adhering to the 3 to 4 out of 10 on the subjective pain scale (see page 92). That means you feel the stretch, but not so much that you trigger a pain response that masks the benefits of downregulating the parasympathetic nervous system. Keep your breathing slow and smooth and pay attention to the signals from your body. You're stretching to relax the muscles, not tighten them back up. If you notice that you're holding your breath, you can't speak without changes in speed, sharpness, and pattern, you're unable to maintain pillar stability, or you start to tension up, then you may be pushing too hard.

STRETCH 1 OR 2 BODY REGIONS

In the Soft Tissue Techniques chapter, you selected a body region based on where you feel pain or are most limited in your movement (linchpin focus), or the area that is most closely correlated with the movement pattern you plan to prioritize that day (key performance indicator, or KPI).

Foam rolling and stretching go together and complement one other. Knowing that makes selecting the body region to stretch straightforward: the area you foam rolled, based on either the linchpin or the KPI, is the area you will stretch.

This isn't just a redundancy; it's a strategic approach to address the areas that are the most prone to chronic tightness and the regional movers that have the biggest influence on movement form.

To achieve the greatest benefit in the shortest time possible, stretch just one or two of these body regions:

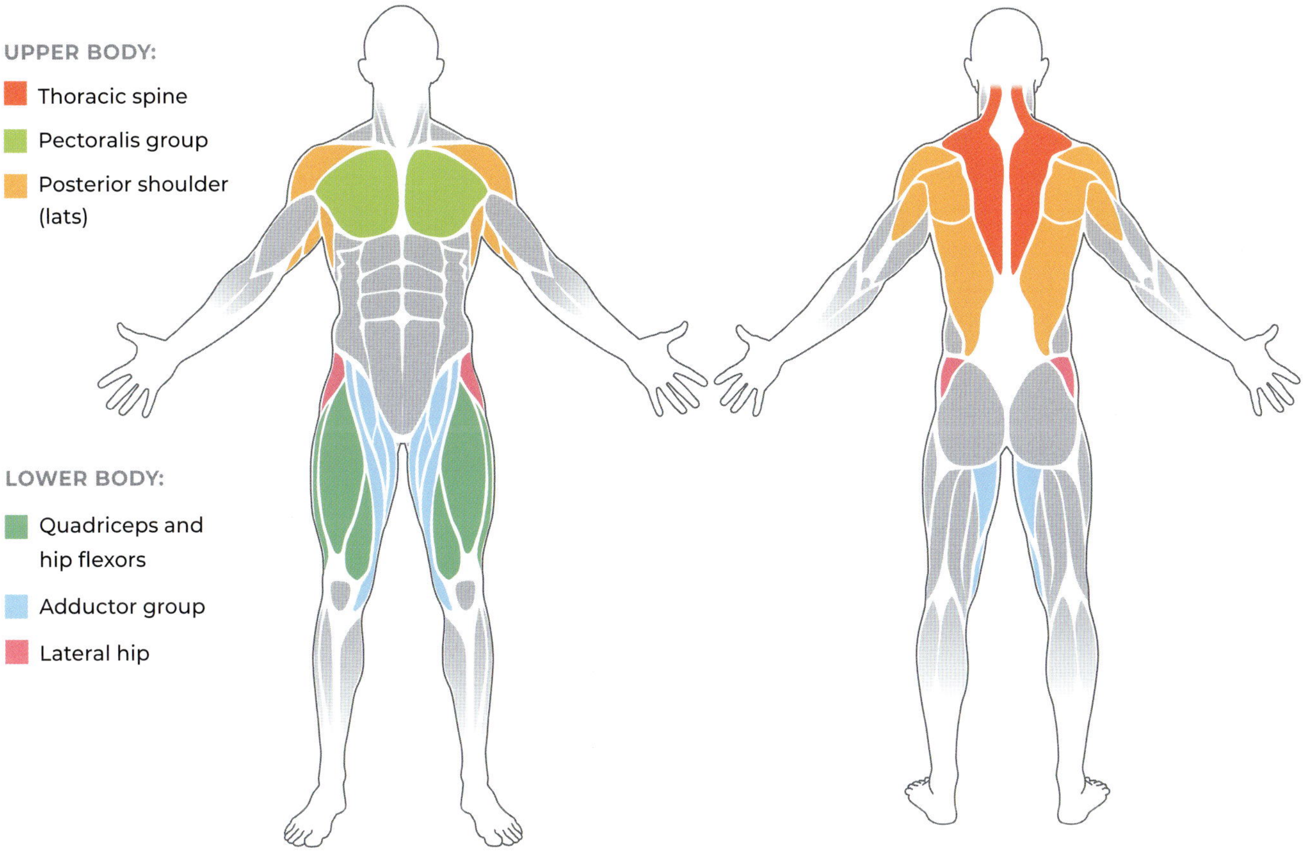

UPPER BODY:
- ■ Thoracic spine
- ■ Pectoralis group
- ■ Posterior shoulder (lats)

LOWER BODY:
- ■ Quadriceps and hip flexors
- ■ Adductor group
- ■ Lateral hip

45 TO 60 SECONDS PER REGION

Research indicates that the duration required to hold a stretch for effective gains in range of motion can vary, but a common consensus is that 30 to 60 seconds can be beneficial, especially for restoring muscles to their functional, resting length.[2] Remember, you're stretching just enough to undo the feeling of tightness created from long bouts of inactivity or repetitive movement, with the goal of reclaiming the end-range positions that you naturally have but rarely access in your daily life. Forty-five to 60 seconds per region is the right amount of time to accomplish that goal.

Outside of the warm-up, such as a post-exercise cool-down or recovery session, longer holds of up to 2 minutes might be more effective for improving overall flexibility. You're not aiming to improve flexibility in the warm-up; you want to improve mobility, period. So resist the temptation to stretch for longer periods in the warm-up. Save that stretching for your recovery session, where the goals shift from doing just enough to doing as much as you want to get the desired stimulus and result (see the Performance Recovery System tenet on page 81 to learn more about how to modify this phase for optimal recovery and to facilitate long-term mobility gains).

THE TIGHT HAMSTRING MYTH

Imagine spending hours stretching your hamstrings every day, only to find them getting tighter and your pain worsening. This isn't just a hypothetical—it's a common frustration that many people experience.

I encountered this exact challenge with an ultra-marathon runner and Ironman athlete who came to me seeking relief from her relentless hamstring tightness and lower back pain.

During our initial consultation, she detailed her intense training regimen, marked by a staggering dedication that few athletes could match. She was in the pool by 3:45 AM, and then from 7 AM to 3 PM she taught an elementary school class. She coached the high school track team from 3 PM to 5 PM, and then she would hit the road for running, biking, or both. Astonishingly, she also revealed spending two to three hours a day static stretching, particularly focusing on her hamstrings.

Her stretching practice began in college when a coach casually commented on her hamstring tonicity affecting her gait. With no further guidance, she took it upon herself to stretch more, eventually escalating to hours of daily stretching, believing it would alleviate her hamstring tightness, resolve her pain, and improve her movement mechanics. Yet by the time I started working with her, she could barely reach her knees during a simple toe touch. After years of endurance training and ritualistic stretching, her flexibility had deteriorated, not improved. Her pain and movement had gotten worse, not better. Overstretching caused lower back pain, hip pinching, general soreness, and central fatigue—common aftereffects of poor stretching techniques performed for long durations and over extended periods.

My approach was both radical and straightforward: I instructed her to stop stretching her hamstrings entirely. Instead, we focused on stretching and strengthening the muscles surrounding her hamstrings (the hip flexors, glutes, and adductors) while placing a heavy emphasis on pillar mechanics and stability. The result? In just two months, her mobility improved significantly, and her hamstrings didn't feel as tight. She was beside herself. Not stretching her hamstrings to alleviate the feeling of tightness and the associated lower back pain went against everything she had been led to believe.

Her experience is not unique.

Most people have tight hamstrings—and we've all been told that simply stretching them will remove the sensation of tightness, improve movement quality, and resolve chronic issues like lower back pain. But that advice, often taken to extremes, seldom delivers on its promise. It's a vicious cycle. We live in a world that encourages sitting. When we sit, we compress our hamstrings and typically round our lower back, which restricts blood flow and exacerbates the sensation of tightness. The more we sit, the tighter we feel. The tighter we feel, the more we stretch. When results don't materialize, we intensify our efforts, mistakenly believing that more stretching is the solution. But it is not.

Contrary to popular belief, resolving tight hamstrings isn't about stretching them more or focusing solely on hamstring stretches. The real solution lies in understanding the root causes—pelvic orientation, reciprocal inhibition, and the lack of regional stability. Often, the issue is not inherently tight hamstrings but the tightness of adjacent muscles that affects the orientation and stability of the hips, creating a perceived sensation of tight hamstrings.

Consider the hip flexors. When they're tight, they prevent full hip extension and tilt the pelvis forward. This misalignment forces the body to compensate by hyperextending through the lower back, often resulting in low back pain. The hamstrings, striving to stabilize the hips and lumbar spine, end up feeling tight—not because they are short or contracted but because they are stretched or inhibited. This is a neuromuscular phenomenon known as reciprocal inhibition, where one muscle's tightness (hip flexors) leads to its opposing muscle's inhibition (hamstrings), creating the sensation of tightness. This was precisely the case with my ultra-marathon client, and it's a common scenario for many with tight hamstrings. This insight also clarifies why hamstring stretches are generally not prioritized in phase 2 of the warm-up—because the solution is not about stretching the hamstrings directly, but rather about stretching the muscles that connect to the hamstrings and hips, influencing pelvic neutrality.

Remember, sometimes the most impactful strategy is eliminating what doesn't work, allowing more time for practices that genuinely improve performance and well-being. When it comes to resolving tight hamstrings—and improving functional hamstring mobility—focus on

- Stretching the muscles that connect to the hamstrings and influence pelvic positioning (hip flexors, glutes, and adductors)
- Prioritizing pillar stability, particularly through the lumbopelvic region (hips and lower back)
- Reducing sedentary behavior—like excessive sitting—by taking movement and stretch breaks
- Engaging in a comprehensive training plan that encompasses the six foundational movement patterns

Now, if your goal is to improve hamstring flexibility or you want to facilitate post-exercise recuperation—say, after an intense deadlifting session—then you should absolutely perform stretches and soft tissue techniques that directly target your hamstrings. But realize that this is different than trying to alleviate the perceived sensation of tightness. In this context, you're trying to reduce muscle soreness, or just stretching and mobilizing the region because it feels good. That's great! Just be sure to stretch your hamstrings with a neutral pelvis, knowing that removing the reciprocal inhibition will have the most benefit.

NEUTRAL PELVIS

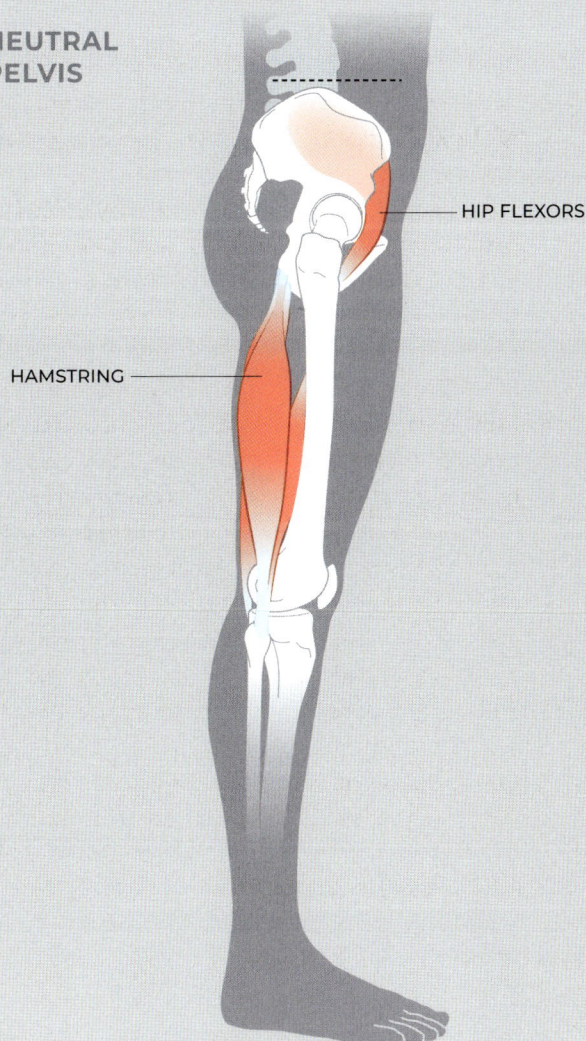

HIP FLEXORS

HAMSTRING

ROTATED PELVIS

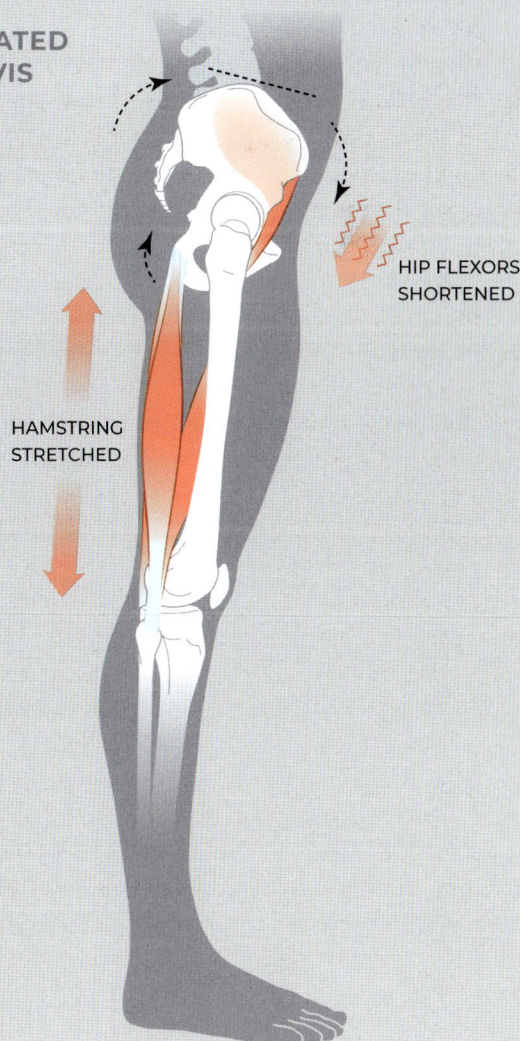

HIP FLEXORS SHORTENED

HAMSTRING STRETCHED

In the 6-phase warm-up, among the myriad of stretching exercises, you will prioritize six techniques. They have proven exceptionally effective— whether for upper body, lower body, or total body workout days—maximizing the gains within the limited time you have allotted to the warm-up.

As previously stated, stretching for recovery, whether post-workout or during an off-day recovery session, offers more freedom than pre-workout stretching. In these sessions, you will still prioritize pillar mechanics and form, but you can hold stretches longer, and you are not limited to the stretches offered here. Feel free to explore and choose variations (such as the supplemental options provided) based on your personal preferences, linchpins, and performance goals.

EXERCISE APPENDIX

PHASE 2: BIPHASIC POSITIONAL STRETCHING

LOWER BODY

HALF-KNEELING HIP FLEXOR STRETCH

SETUP AND BODY POSITION: Start in a half-kneeling (90/90) position with your feet hip-width apart for stability, and position your back foot so that your toes are flexed and in contact with the floor. To find a neutral pelvis, tilt it slightly so that your hip points more toward the bottom of your rib cage ("belt buckle to chin"). Lightly squeeze your glutes and adductors to stabilize your pelvis. Place your hands on top of your front thigh near your knee, and gently engage your pecs and lats to stabilize your shoulders. With a light brace, your pillar will stay solid as you oscillate.

EXECUTION: To initiate the stretch, push forward slightly with your back foot, or imagine your front hamstring pulling you forward. The goal is a strong, pillar-focused position, so even if you don't feel a deep stretch, that's okay. Over the next 30 seconds, perform small oscillations—about 1 inch forward and ¾ inch back—repeating 6 to 8 times to gradually increase range. Once you reach your end range without compromising your pillar, hold for 15 to 30 seconds with smooth, steady breathing.

As you progress, you can add a gentle isometric contraction. For example, if you're stretching your right quad/hip flexor with your right knee on the ground, lightly squeeze your right glute during the hold (10 to 30 percent effort) and continue breathing.

CONSIDERATIONS: If your squat assessment (page 240) indicates a preference for a wider stance, you may feel more comfortable positioning your front leg slightly outward. If you have greater flexibility, consider placing your front foot a bit farther forward to prevent your knee from excessively tracking beyond your toes. Remember, always prioritize maintaining pillar stability over chasing a deeper stretch.

Scan the QR code to access demos of each exercise.

DYNAMIC OSCILLATORY STRETCH

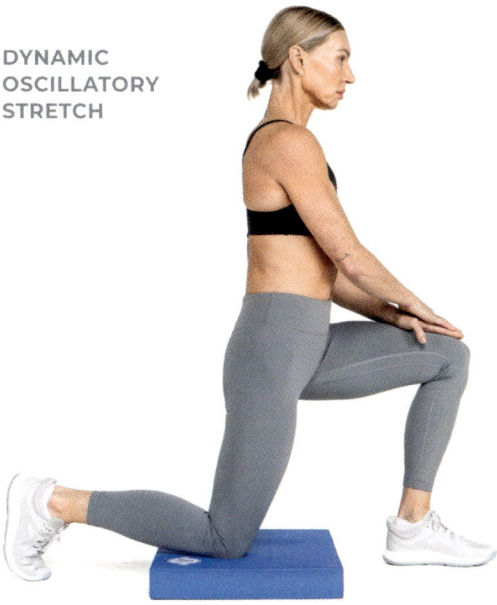

PROGRESSIONS: Once you're comfortable with the bodyweight position, you can try adding a band behind your femur just under your glute to create gentle hip joint distraction. Use a light to moderate band, ensuring the tension doesn't force you to over-brace to stay balanced. Another option is to elevate your rear foot, which increases stretch in your quads and hip flexor. All the same rules apply as in the half-kneeling hip flexor stretch: Maintain a gentle glute squeeze on the stretching leg and keep a neutral pelvis. The key focus here is to avoid hyperextending or arching through your lower back in an attempt to get your torso upright—this compensation reduces the effectiveness of the stretch and places undue strain on the lower back. Instead, prioritize keeping a neutral spine throughout. If needed, place your hands on an elevated surface for support or keep them on the ground, whichever allows you to hold proper alignment and focus on the hip flexor stretch.

REAR-FOOT-ELEVATED VARIATION (PROGRESSION)

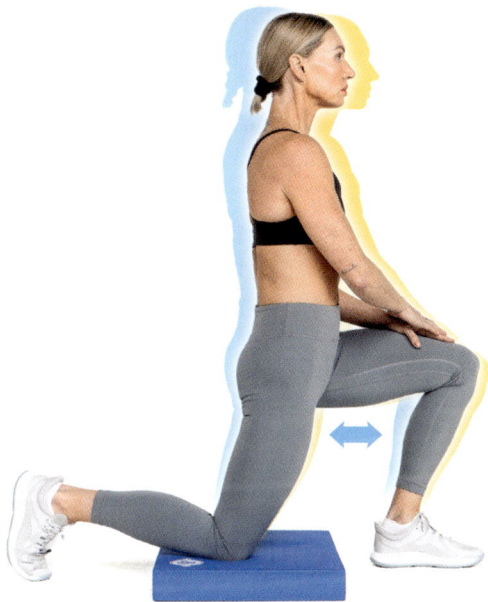

STATIC END-RANGE STRETCH

BANDED DISTRACTION VARIATION (PROGRESSION)

ADDUCTOR ROCK-BACK

SETUP AND BODY POSITION: Begin in a quadruped position with hands under your shoulders and knees under your hips. Extend one leg out to the side. While the example shows the leg perpendicular to the body, feel free to adjust the angle if that's more comfortable within your range of motion. The key is to keep your pelvis level, avoiding excessive tilt up toward your armpit on the stretching side.

Press into the floor with your hands and gently draw your head back to lengthen through your upper back and neck. If possible, lightly press the bottom of your extended foot into the ground. If that activates the outside of your lower leg too intensely, switch to pressing the inside edge of your foot down instead.

EXECUTION: If you don't feel a level-3 to -4 stretch, rotate your pelvis slightly so that the front of the hip on the stretching side angles toward the floor. Engage your quad by drawing the kneecap up toward your hip and adjust the pressure through your outstretched foot for additional activation. Taking a moment to establish this active stretch before oscillating can make a significant difference for this stretch.

Begin oscillating by gently shifting your hips back. While the example shows the hips nearly reaching the heel, that depth isn't necessary. What matters most is maintaining a neutral spine, avoiding any rounding or "tucking" of the tailbone. Move in small, controlled increments of about ½ to 1 inch with each oscillation. Even minor gains here can have a positive impact on your workout.

After about 30 seconds of oscillation, hold at the active end range for another 15 to 30 seconds, maintaining steady diaphragmatic breathing. Use this hold to check in with your jaw and shoulders, ensuring your jaw stays relaxed and your shoulders aren't creeping up toward your ears. This promotes a parasympathetic response, which is the goal.

CONSIDERATIONS: If this position causes discomfort in your wrists, you can perform the exercise on your forearms using a low box or step. This modification maintains shoulder alignment and keeps your back relatively parallel to the ground.

DYNAMIC OSCILLATORY STRETCH

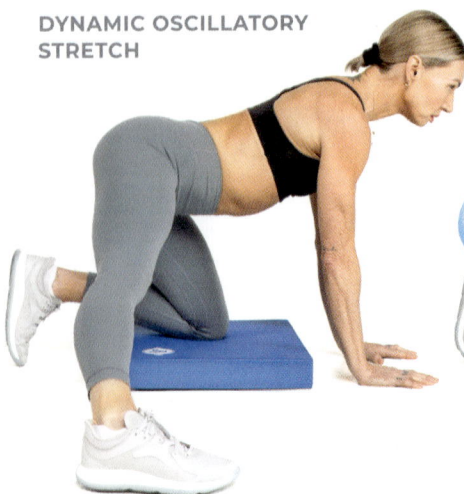

STATIC END-RANGE STRETCH

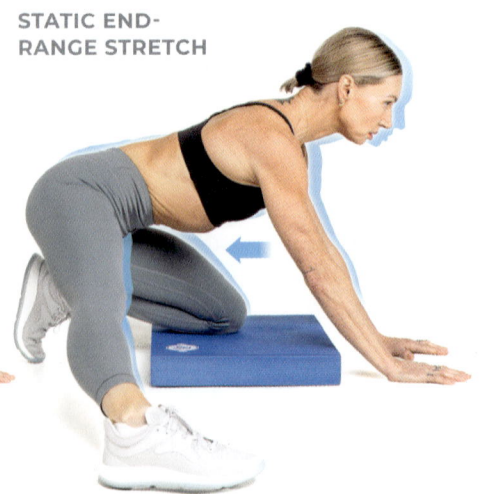

DYNAMIC PIGEON STRETCH

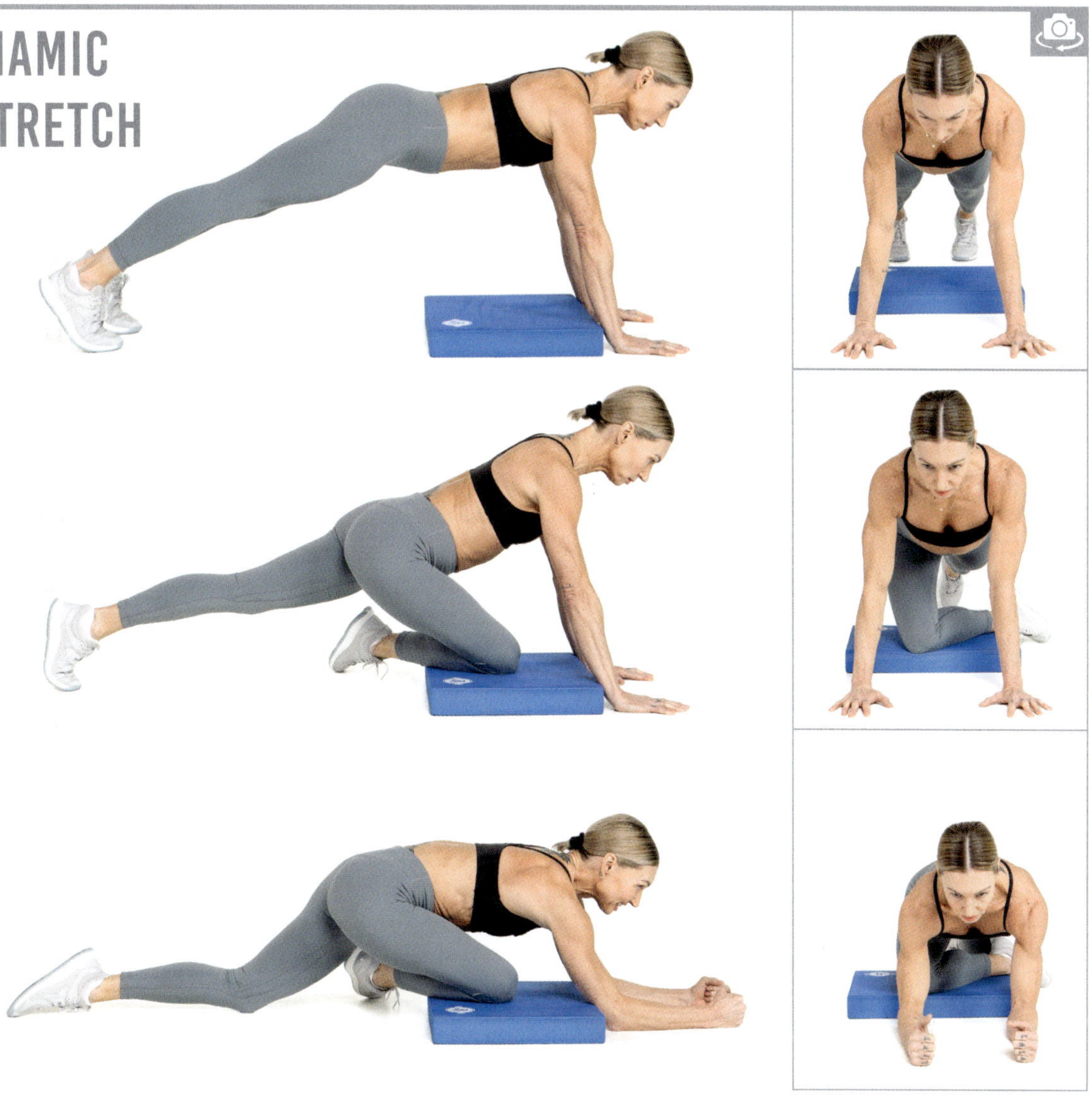

SETUP AND BODY POSITION: Say you're stretching your right glute. Start in a push-up position, with your core braced to keep a neutral spine. Pull your head back slightly to lengthen your upper back and neck. Bring your right knee forward toward your chest, keeping it aligned with your belly button. Place your right knee on the ground and rotate your right foot toward your left hand, moving it as far as is comfortable.

EXECUTION: If you feel a moderate stretch (3 to 4 intensity) in your right glute, proceed to the next steps. If not, shift your left toes back slightly until you feel that level of stretch.

This is an active stretch, meaning you should be able to lift your hands a couple of inches off the ground without losing balance—this ensures your muscles are engaged and stable, rather than just hanging off connective tissue.

Begin oscillating with small movements in one of two directions:

1. Deepen Hip Flexion: Gently pull your hips back and lower your chest slightly. You can lower your back knee to the ground, adjust your foot back, then lift the back knee again and repeat this sequence for 6 to 8 oscillations. Avoid fully resting down; keep control of each movement, ensuring you can still lift your hands without losing stability.

2. Add Rotation: With a long spine, rotate your left shoulder and torso toward your right hand, creating a rotational stretch (not pictured). This utilizes the fascial line connecting your left shoulder to your right hip, helping you access a deeper stretch. Perform 6 to 8 gentle rotational oscillations, keeping your pillar stable and avoiding any side bending.

After 30 to 60 seconds of oscillation, hold at your end range for another 15 to 30 seconds, breathing smoothly. This is also a chance to relax any unnecessary tension in your jaw or shoulders, supporting a parasympathetic response.

CONSIDERATIONS: This stretch can be challenging if you're new to mobility work or dealing with low back, hip, or knee pain. An effective regression is performing the stretch on a bench. Stand facing the bench and place your front leg on top, maintaining the 90-degree angle in your knee. Your back leg remains straight, foot on the floor for stability. For added comfort, you can place a pad underneath your knee on the bench. Keep your spine long and hinge gently from the hips to intensify the stretch, focusing on controlled breathing throughout.

PROGRESSION: Once comfortable with the basic position, try adding a band around the inner thigh/ high hip crease. This creates a slight distraction in the hip joint, helping alleviate any pinching sensation as you move deeper into flexion. Maintain a stable and active position, as this activation will transfer into your training session.

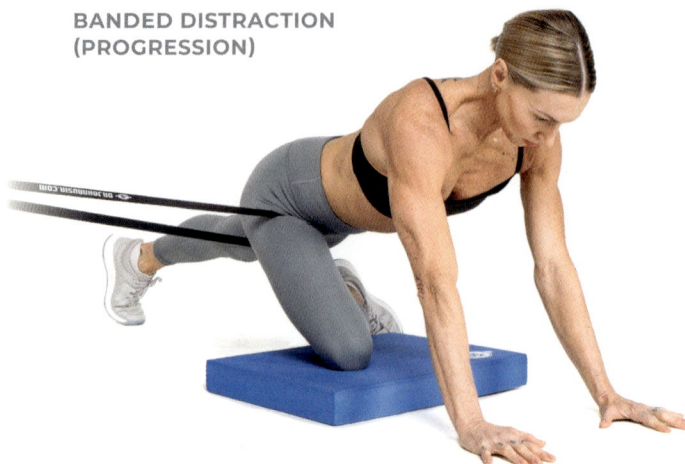

BANDED DISTRACTION
(PROGRESSION)

UPPER BODY

90/90 CHEST STRETCH

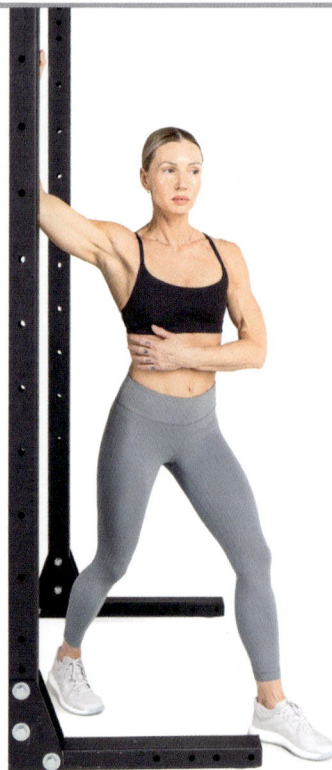

DYNAMIC
OSCILLATORY
STRETCH

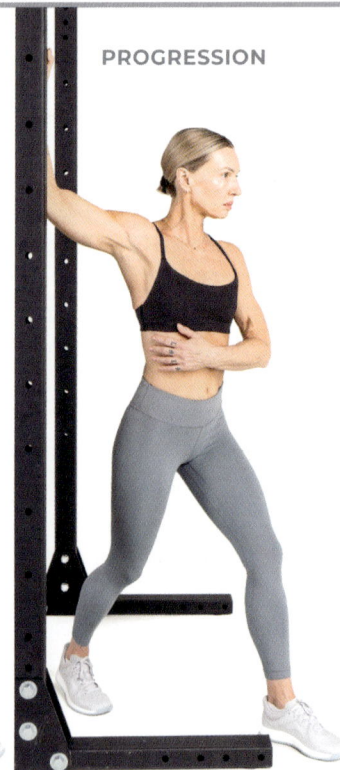

PROGRESSION

SETUP AND BODY POSITION: Stand beside a rack or a wall, placing your forearm on the surface with your elbow bent slightly above 90 degrees. If your right arm is on the wall, step your left foot forward, keeping your hips level and your ribs stacked over your pelvis. Engage your core to maintain a stable pillar, and gently draw your head back to keep your spine in neutral alignment.

EXECUTION: To find a moderate 3 to 4 stretch sensation in your chest, keep your shoulder down and back as you take small steps forward. Avoid simply leaning forward, as this can place the shoulder in an unstable (internally rotated) forward position and shift the stretch onto connective tissues in the front of the shoulder.

For the oscillations, gently press your forearm into the rack (at about 10 to 30 percent effort) while inhaling. As you exhale, relax the push, using this release to move your chest slightly forward. Like the lower body stretches, maintain a constant, gentle stretch on the muscle. You should feel subtle movement into new range of motion with each oscillation. To help shift forward, consider coming up onto the ball of your back foot.

After oscillating for 30 seconds, hold the new end range for another 15 to 30 seconds while breathing steadily. Keep the intensity moderate, between 3 and 5 out of 10.

CONSIDERATIONS: If the 90-degree arm position causes discomfort in your shoulder, adjust by raising or lowering your elbow slightly to find a pain-free position.

PROGRESSION: If the stretch feels minimal with the standard oscillations, you can add a torso rotation. After finding the initial stretch and completing a few push-relax oscillations, try rotating your torso and head away from your elevated arm. For example, if your right arm is stretching, turn your torso and look over your left shoulder. This rotation increases the stretch across the pec fibers that attach to the sternum, enhancing the effectiveness of the stretch.

HINGED T-SPINE EXTENSION / BILATERAL LAT STRETCH

SETUP AND BODY POSITION: Stand upright, holding the handles or rings with your arms at shoulder height. Pull your hips back into a hinge position, adjusting your feet as needed to ensure a long, neutral spine in your lower back. Trust your grip and allow your weight to settle back, letting your shoulders slide slightly toward your ears to create a gentle stretch in your lats. Keep your ribs aligned over your hips, and draw your head back so your ears are positioned between your biceps.

EXECUTION: To improve thoracic spine extension, gently round your upper back, allowing your shoulder blades to wrap around the sides of your ribcage. Then stretch your chest forward and down slightly toward the floor as your shoulder blades retract.

After 30 seconds of this movement, hold the extended position and apply a gentle pull on the rings or handles to deepen the stretch.

CONSIDERATIONS: If you feel any pain or pinching in your shoulders with your arms overhead, adjust by hinging less and bringing your arms slightly in front of your head until you find a comfortable position. Rotating the handles so your thumbs point toward the ceiling can also help reduce discomfort.

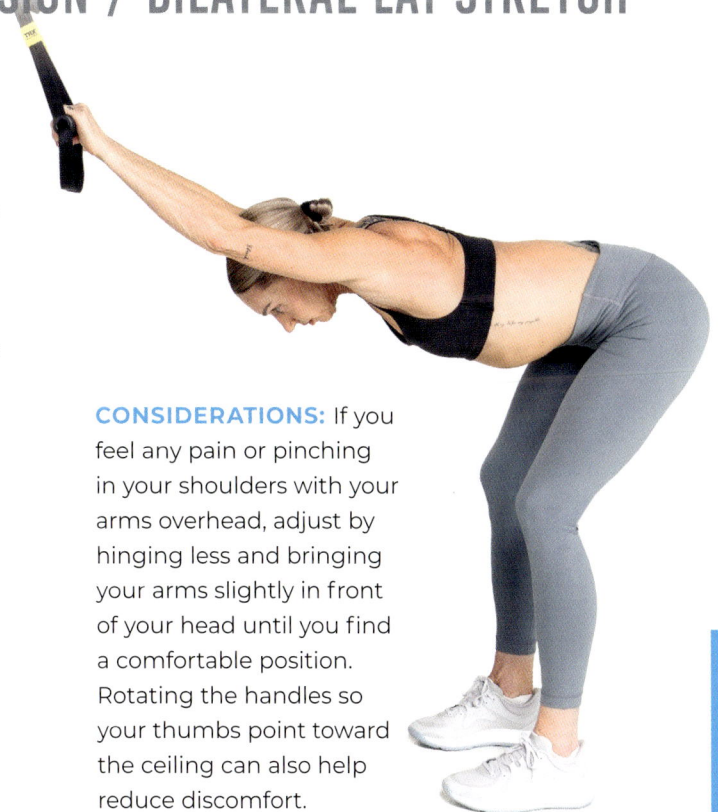

POSTERIOR SHOULDER STRETCH

SETUP AND BODY POSITION: Stand upright and hold the suspension trainer handle with one hand, with your arm extended at shoulder height. Pull your hips back into a hinge position, adjusting your feet as needed to keep your lower back lengthened and neutral. Relax slightly, allowing your weight to settle back so your shoulder moves slightly toward your ear. Keep your ribs stacked over your hips, and draw your head back so your ear aligns with your upper arm.

EXECUTION: For this stretch, you can perform two types of rotational oscillations:

1. Global Rotation: If your right hand is holding the handle, place your left hand on your right ribs. Slowly rotate your torso and head to the left, then to the right, moving through the thoracic spine while keeping your knees level and lower back stable. Perform this rotation for 20 to 30 seconds, noting which side creates a deeper stretch, and pause briefly on that side.

2. Local Rotation: This variation places more emphasis on the shoulder joint. With your right hand on the handle, rotate your thumb down toward the floor and then up toward the ceiling. Aim to create this rotation from the shoulder, moving the humerus bone through a pain-free range of internal and external rotation. Continue for 20 to 30 seconds.

Once you've completed the oscillations, hold the position with the most stretch sensation for 15 to 30 seconds, breathing deeply to help your intercostal muscles (between your ribs) relax and expand, which can improve both range of motion and breathing capacity.

CONSIDERATIONS: If you experience pain or pinching in your shoulder with your arm overhead, reduce the hinge and keep your arm slightly in front of your head to find a comfortable position. Rotating the handle so your thumb points toward the ceiling can also relieve tension.

Note: If you lack shoulder stability—you have hypermobile shoulders, for example—consider skipping this stretch. Instead, focus on the strengthening exercises in phases 3 and 4.

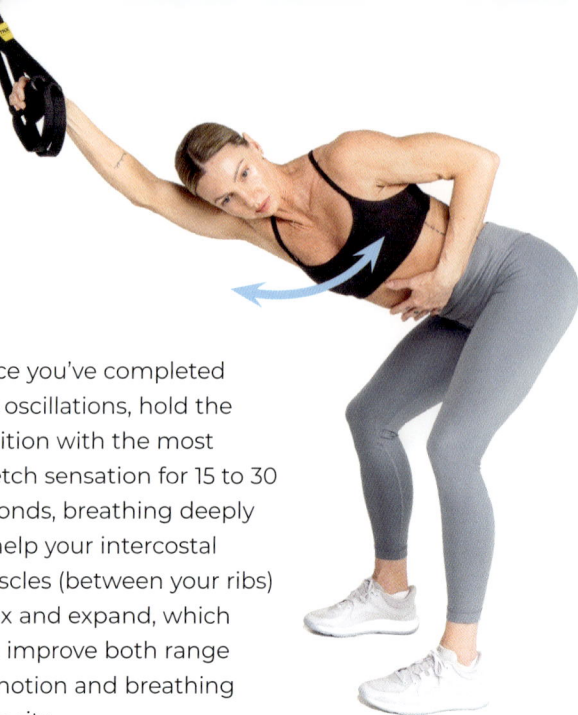

SUPPLEMENTAL OPTIONS

HALF-KNEELING SOLEUS STRETCH

SETUP AND BODY POSITION: Start in a half-kneeling (90/90) position with your feet hip-width apart for stability, and position your back foot so that your toes are flexed and in contact with the floor. To find a neutral pelvis, tilt it slightly so that your hip points move toward the bottom of your rib cage, creating a "belt buckle to chin" alignment. Lightly squeeze your glutes and adductors to stabilize your pelvis. Place your hands on top of your front thigh near the knee, and gently engage your pecs and lats to stabilize your shoulders. With a light core brace, maintain a solid pillar position.

EXECUTION: Press down with your hands as you slowly move your front knee forward. You may or may not feel a strong stretch sensation, which is fine. Focus on achieving as much range as possible while keeping these key points intact: Keep your heel on the ground, maintain an active arch and stacked ankle, align your knee with your middle toes, and keep your pelvis square (e.g., if stretching the right side, avoid letting the pelvis rotate open to the left).

CONSIDERATIONS: The goal is to achieve "good enough" range, such as passing a knee-to-wall test (page 247), since this will support fundamental squat variations. When squatting, you need stability and control, so avoid collapsing the arch, ankle, knee, or hip just to achieve extra range in the stretch. This collapsed range won't translate to usable, trainable mobility.

If limited forward knee movement (knee flexion) is an issue—knee pain, for example—try placing a wedge under your front foot. This adjustment allows for more ankle range of motion without requiring excessive forward knee movement.

PROGRESSION: For an increased range of motion, place your front foot on a wedge to elevate the dorsiflexion angle (toes to shin angle). Unlike the previous option, the goal here is to maximize both forward knee movement and ankle range, building up toward greater mobility in the soleus and ankle complex.

STANDING WEDGE CALF STRETCH

SETUP AND BODY POSITION: Place your entire foot on the wedge, pointing it straight forward.

EXECUTION: Shift your weight onto your elevated foot and begin to slowly step your opposite foot forward. Aim for a moderate stretch sensation (around 3 to 4 out of 10). Depending on your range of motion, you may feel a sufficient stretch with your foot behind, beside, or on the floor in front of the wedge, or even on the wedge itself. The more you lean your body forward, the greater the dorsiflexion angle at the ankle, and the deeper the stretch.

CONSIDERATIONS: If balance is challenging, hold onto a squat rack or wall to maintain stability. Focus on the quality of the stretch rather than managing balance.

PROGRESSION: To deepen the stretch and make it more active, gently press the knee of the stretching leg back, which may activate the quad slightly. Alternatively, create end-range activation by trying to lift your right foot off the wedge (though it won't actually move), which activates the shin muscle and encourages further relaxation and lengthening of the calf.

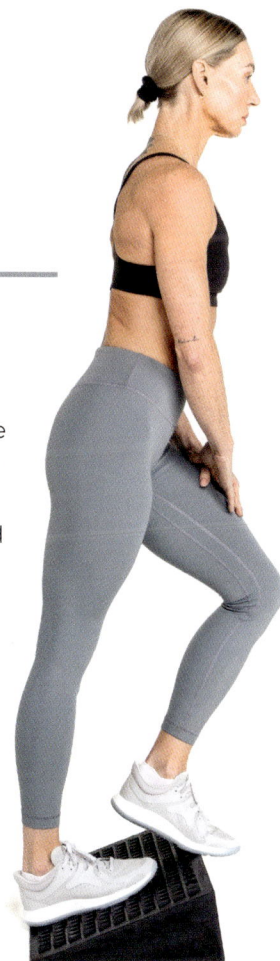

PRONE QUAD STRETCH WITH STRAP (OR LONG BAND)

SETUP AND BODY POSITION: Lie on your stomach with legs hip-width apart. Draw your tailbone down toward your heels to lengthen your lower back and bring your pelvis to a neutral position. Bend the stretching leg and loop the strap around your laces, drawing the length of the strap over your same-side shoulder.

EXECUTION: Pull on the strap to bring your heel closer to your glutes, aiming for a gentle stretch sensation (3 to 4 out of 10). Staying propped up on your elbows will enhance the stretch along the front line of your body, including your abdominals. Breathe deeply and calmly as you hold the stretch.

CONSIDERATIONS: If propping on your elbows causes discomfort in your lower back, rest your chest and forehead on the ground. If the strap is long enough, you can also extend your arms forward on the ground to make the position more restful.

PROGRESSION: If your heel touches your glutes and you don't feel much stretch, place a pad under your bent knee. This adds a bit of hip extension, intensifying the stretch at the top of the quad and hip flexor. As you progress, keep your tailbone down and lower back long to avoid arching, as this spinal compensation does not contribute to functional range in the hip flexors or quads.

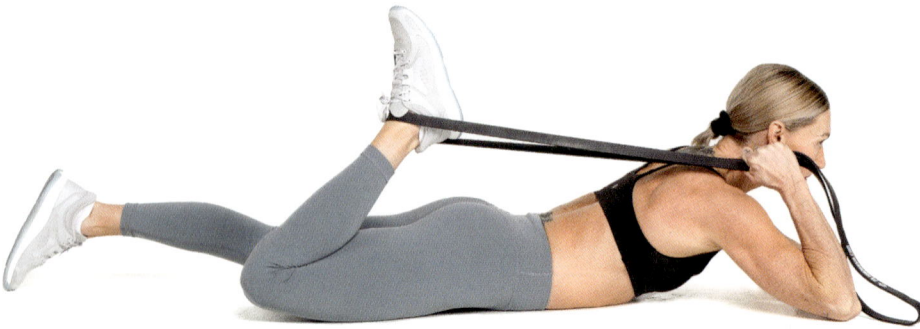

STANDING QUAD STRETCH WITH STRAP

SETUP AND BODY POSITION: Stand close to a wall or rack for support. Bend one knee and loop the strap or long resistance band around your laces or the top of your foot. Placing the strap on the laces can provide an additional stretch through the shin muscles and tendons; however, if this feels uncomfortable or the strap slides, positioning it over the top of your foot is also effective. Alternatively, if you have the flexibility, you can hold the top of your foot or laces with your hand.

EXECUTION: Using either the strap/band or your hand, pull your heel toward your glutes until you feel a gentle stretch (3 to 4 out of 10) along the front of your thigh. Keep your thigh pointing straight down from your hip (avoid letting it drift outward), and maintain a slight bend in your standing leg with your pelvis in a neutral position. Breathe calmly and steadily as you hold the stretch.

CONSIDERATIONS: If this position causes knee discomfort, try the prone quad stretch instead. The prone position allows you to relax on the ground, avoid balance issues, and adjust the knee bend comfortably without the weight of your leg increasing the stretch.

PROGRESSION: For a deeper stretch, incorporate a contract-relax technique. Start with a 15- to 20-second hold at a gentle stretch intensity (3 to 4 out of 10). Then hold the strap steady and inhale as you press your foot into the strap, creating an isometric contraction of the stretching quad at 20 to 30 percent effort. Maintain this contraction for 5 to 7 seconds, then exhale, relax, and see if your heel moves slightly closer to your glutes. Pull the strap a bit more over your shoulder to support this new range and hold it for another 20 to 30 seconds. You can repeat this sequence once more if desired.

HALF-KNEELING HIP FLEXOR STRETCH WITH LATERAL REACH

SETUP AND BODY POSITION: Start in a half-kneeling (90/90) position with your feet hip-width apart for stability, and position your back foot so that your toes are flexed and in contact with the floor. To establish a neutral pelvis, tilt it slightly so that your hip points move toward the bottom of your rib cage, as if drawing a "belt buckle to chin." Lightly squeeze your glutes and adductors to stabilize your pelvis.

EXECUTION: Maintain focus on your pillar with a light core brace and gently shift your hips forward until you feel a mild stretch (around 3 to 4 out of 10) in the hip flexor of your back leg. Inhale as you reach the arm on the same side as the stretching hip straight up toward the ceiling, keeping your ribs stacked over your hips. On the next exhale, reach that arm over your head to create a stretch along the lateral side of the hip and torso. Stay tall, avoid collapsing at the waist, and make sure you can continue to breathe calmly while holding the stretch for 30 to 60 seconds. If you feel strained in your breathing, ease off slightly to maintain a tall posture and use your breath to help relax into a deeper stretch gradually.

CONSIDERATIONS: As with the standard half-kneeling stretch, if your squat assessment indicates that you benefit from a wider stance, adjust by taking your front foot wider or opening the hip angle slightly for added comfort and stability.

SUPINE HAMSTRING STRETCH WITH STRAP

SETUP AND BODY POSITION: Lie on your back with your knees bent and feet flat on the floor to establish a neutral spine and rib cage alignment. Bring one knee up and loop a strap around the bottom of your foot. Extend this leg up toward the ceiling and walk your hands up the strap until your arms are straight and your shoulders can relax down onto the ground. This allows you to use the weight of your arms to support your leg rather than relying on grip strength or biceps engagement.

EXECUTION: Gently pull your leg closer to your chest or move your foot slightly toward your head, aiming for a mild stretch (3 to 4 out of 10). The goal is to keep your leg extended without locking or hyperextending the knee; a slight bend in the knee is preferred. If it feels manageable within your stretch tolerance, you can extend your opposite leg fully along the ground to increase the stretch.

CONSIDERATIONS: If it's difficult to keep your elevated leg straight or if using your arms makes the stretch feel overly strenuous, try using a rack or doorway. This setup supports your leg and allows your arms to relax on the ground, making it easier to hold the position comfortably.

PROGRESSION: To deepen the stretch, use the contract-relax protocol. Set up as described, and hold the initial stretch for 15 to 20 seconds. Then inhale and press your elevated leg gently into the strap as if trying to bring it back down to the floor, creating an isometric contraction in the hamstring. Use 20 to 30 percent effort for 5 to 7 seconds, then exhale and relax. You may notice your leg moves slightly further toward your head. Adjust your grip on the strap to hold this new end position for an additional 20 to 30 seconds. Repeat the sequence if desired.

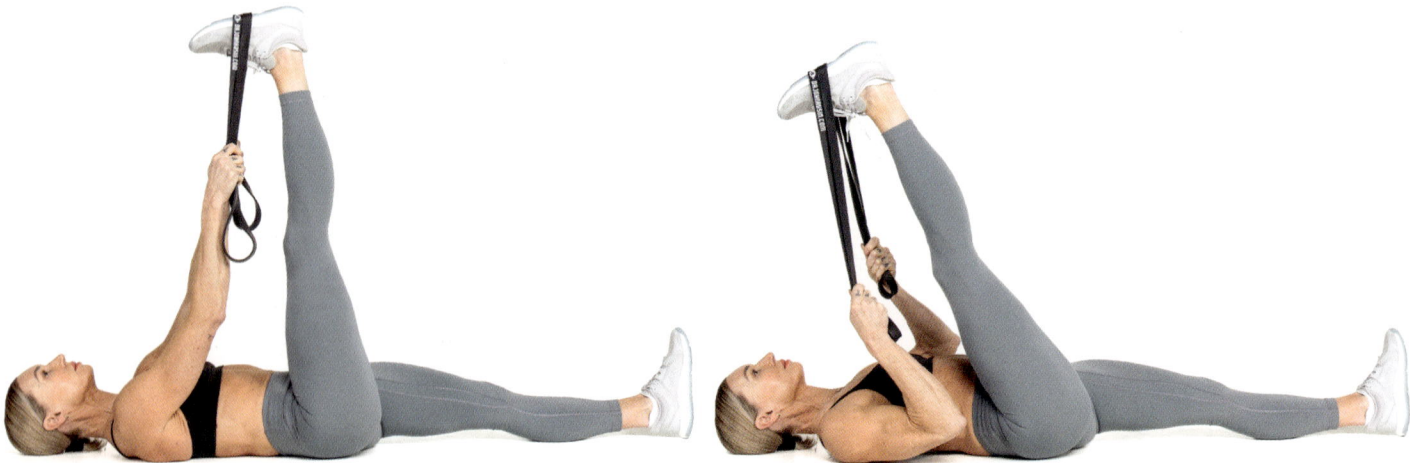

WORLD'S GREATEST STRETCH

SETUP AND BODY POSITION: Start in a quadruped position with hands spread out, shoulders stacked over wrists, and knees under hips. Press into the floor to stabilize your shoulders and gently draw your head back to align your neck with your spine.

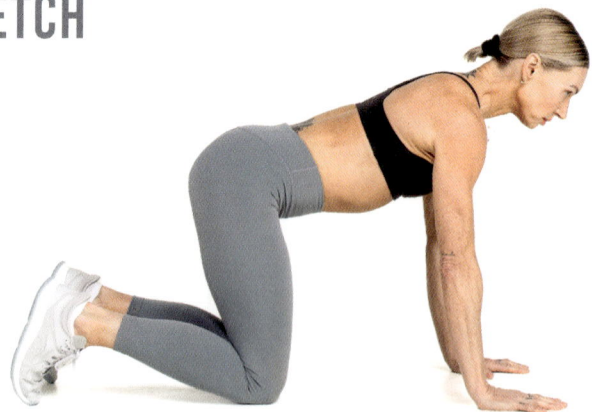

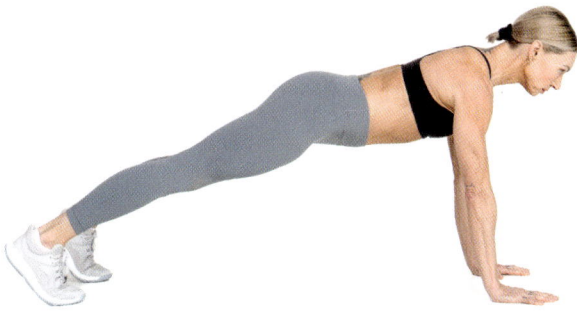

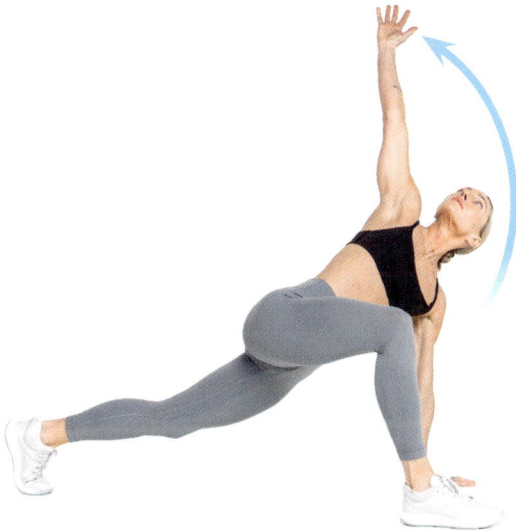

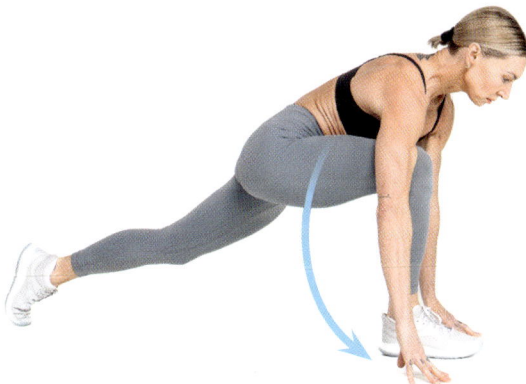

EXECUTION: Follow these steps to flow through the full stretch, opening up the hips, hamstrings, and chest:

1. Step one leg back, tuck your toes under, and fully extend your leg, engaging your quad.

2. Step the other leg back to enter the top of a push-up position.

3. Inhale as you step your right foot forward to the outside of your right hand. If necessary, take a few smaller steps or use your right hand to assist in bringing the foot forward.

4. Keep your back leg long, extend your chest forward, then exhale as you press through your left hand and reach your right hand up toward the ceiling, opening through the chest and shoulders.

5. Inhale to bring your right hand back down beside your right foot.

6. Exhale as you pull your hips up and back, straightening your right leg to stretch the hamstring.

7. Inhale to return to the low lunge position. You can repeat the sequence on the same side or step your right foot back and switch to the other side.

CONSIDERATIONS: This stretch is excellent for enhancing overall mobility, but if you're working on flexibility, you can modify it with shorter levers. From the push-up position, lower your left knee to the floor, shift your torso left, and lift your right hand to help bring your right foot forward into a 90/90 position. From here, reach your right hand up, then place it on your thigh to help pull your hips back for the hamstring stretch. Adjust your torso angle to find a comfortable stretch level (3 to 4 out of 10).

PROGRESSION: As you become more comfortable with this flow, focus on increasing your range of motion and making the transitions smoother. When you feel stable and mobile, add another rotation at the start of the long lunge position. With your right foot beside your right hand, bring your right elbow down toward your ankle, then push the floor away as you reach that hand back up toward the ceiling. Continue with the rest of the sequence from there for added depth and mobility.

PHASE 3: CORRECTIVE EXERCISE

Foam rolling and stretching are the keys that unlock your mobility and movement potential. Phase 3, corrective exercise, harnesses this newly acquired range through exploratory, restorative movements. Utilize the corrective exercise progressions in this chapter to improve motor control and movement quality—the sequencing, stability, and smoothness of your movement patterns—locking in the ranges and regions opened up in phases 1 and 2.

It's so easy to major in the minor aspects of exercise that we often lose sight of the main goals for training, which are fundamentally about

- Building strength for a resilient and functional physique

- Enhancing mobility through full-range-of-motion exercises

- Prioritizing foundational movement patterns for better performance

- Cultivating functional abilities that will help you navigate the physical demands of life

- Improving mental, physical, and emotional well-being

- Ensuring steady progress for lasting health benefits

These core goals form the foundation of the pain-free performance training system, where the emphasis is on holistic development and continual progress, and where each warm-up and training session provides compounding returns on your physical health.

Yet the path to achieving these goals isn't always straightforward. In the pursuit of pain-free performance, it's crucial not to get sidetracked by the minutiae of training—the "minor aspects" that, while potentially beneficial, can siphon precious time and energy from what matters most.

I know this all too well because I've made this mistake myself. For years, I was what you might call a corrective exercise specialist. My coaching sessions were filled with screens and assessments to pinpoint specific movement and mobility dysfunctions. From there, I prescribed precise exercises to address these so-called problems. This method had a certain allure, promising quick fixes and targeted solutions. Identifying an issue and applying a precise exercise to correct it felt incredibly satisfying. It gave me a sense of control and expertise, making me believe these interventions were essential to improving performance and reducing injury risk. But there was a catch.

In my constant quest for perfection, I found myself ensnared in an endless loop of assessments and corrections. Each time I fixed one problem, five more emerged. While the corrective exercises did offer some benefits, the practice had morphed into pseudo–physical therapy, where the pursuit of perfect movement eclipsed the broader goals of training. This realization marked a turning point for me, and I began to understand that striving for perfection in movement was not only unrealistic but also counterproductive.

Unintentionally, I had created an environment where my clients felt they were never good enough, always needing to fix something before they could truly engage in their workouts. This mindset proved detrimental, as it shifted attention away from the core goals of training and placed too much emphasis on minor details. Rather than empowering them to push their limits and embrace the challenges of training, they became overly cautious, worried that any misstep would lead to injury or further issues. Instead of feeling motivated and confident—which is what every trainer should impart to their clients—they felt anxious and discouraged, believing that their ability to train and perform was contingent on achieving perfect form, an inherently unattainable goal due to the subjective nature of human movement.

Recognizing the pitfalls of the traditional approach to corrective exercise as well as the benefits they provide, I put the main goals back in focus by shifting the emphasis of the practice to the major aspects of exercise: enhancing motor control, improving mobility, and developing functional movement patterns. I acknowledged the utility of assessments and corrective exercises but geared them toward the individual and aligned them with the overarching goals of pain-free performance. By prioritizing the elements that truly matter and letting go of the minor aspects, I was able to tap into greater potential and promote meaningful progress in training.

Here's the point. Even within the 6-phase warm-up, where corrective exercises will always have a place, they are employed with the intention of making continuous improvements that provide accumulative benefits. Instead of addressing a specific movement limitation, they are tools to enhance overall movement quality. This way, they serve their true purpose: to facilitate more effective training, not become the training. So, while you will incorporate corrective exercises, you will do so with a movement mastery mindset—always aiming to move the needle forward while keeping your focus on the primary goals.

By strategically incorporating and progressing the corrective exercises in this chapter, you can significantly enhance a workout, unlocking new positions for training. You will improve your motor skills, allowing you to perform movements and exercises with better form and efficiency. You may even get that lightbulb moment, a revelation of newfound abilities that feels almost instantaneous.

However, the common misconception lies in believing that merely gaining access to a new position or skill through correctives is the ultimate goal. This is only the beginning. True value comes not just from accessing new positions but from the ability to train within them, challenging them under load or speed. This progression is crucial; without it, you cannot "hit the save button" on your gains, nor can you fully develop or demonstrate your functional abilities. This becomes particularly relevant as you advance into phase 4 and beyond, into the core of the training session, where the aim is to harness these expanded ranges and skills to the foundational movement patterns.

In the coming pages, we'll delve deeper into corrective exercises, their intended purpose, and how to integrate them effectively into your training without losing sight of the big-picture goals that drive us to train in the first place.

THE GOALS OF CORRECTIVE EXERCISE

It's natural to assume that corrective exercises are solely about correcting some aspect of your movement that is wrong or faulty. After all, they're called corrective exercises for this very reason. But correction is not the sole focus or the intention that we attach to them in phase 3 of the warm-up.

First off, I don't want you to start with the assumption that you are dysfunctional and broken—that unless you correct what is dysfunctional and broken, you are destined for pain and poor performance. That's fearmongering, and that type of thinking will limit your progress because you're fixating on achieving perfect movement before actual training can begin. I want corrective exercises to empower your training, not discourage it.

To that end, the role of corrective exercise in phase 3 isn't about fixing anything that is wrong; it's about exploring new ranges of motion, progressing your functional abilities, and refining your movement quality. It's a process for learning something new about your movement capabilities, whether it's moving into a previously inaccessible range or coordinating your body in ways that feel better or more functional.

Yes, the movements in phase 3 are indeed corrective exercises. Yes, they are the same corrective exercises typically used in physical therapy and other corrective models. But this is not physical therapy. This is training. As such, your central goal is not to remedy a movement dysfunction but rather to enhance your overall movement skill for better performance.

This phase is less about *correcting* minor limitations and more about *improving* major aspects of movement that can be better.

In other words, this phase is less about *correcting* minor limitations and more about *improving* major aspects of movement that can be better.

You achieve this by focusing your efforts on the linchpins—the qualities of movement that require constant maintenance and attention. That, when neglected, potentiate compensations that can compromise performance and movement health. The compensations perpetuated by our modern lifestyle, that we all deal with, that we all need to improve...always and forever.

With this in mind, every corrective exercise in phase 3 aims to improve one or more linchpin by enhancing the following:

PILLAR FUNCTION AND SYNERGY:

To amplify and refine your movement capabilities—and avoid unwanted compensatory movements—you must begin with control over the pillar, which is the cornerstone goal of every corrective exercise. It's from this stable, neutral starting point that you can unleash the full potential of your limbs. This concept is encapsulated in the principle of proximal stability fostering distal mobility. When the pillar is stable, the extremities can move with freedom and precision, allowing for that coveted, effortless-looking execution. With each corrective exercise, focus on connecting your shoulders, hips, and core. Then feel how this opens up your movement, creating synergy between the proximal stability through the pillar and the distal mobility through your limbs.

ANTERIOR CORE FUNCTIONAL STABILITY:

Your anterior core is the locking mechanism of the pillar. You must engage your midsection to brace and stabilize your shoulders, hips, and spine while also scaling tension to allow for controlled, dynamic movement. However, daily habits, particularly prolonged sitting, can turn off the switch that lights up your midsection. Your goal is to turn that switch back on and carry that feeling into the subsequent phases and workout. Corrective exercises, such as the dead bug progression, are designed for this purpose—to reignite and maintain your core's activation.

THORACIC SPINE MOBILITY:

Modern life places us in positions that compromise thoracic mobility. We sit with our upper back hunched for prolonged periods. We hold our phone out in front of our body, rounding our shoulders with our head craned forward over our neck. Spend enough time in these positions—which many of us routinely do—and it becomes much harder to extend your thoracic spine into an upright position and rotate. To counteract these pervasive daily postures, you will employ corrective exercises, such as the quadruped T-spine rotation, to reverse these positions—essentially undoing the mobility restrictions that have the potential to compromise your pillar and movement capabilities.

SCAPULAR DYNAMIC STABILITY:

The same forward-rounding positions that inhibit movement through the thoracic spine can also compromise shoulder mobility and function—more specifically, your ability to stabilize and move your shoulder blades dynamically through the six types of movement: protraction and retraction (forward and backward), depression and elevation (downward and upward), and rotation (inward and outward). So, in addition to opening up extension and rotation through the thoracic spine to facilitate pillar neutrality and mobility, you will improve scapular dynamic stability, which is the ability to control your shoulder blades through all of their ranges of motion as you rotate and move your upper body.

REGIONAL UPPER AND LOWER CROSS-BODY INTEGRATION:

Daily activities and movements often tap into the complex synergy of the body's posterior and anterior oblique slings, which play a pivotal role in transverse (cross-body) actions. From the rhythmic stride of walking to the seemingly simple task of opening a door, these actions are not isolated to single limbs but rather engage a dynamic cross-body link. For example, the posterior oblique sling connects the latissimus dorsi on one side to the opposite gluteus maximus through the thoracolumbar fascia, mirroring the anterior oblique sling that links the external oblique to the opposite internal oblique and adductors. This intricate connectivity across the body, from right shoulder to left hip and vice versa, epitomizes our natural movement patterns where opposite sides of the body work in concert, not in isolation. This coordination not only refines our physical movements but also ignites our neurological pathways, creating a more integrated and responsive system. Corrective exercises such as the bird dog aim to synergize this left-to-right and right-to-left connection, promoting fluid and efficient movement through regional upper and lower body cross-integration.

DEAD BUG

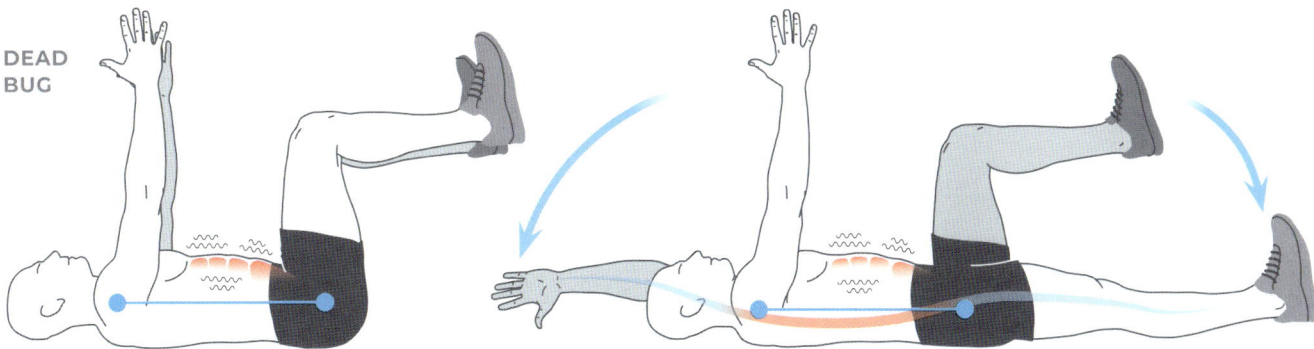

The dead bug exercise reinforces anterior core functional stability, helping you connect your shoulders, hips, and core. This synergy between core stability and limb mobility allows for controlled, precise movement, reducing compensatory patterns and enhancing overall movement efficiency.

QUADRUPED T-SPINE ROTATION

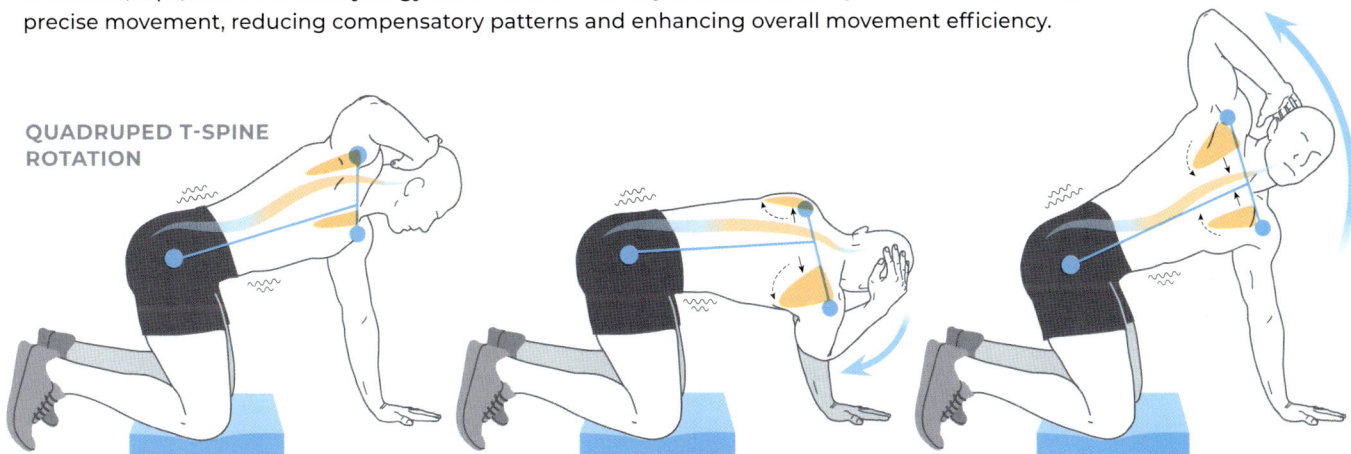

The quadruped T-spine rotation exercise improves thoracic mobility and scapular stability, allowing for greater freedom of movement. This exercise counteracts daily postures that restrict movement, promoting balanced and efficient upper body mechanics.

BIRD DOG

The bird dog exercise enhances cross-body coordination by integrating the upper and lower body through dynamic opposing-limb movements. This exercise strengthens the connection between the right and left sides, promoting balanced and efficient movement through a stable pillar.

POSTERIOR AND ANTERIOR OBLIQUE SLINGS

Improving the linchpins—pillar stability, thoracic spine mobility, and cross-body slings—is central to getting the most out of the corrective exercises. However, to harness the improvements, you're not running screens and assessments to determine which corrective exercise to implement with the hope that it will somehow transfer to the workout. You're simply choosing one corrective exercise to progress, leveraging the strategic placement within the 6-phase sequence to actualize and maximize the benefits. Here's how it works:

1. You open up your body in phase 1 with soft tissue techniques to promote a parasympathetic response and reduce muscle tonicity (tightness).

2. Then you stretch in phase 2, further potentiating the parasympathetic response, to improve joint and tissue range of motion.

3. Now, in phase 3, you perform corrective exercises to enhance motor control (the ability of the nervous system to coordinate and regulate movement) and facilitate motor learning (the process of improving the fluidity and accuracy of movements) in the newly gained ranges made accessible in the initial phases. In essence, you're building on the momentum from phases 1 and 2 to potentiate the mobility and movement that you're working to improve in phase 3 and beyond.

MOTOR CONTROL GAP THEORY

PASSIVE HAMSTRING LEG RAISE

PASSIVE ROM

ACTIVE HAMSTRING LEG RAISE

ACTIVE ROM

MOTOR CONTROL GAP

Flexibility is the range that you can get into passively—someone raises your leg into a hamstring stretch while you remain relaxed or you pull your leg into a hamstring stretch using a strap, for example. Because your muscles are relaxed, you have greater range of motion, but you don't have control or stability in the end-range position.

Mobility is the range that you can get into actively—you raise your leg using your muscles to power the motion, for example. Because your muscles are active, you have less range of motion, but you have control and stability in the end-range position.

The difference between your passive range of motion (flexibility) and your active range of motion (mobility) is the motor control gap—the range that you don't control, that hasn't been developed or trained.

Now, it's important to note that there will always be a gap between what you can passively access and what you can actively control. A normal gap is roughly 10 to 15 percent. Anything more than that, and the incidence of pain and injury rises. The goal, then, is to close any glaring gaps that exceed that range or any discrepancies between your right and left sides. To accomplish this, the key is to expand your authentic active range of motion, enhancing your motor control within a range as close as possible to your passive limits. That is exactly what you are trying to achieve with the corrective exercises in this chapter.

PASSIVE ROM — ACTIVE ROM = MOTOR CONTROL GAP

This is the primary goal—the main focus when performing corrective exercises.

▼
To feel a little bit better moving into ranges that normally feel restricted and tight

▼
To explore and exhibit control within those newly gained ranges

▼
To carry that deliberate and purposeful motor control sequencing into the foundational movement patterns

▼
To close the motor control gaps

Recall from the stretching chapter that just because you have access to a range of motion (flexibility) doesn't mean you can control the range of motion (mobility). This is important to understand because the exercises in phase 3 aim to close the motor control gap—the zone between your passive flexibility and your active mobility.

You measure progress in phase 3 by your ability to close the gap between passive and active ranges of motion. With each repetition, the goal is to reduce the disparity between what your body can do passively and what you can actively control. This is what preps you to move better, ensuring that you're not just passively flexible, but actively in command of your movements.

How do you improve motor control and effectively close the motor control gap? Simple. You home in on the sequencing, stability, and smoothness of the movement.

SEQUENCING

Sequencing refers to the order or arrangement of the movement and the coordinated action of muscles firing to power efficient movement. Ask yourself: What is the defined sequence for this movement? Are my muscles turning on in the correct order? Does it feel right? Take the pillar, for example. There is a defined bracing sequence to stabilize the hips, shoulders, and core: set the pillar, amplify the pillar, breathe in, brace, and scale tension (see pages 34–35). This sequence—the order in which you turn on the pillar—determines the effectives of your stabilization efforts. If any of these steps are out of sequence, say you brace before setting your neutral position, then you will likely compensate, compromising your stabilization capabilities.

The key takeaway is this: When muscles are firing in the right order, movement occurs fluidly and efficiently. "The First Line of Action" principle states that the first muscle to kick on during a compound movement will most likely become the primary mover of the exercise. If the wrong muscles activate first, it can lead to inefficient movement patterns, increased risk of injury, and suboptimal performance. One of the primary goals with corrective exercises is to improve the universal sequencing—the motor control—that influences global movement patterns. In the exercise descriptions, you will learn the proper sequencing for each corrective exercise, with the aim of carrying that coordination into the foundational movement patterns.

STABILITY

Stability relates to the pillar and the ability to maintain neutral shoulder, hip, and spinal alignment during movement. It can also be defined as the ability to avoid unwanted movement at specific segments of the body (compensations)—specifically at the hips and shoulders. For instance, let's say you habitually dump your pelvis forward (anterior pelvic tilt) and round your shoulders. The former transfers force into your lower back while the latter promotes forward rounding of the spine that transfers force into the neck. Both actions can be contributing factors to pain and can limit your ability to stabilize your hips and breathe and brace effectively. The same can be said for the shoulders. When the humeral bones are not centered in the joint, it's nearly impossible to stabilize the shoulders in a safe and effective position.

The aim of each corrective exercise is to create stability through the pillar complex by achieving and maintaining a neutral position. As you've learned, this is essential not only to move pain-free but also to optimize overall movement performance.

SMOOTHNESS

Smoothness is the fluidity of motion. How does one achieve fluidity, the kind that even a novice observer would deem beautiful? It's in the sequencing and stability of the movement. Picture the grace of an Olympic weightlifter, especially those in lighter weight classes. Their movements are devoid of excess, each motion flowing into the next, a harmony of strength, stability, and mobility. This grace is born from the precise timing and coordination of muscle engagement, the appropriate gradation of tension, and the control of key joints and segments of the body.

It's a concept that, when witnessed, needs no expertise to appreciate—flawless motion is universally captivating. But achieving this seamless orchestration is no small feat. It's not merely about having the components of the movement; it's about the order in which they're activated. The kinematics of movement rely on the action that precedes it. For instance, if the thoracic spine extends too soon or flexes too late, the rhythm is disrupted.

Sequencing, stability, smoothness—these are the qualities that make movements safe and efficient, and more often than not serve as our first line of defense for pain-free training.

When muscles turn on in the right order, the pillar is stable, and the movement is smooth, compensatory patterns are minimized and acute pain sources around vulnerable regions such as the lower back, neck, shoulders, and hip tend resolve automatically. If improvements in mechanics don't alleviate the issue, the next step might involve addressing clinical sources of pain, which falls into the realm of physical therapy. However, it's worth noting that the majority of people—say, nine out of ten—can reduce pain simply by moving better, which, again, is the focus that underpins the overarching corrective exercise goals.

CAUTION WITH CORRECTIVE EXERCISES

It's tempting to overemphasize corrective exercises, especially when the results can seem miraculous. Especially when we're often told that we are dysfunctional and broken. That the only way to train pain-free and perform at our best is to identify and correct every nuanced detail of our faulty movement and mobility.

While it's true that we need to adopt a movement mastery mindset by continuously working to improve and individualize our movement and mobility, it should never replace a progressive model for training. Corrective exercises are part of the solution, not the entire solution. When you obsess over minor imperfections, the training session can become overwhelmed by corrective measures, stalling genuine progress.

So don't be swayed by the so-called corrective exercise gurus who advocate for an endless cycle of assessments and fixes, potentially trapping you in a "rehab purgatory" where real training and improvement are sidelined for the sake of achieving the unattainable standard of perfect movement.

Your movement and mobility will never be as good as they could be. They will never be perfect. But with the right intent and focus, **you can always get better.** This is why you are training. This is the purpose of the corrective exercises in phase 3.

RECOMMENDATIONS AND GUIDELINES

To reach any goal, it's crucial to first identify the outcomes that will signify success and then follow a systematic approach—and diligently stick to it—to guide your journey toward the goal.

Now that we've established the aims of corrective exercises, let's specify the success indicators and present a clear set of guidelines for accomplishing these goals during phase 3 of the warm-up.

Movement mastery is the guiding principle that will ultimately enhance motor control, facilitate motor learning, and close your motor control gaps—the major goals—not only with the corrective exercises but also your ability to transfer those newly expanded skills into the foundational movement patterns. You will know success because you will feel it when

▶ You move into a range that was previously inaccessible.

▶ You are less apprehensive.

▶ You alleviate pain.

▶ You improve the sequencing, stability, or smoothness of the movement.

▶ You're able to progress to a more challenging variation of the exercise.

Remember, corrective exercise is the phase where you start to lock in the gains from the initial phases. It's a process of accumulation, where the cumulative improvements mark progress. Here's how to accomplish that in the short time available in phase 3.

CHOOSE ONE CORRECTIVE EXERCISE

When the goal is to improve motor control, it doesn't matter which corrective exercise you choose or which aspect of your movement you improve. All of them will have a transference effect to every foundational movement pattern, complementing any key performance indicators (KPIs) guiding your warm-up.

Knowing this, choose one corrective exercise to progress based on the linchpin focus: pillar function and synergy/anterior core functional stability (dead bug), thoracic spine mobility/scapular dynamic stability (T-spine rotation), or regional upper and lower cross-body integration (bird dog). As you've learned, certain corrective exercises emphasize specific aspects of a linchpin. However, there is significant overlap—they all improve pillar stability, for example. So don't overthink the process. Choose one, only one, and get to work.

Also, don't get locked in on one corrective exercise, repeating it over and over, without progressing or experimenting with other variations. Certain corrective exercises may offer the most benefit for addressing your biggest linchpin, and those should get prioritized for several weeks. Just don't get trapped in a rigid, ritualistic practice. Challenge yourself by cycling through and advancing skill with the other corrective exercises to strengthen all your linchpins.

1 TO 2 MINUTES TOTAL: FOCUS on PLAY, EXPLORATION, and DISCOVERY

When it comes to acquiring new motor skills, research shows that the most effective and efficient method is unrestricted play.[1] This approach allows for discovery and exploration, far removed from the pressure of right or wrong techniques. In graduate school, I took part in a research project that investigated this hypothesis by comparing two groups. One received precise instructions from a coach on kicking a soccer ball, and the other simply experimented with the task. Interestingly, the group that kicked freely performed better than those coached with step-by-step instructions.

This principle also applies to corrective exercise, where the focus is on play, exploration, and discovery. You're playing with the sequencing of the movement. You're exploring novel ranges of motion. You're discovering new abilities. And you're learning along the way.

To create an environment that fosters play, you must remove pressure and reduce restrictions. You want to open up your mind so that you can focus on the quality of the movement rather than the quantity of the reps. You do that with a block-based practice of 1 to 2 minutes. Instead of mechanically counting reps—1, 2, 3, with your mind already on number 4—focus on how the movement feels. You might think, "That felt good; let's push a bit more this time. Ah, there it is. I'll try breathing out this time to see if I can go farther. Oh, that's a new sensation." That represents progress.

In other words, it's about slow, deliberate practice, focusing on the sensation and function of the movement in a low-stress environment without the added variables of sets or reps.

Don't worry about matching time on each side. You don't even need to set a timer. A movement needs to be good enough to switch sides or move on to the next phase. How do you know when a movement is "good enough"?

It's about forward progress—whether that's an improved range of motion, smoother execution, or a reduction in pain.

Ask yourself:

▶ **Are my muscles turning on in the right order?**

▶ **Are my hips, shoulders, and spine neutral and stable?**

▶ **Is the movement fluid?**

Once there's a noticeable improvement, even if it's just a single rep that changes your perspective or alleviates discomfort, that's your cue to move on.

KEEP A PROGRESSIVE MINDSET: IMPROVE ONE THING at a TIME

When it comes to corrective exercises such as the dead bug, side plank, and bird dog, most people go through the motions, with no goal in mind. They think: This will help me in some way as long as I do it. No, it will only help you if you attach an intention to the movement—a singular focus that will progress your motor skills.

To accomplish this, narrow your attention to one aspect of the movement that you're aiming to improve. Trying to make multiple improvements simultaneously usually backfires, especially when you're tapping into the sensation of a movement. So focus on just one of the key components of enhancing motor control: sequencing, stability, or smoothness. Once you experience a benefit, shift your focus to another aspect. This is how you progress skill with the exercises and enhance your overall movement quality.

Advancing the difficulty of exercises is another way to promote continual progress. Eventually, you'll reach a point where the exercise no longer provides a noticeable improvement, and the sequencing, stability, and smoothness of your movements are consistently solid. This is a positive milestone! At this juncture, it's time to increase the challenge of the movement to sustain your development. You do that by

▶ **Moving slower**

▶ **Increasing time under tension (think pillar stability)**

▶ **Removing points of contact, such as an arm or leg that is supporting your body weight**

▶ **Adding a band or increasing the complexity, such as adding a secondary movement like a crawl**

The key takeaway is this: with a mindset geared toward movement mastery, the progression through corrective exercises becomes limitless—because there is always some quality of your movement that you can develop, improve, and advance.

As previously stated, there is a sequential progression for the corrective exercise sequences. Start with the first exercise and then advance from easier to harder variations as you develop the proper sequencing, stability, and smoothness for each.

Remember, when it comes to corrective exercise, the concepts and the system allow for endless possibilities. The progressions featured here are your starting point—the minimums you need to get started and correctives that damn near everyone needs. Once you get a feel for the progressions, play around with the different variations, prioritizing correctives that address your goals and movement patterns, understanding that while the specific exercises might change, the principles remain the same.

One of the most rewarding aspects of this phase is the "aha" moment—the sudden realization and new feeling in your body when something clicks. You might experience a newfound range of motion or a level of movement that you've never achieved before. It's that lightbulb moment where you think, "Oh, I've never felt that or moved into that range." This is what you're striving for with every corrective exercise. It's about learning something new, experiencing a breakthrough, and gaining abilities. When this happens, it's a sign that you're on the right track.

We see these moments with our clients every single day. There's a visible change in their faces when they experience that epiphany. They don't need further explanation—they just get it. It's a powerful feeling when someone realizes, "Oh, I've been doing this for twenty years, and now I get it." That's what you're looking for: those transformative moments that drive progress.

So, as you work through these exercises, stay open to experimentation. Tailor them to fit your unique needs while keeping the core principles in mind. Embrace the process of continual improvement and let those "aha" moments guide you toward better performance.

EXERCISE APPENDIX

PHASE 3:
CORRECTIVE EXERCISE

Scan the QR code to access demos of each exercise.

DEAD BUG

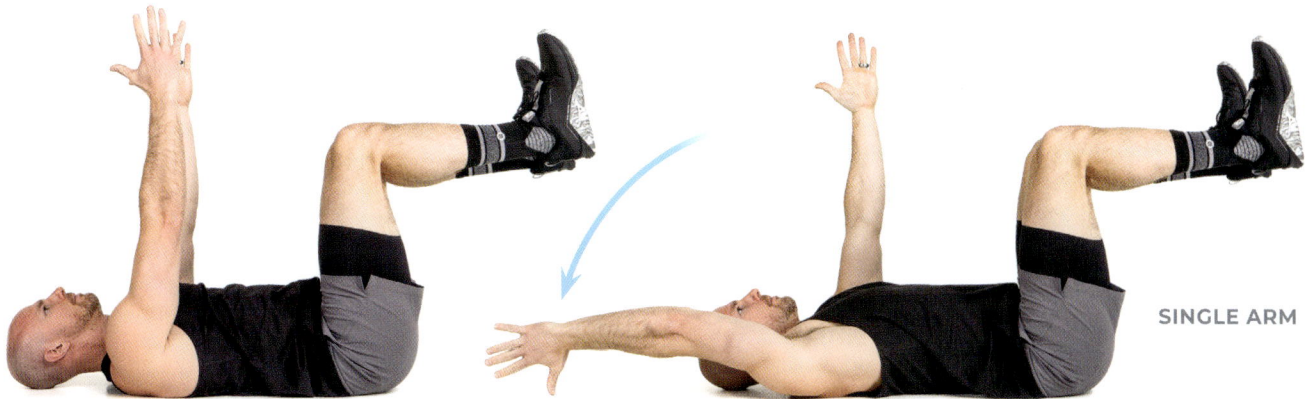

SINGLE ARM

PURPOSE: The dead bug is an excellent exercise for improving pillar function and synergy, enhancing core stability, and supporting pain-free movement across all six foundational movement patterns and many daily activities.

In the supine position, the ground provides proprioceptive feedback, helping you maintain pelvis and spine alignment, as well as rib cage stability during upper and lower extremity movement. The progressions reveal key linchpins that include

- **Core Stability:** Can you maintain pelvis, spine, and rib cage position in all variations?

- **Functional Anterior Core Engagement:** Can you brace effectively and hold it while breathing?

- **Overhead Mobility:** Can both arms fully extend beside the ears with straight elbows?

- **Hip Extension Mobility:** Can both legs extend with straight knees without rocking the pelvis forward?

- **Upper/Lower Cross Integration:** Can you perform the opposite arm and leg movement without losing pillar stability?

SETUP AND BODY POSITION: Before adding movement to the dead bug, it's crucial to master the setup, brace, and breathing. These fundamentals create a stable pillar, protect your spine, and build a strong foundation for safe and effective progress.

1. Start Position: Lie on your back with knees bent, feet flat, and arms at your sides. Begin by finding a neutral pelvis—imagine your pelvis as a bowl of water. Tilt it forward and back until you reach a balanced "middle" where the water would stay level.

2. Align Rib Cage and Pelvis: Stack your ribs over your hips to prevent flaring. Think "ribs to hips" to create a strong, stable core. This position helps distribute load evenly and prevents arching.

3. Brace Your Core: Place your hands around your waist, fingers spread along the sides of your lower ribs and hips. Take a deep breath and feel 360-degree expansion around your waist—not just your belly. Try a gentle cough to feel the core muscles tighten; this is the brace you want.

4. Visualize Core Stability: Picture your core like a pressurized soda can. When fully pressurized, even the thin aluminum walls become strong and stable. Likewise, by maintaining this "pressure" in your core, you're creating a stable pillar of support.

5. Practice Bracing with Breath: Hold this brace while breathing naturally, avoiding breath-holding. This skill of bracing and breathing is essential for pain-free, controlled movement.

6. Progress to Dead Bug Hold: Once you're stable, lift one leg at a time to 90 degrees with knees over hips, then raise your arms above your shoulders. Hold this position with a strong brace and steady breath for 30 to 60 seconds. This basic hold is an effective core stability exercise for beginners. Once you can brace and breathe with a solid 30-to-60-second hold, progress sequentially through the exercises.

EXECUTION AND PROGRESSIONS: Begin with the single-arm variation to isolate core engagement, then progress to single leg for added stability challenge, and finally, advance to opposite arm and leg to develop full-body coordination and control.

- **SINGLE ARM:** This variation is excellent for testing and improving your overhead range of motion while maintaining tension through the pillar—key skills for any vertical pressing or pulling exercises. Keep your elbow straight and palm facing in toward your ear as you extend your arm overhead. Alternate arms, focusing on keeping your "ribs to hips" position stable throughout.

SINGLE LEG

It's helpful to exhale as you extend your arm and inhale as you bring it back, though it's not essential to sync every movement with your breath, especially in slower or advanced progressions. The primary goal is to maintain a solid brace and steady breathing.

If you struggle with overhead mobility, incorporate soft tissue work for your lats and a thoracic spine/lat stretch before performing this variation. By consistently following this warm-up blueprint, you should notice improvements in your range of motion over time.

- **SINGLE LEG:** This variation is a core stability challenge that emphasizes hip extension and pelvic control. Start in the dead bug hold position with knees bent, shins parallel to the ground, and arms reaching toward the ceiling. Keep your core braced and breathing steady, then extend one leg out and down until your heel hovers just off the floor. Bring that leg back in, then extend the other.

For added engagement, flex your feet by pulling your toes toward your shins—this mimics the standing position of your feet. Also, watch for the tendency of the non-working knee to drift closer to your chest as you extend the opposite leg. While not necessarily "wrong," this can indicate a need for improved hip stability or cross-body coordination.

- **OPPOSITE ARM AND LEG:** The opposite arm and leg variation brings together everything from the previous single-arm and single-leg progressions, adding an extra challenge to core stability by introducing movement from both ends of your body. As you extend one arm overhead and the opposite leg toward the floor, keep your chin tucked to lengthen the back of your neck. Reach through your fingertips to maximize shoulder range. Flex your feet (toes to shins) up to ensure controlled movement in the extended leg. Focus on maintaining the "ribs to hips" alignment to keep your pillar stable.

With these familiar cues in place, remember that pillar stability will be additionally challenged in this variation, so keep your breathing steady to support your brace and optimize oxygen flow.

CONSIDERATIONS: The dead bug may look simple, but many struggle to hold a strong brace while breathing for even 30 seconds, especially if they have a history of low back pain, tight hips, or post-natal conditions. If you're finding it challenging to maintain the dead bug hold, don't worry—bracing is a skill, and mastering it is key to progressing effectively in your training. Here are some effective modifications to help you "find a way to win."

1. **Dead Bug March:** With knees bent and feet flat on the floor, place your hands on your waist to monitor your brace. Slowly lift one knee over your hip, lower it, and repeat on the other side. This helps ensure the brace stays strong and your pelvis remains stable.

2. **Dead Bug Heel Drops:** If you can hold the dead bug but struggle with full leg extensions, try heel drops. Keep both knees bent at 90 degrees and tap one heel to the floor at a time, maintaining core control.

3. **Arms-Banded Heel Drops or Leg Extensions:** Adding a band to the arms may seem like it increases the difficulty, but it actually enhances lat and core activation, which can improve pillar stabilization. Anchor the band behind your head and loop it around your palms or wrists so that you need to "pull" against the band to keep your arms in a straight-up position. With the band in place, perform heel drops or leg extensions, focusing on keeping your core stable and your spine neutral. Progress as your stability and control improve.

4. **Self-Resisted Opposite Arm and Leg Dead Bug:** For this variation, press your right hand into your left knee and pull that knee into your hand, creating isometric tension on one side while moving the opposite arm and leg. You can also use a physio ball between the static arm and leg for added resistance.

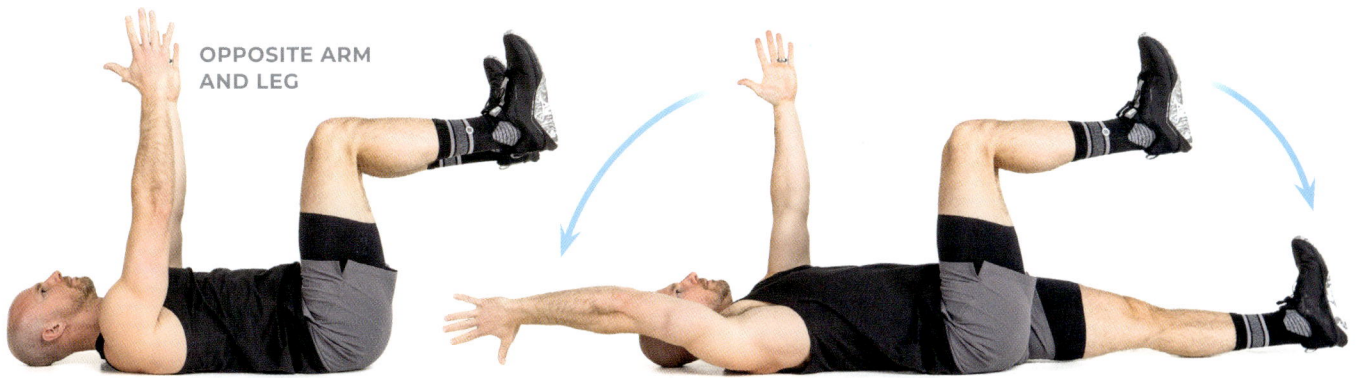

OPPOSITE ARM
AND LEG

5. Dead Bug with Kettlebell Internal/External Rotation: This progression adds shoulder stability. Pick up a kettlebell safely by sliding your hand into the handle at an angle, then press the kettlebell to the ceiling. With your knees up over your hips, either hold the leg position, extend the leg opposite to the kettlebell, or alternate leg extensions for a greater challenge. Rotate the kettlebell at the shoulder joint (internal/external rotation) while keeping it stable above your shoulder, focusing on humeral rotation rather than just the wrist.

6. Band-Resisted Dead Bug Variations: Adding bands in various directions can target specific muscles and provide different challenges:

• *Band around both feet*—challenges the hip flexor of the stationary leg.

• *Band below the foot, anchored overhead*—unloads the weight of the leg as it extends, making it a useful middle step between heel drops and the full leg extension variation.

• *Band in both hands, anchored above head*—integrates a lat pullover into the dead bug.

• *Band on opposite foot and hand*—challenges the arm and leg extension, firing up posterior shoulder and glute.

• *Band on one foot and both hands*—tests shoulder stability as the banded foot extends.

• *Lateral band pull*—hold a band anchored to the side to create lateral tension, increasing oblique stability.

QUADRUPED T-SPINE ROTATION

PURPOSE: The thoracic spine (T-spine) is crucial for both extension and rotation, but these movements can be limited due to prolonged sitting or poor posture from computer work and texting. This corrective exercise should be a staple in your warm-ups and regular movement practice, helping you open up your posture and maintain pain-free function in your back, neck, and shoulders. The goal is not only to achieve sufficient range of motion on each side but also to establish symmetry between them.

This exercise helps identify and target key linchpins:

• **Pillar Function and Synergy:** Can you rotate through the length of your spine without arching the lower back or flaring the ribs?

• **T-Spine Mobility:** Do you have adequate extension and relatively symmetrical rotation on both sides?

• **Dynamic Scapular Stability:** Can the stabilizing arm maintain proper scapular movement (protraction/retraction) without elevating or winging?

SETUP AND BODY POSITION: Unlike lumbar-locked variations (where your butt sits on your heels), this drill is performed from a quadruped position. This setup allows you to integrate pillar stability and lumbopelvic control with the extension and rotation movement—similar to positions used in exercises like seated or half-kneeling rows, as well as unilateral push, pull, and press movements.

To get set up in the quadruped position, align your knees directly under your hips and your hands under your shoulders. Follow these steps to achieve optimal, pain-free form:

1. Pay special attention to the positioning of your hands and arms. Although it may seem like the main focus is on the moving arm, the stability and engagement of the grounded arm is key. Start by tenting your fingers, then spread them wide and press the pads of your fingers into the floor, creating a subtle grip. This not only enhances hand and wrist mobility but also shifts weight into your muscles, preventing strain on the wrists.

2. Check your elbows next. Aim for a slight bend with your elbow pits facing each other or slightly forward. If you're naturally flexible or hypermobile, avoid locking out your elbows. Locked elbows place stress on your bones and tendons, rather than activating stabilizing muscles like the lats. Instead, keep a slight bend, engage your hands, press the floor away, and slightly lift your rib cage and collarbones toward the ceiling to bring your shoulder blades and rib cage into alignment. Think about sliding your armpits toward your waist to further engage the lats. It may feel like more work initially, but this setup will support better performance in movements like push-ups, dumbbell presses, and rows.

3. Now check your spinal alignment. Aim for a neutral spine, just as you would in the dead bug exercise. Imagine reaching the crown of your head forward while pointing your tailbone back, keeping your pelvis and rib cage aligned. Your torso may or may not be parallel to the ground, depending on your body proportions—the key is maintaining your natural spinal curve.

EXECUTION: To begin the movement, place your right fingertips lightly behind your right ear, avoiding any pressure on your neck. Rotate your right elbow down toward your left forearm or wrist, allowing your chest to turn toward your left arm and your left shoulder blade to wrap around your rib cage. If you struggle with hip stability or feel your hips shifting sideways during the movement, try widening your knees for a more stable base.

To open up, push the floor away with your left hand as you rotate your right arm upward, reaching your chest forward to extend your thoracic spine. Continue pushing into your left hand as you lift your right elbow and look slightly to the right and forward, following the rotation with your gaze to maximize range of motion.

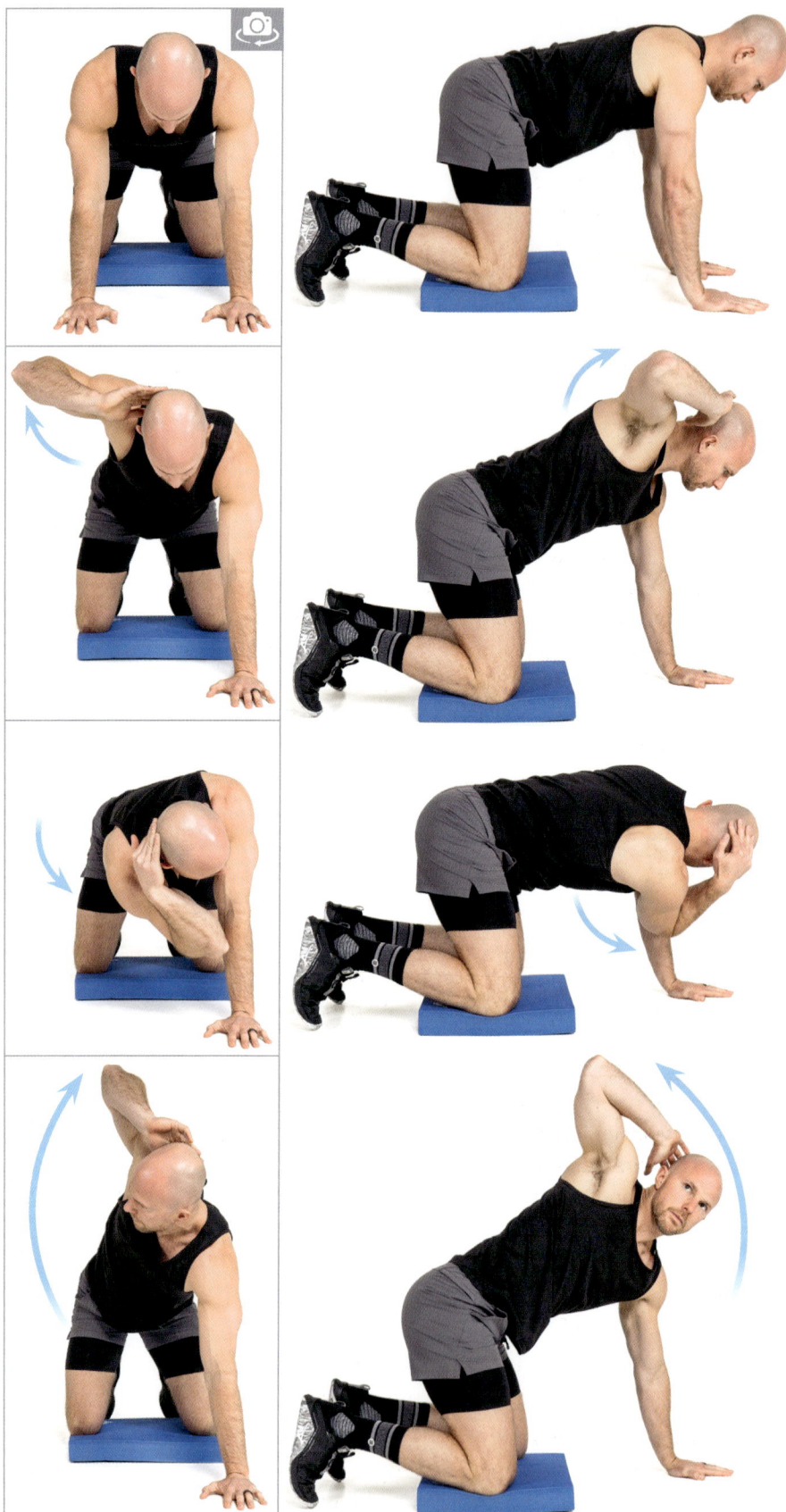

Perform slow, controlled reps, maintaining a smooth rhythm. For an added breathing pattern, try inhaling as you rotate down and exhaling as you open up. Repeat on the other side, keeping each movement fluid and intentional to get the most out of this corrective exercise.

CONSIDERATIONS: Here are some modifications to address common compensations and pain during the T-spine rotation.

If you notice your hips shifting to the side, it means you're compensating and limiting the desired movement at the T-spine. To help manage this, place a foam roller between your knees and lightly squeeze it. This will engage your adductors to stabilize the pelvis. You may notice a reduced range of rotation in the spine or a lower elbow height at first, but the movement will be more authentic to the T-spine and will likely improve with practice.

If your lower back is arching or your rib cage is flaring open, you're losing pillar stability, which limits the T-spine mobility gains you're after. To fix this, start in a neutral quadruped position, finding a gentle "ribs to hips" connection and core brace. Imagine a wide, flat belt wrapped around your waist—not a heavy brace like a deadlift, but enough tension to keep your torso stable. Maintain this low-threshold tension throughout the T-spine rotation, keeping shoulders, ribs, and hips aligned like a cylinder.

If your top arm rotates up while your chest stays facing the ground (a "chicken wing" effect), you

may be overly mobile in the shoulder. Remember, the focus here is T-spine rotation and scapular integration. Emphasize the grounded arm and focus on dynamic scapular movement, using your obliques to twist your torso as if gently wringing out a washcloth.

For wrist pain, place your down hand on a squat wedge to reduce wrist extension, or hold a dumbbell (preferably a hex dumbbell for stability) to keep your wrist neutral.

For knee discomfort in the quadruped position (even with a mat or pad under your knees), perform this exercise standing with your hands on a barbell or wall at shoulder height. Be mindful to resist hip rotation—when your right elbow rotates open, actively push your right hip forward to prevent it from turning out.

For neck pain, if you experience shooting pain, dizziness, visual changes, or headaches, consult a rehab professional. However, if your neck pain feels more like tightness or stiffness, this movement may help. Start with a smaller, pain-free range and explore the motion gently over a few weeks, focusing on gradual improvement in T-spine and shoulder mobility.

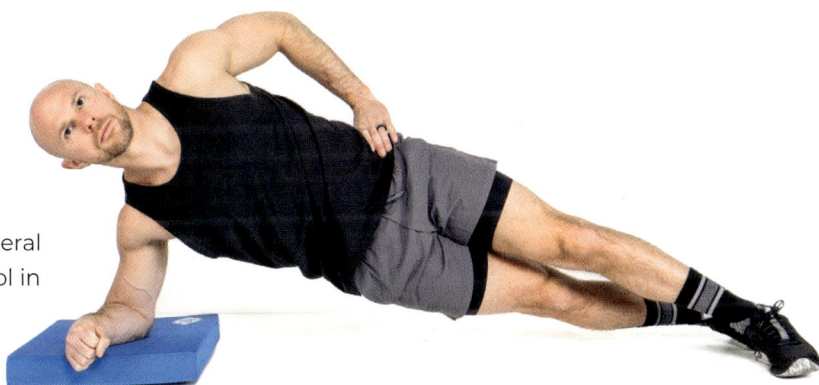

SIDE PLANK

PURPOSE: Stability in the frontal plane (lateral movement) is crucial for maintaining control in foundational movement patterns like the squat, hinge, and lunge. It also enhances shoulder stability, which improves performance in push and pull exercises. If you're experiencing pain or noticing asymmetries between sides, working through the side plank correctives can lead to significant improvements in pain-free function.

Here, you'll learn how to identify linchpins and address common issues associated with pillar function and scapular stability:

- **Pillar Function and Synergy:** Can you maintain a neutral spine with your pelvis and ribs stacked?

- **Scapular Stability:** Does your supporting arm stay stable with the scapula flush against the rib cage, avoiding elevation or winging throughout the hold and movement?

SETUP AND BODY POSITION: Lie on your side with your body in a straight line, hips extended, and your top foot positioned in front of the bottom

foot. Anchor the inside edge of your front foot and the outside edge of your back foot to the ground, keeping your ankles neutral, as if standing. Place your elbow directly beneath your shoulder. Avoid positioning your arm too far out or under your ribs, as this can compromise shoulder stability and comfort.

Push the floor away through your forearm to lift your rib cage and support your scapula. At the same time, pull your bottom shoulder down away from your ear to engage your lat and upper rib muscles (serratus).

As you lift your hips, press the edges of your feet into the ground and squeeze your glutes and inner thighs to stabilize your hips. To increase engagement in your obliques, think about pulling your top foot down, keeping your top hip stacked or rotated slightly forward.

Many people face challenges with the side plank, like shoulder discomfort or difficulty engaging the obliques. Common compensations include flaring the ribs, pushing the hips back, or letting the top hip rotate backward.

To prevent and correct these issues, apply the following setup cues to improve stability, alignment, and muscle engagement:

· Squeeze your glutes to keep your hips extended.

· Think "ribs to hips" to engage your core and maintain a strong, stable torso.

· Press the floor away and draw your head back to align your spine.

EXECUTION AND PROGRESSIONS: The side plank corrective begins with a strong isometric hold. As a high-effort, high-intensity drill, tension steadily builds across the body. The goal is to amplify this tension by actively engaging your core, shoulders, and hips until the tension reaches its peak—then holding for 3 to 5 seconds. This heightened tension signals the end of one set, which typically lasts up to 30 seconds.

Once you can hold a stable isometric side plank on both sides for 30 seconds, you're ready to progress by incorporating movement. In this next phase, start from the floor, press up into a side plank, and then lower your hips back down to complete the rep. Focus on maintaining pillar alignment and stability throughout each repetition, targeting the lateral chain (hips and obliques).

The final progression is the starfish variation, where the top arm and leg extend away from the body. This advanced position challenges balance and pillar engagement, further enhancing the stability demands.

PROGRESS CHECK: Side plank variations, such as side plank hip drops and side plank to starfish, prioritize quality over quantity. Aim for 3 to 5 controlled reps per side, focusing on maintaining proper form and alignment. These movements are more fatiguing than standard correctives, so incorporate brief rests between reps to avoid compensations and improve control. Advanced exercises like the starfish variation require significant strength, skill, and full-body synergy. Progress to these only after holding an isometric side plank for 30 seconds with optimal form. Mastery is demonstrated when you maintain pillar alignment, control movements fluidly, and breathe steadily throughout each repetition.

CONSIDERATIONS: For those experiencing common side plank issues, such as shoulder discomfort or difficulty holding form, the best way to modify the exercise is to keep its key elements intact while making it accessible. A great initial regression is the incline side plank: Place your forearm on a box or bench, keeping your legs straight and feet on the floor. This setup reduces load on the shoulders while preserving the engagement of your glutes, adductors, and quads.

If you have limited equipment, have shoulder pain, or find the incline side plank too challenging, try performing the side plank with your knees bent. While the bent-knee option provides a more accessible starting point, it does reduce lower body engagement. For this reason, I recommend prioritizing the incline side plank with straight legs if possible, as it better engages the glutes, adductors, and quads, helping you progress more effectively and transition smoothly toward the full side plank.

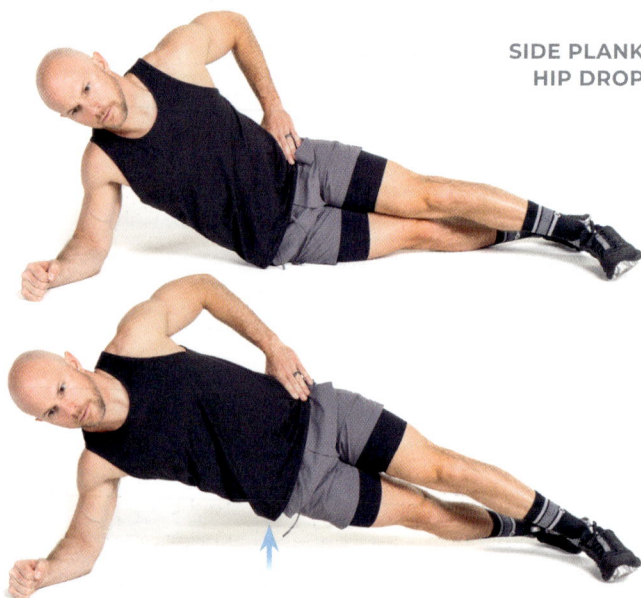

SIDE PLANK HIP DROP

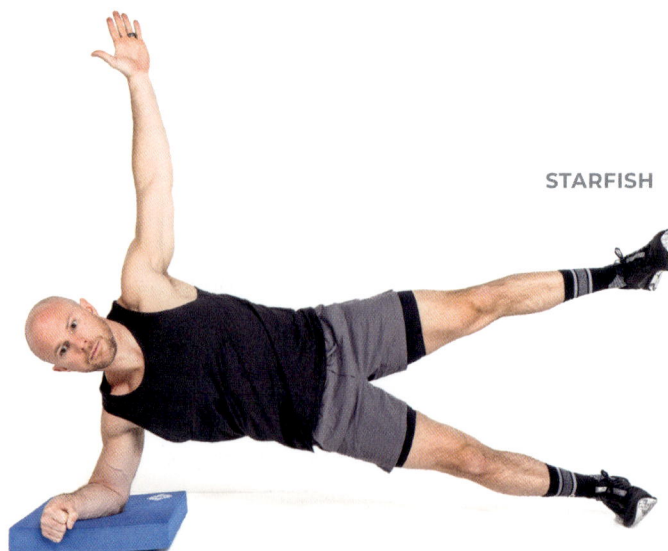

STARFISH

QUADRUPED ARM-LEG OPPOSITES (BIRD DOG)

PURPOSE: With substantial research supporting its effectiveness, this corrective exercise is a powerful tool for managing low back pain—a condition impacting over 90 percent of adults at some point in their lives.[2] Not only does it offer relief, but it also reinforces foundational postural stability by targeting the muscles along the back of the body, including the posterior shoulder and glutes.

In addition to these benefits, you're also gathering powerful insights about your body's movement mechanics and capabilities:

- **Pillar Function and Synergy:** Are you able to maintain a neutral spine with stacked pelvis and ribs?

- **T-Spine Mobility:** Can you achieve good upper back extension with the head aligned?

- **Dynamic Scapular Stability:** Is the supporting arm stable, with the scapula flush against the rib cage throughout the movement?

- **Anterior Core Stability:** Can you brace the core and maintain this engagement while breathing?

- **Upper/Lower Cross Integration:** Can you perform the opposite arm and leg reach without losing core stability or rotating out of alignment?

SETUP AND BODY POSITION: Set up in the quadruped position as you would for the T-Spine Rotation (see page 145 for setup instructions): knees positioned directly under the hips, hands spread under the shoulders, and maintain a neutral spine.

EXECUTION AND PROGRESSIONS: Begin with the basic quadruped setup and progress when each movement feels stable and controlled.

- **SINGLE ARM:** With your hands and knees grounded, this variation challenges your shoulder stability and overhead range of motion. Tuck your toes under and gently squeeze your inner thighs to stabilize your hips. Push the floor away, pull your head and chin back to align your neck with your spine, and create tension by making a fist with your right hand—this increases irradiation and stability that will carry over to push and pull movements later in the workout.

To start, pull your right elbow back past your ribs, as if doing a row, then slowly, with controlled tension, punch your fist forward until your biceps is beside your ear. Return your elbow to your ribs, then extend it forward again. Keeping your thumb pointing up can be more comfortable, but you can also rotate your palm down during the press to follow your shoulder's natural rotation.

> **PROGRESS CHECK:** When you can reach higher beside your ear, extend your shoulder and elbow more fully, or feel increased engagement in the back of your shoulder and upper back, it's time to end the set and switch sides.

SINGLE ARM

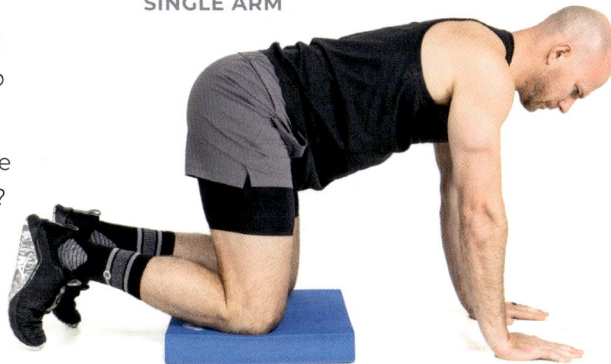

If you notice your hip or toes rotating outward, try pointing your toes toward the floor and gently squeezing your inner thighs together. This slight adductor engagement on the grounded knee will help stabilize your pelvis in a neutral position.

PROGRESS CHECK: When you can maintain a stable, neutral spine with minimal pelvic rotation, feel strong engagement in the glutes, and steady pillar tension as you extend and lift your leg, it's time to end the set and switch sides.

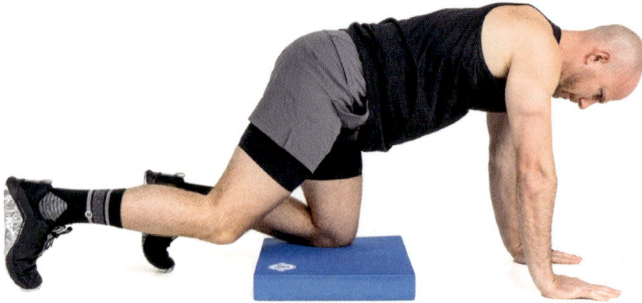

OPPOSITE ARM AND LEG

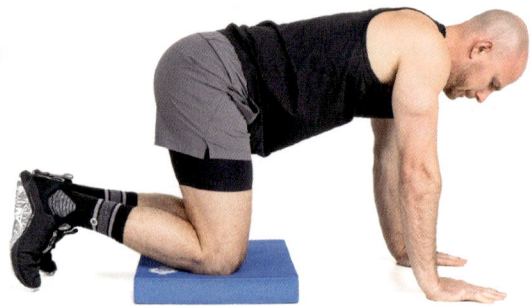

- **SINGLE LEG:** This variation explores hip extension, core stability, and your ability to resist unwanted pelvic rotation—whether tilting forward into a low back arch or rotating open—and offers a great opportunity for glute activation. In common practices like Pilates or yoga, the exercise often focuses on mobility, but here, our purpose is corrective: you're building pillar strength, refining motor control, and supporting progression toward loaded movements. While the spine naturally flexes, extends, and rotates, in this exercise, the goal is to maintain a neutral spine, allowing you to explore joint range of motion with controlled stability.

To begin, set up in the quadruped position with your toes tucked. Push the ball of your foot along the ground until your knee and hip are extended. Then lift that back foot 1 to 2 inches off the ground, keeping it dorsiflexed to increase lower limb sensation and promote proper alignment. Imagine pressing your heel into an invisible wall behind you to feel controlled tension and engagement. As you bring your knee back in, avoid resting it down; simply bring it under your hip, then push it back out again.

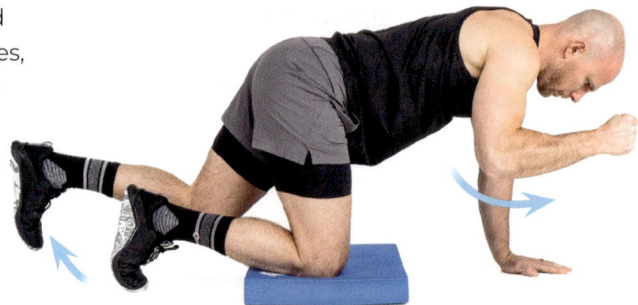

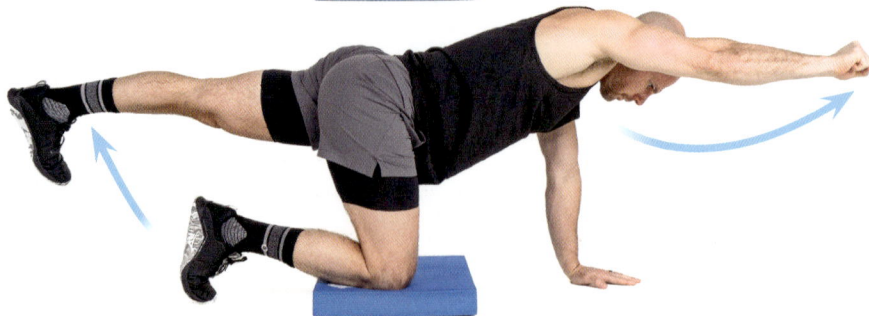

- **OPPOSITE ARM AND LEG:** Now, you'll combine the arm and leg variations, extending the opposite arm and leg simultaneously. Everything about the arm and leg extension remains the same, but with fewer points of contact, the grounded hand and knee will be essential for stability.

To enhance control, press your grounded hand and opposite knee into the floor and gently squeeze them toward each other to activate the front functional line connecting those limbs. This exercise demonstrates the power of the body's spiral effect—"screwing in" the arm and leg to create torque, irradiation, and tension from the ground up through the joints, generating stability that supports controlled, distal mobility.

> **PROGRESS CHECK:** Watch for improvements in your ability to keep a steady, neutral spine without shifting or rotating through the hips and shoulders. Increased control and muscle tension through the back of the shoulders, glutes, and core will indicate effective engagement and stability.

CONSIDERATIONS: If you experience wrist or knee pain during this exercise, try these modifications to improve comfort and maintain alignment.

- **Wrist Pain:** Place your "down" hand on a squat wedge to reduce the wrist bend needed, or use a dumbbell or handle to keep your wrist neutral. (A hex dumbbell with flat sides is ideal, as a round dumbbell may roll, causing your wrist to flex or extend as you rotate.) Another option is to use a low plyo box or step, setting up on your forearms instead of your hands. If you choose this setup, adjust the box or step height so your spine remains relatively parallel to the floor.

- **Knee Pain:** If the quadruped position is uncomfortable, even with a mat or pad under your knees, try performing this exercise from an incline plank. Widening your feet will help stabilize the hips during arm extensions. When doing hip extensions, avoid lifting the leg too high, as this often leads to a common error of tilting the pelvis up and arching the lower back, which reduces core stability.

CRAWL

PURPOSE: Crawling is an innate movement pattern that all humans are hardwired to perform—even without guidance, babies instinctively start to crawl as part of their development. Yet many adults experience limited mobility or discomfort in areas like the knees, lower back, shoulders, or wrists, making it challenging. By reintroducing crawling as a corrective exercise, you can build joint resilience and restore functional movement, strengthening the foundation for all other movement patterns.

In this exercise, you'll challenge and identify key linchpins, such as

- **Pillar Function and Synergy:** Can you maintain a neutral spine with a stacked pelvis and ribs?

- **T-Spine Mobility:** Are you able to achieve sufficient upper back extension with the head aligned?

- **Dynamic Scapular Stability:** Is your supporting arm stable, with the scapula flush against the rib cage throughout the movement?

- **Anterior Core Stability:** Can you brace your core and maintain this engagement while breathing?

- **Upper/Lower Cross Integration:** Can you perform opposite arm and leg movements without losing core stability or rotating out of alignment?

SETUP AND BODY POSITION: Begin in a quadruped position with your spine long, knees under your hips, and hands under your shoulders. Tuck your toes under and spread your fingers wide, pressing as much of your palm into the ground as possible. "Grip" the floor with your fingertips to reduce pressure on the wrists. Keep elbows slightly bent with elbow pits pointing toward each other or slightly forward. Push the floor away, gently extending your upper spine, and pull your head back to align with the spine. Engage your inner thighs with light tension, breathe, brace, and lift your knees about one inch off the ground—this is your hover position.

HOVER

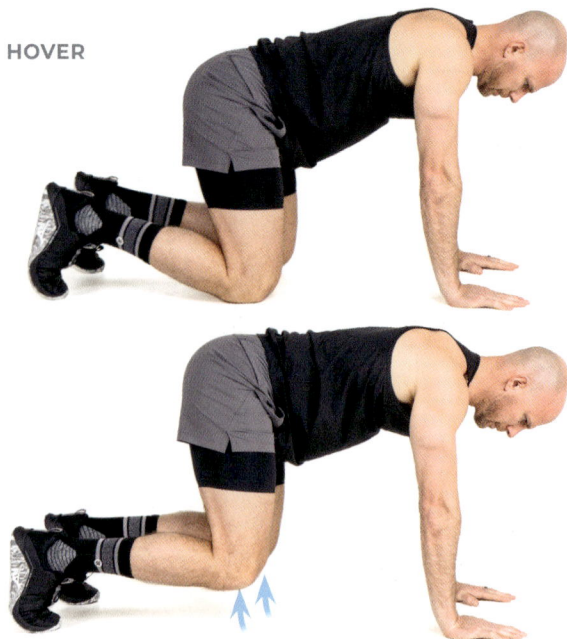

HOVER WITH OPPOSITE HAND AND FOOT LIFT

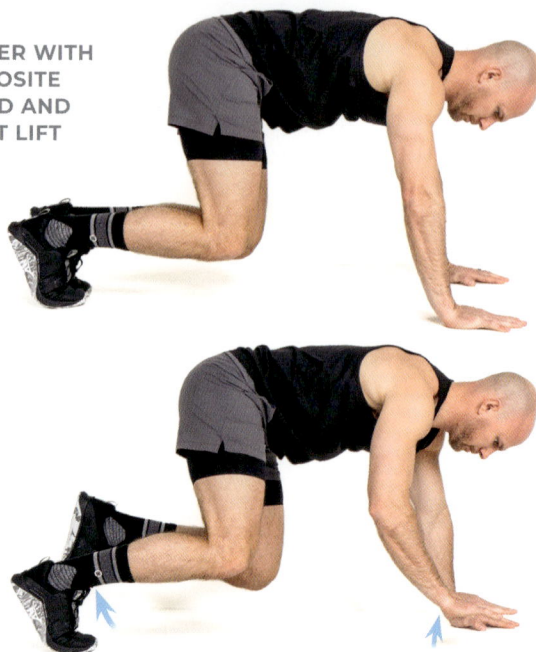

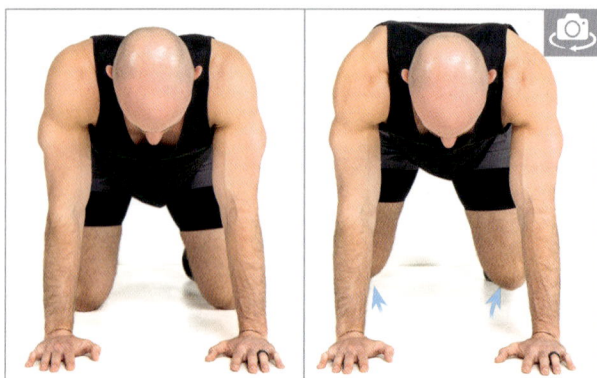

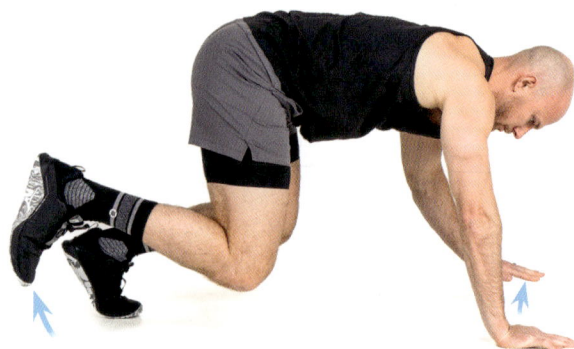

EXECUTION AND PROGRESSIONS: This sequence of progressions will help you build stability, core strength, and coordination for crawling. Start with a basic hover hold, then gradually reduce points of contact for increased challenge. Once stable, progress to forward and backward crawling to improve full-body control and joint strength.

- **HOVER HOLD:** Begin by holding the hover position for 30 to 60 seconds, focusing on maintaining stability throughout.

- **AROUND THE WORLD (ISOLATED LIMB LIFTS):** Start in a hover position. Press your left hand into the floor, making your right side slightly lighter, and lift your right arm to tap the front of your left shoulder. Lower your right arm back down and repeat on the other side, pressing down into your right hand and lifting your left arm to tap the front of your right shoulder. Next, shift your weight slightly to lift each foot one at a time. This sequence of single-limb lifts challenges your stability and is known as "around the world." Focus on maintaining a neutral spine and avoiding any hip pike or torso rotation.

- **OPPOSITE HAND AND FOOT LIFTS:** Once you're able to perform the single-limb lifts with control, progress to lifting the opposite hand and foot simultaneously, similar to a bird dog but with a higher core engagement since only two diagonal points remain grounded. From the hover, lift your right hand and left foot together, then return to the starting position before lifting your left hand and right foot. This progression places greater demands on core stability and shoulder control, enhancing balance and anti-rotation strength.

PROGRESS CHECK: Transitioning from four points of contact to three, and eventually to two, places significant demands on core and shoulder stability. As you perform these progressions, aim to keep your body as steady as possible—imagine balancing a tray of full glasses on your back. At first, minor shifts or "spills" are natural, but with practice, you'll work toward complete stability. Mastery is indicated by maintaining this control with consistent, calm breathing throughout the movement.

FORWARD
CRAWL

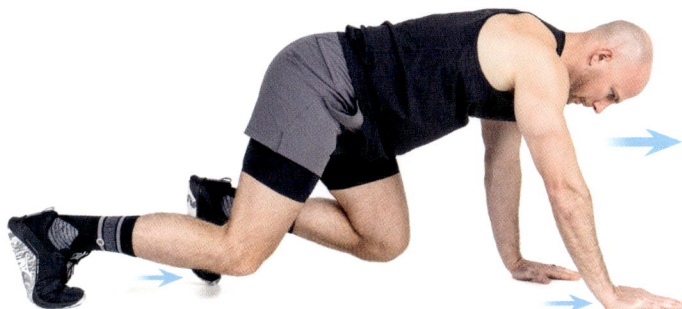

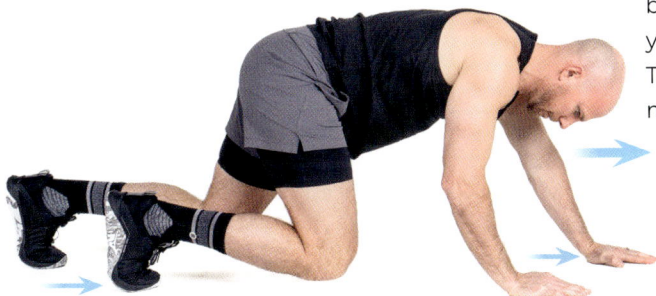

PROGRESS CHECK: You'll know you've made meaningful progress with forward and backward crawling if you can maintain stability and body alignment without straining. Ideally, your hips stay level and your core remains engaged throughout. You can stop the set when you can keep your movement smooth and controlled, breathing easily while maintaining form for the duration of each crawl.

CONSIDERATIONS: If you experience wrist pain, try substituting a plank (or incline plank) on your forearms and perform shoulder taps. This variation mirrors the stability focus of the around the world exercise. Start in a stable plank position, pressing down into your left forearm to lighten the right side. Lift your right arm and tap the front of your left shoulder. Return your right forearm to the ground or bench, then shift your weight to the right side, lift your left arm, and tap the front of your right shoulder. The goal is to maintain a strong pillar position and minimize rotation throughout the movement.

BACKWARD
CRAWL

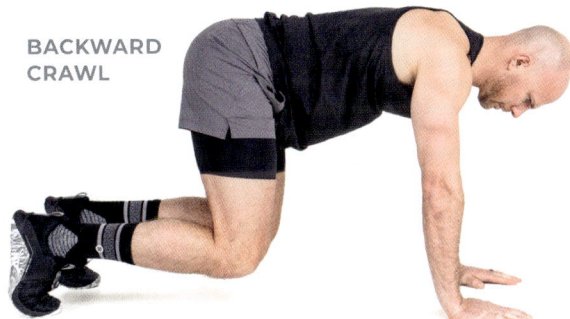

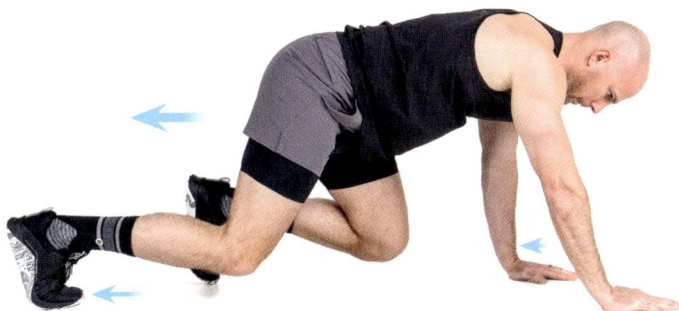

- **FORWARD CRAWL:** Begin crawling by stepping the opposite hand and foot forward (e.g., left hand and right foot), lightly "pulling" the grounded hand and foot toward each other for stabilization. Alternate with the opposite side, taking small steps to ensure your shoulder and hip stay aligned over your hand and foot.

- **BACKWARD CRAWL:** For backward crawling, focus on "pushing" yourself back with each step, engaging more shoulder muscles (especially the deltoids) as you push your body weight back rather than pulling forward with your lats.

PHASE 4:
ACTIVATION DRILLS

The culmination of the previous phases opened up new ranges of motion, easing pain through movement and achieving a higher level of skill around a solid pillar. Now, in phase 4, the objective shifts to stabilizing this expanded range or skill. Think of it as "saving" your progress by activating the muscles that stabilize the joints involved in the ranges you've just improved. Choose one or two areas of emphasis. Consciously focus on muscle engagement from authentic positions. Activate, don't annihilate.

The burn was so deep it felt like my shoulders were about to burst into flames. Midway through a set of band face pulls, I was struck by the intensity of what was a mere activation exercise. My muscles were signaling their limits in a language of fiery pain, different from anything I had experienced before.

"You want me to do how many?" I asked between breaths, trying desperately to recover, knowing that I had many more reps to complete.

My training partner, the late John Meadows, known in the bodybuilding world as "Mountain Dog," replied with a characteristic grin. "100, then we do it again. Keep going. Embrace the burn!"

We powered through 6 sets of 100 reps, a volume that would seem excessive by any standard. By the end of it, my shoulders swelled with such an extreme pump that moving my arms felt like a Herculean task. And this was just the warm-up. We hadn't even begun the workout. The so-called activation exercise was only a preamble to the main lift of the day—the bench press.

"We just annihilated those tissues!" Meadows proclaimed, his voice a mix of enthusiasm and satisfaction after completing one of his notoriously intense warm-ups. "Now it's time to train."

John Meadows was an extraordinary athlete and trainer. Highly respected in the world of bodybuilding, he gained prominence not just as a competitor but also as a visionary coach, nutrition expert, and beloved mentor to many in the fitness community. Training and working with him, I was privy to his unique preparation methods and philosophy, which centered on the principle of muscle stimulation. He believed that completely fatiguing the muscles through activation exercises—particularly those targeting the posterior chain—before performing the main compound lifts would help safeguard the body against pain and injury while amplifying the central physique goals of a bodybuilding workout.

It was an interesting divergence from the traditional physical therapy approach I had been taking to activation exercises. For nearly a decade, I had been incorporating the same exercises with my athletes, yet Meadows was getting better results at reducing and managing training-related pain, despite programming sets that on paper seemed pathologically insane. How could this be?

Looking for answers, I dug deeper into Meadows's approach. I examined the central goals driving the practice, the way he executed the exercises, and the precise methods underpinning the stimulatory effect he was able to achieve. Through that process, I uncovered several benefits, which ultimately reshaped my understanding of activation exercises and the important role they play in training preparation.

• **Injury Prevention:** John understood firsthand the toll that years of heavy lifting could take on the body. He had endured numerous injuries and chronic pain, and many of the athletes he worked with were in the same camp. The purpose behind the stimulation techniques revolved around increasing blood flow to lubricate the joints, strengthening weaker muscle groups that were often neglected in training, and pre-exhausting muscles to reduce the amount of load needed for hypertrophic (muscle-growing) gains. For John, if benching 185 pounds could achieve what benching 275 pounds did, that was a strategic win. It was about balancing load and volume for long-term joint health and muscular development, with the goal of reducing susceptibility to pain and injury.

• **Enhanced Muscle Engagement:** *By pre-exhausting muscles, John ensured that every rep of the workout counted. This technique forced muscles to work harder, leading to potential gains in strength and size—again without the stress of heavy lifting. This approach not only reduced joint strain but also optimized hypertrophic outcomes with a focus on volume, particularly in key areas like the shoulders, back, glutes, and hamstrings.*

• **Improved Mind-Muscle Connection:** *Like most bodybuilders, John was a staunch advocate of developing a strong mind-muscle connection— the conscious, focused engagement of a targeted muscle group or body region. His exercises were crafted to sharpen body awareness, leading to more effective and improved muscle contractions. This focus on engagement ensured that the target muscles were thoroughly fatigued during the exercise and used to their maximum capacity.*

• **Increased Blood Flow:** *John's methodology was particularly mindful of joint health, emphasizing the importance of using low-load muscle engagement to drive blood flow to vulnerable areas. The idea was to saturate the joints with synovial fluid, essentially lubricating them like motor oil in a machine. This focus on blood flow was crucial, especially for joints like the shoulders, where muscular and tendinous attachments are most susceptible to pain and play a pivotal role in movement.*

• **Posterior Chain Emphasis:** *John's training placed heavy emphasis on the posterior chain (the muscles on the back side of the body), recognizing that these muscle groups tend to be slow-twitch dominant and require more volume through activation. By engorging these often undertrained areas with increased blood flow, he took advantage of their diverse three-dimensional musculature to promote more effective synovial fluid production around the muscles, tendons, and bony joints—essentially greasing the wheels for smoother movement.*

The Mountain Dog's distinct approach transcended traditional preparation and redefined the very nature of the workout. Each grueling set was designed with specific goals, which centered around pain management, injury prevention, and hypertrophic physique gains. That's why he was getting results that I was unable to achieve. There was an intention—a goal, a focus—powering the execution.

Meadows's programming wasn't for everyone, and it certainly didn't fit into the larger framework of my training goals. But those fatiguing sets gave me a new understanding of what it means to truly stimulate muscles. I realized that before meeting Meadows, I had been going through the motions, performing the same exercises out of habit rather than strategy. This mindless repetition kept me from experiencing the true benefits of those exercises, which is why I never achieved the same level of results. Training with Meadows reinforced a crucial principle that would become a cornerstone of pain-free performance: It's not just about doing the exercises; it's about doing them with intention and purpose.

The activation drills employed in phase 4 of the warm-up are a direct homage to the Mountain Dog's methods. However, while the underlying philosophy and techniques are similar, our goals and the intent underpinning the application are very different.

THE GOALS OF ACTIVATION DRILLS

John Meadows's utilization of activation exercises in the warm-up worked great for bodybuilders who cared mostly about aesthetics and muscle development. It was less about activation and more about pre-fatiguing the muscles. As such, the focus and process revolved around counteracting the dangers of heavy weight training that taxes the body, exhausting muscles for a hypertrophic stimulus, and achieving high levels of muscular engagement in areas that are generally weaker and imbalanced.

While the role of activation drills in phase 4 are based on the same tenets that I extracted and defined for Meadows, pain-free performance is not isolated to the realm of bodybuilding. We want the option to lift heavy, without risking harm, when the aim of the program is to develop strength. We don't want to exhaust muscles to the point of failure; we want just enough activation—the minimum effective dose—to "wake up" the muscles and drive blood into the joints.

Similar to Meadows's warm-up, we keep activation efforts focused on the posterior chain, not just because these regions are often neglected and underdeveloped, but also because they are functional stabilizers for the primary movers of the body. Take, for instance, the upper back, with its 16 intrinsic muscles enveloping the shoulder blade. The main action of these muscles is to stabilize the shoulder joint as the arm moves dynamically. We also avoid activating the anterior chain, such as the pectoralis muscles at the front of the shoulder, because they are typically overemphasized in training and function as primary movers. They don't stabilize the joints, but rather move the limbs attached to the joints.

Activating the body regions responsible for stabilization brings awareness to the pillar and offsets the pervasive postures that tend to compromise safe and effective movement: forward rounding of the back, internally rotated shoulders, forward head position, and posteriorly tilted pelvis coupled with spinal flexion. Once these regions are activated, getting into and maintaining proper alignment is much easier. You can feel the muscles that support your authentic neutral positioning turn on. That, in turn, brings greater awareness not only to your position but also to the feeling required to stabilize the position.

But you're not annihilating the tissues, as Meadows would say, because fatiguing muscles can compromise the stabilization properties that you will depend on as you transition into the main lifts of the workout.

You're also adding an element to the mind-muscle connection. As Meadows proposed, conscious, focused engagement of a targeted muscle group is necessary for maximizing activation. However, one of the most challenging aspects of training is developing the ability to integrate certain contraction types into movement patterns—especially those contractions you can't easily feel or control. When you're working through an activation exercise, it's not about feeling each muscle in isolation; it's about sensing the tension and recruitment from the entire region and then carrying that feeling into a global pattern of movement.

Consider an activation exercise like the band face pull. Your aim here isn't to target a single muscle such as the teres minor, but rather to activate the entire posterior shoulder region. This approach ensures that there is a connection point between the muscles being activated and the feeling of tension required to stabilize the joint in a safe and strong position when performing a foundational movement. So you feel the muscles that stabilize the shoulder region activate with a band face pull. Then, when you stabilize your shoulders during a movement such as the barbell back squat, you can connect the sensation you felt during the activation exercise to better fortify the stabilization requirements needed to perform the lift. This is the mind-muscle-movement connection—it's the entire chain lighting up, creating a unified point of tension and recruitment that stabilizes the body during movement.

Lastly, by utilizing activation exercises that target the functional stabilizers and enhance your exercise form, you build resiliency against pain and injury. In other words, you protect and enhance the integrity of the pillar complex, helping to avoid the compensatory patterns that wreak havoc on your movement quality. And by doing just enough, you get adequate blood flow without fatiguing the muscles so that you feel good and have plenty of reserves in the tank to maximize performance with your big lifts in the workout.

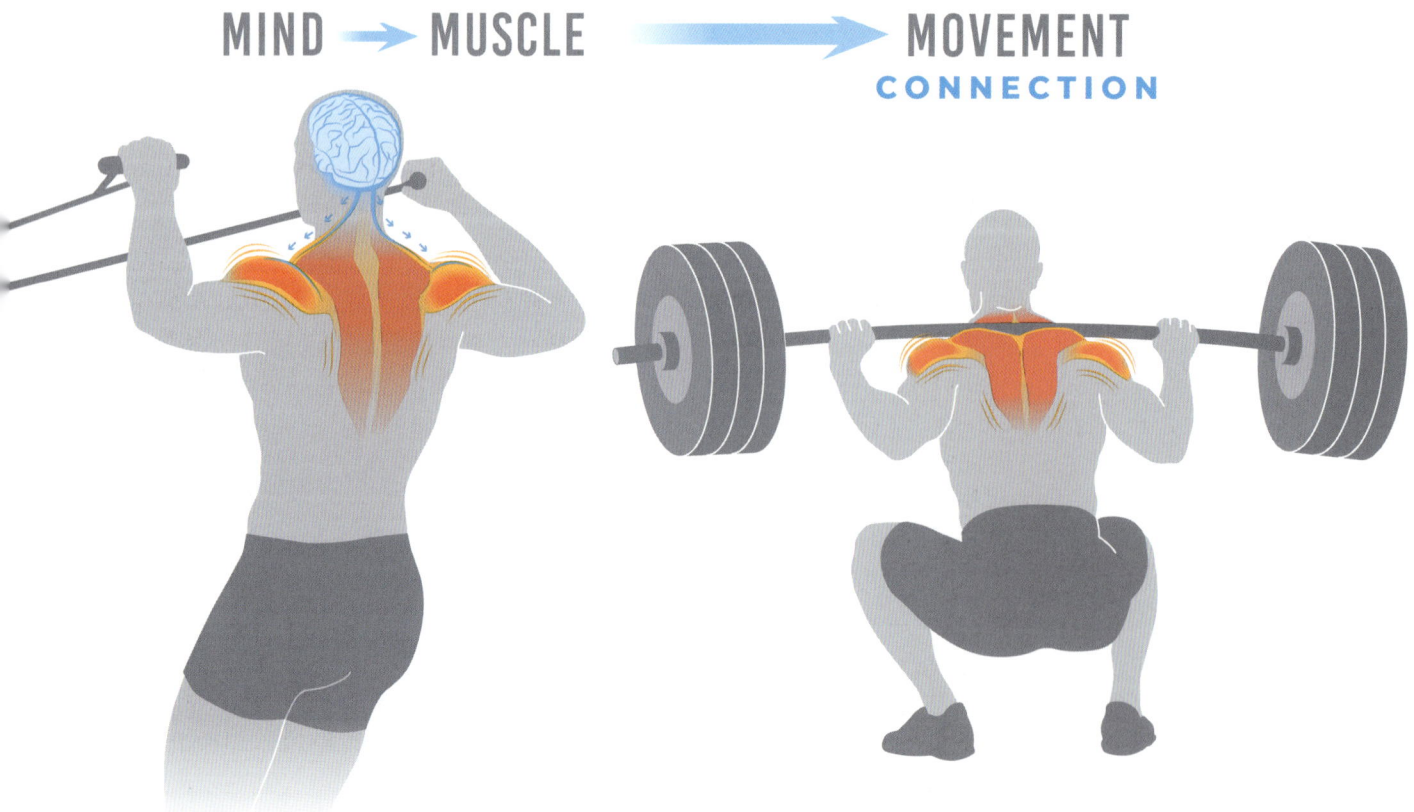

MIND → MUSCLE → MOVEMENT
CONNECTION

RECOMMENDATIONS AND GUIDELINES

In phase 3, you harnessed the new range of motion achieved in phases 1 and 2, alleviating pain with movement or simply moving with a higher level of executional skill around a stable pillar. Phase 4 is all about stabilization through activation. Think of it as hitting the save button, or locking in the movement skill you just acquired. To put it another way, you're activating the muscles responsible for stabilizing the joints in the ranges you just unlocked.

To achieve that, you need to feel the muscles that stabilize the joints turn on so that you can carry that sensation of tension into each movement. It's important to find that sweet spot—a minimum effective dose of engagement that preserves your stabilization capacity, ensuring that your exercise form remains pristine as you transition into the foundational movement patterns in the subsequent phases and workout. Adhere to these guidelines to achieve this balance.

POSITION FOR AUTHENTIC ACTIVATION

This guideline is based on the principle of movement mastery—prioritizing your exercise form to achieve quality activation through authentic muscle engagement. Again, it comes down to pillar alignment and stabilization. You not only need to set the pillar, but also must maintain enough tension through your hips, shoulders, and core to prevent unwanted movement.

Remember, anytime you compensate—move outside your neutral centration zone—tension is redirected and force leaks into non-mechanical structures, such as your ligaments, tendons, and bones. When it comes to activation exercises, this translates to less muscle engagement, which is the opposite of what you're trying to achieve.

Here are some strategies and recommendations that will help you maximize contraction quality while minimizing compensatory movement:

▶ **Prioritize Pillar Stability:** From setup to execution, ensure that the heads of your humerus and femur are centered in the joint sockets. If necessary, revisit the step-by-step cueing sequence on page 34, and then apply the alignment principles to the positions and movements that power the activation exercises. Equally crucial is to keep enough internal tension, sequencing your breath with bracing, to sustain a stable pillar. This will prevent undesirable movement that decreases the quality of muscle activation.

▶ **Apply the Mind-Muscle-Movement Connection:** The quality of your muscle engagement is directly linked to pillar stability and the focus you pour into each rep. Research demonstrates that when you consciously think about engaging the muscles you're targeting, you get higher levels of activation. So place your focus into the region you are activating, realizing that your form dictates muscle engagement quality.[1]

> It's important to find that sweet spot—a minimum effective dose of engagement that preserves your stabilization capacity, ensuring that your exercise form remains pristine.

As you get a feel for the sensation of tension enveloping the entire region, I want you to take it one step further. Instead of simply feeling the regions light up with tension, connect that level of tension to the movement patterns that rely on those regions for stability. So, rather than just producing the tension, you're focusing on the bigger picture—the role that tension plays in safe, efficient movement.

▶ **Follow the Exercise Cues:** Achieving maximal activation requires precise form. While you may need to make small tweaks to the exercises, personalizing them to suit your unique movement, there are universal cues that will help you get the most from them. In the exercise appendix beginning on page 162, pay special attention to the setup and execution. Simply placing the band in the right location and directing focus into the key aspects of the technique will drive engagement to the desired locations.

▶ **Maintain Tension Through the Entire Range:** Most activation drills utilize a resistance band. With these exercises, the resistance increases as you move from the start position to the finish position. However, the goal is to keep tension in the band from beginning to end, from the first rep to the last. That means you need to start with some resistance in the band. Take the slack out of the band so that there is tension from the start, and then maintain tension throughout the entire set.

▶ **Control the Tempo:** Initiate the movement with a dynamic concentric contraction (quick but controlled), a peak flex with a maximal isometric contraction in the finish position, and then a slow, accentuated eccentric returning to the start position. The quicker concentric phase activates motor unit recruitment, the flex amplifies motor unit recruitment, and the slow eccentric creates more total time under tension, maximizing muscle activation through the entire range of motion.

CHOOSE 1 OR 2 AREAS OF EMPHASIS

Choosing which area to target with activation ties in with the previous phases (your linchpin or KPI focus). Much like how phases 1 and 2 of the warm-up are synchronized—pairing foam rolling and stretching to target the same region—phases 3 and 4 are aligned to achieve a seamless transition from learning to move through a new range of motion to actively restabilizing that range with phase 4 activation drills. This synergy is crucial for reaping the maximum benefits of the program.

Sure, you could mix and match different exercises, but without a strategic pairing, the benefits aren't assured. Experience has shown us that when the objectives of each phase are in sync, we amplify the results. It's about efficiency and efficacy, ensuring that every minute of the 10-minute warm-up is optimized and purposeful.

So stick with the theme that you started with and carry it through to this phase. If you're following the linchpin and KPI blueprints, the work is done for you. Simply mirror the exercises included in the program (pages 464–475).

PERFORM 3 TO 5 SETS OF 3 TO 5 REPS WITH SHORT REST PERIODS

When it comes to programming, our mantra is simple: activate, don't annihilate. This approach ensures that you activate muscles effectively without annihilating their stabilization roles.

The biggest pitfall in the activation phase is taking the exercises to exhaustion. You're not seeking a hypertrophic stimulus, like the Mountain Dog's approach. What you're looking for is a sweet spot of volume that actualizes the neural and mechanical activation benefits while avoiding pre-fatigue. I can't emphasize this enough—you're warming up, not wearing down. Usually, you want to stick in the range of 3 to 5 sets of 3 to 5 reps, and to avoid fatigue, you break up the sets and reps with short rest periods of 15 to 20 seconds. Think of it as a finely tuned cluster set. You're doing just enough to feel regional activation at 5 reps, but you are able to recover within the short 15- to 20-second recovery window. Here's an example of how it would work for the hip and back emphasis exercises:

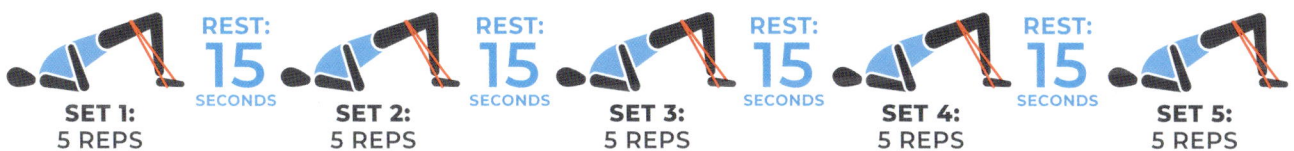

SET 1: 5 REPS — REST: 15 SECONDS — **SET 2:** 5 REPS — REST: 15 SECONDS — **SET 3:** 5 REPS — REST: 15 SECONDS — **SET 4:** 5 REPS — REST: 15 SECONDS — **SET 5:** 5 REPS

The notable exception is the Rusin Tri-set, which includes 3 consecutive exercises, where 15 total reps across all 3 exercises might constitute a single set. But again, you want to go just shy of a sustained burn by treating it as a circuit.

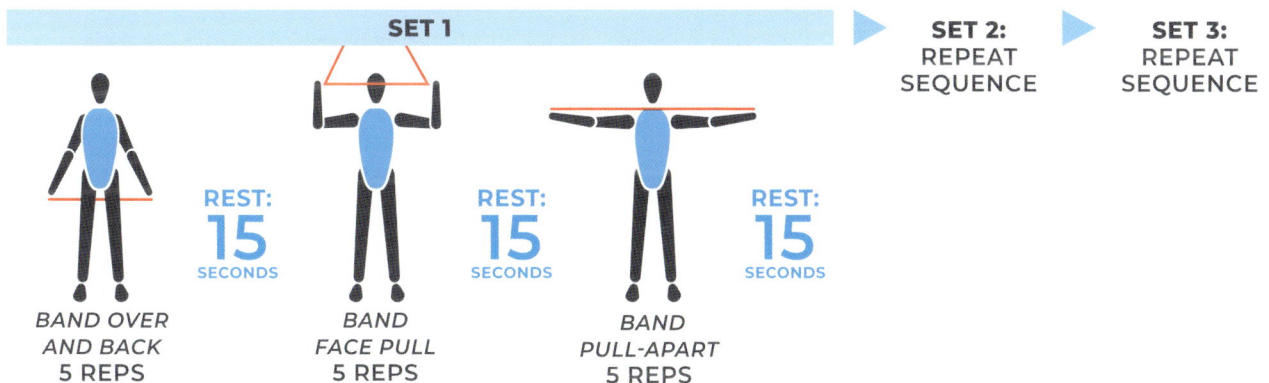

SET 1

BAND OVER AND BACK 5 REPS — REST: 15 SECONDS — BAND FACE PULL 5 REPS — REST: 15 SECONDS — BAND PULL-APART 5 REPS — REST: 15 SECONDS

SET 2: REPEAT SEQUENCE ▶ **SET 3:** REPEAT SEQUENCE

The activation exercises are not that difficult in terms of effort, especially when you break up the sets and keep the reps below five. Given that, many people feel inclined to combine the reps into a single set to make it a challenge—knocking out 25 glute bridges and calling it a day, for example. The problem is that fatigue accumulates quickly.

To reiterate, you're not trying to build strength or grow muscle here. While pushing sets to mechanical failure is where the magic happens, it's counterproductive in a warm-up where the goal is to ramp up to your key performance indicators. So tread the line carefully, aiming for just enough to progress, feeling energized and ready to tackle the more demanding tasks ahead without pre-exhausting the tissues.

To help you navigate this section, the activation exercises are organized by body region of emphasis: hips, back, and shoulders. Simply go to the region that aligns with your KPI or linchpin and choose an exercise to perform. While I do provide specific instructions for setting up and executing each exercise, achieving optimal activation may require making specific modifications. Make sure to review the considerations and modifications to customize each exercise to your unique body mechanics, guaranteeing that the right muscles are firing as intended.

It's also important to note that many of these activation exercises involve using short and long resistance (loop) bands. Selecting the correct resistance is crucial for effective activation, and finding the right level may require some trial and error. Different exercises demand varying levels of resistance, and while I provide some general recommendations, it's essential to follow the guidelines and cues closely. This will help you determine the resistance that best suits your strength level and experience, ensuring you get the most out of each exercise.

EXERCISE APPENDIX

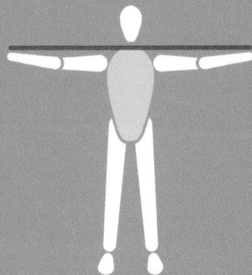

PHASE 4:
ACTIVATION

HIP EMPHASIS

BANDED GLUTE BRIDGE

SETUP AND EXECUTION: For this exercise, use a light or moderate resistance band. Get set up by following these steps:

1. Hold the band in the center to create two loops and place each loop over the tops of your feet, positioning them under your arches. Then pull the middle of the band over your knees to mid-thigh height. This setup activates more glute muscles compared to banding around the knees, which primarily encourages abduction.

2. Lie on your back with your feet positioned hip- to shoulder-width apart and slightly turned outward. Bring your feet in close enough that the entire bottoms of your feet press firmly into the ground. Over multiple sets, you can experiment with foot width and turnout to find the best position for glute activation.

3. Align your spine in a neutral position with ribs stacked over your hips. Position your upper arms about 45 degrees from your torso, elbows bent and knuckles pointing up. Create a slight posterior pelvic tilt (like tipping water toward your chin) to fully engage your glutes. Ensure full foot contact (big toe, little toe, and heel) with an active arch. Push your knees outward into the band to engage your glutes, but keep them aligned with your feet.
   Maximize glute activation and hip stability for each rep by

- Pressing your upper arms into the ground to stabilize your upper body.

- Breathing in, bracing your core, and pushing through your feet to lift your hips to full extension.

- Holding the top position for 1 second, focusing on squeezing your glutes.

- Lowering your hips slowly without resting at the bottom, lightly touching down while maintaining muscle engagement for maximum activation throughout the set.

Scan the QR code to access demos of each exercise.

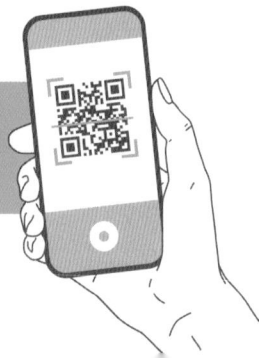

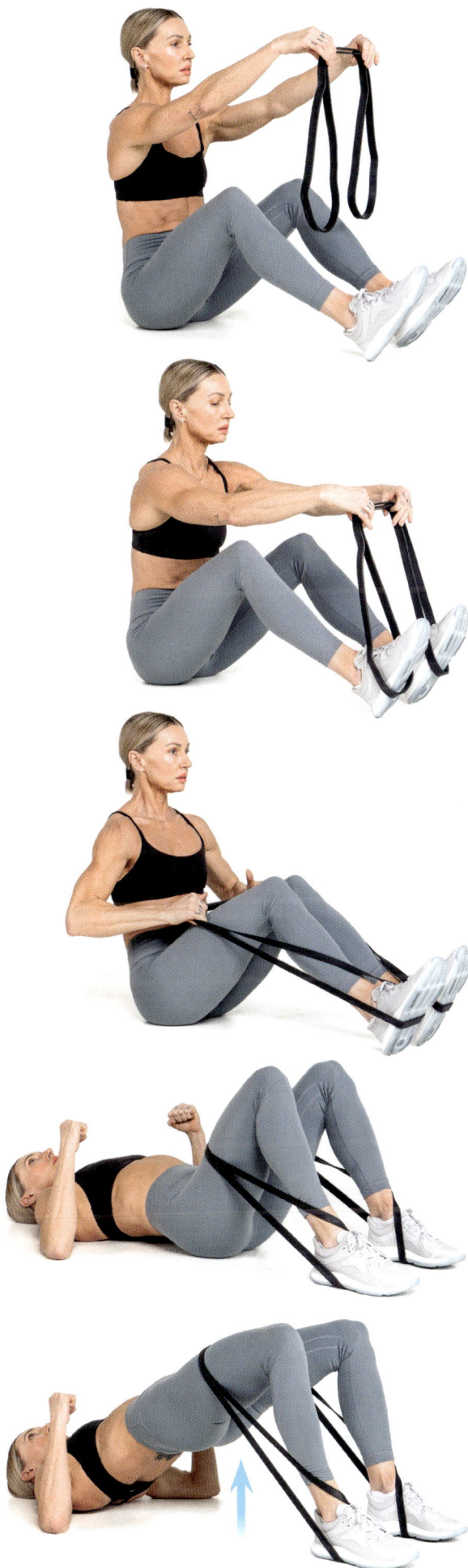

CONSIDERATIONS AND MODIFICATIONS: When performing the banded glute bridge, adjusting your form and positioning can make a significant difference in comfort and effectiveness. Below are a couple key considerations to help you maximize glute activation and avoid compensations from other muscle groups.

- **Hamstring Cramping or Lower Back Tightness:** If you're feeling tightness in your lower back, move your feet slightly further away from your body to reduce strain. If your hamstrings are cramping, move your feet closer toward your body to ease tension on the hamstrings. The ideal foot position should create a slight backward angle of the shins toward your body. Avoid positioning your knees excessively forward beyond your toes. If these adjustments don't resolve your hamstring cramping or lower back tightness, you may be tilting your pelvis forward (anterior pelvic tilt). This position can inhibit the glutes, causing your hamstrings or lower back muscles to compensate and take over the movement. To correct this, reset your position with a slight posterior tilt (pelvis tipping toward your chin) before each rep. You may also benefit from a reduced range of motion until you build strength and mobility, allowing for gradual improvement without straining your stabilizer muscles.

- **Line of Drive:** If you're feeling this exercise more in your quads or hamstrings, check the direction of your drive. Pushing your feet away from you creates an isometric contraction in the quads, while pulling them toward you activates the hamstrings. Instead, focus on pushing your feet directly down to drive your hips up. Using a slant board or wedges to elevate your toes can also help if tightness in the shins or foot position makes it difficult to connect your full foot to the ground. This modification places your feet at a more comfortable angle, encouraging better glute activation.

SINGLE-LEG GLUTE BRIDGE

SETUP AND EXECUTION: Begin in a similar starting position to the banded glute bridge, but without the band. Lie on your back with your spine in a neutral position, ribs stacked over your hips, and your upper arms pressed down at about a 45-degree angle from your torso. Maintain a slight posterior pelvic tilt to engage your glutes from the start, and ensure full foot contact with the ground—big toe, little toe, and heel pressing down.

To set up for the single-leg variation:

1. Position your grounded foot hip-width apart, pointing slightly outward for optimal stability.

2. Lift your opposite leg off the ground, keeping it bent at roughly 90 degrees.

SINGLE-LEG GLUTE BRIDGE

BANDED SINGLE-LEG GLUTE BRIDGE VARIATION

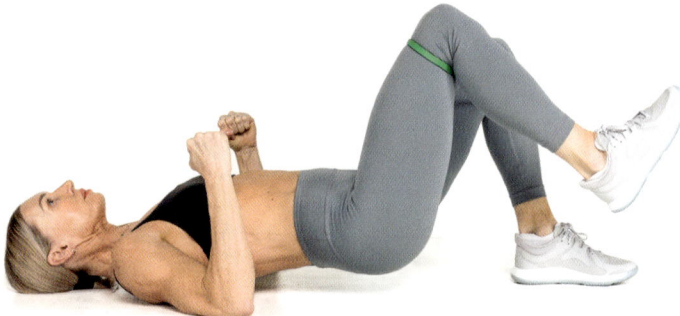

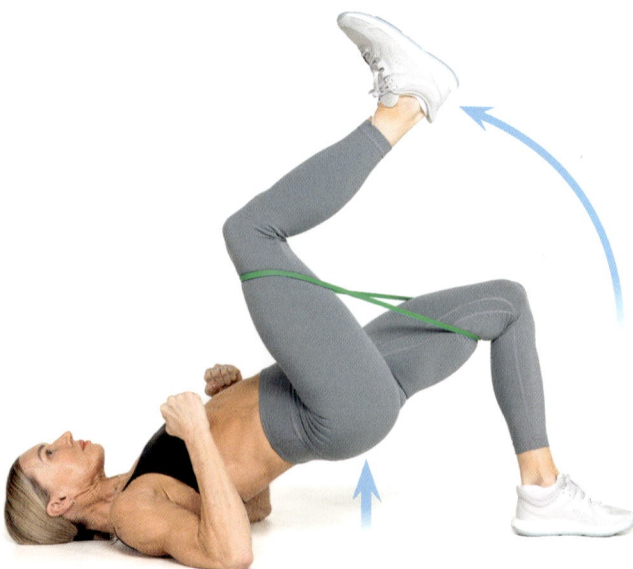

As you initiate the movement, focus on the breathe-brace-move sequence:

- Breathe in to stabilize, brace your core, and then press through your grounded foot to lift your hips.

- At the top of the movement, imagine gently squeezing your legs together to engage the inner thigh muscles (adductors) on both sides. This is an isometric contraction that helps stabilize the pelvis without visible movement.

- Lower your hips back down with control, keeping the lifted leg in position and avoiding any collapse in your core.

- Since you're working with a narrower base of support, you may notice a reduced range of motion in hip extension—this is normal. The adductors, which stabilize the pelvis, play a crucial role here, building strength that supports squats, hinges, lunge patterns, walking, running, and various sports.

CONSIDERATIONS AND MODIFICATIONS: These modifications for the single-leg glute bridge can help you progress gradually or increase activation and stability, making it easier to find the ideal setup and execution for your body and goals.

- **Slant Board or Wedges:** Similar to the standard glute bridge, using a slant board or wedge under your foot can be a helpful modification, allowing for greater stability and range of motion.

- **Kickstand Variation:** This variation is a midpoint between the two-foot glute bridge and the single-leg version. Place one foot flat on the ground for the primary support, while the opposite heel lightly touches down. This setup allows for a single-leg emphasis while using the heel of the non-working leg to prevent unwanted pelvic rotation.

- **Self-Resisted Variation:** For this variation, press your hands against the raised knee to create tension through the core and hips. This push-pull action stabilizes your pillar and reinforces hip alignment, enhancing muscle activation.

- **Banded Variation:** Adding a short resistance band or miniband above your knees creates more challenge and activation, including direct engagement of the hip flexors.

SIDE PLANK HIP THRUST

SETUP AND EXECUTION: This advanced activation drill is excellent for functional integration, reinforcing pillar-wide stability.

1. Begin in a side plank position with your hips stacked and your elbow directly under your shoulder. Push the floor away with your forearm to stabilize your shoulder.

2. Bring your knees forward so your thighs form a 45-degree angle from your torso. Stack your feet in line with the back of your body, and gently pull your head and chin back to align your neck with your spine.

3. To start the movement, reach your top arm under your ribcage, keeping your bottom arm actively pressing into the floor. Then press your bottom knee into the ground to lift your hips up and forward. As you reach the top, open your top arm and knee together.

To properly execute this exercise, focus on these key cues:

- Squeeze your glutes to drive your hips forward.

- Maintain "ribs to hips" alignment for a strong core.

- Keep your head and chin pulled back to align with your spine.

- Engage your top arm and leg to avoid any "floppy" movement.

- Drive your hips up with intention, pause for a second at the top, and lower with control.

- As you descend, focus on pushing your hips back into flexion rather than simply lowering to the ground.

CONSIDERATIONS AND MODIFICATIONS: The side plank hip thrust is an advanced activation drill that requires coordinated integration between the hips, core, and shoulders. If you find it challenging to keep the movement smooth or struggle to engage your glutes effectively, try building up with the following progression of simpler exercises. This road map will help you develop the stability and strength needed for the full side plank hip thrust. Progress only when an exercise feels manageable—this may take days, weeks, or even months, so focus on quality movement rather than speed.

- **Side-Lying Banded Clam:** Lie on your side with your bottom arm under your head, knees bent, and a miniband looped around your legs just above the knee joint. Position yourself against a wall so that your head, back, pelvis, and feet are all in contact with it. The wall serves as a guide, helping you resist the tendency to roll your pelvis back as you lift your top knee. Keeping your feet together, lift and rotate your top knee upward. As you do this, gently press your hips forward, slightly away from the wall, to activate your glutes more effectively.

- **Elevated Banded Clam:** By propping yourself up on your elbow and forearm, this variation begins to incorporate shoulder stability and core control, challenging you to maintain a steady pillar without sinking into your side.

- **(Short Lever) Side Plank Iso with Banded Clam:** In this progression, lift your hips into a side plank hold, activating the bottom leg glutes to support the plank while the top leg moves. This combines core stability with targeted glute engagement.

- **Side Plank Hip Flexion/Extension:** This exercise prepares your hip for the flexion and extension movement needed in the side plank hip thrust. Set up as you would for the hip thrust, keeping your feet and knees together. Push your hips back to touch down and then drive them forward into extension. For added resistance, anchor a band behind you, looping it around your hips.

- **Side Plank Hip Thrust (Feet Together):** This step is nearly identical to the original side plank hip thrust, but with feet together for added stability. This extra contact point supports the integration of hip flexion/extension with side plank hip drops and top leg movement. To increase the challenge, you can add a long band anchored behind you around your waist, and a miniband around your knees for extra resistance.

BACK EMPHASIS

BENT-OVER LAT PULLDOWN

SETUP AND EXECUTION: Anchor a moderate resistance band to above head level, then follow these steps:

1. Stand with your feet hip- to shoulder-width apart, holding the band at shoulder height with hands 4 to 6 inches apart. Pull your hips back into a hinge position, maintaining a long spine. Extend your arms fully overhead, with biceps beside your ears. If full extension causes discomfort, adjust to a pain-free angle.

2. Focus on keeping your ribs stacked over your hips, bracing your core to avoid arching your lower back as you pull down.

3. From the hinge position, pull your arms straight down and slightly apart, aiming for your hands to land beside your legs at or just above knee height. Keep your elbows straight throughout the movement to ensure the lats are engaged, avoiding elbow bending, which would shift the work to your triceps.

With all the upper body banded activation drills, it's crucial to maintain resistance in the band throughout the exercise. If there is slack in the band when you hinge, you may need to step back to create tension. Also, you may need to widen your grip on the band to ensure a slight stretch between your hands.

CONSIDERATIONS AND MODIFICATIONS: If core stability is a linchpin, maintaining pillar alignment during the standing banded lat pull-down may be challenging. For increased lat activation with additional core support, consider performing this exercise in a supine position:

- **Supine Position Modification:** Lie on your back with your knees bent and feet flat on the floor. Anchor the band behind you—either low to the ground if you have full overhead range of motion or higher up if you prefer to keep your arms in front of your ears for a pain-free setup.

EXECUTION: Start with your arms overhead and pull the band down until your hands are stacked above your shoulders, similar to a dead bug hold. Although this variation provides less range of motion than the standing version, it allows you to engage your lats while integrating upper body movement into a core stability–focused exercise.

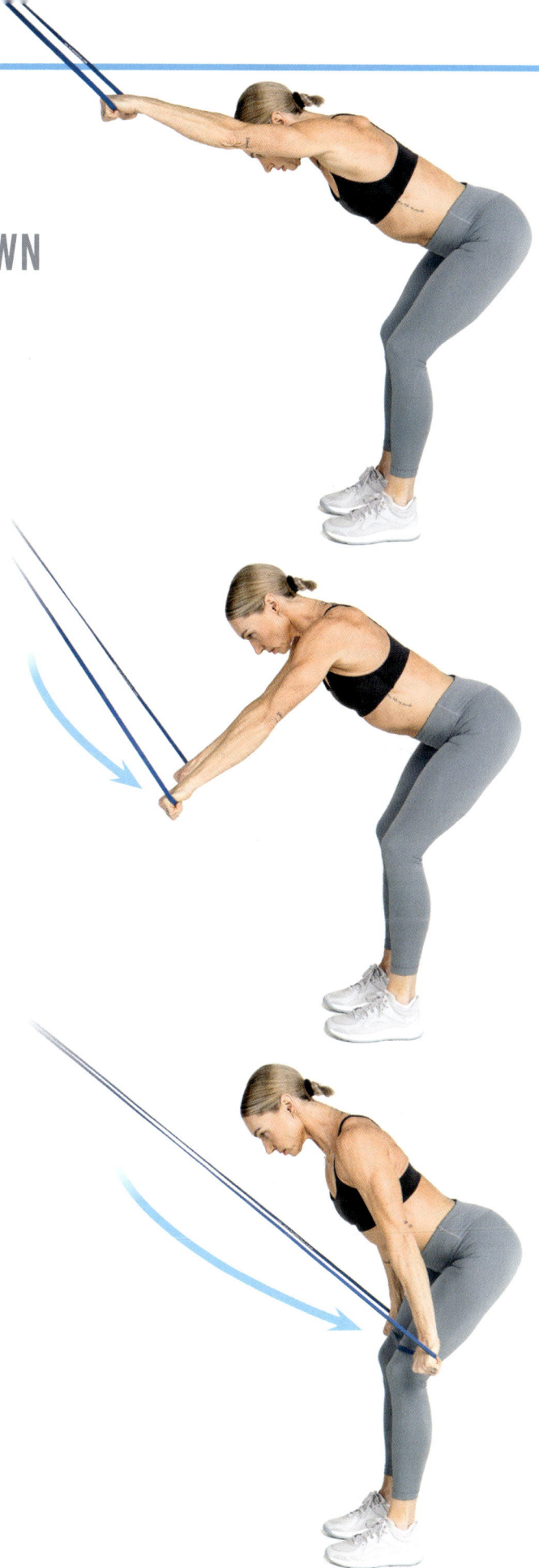

SHOULDER EMPHASIS

RUSIN TRI-SET

The Rusin Tri-set is a structured sequence of movements designed to be completed in order. It's a foundational component of the pain-free training system, supporting shoulder mobility and stability. Given that the shoulders are the body's most mobile joint and a common pain-point for many people, this warm-up is beneficial for nearly everyone. Whether your goal is to address a specific linchpin or to counteract the effects of prolonged sitting and forward posture, this activation sequence should be a regular part of your training.

BAND OVER AND BACK

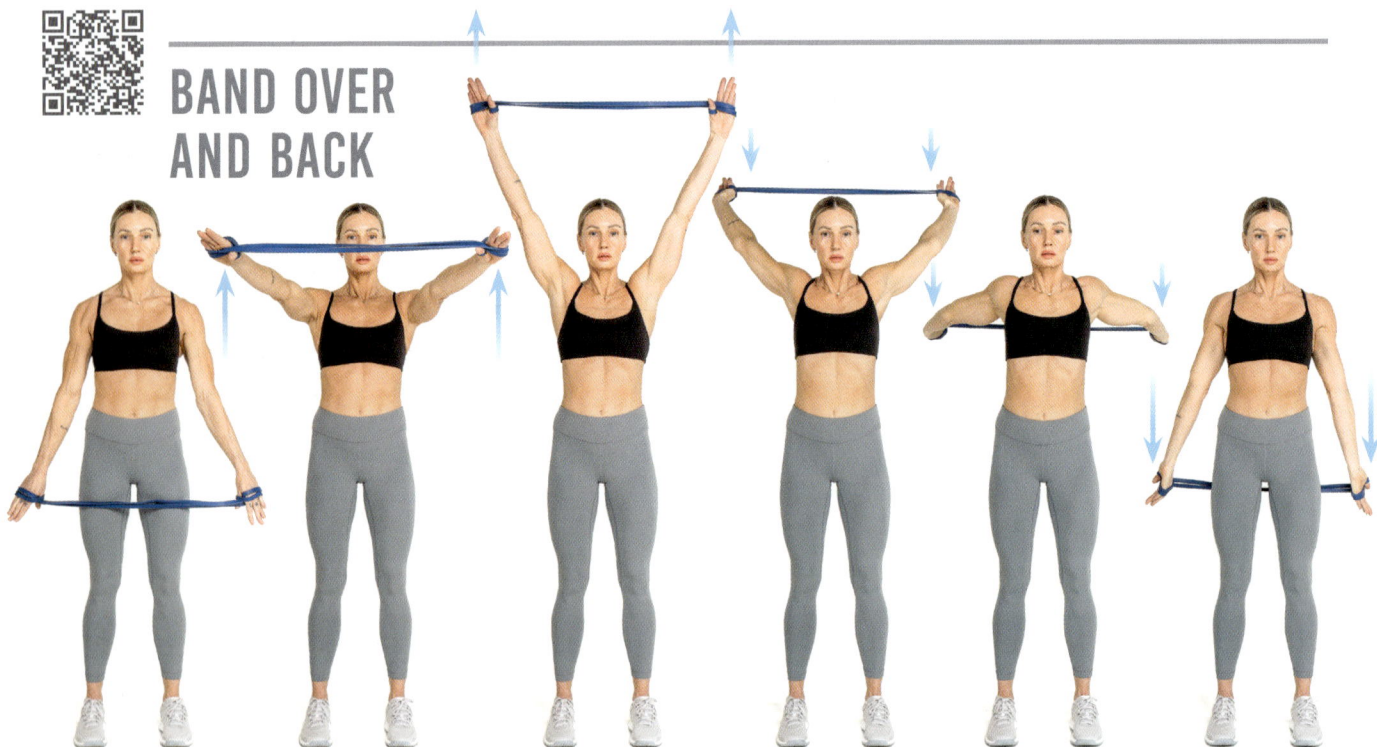

SETUP AND EXECUTION: Select a light resistance band, and then follow these steps:

1. Place your hands inside the band with palms facing away from your thighs, thumbs pointing behind you. In this starting position, your shoulders and scapulae will be slightly elevated, protracted, and internally rotated.

2. Keeping your palms facing away and arms mostly straight, lift the band up and over your head, continuing to move it behind your head until it reaches down toward your glutes. At this point, your shoulders and scapulae should now be in a depressed, retracted, and externally rotated position. This creates a full range of motion for the shoulders.

3. To return, reach your hands away from your glutes or lower back, maintaining palm orientation. Bring the band back up and over your head, returning to the starting position in front of your thighs.

CONSIDERATIONS AND MODIFICATIONS: When first starting the banded over and back, you may feel tightness as your arms move into the overhead "Y" position. If you experience any pain, stop just before the painful range and bring your arms forward and down. You can widen your grip on the band to help ease through tight spots—discomfort is okay, but don't push through pain.

With consistent practice, as you complete the 6-phase dynamic warm-up and train effectively, your range of motion will improve.

To maximize the benefits of this movement:

- Allow your scapulae to move freely. As you bring the band overhead, let your shoulders shrug slightly, and let your shoulder blades glide naturally—this mobility is one reason why the band is preferred over a rigid dowel.

- Keep your hands open on the band rather than gripping it. Holding the band tightly creates tension through the forearms and shoulders, which can limit the range of motion you're aiming for.

If the band feels too long or loose and you aren't feeling much stretch, try wrapping the band once around one or both hands. This adjustment shortens the band, bringing your arms more overhead instead of wide in the "Y" shape, creating a steeper angle and greater stretch. (The model in the pictures demonstrates this by wrapping the band around both hands.)

BAND FACE PULL

SETUP AND EXECUTION: The band face pull emphasizes coordinated external rotation, engaging the smaller muscles in the back of the shoulder that work together to stabilize the scapula and shoulder joint. Unlike a traditional row, which focuses on pulling the shoulder blades back, this movement targets the external rotators to promote better shoulder alignment and stability.

To set up, choose a light or very light band and anchor it just above head height. From there, follow these steps to ensure proper form:

1. **Grip and Stance:** Hold the band about 4 to 6 inches apart using a hook grip, where only the first knuckles of your fingers rest on the band. Avoid a full grip that wraps the band into your palms, as this creates unnecessary tension in the forearms. Step back into a hip-width stance to create light tension on the band, with your arms at shoulder height.

2. **Pillar Position:** Set your posture by aligning your pelvis neutrally, stacking your ribs over your hips, and lengthening through your upper back and neck. Breathe deeply and brace your core to establish stability.

3. **Movement Execution:** Pull the band toward the bridge of your nose, forehead, or hairline, simultaneously pulling the band apart slightly as you do so. Imagine "wiping" your cheeks with your thumbnails for a helpful visual cue. At the top of the movement,

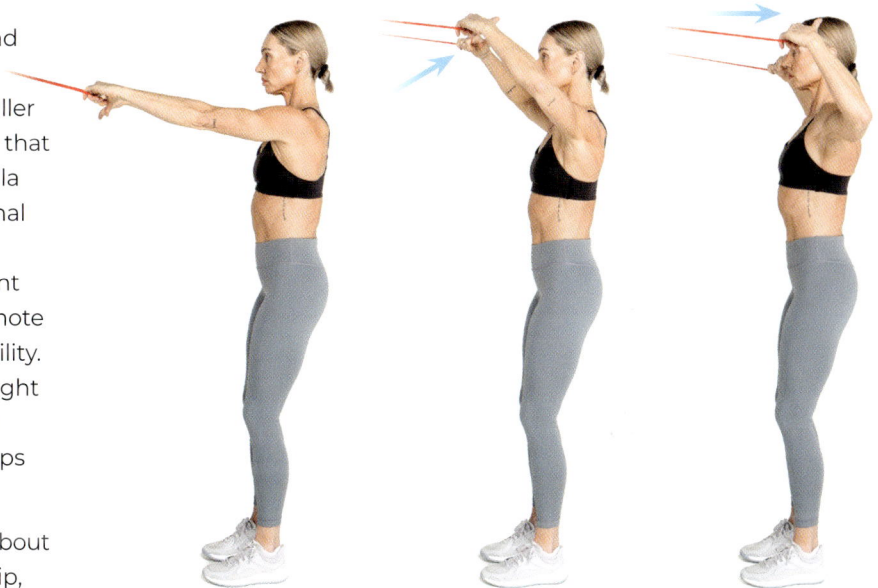

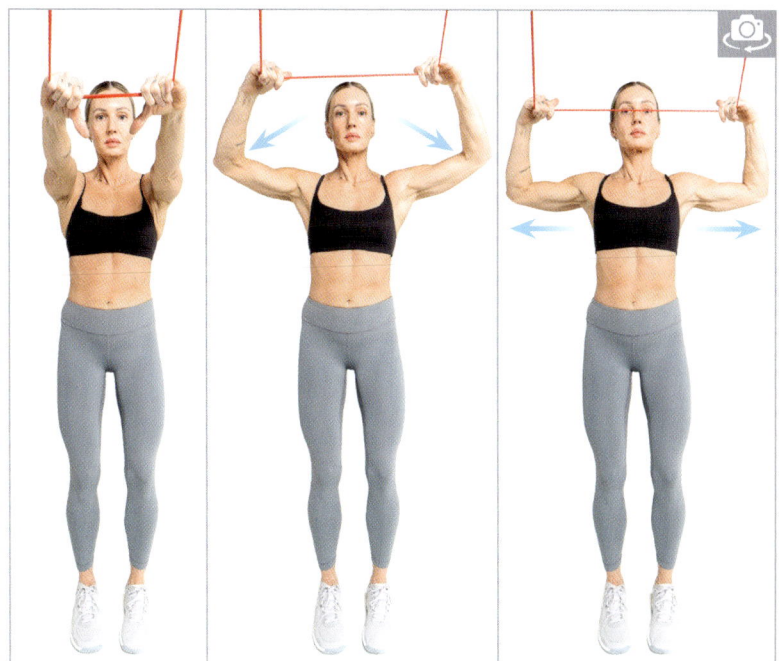

your elbows should be at approximately 90 degrees and in line with your shoulders (not pulling behind your body). Your forearms should remain slightly angled with wrists positioned just in front of the elbows.

4. Control and Tempo: Execute the concentric pull with purpose (slow and smooth), pause briefly at the top, then return to the starting position with control.

CONSIDERATIONS AND MODIFICATIONS: A common issue with face pulls is the tendency for the upper trap muscles to dominate the movement. This often happens when the upper traps are tight or overactive, while the mid traps and smaller posterior shoulder muscles—such as the rhomboids, infraspinatus, and rear deltoids—are relatively weak. This imbalance can make it challenging to effectively engage the intended stabilizing muscles, leading to excessive shoulder elevation and reduced activation of the muscles that support scapular stability and shoulder alignment. Here are some modifications to address this issue, along with other pain and performance challenges, ensuring you target the intended muscles and avoid compensations.

- **Higher Anchor Point:** If you find your upper traps taking over, try anchoring the band slightly higher so that you're pulling downward. This encourages shoulder blade depression rather than elevation, helping to engage the correct muscles.

- **Supine Position:** For added stability, perform the face pull lying on your back with your knees bent and feet flat on the floor. This position stabilizes your shoulder blades against the floor and prevents your elbows from traveling too far back. Anchor the band above you, ideally on a barbell rack, pull-up bar, or similar secure point.

- **Kneeling Variations:** Performing the face pull in a full or half-kneeling position can help if you're working on core stability and tend to arch your lower back. This position encourages a more stable core and neutral spine throughout the movement.

- **Hands-Free Face Pull:** If you experience pain or discomfort in your elbows, wrists, or hands, try placing the band around the backs of your wrists or hands. Keep your fingers open and gently extend your wrists backward (wrist extension) as you perform the movement.

BAND PULL-APART

SETUP AND EXECUTION: This movement emphasizes scapular stability and external rotation, providing a focused activation for the shoulder and upper back muscles. Follow these steps and guidelines to maximize form and effectiveness:

1. Starting Position: Begin with your feet hip-width apart, maintaining a strong pillar position with your spine neutral, ribs stacked over hips, and arms raised to shoulder height with a slight bend in your elbows. Hold the band with your hands shoulder-width apart, palms facing down.

2. Grip Option: Wrap your hand fully around the band, but keep your grip light rather than gripping tightly.

3. Band Setup Tips:

- If using a very light band, you can double it up for more resistance (option 1).

- If using a light band, loop it around your neck so one end hangs down behind you, and hold the other end in front (option 2). This prevents the loose end from snapping back.

4. Movement Execution: Pull the band apart, opening your arms while keeping your elbows slightly bent. As you reach the wide position, rotate your arms so your thumbs point toward the ceiling. Focus on externally rotating from the shoulder joint rather than just twisting your wrists.

5. Control and Range of Motion: Pull with intent, pause for a moment when the band touches your chest (arms aligned with shoulders), then return to the start position with control. Avoid pulling your hands too far back; instead, aim for shoulder-width to maximize activation of the target muscles. Think of "reaching your hands away from each other" rather than pulling them back.

6. Wrist Position: Maintain a neutral wrist, similar to the alignment you'd use for a punch, avoiding any backward bending.

BAND PULL-APART (OPTION 1)

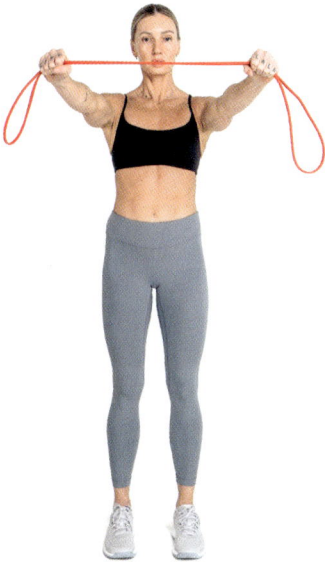

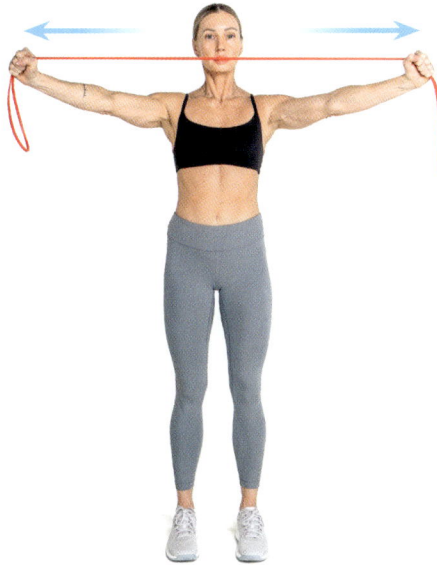

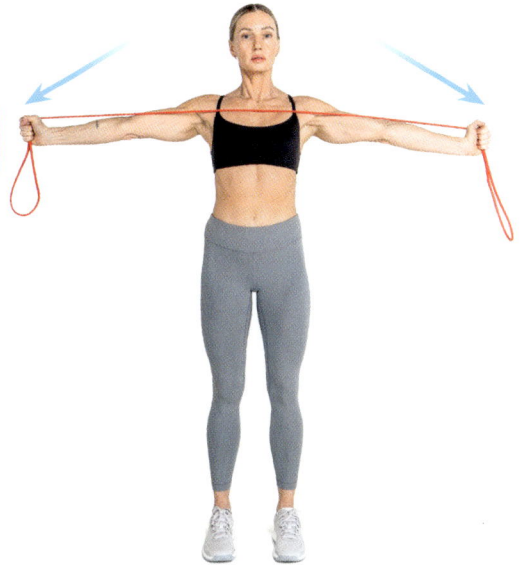

BAND PULL-APART (OPTION 2)

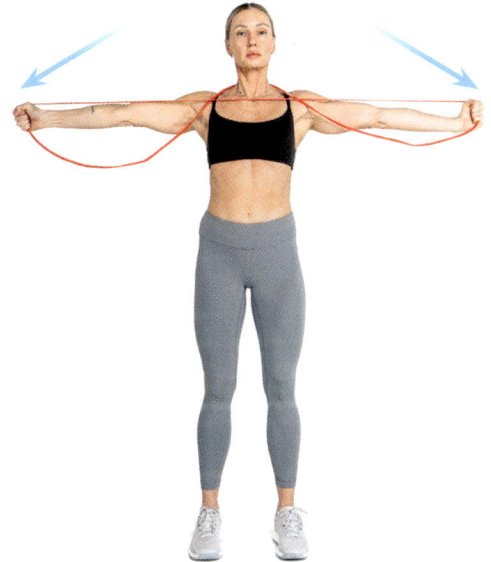

BAND PULL-APART VARIATION

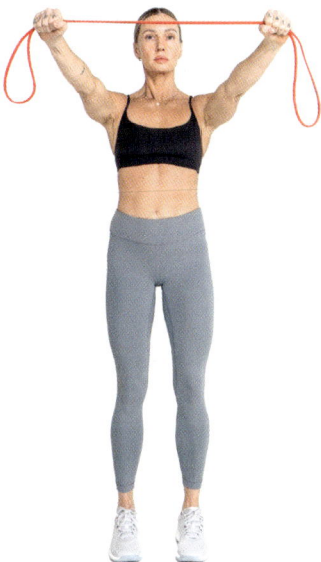

CONSIDERATIONS AND MODIFICATIONS: If you find that your upper traps are overly engaged during this exercise, try adjusting to a slight downward pull. Start with your hands at forehead height and pull the band down to just below your chest while pulling it apart. This motion helps engage the lower traps, reducing the involvement of the upper traps and promoting better shoulder stability.

Another modification is to perform the pull-aparts lying on your back, similar to the supine face pull variation. This position provides additional stability and is particularly useful if you're addressing a limitation in scapular stability.

PHASE 5:
MOVEMENT PATTERN DEVELOPMENT

Phase 5 is where the culmination of synergistic benefits from the previous phases are channeled into the foundational movement patterns. This is your time to practice and refine your executional skill with the exercises that you will perform in the workout to promote and develop movement mastery. Pick one or two exercises. Move slowly, with intent and precision, optimizing and improving with every set and rep.

My hands are gripping a barbell loaded with 405 pounds as I get ready to squat for the first time in months. Suddenly, the coach, who I just met, starts in on me with this booming voice, "Alright, let's get your feet set! Get that bar on your back! Drive into it!"

I'm totally thrown off my game. This is a different style of coaching, intense and in my face, unlike anything I've experienced.

As I position the bar on my back and stand up with the weight, my mind races, distracted by the chaotic and untenable instructions. I descend into the squat, something I've done countless times before, but I struggle to maintain my typical form. The coach, unrelenting, continues his slew of commands, "Keep your back flat! Push your knees out! Breathe with it!"

I try my best to make in-the-moment corrections, but it's impossible. I'm thinking about all the things I need to do, and as a result, I make the exact errors I'm trying to prevent. I feel my body give way to my thoughts and the technique I'm trying to will into action. I completely lose it. My spine reacts in a way I've never felt before. Like an accordion folding, it buckles.

The coach's commands get even louder and more frantic, though I can't make sense of what he is saying. He's probably telling me to straighten my spine, which now resembles a fishhook, my shoulders rounding forward over my chest. Struggling, I finish the rep and heave the bar back into the rack. My heart pounding. Legs trembling. For a moment, I'm convinced I've broken my back. Miraculously, I'm not injured, but the truth hits me hard: I was ill prepared.

Prior to this experience, I hadn't touched a weight in nearly five months. Yet there I was, attempting a max-effort lift under the scrutiny of my teammates in a collegiate weight room. All the while getting aggressively coached.

We didn't warm up. We didn't do any ramp-up sets.

My focus was scattered. My body cold.

Even though I had performed the same lift with the same weight (and more) on numerous occasions, the chaos of the room, my lack of preparation, and the delivery of the cues shifted my mindset. Instead of focusing on the task of squatting, I was thinking about my technique. I was in a practice mindset when I needed to be in a performance mindset.

This is how injuries happen in the weight room, and why there are high occurrences of training-related pain. People make the same movement-compromising and performance-hindering errors again and again, doing exactly what I did—not warming up or taking time to practice—and lowering their executional skill to the level of their preparation.

There is a time for practice and a time for performance. Each is distinct, with different intents, goals, and strategies. During practice, you are thinking about the specific actions that make the movement safer, smoother, and more effective. You dial up internal tension, tapping into the feeling that creates and maintains pillar stability. You make small tweaks to the movement that help you avoid catastrophic mistakes that result in injury and avoid aggregate compensations that result in training-induced chronic pain.

When you are performing, your focus is on completing the movement, applying the technique that you patterned in practice. If you are thinking about all the nuanced aspects of the technique or which muscles are firing, then your focus will fray. And once that happens, the dominoes that hold your form together start falling.

The time for practice is in the warm-up, not during the workout. The time for learning and coaching is during practice, not while under a maximal load. You need to separate practice from performance— which is where phase 5 comes in.

GOALS OF MOVEMENT PATTERN DEVELOPMENT

PRACTICE is for feeling, learning, and refining the components of the skill.

PERFORMANCE, on the other hand, relies on the foundation built during practice to execute the skill efficiently and effectively without thinking about the technical nuances.

Picture a basketball player laser-focused on mastering their free-throw technique. To achieve proficient execution, they deconstruct each phase of the shot: positioning feet with precision, ensuring body balance, gripping the ball just right, bending knees at the optimal angle, extending the arm smoothly, flicking the wrist accurately, and completing with a consistent follow-through. Each repetition is an exercise in meticulous attention to detail, fostering a deep mind-body connection with the goal of patterning a repeatable and individualized routine. This process, known as "internal attentional focus" or "internal cueing," involves an intense awareness of every movement, gradually embedding the correct mechanics into the player's muscle memory.

Now, imagine that same player in the heat of a game, standing at the free-throw line with the crowd's roar fading into the background. In this high-pressure moment, their focus shifts outward—the goal is no longer about the mechanics but about landing the ball in the net, embodying "external attentional focus" or "external cueing." The hours of detailed practice recede, allowing instinct and training to take over. Here, the player doesn't dissect the shot into its constituent parts. Instead, they execute it as a singular, fluid motion, trusting their body to recall the precision honed during practice.

This pivotal shift from a conscious, internal focus during practice to a more subconscious, external focus during performance illustrates how athletes manage to perform complex tasks under pressure. It exemplifies the profound impact of where and how focus should be applied.

Practice is for feeling, learning, and refining the components of the skill.

Performance, on the other hand, relies on the foundation built during practice to execute the skill efficiently and effectively without thinking about the technical nuances.

This is as true for exercise as it is for sport.

Phase 5 is where you apply the concepts of deliberate practice and motor control development to improve exercise form and promote movement mastery—as covered in the Movement Mastery Mindset chapter. More specifically, the aim is to

▶ Practice your technique

▶ Improve your form

▶ **Feel, learn, and refine**

You focus on the quality of movement and the muscles that power the motion (feeling). You pinpoint and correct weaknesses (learning). And you make technical adjustments to groove the pattern (refining). Then, when it comes time to perform (the workout), you turn on your reliable autopilot, allowing the technique you developed during practice to power your performance in training.

To accomplish this, however, you must mimic the pattern that you plan to train, without the challenges of load and speed. In phase 5, for example, you move with just your body weight or a very light weight.

You also move slowly. This allows you to control every aspect of the movement and make refinements that improve the range, smoothness, symmetry, and quality of the pattern.

Lastly, there is no pressure to perform. You're not trying to hit a PR or a specific performance metric. This allows you to direct your attention into the mechanical and technical aspects of the movement, fine-tuning with every set and rep.

As you transition into your workout and the key performance indicator (KPI)—the heaviest or hardest movement or lift of the training session—you can transfer what you learned and felt in phase 5 into the movement pattern that you are training. More than that, you can accurately direct your focus into the task, drowning out the environmental noise and the minute details underpinning the execution of the movement. Put simply, you will be able to perform to your true abilities, automatically.

INTERNAL VS. EXTERNAL FOCUS/CUES

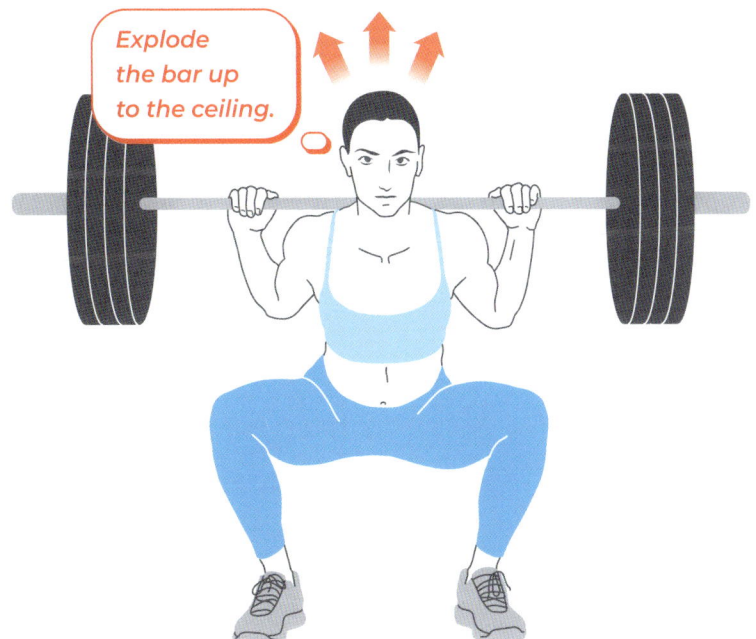

The mind-muscle connection is fundamentally an internal cue—focusing on tension and torque within the pillar, for example—which is especially effective in phase 5. Here, when the emphasis is on the quality of movement or viewing movement as an input skill, internal cues prove very effective. Conversely, when the goal shifts toward strength or power, external cues that involve moving the body through space become more relevant. For example, "drive your back through the bar" and "throw the bar through the ceiling" are external cues for a one-rep max back squat, whereas "screw your feet into the floor" and "create tension and torque within the pillar" are internal cues focusing on muscle engagement rather than the movement from point A to B.[1]

INTERNAL FOCUS

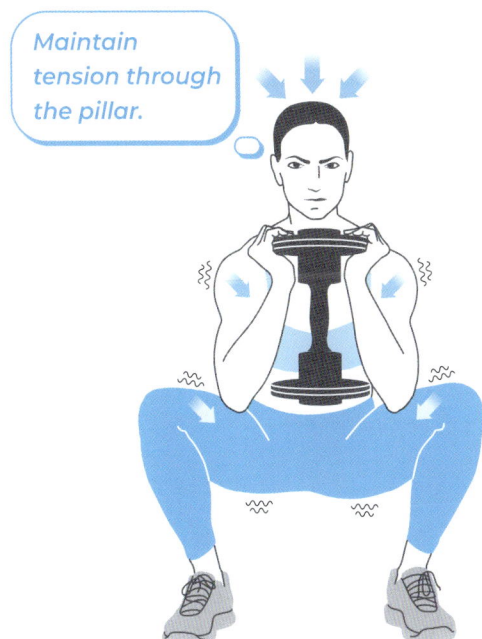

Maintain tension through the pillar.

EXTERNAL FOCUS

Explode the bar up to the ceiling.

RECOMMENDATIONS AND GUIDELINES

Have you ever been under a heavily loaded barbell, your mind racing with the checklist of what you need to do to execute the lift flawlessly? Or found yourself hesitating before a deadlift, doubting your readiness? Perhaps you've experienced an injury that could have been prevented with adequate warm-up and practice, or maybe you've reached a standstill in enhancing your mobility and movement due to inconsistent focus and preparation.

If any of these scenarios resonate with you, then the recommendations and guidelines outlined in this section will be immensely valuable. Think of them as your practice blueprint—actionable strategies that ensure you're not just going through the motions but actively progressing toward pain-free movement and performance mastery.

CHOOSE 1 OR 2 EXERCISES, MATCHING the PHASE 5 EXERCISE with the PRIMARY MOVEMENT (KPI) of the TRAINING DAY

Before you start the 6-phase warm-up, you will pick one foundational movement pattern as your KPI to prioritize in the workout. This makes selecting an exercise in phase 5 straightforward because you will have already chosen a movement pattern focus before starting phase 1. If your KPI is a barbell back squat, for example, pick a blueprint for the warm-up that addresses your squat or lower body linchpin, and then choose a squat exercise from phase 5, like a goblet squat.

It's important to note that you need to pick only one exercise in this phase to get a movement-enhancing benefit. However, I typically encourage choosing two exercises because, again, this is the best time to practice and refine your movement patterns.

AVOID THINKING (AND COACHING) WHEN IT'S TIME TO PERFORM

Skipping the warm-up and neglecting practice often leads to an unnecessary focus on technique during crucial performance moments. When the pressure mounts, your instinct should take the helm, not a conscious analysis of every movement detail. In high-stakes situations, such as executing a max-effort lift or movement, your mind should be clear of technical minutiae. Consider a barbell back squat at a challenging weight: pondering muscle engagement or form corrections mid-lift can disrupt your flow and increase the risk of failure, as my story elucidated.

Form matters, as you've learned, but errors will inevitably surface. These missteps provide invaluable feedback, shaping future training priorities without hampering performance in the moment. For instance, noting knee valgus during a heavy squat pinpoints what to address in subsequent phase 5 sessions (you should work to align your knees over your toes in this example), refining focus without overburdening the mind during execution.

Coaches play a pivotal role in this scenario. While well-intentioned, issuing a barrage of instructions mid-lift can do more harm than good, diverting attention from the task at hand. Effective coaching synchronizes with an athlete's goals and execution, offering guidance that enhances, not detracts from, performance.

The foundational work—instilling proper technique and responding to feedback—occurs in the preparatory stages: phase 5 of the warm-up and incremental priming sets (more on priming sets on page 442).

Again, internal cues are for refining technique, which occurs during practice. When it's time to perform, shift to external cues that direct focus outward, anchoring attention on the objective.

If you're following a body part split routine, where you focus solely on either upper or lower body movements, choose exercises that target the regions you plan to train. For instance, if it's an upper body workout, perform a push and/ or a pull exercise. If it's a lower body workout, choose one or pair two exercises from the squat, hinge, or lunge categories.

If you are doing a full-body workout, choose one upper body and one lower body exercise, matching the exercise to the main movement patterns or KPIs for the training session.

When you perform two phase 5 exercises—whether it is two upper body movements, two lower body movements, or one upper body and one lower body movement—I recommend combining them into a superset: perform one set with the first exercise, one set with the second exercise, and then repeat.

EMPHASIZE AND ACCENTUATE: ECCENTRIC PHASE, ISOMETRIC PAUSES, and CONTROL

To develop a movement pattern that emphasizes conscious engagement and learning, it is crucial to slow down and focus on specific segments of the movement. This approach involves extending the duration of the eccentric or lowering phase, pausing at challenging points, and controlling your body through the entire range of motion. Let's break down each aspect, focusing on the tempo and what you're trying to achieve in each stage.

1. **Accentuate the eccentric phase of the movement.** It normally takes 1 to 2 seconds to lower into the bottom position of a movement. I want you to extend it to 3 to 5 seconds. This slower pace fosters improved movement quality and heightens body awareness, contributing to better form and potentially reducing the risk of pain and injury by promoting mindful, deliberate movement.

2. **As you descend, pause when you feel your form falter, or at points requiring additional focus.** Typically, this is the bottom or lowest point of the movement. By performing an isometric hold—where muscles are contracting without any visible movement in the angle of the joints—you can home in on specific aspects of your form with a directed cue. If you lower into a squat and you feel your knees start to cave inward, pause and drive your knees out. If you are lowering into a hinge and you feel tension move from your hips to your back, pause to recalibrate by adjusting your knee position and shin angle, shifting tension into your hips and hamstrings. It's important to note that any stage of a movement—be it the top, midpoint, or bottom—can benefit from this strategic pause. Think of it as a positional checkpoint to verify and adjust your form.

3. **In the concentric or rising phase, maintain a consistent, controlled pace.** You're not exploding here; it's a similar tempo to your normal execution with a heavy load. This deliberate approach demands focus, as lighter weights can tempt you to accelerate, masking true control over the movement. To maintain an authentic concentric rhythm, approach the lighter weight as if it were a maximum-effort lift.

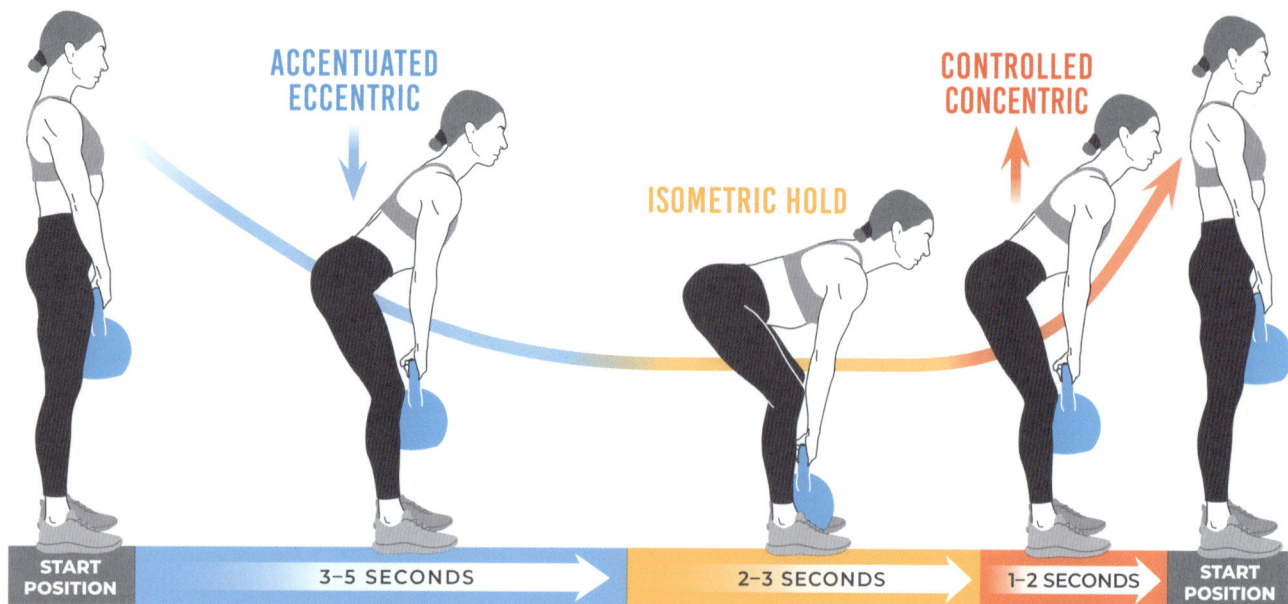

ACCENTUATED ECCENTRIC

ISOMETRIC HOLD

CONTROLLED CONCENTRIC

| START POSITION | 3–5 SECONDS | 2–3 SECONDS | 1–2 SECONDS | START POSITION |

In the military, there's a saying: Slow is smooth; smooth is fast. This mantra perfectly captures the execution that you're aiming for. Similar to the corrective exercises, focus on sequencing, stability, and smoothness. If the movement is clunky or you lose tension, you're probably moving too fast.

Speed negates tension. When you rush through a movement and lose tension, especially at the bottom position, you're not setting yourself up for success when managing load at that depth. Similarly, moving too quickly and losing pillar integrity at the top undermines control and essentially wastes the effort you put into setting up before starting the set. To stay in control and avoid moving too fast, it's crucial to be mindful and maintain the mind-muscle connection throughout each movement.

In phase 4—the activation phase—you focused heavily on establishing that mind-muscle connection. You directed your attention to activating the specific muscles targeted by each exercise. However, the activation exercises in phase 4 are region-specific and don't mimic the full foundational movement patterns. In phase 5, the goal is to apply that same mind-muscle connection, but now you're carrying over the muscle activation from phase 4 into the exercises of phase 5.

Say you performed a glute bridge in phase 4. In this scenario, your focus was on feeling your glutes and the surrounding muscles activate during the exercise. Here, you transfer the activation you felt in phase 4 into the phase 5 lower body movements—feeling tension in your posterior chain that stabilizes and powers the squat, hinge, or lunge patterns.

MAXIMIZE INTERNAL TENSION (MAKE LIGHT WEIGHT FEEL HEAVY)

In the Pillar chapter, you learned how to stabilize your hips, shoulders, and core using co-contractions and the irradiation effect. Then you followed it up in the Breathing Strategies chapter by learning how to coordinate your breath to maximize and maintain tension and stability during movement. Now it's time to put these concepts into practice.

The idea is simple: brace your pillar and move as if you were performing a one-rep max lift. If you're goblet squatting with a 35-pound dumbbell, for example, pretend that you're holding a 150-pound dumbbell.

To make it realistic, dial up internal tension through the pillar by

1. Co-contracting the main muscle groups surrounding your hips and shoulders. Contract your pecs and lats, and glutes and adductors maximally.

2. Creating a rotational force (torque or irradiation) with your hands and feet. Press your hands into the dumbbell, gripping it as tightly as possible, while simultaneously rotating your feet into the floor—driving your big toes into the ground, creating arches in your feet, and turning your knees outward without moving your feet. You should feel the tension in your hips and shoulders increase.

3. Bracing with the Double Breath Technique (page 49). Begin with a deep nasal inhalation, holding your breath momentarily at full lung capacity, and then take a second, shallower mouth breath to fully expand your lung capacity and core, followed by a contraction of the muscles around your trunk.

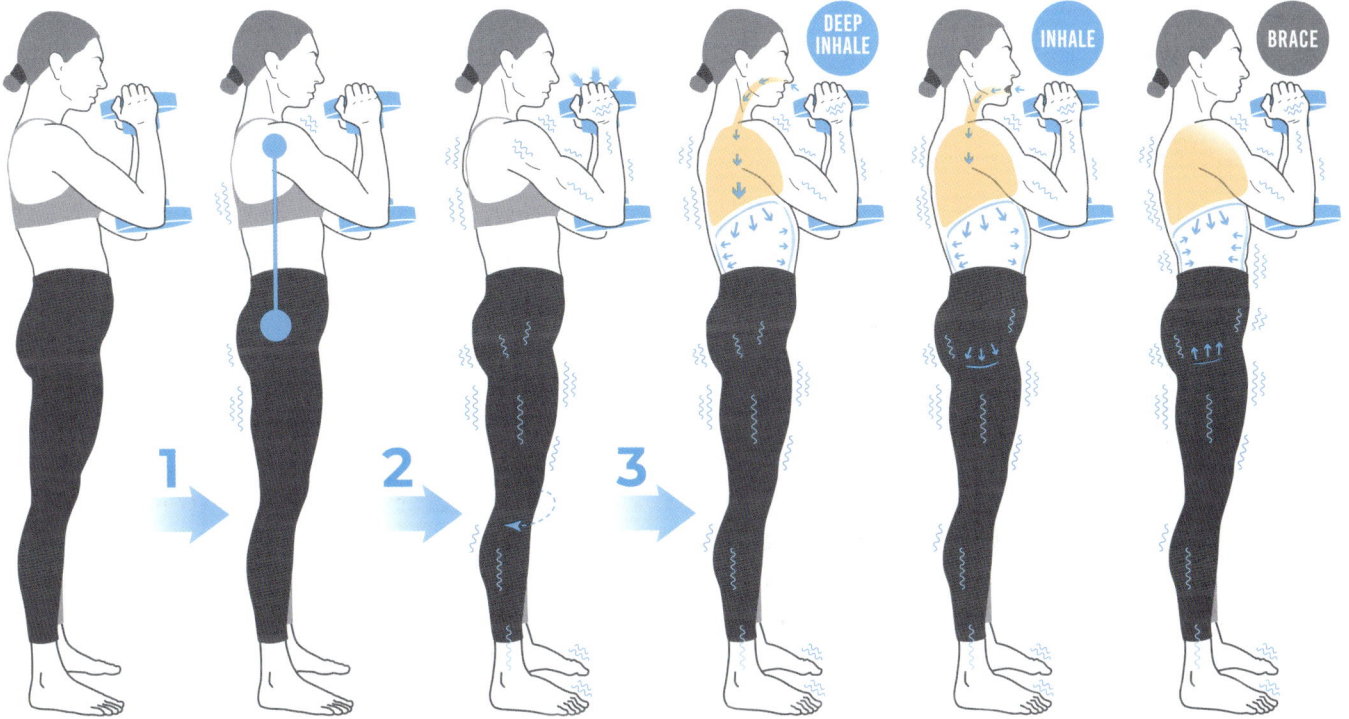

4. Perform the goblet squat while maintaining maximum internal tension. Hold your breath during the descent, push air out slightly and slowing during the concentric phase, and then sip air at the top as if "sipping through a straw." Remember, you will never take a full breath between reps (revisit pages 34–35 for a more precise breakdown on breathing and bracing).

It doesn't matter which phase 5 exercise you are practicing—the goal is to make light weight feel heavy. This approach is designed to mirror the level of engagement you would apply in heavier, performance-focused training, emphasizing maximum internal tension and pillar stability.

This takes effort, which is the point. Phase 5 should feel like training. You're preparing to perform, doing just enough to simulate a max-effort lift without the stress or danger of lifting a max-effort load.

Think of this process as a mental and physical rehearsal to optimize the movement pattern for that day, aiming to refine it to its best form before you launch into the workout where the focus shifts from practice to performance.

PERFORM 3 TO 5 SETS OF 3 TO 5 REPS, ADJUSTING and IMPROVING with EACH SET and REP

The number of sets and reps you perform depends on two things: the number of exercises you are practicing and the quality of your movement.

For a single exercise, aim for 3 to 5 sets. When incorporating two exercises, a total of 4 sets—2 sets per exercise—is enough. Again, I recommend alternating between exercises in a superset format for efficiency and focus.

Whether it's one exercise or two, the sets shouldn't push you to fatigue, so extensive rest periods aren't necessary—just enough time, 15 to 30 seconds, to reset, refocus, and concentrate on the specific cue that will refine your movement.

FOCUS ON ONE CUE THAT WORKS FOR YOU

The essence here is personalization—finding the one cue that resonates with your technique and consistently applying it to sharpen your execution. The pitfall many fall into is trying to manage and improve every aspect of their form in one training session, toggling their attention from one cue to another. Such scattered focus can dilute the potency of this phase, leading to numerous reps executed without meaningful improvement.

The key is to concentrate on your most significant linchpin, utilizing a cue that helps improve the weakest or most pain-potentiating aspect of the movement. For example, if your lower back flares up during hinge exercises, then you should utilize a cue that emphasizes pillar stability, such as "stay tight," or perhaps a cue that directs your attention to the sequencing of the hinge pattern, such as "push your hips back."

By focusing on one cue specific to your form, you create a foundation for consistent, targeted development. This singular focus not only simplifies your process but deepens the effectiveness of each set and rep, turning practice into progress. As you home in on this one cue, you ingrain it into your muscle memory, building a movement pattern that becomes second nature. Over time, this approach cultivates a resilience that translates to more complex movements and heavier loads, enhancing both your performance and your resilience against injury. In essence, by narrowing your focus to one transformative cue, you amplify the benefits of your training, propelling yourself closer to movement mastery.

TREAT PHASE 5 AS A MOVEMENT SCREEN

A movement screen is a systematic evaluation process used to assess and develop the quality of the movement, identify and address imbalances or limitations, and inform training for the pattern.

Before introducing load or speed to a movement, it's crucial to conduct a movement screen to tailor its implementation in your workout, acknowledging that your performance will fluctuate from day to day. On some days, movements may feel strong and smooth, while on others, they might feel weak and labored. Phase 5 provides a consistent, automatic screening within every training session, giving you an opportunity to adapt to the variable conditions of your life—be it pain, poor sleep, or other stressors—that might influence how you move.

In other words, this phase involves assessing your movement quality and your subjective readiness during its execution to determine appropriate modifications in load, effort, volume, or the exercise itself.

For example, say your KPI is a barbell back squat—the most challenging squat variation in terms of loading potential. In this scenario, you perform the goblet squat in phase 5, matching the pattern to your KPI.

Now, let's say on this particular day your knee hurts every time you descend into the squat—and cuing proper mechanics doesn't resolve the issue. Do you power through the pain and stick to the plan? Absolutely not. You should use this valuable insight to adapt your KPI, either by reducing the intensity of the exercise (load, range, etc.) or by regressing to a pain-free variation.

On the flip side, if you're moving pain-free and the pattern feels stable and smooth, you can confidently advance, assured that you're primed for the KPI.

Realize the objective: It is not to highlight deficiencies, but to empower and improve. By examining and refining movement patterns in a supportive manner, you set the stage for either progressing or regressing exercises based on your current condition. This adaptive approach is fundamental to pain-free performance, confirming that before you apply load or speed, you screen and optimize the movement, readying yourself for safe and effective training.

When you are learning how to perform the foundational movement patterns, you start with the basics: stance, body position, and pillar stability. Then you gradually add internal cues—concise directives—that guide the technique and execution of the movement.

With each cue, you cultivate a deeper connection with the pattern, allowing you to think and feel your way through it. Maybe you need to reduce the range of motion to maintain pillar neutrality, or perhaps you need to adjust the width of your stance to achieve greater control. Phase 5 is where you make those corrections and modifications and home in on the cues that serve your unique needs.

In the next section, you will learn how to execute the six foundational movement patterns, which, again, are the functional movements integral to human biomechanics. More specifically, you will learn the cues that guide optimal form and execution and how to customize the movement to suit your individual skill set and needs. The exercises in this chapter introduce the universal internal cues. But it's your job to apply those cues to your unique stance, range, and technique.

EXERCISE APPENDIX

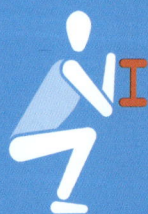

PHASE 5:
MOVEMENT PATTERN DEVELOPMENT

WHAT ABOUT THE CARRY PATTERN?

You might be wondering why the carry pattern—that is, locomotion (walking, running, crawling, etc.)—is missing from phase 5. There are a couple of reasons for this omission.

First, the carry isn't considered a KPI and is generally performed at the end of a workout as a finisher. Even when the carry is the focus of a training session—during a conditioning or cardio workout, for example—you'd still prioritize a more complex lower body exercise in phase 5 because it expresses the full movement potential of your joints, which better prepares your muscles and body for the demands of the workout.

Second, the carry pattern is relatively simple compared to the squat, hinge, lunge, push, and pull. This ties into the first reason—it's not typically a KPI or prioritized in phase 5 because it doesn't require as much practice. Unlike exercises that involve complex movement patterns and full joint articulation, the carry doesn't challenge your body's full range of motion in the same way. Movements that require you to work through a greater range are inherently more complex, demanding more practice to refine and focus on maintaining form under load. That's why these more intricate patterns take precedence in phase 5, allowing you to master the essential skills needed to advance to more complex variations.

You'll find more about how to effectively incorporate the carry pattern into your training in the dedicated Carry chapter.

Scan the QR code to access demos of each exercise.

SQUAT

GOBLET SQUAT

PURPOSE: The goblet squat is a foundational exercise for practicing and screening the squat pattern. Unlike the bodyweight squat, the goblet squat's anterior load—holding a weight in front of the body—naturally encourages a neutral spine and a stable torso, making it easier to reinforce proper pillar mechanics and shoulder stability. The weight in front shifts your center of gravity slightly forward, which helps keep your torso more upright and reduces the tendency to lean forward excessively. This positioning also promotes greater engagement of the core and shoulders, adding stability to the entire movement.

While the bodyweight squat is a useful regression (see the squat pyramid on page 260), the goal here is to enhance pillar mechanics by creating torque and irradiation. Holding a light weight in front allows you to engage these stabilizing forces more effectively, increasing tension throughout the body.

SETUP AND EXECUTION: For the goblet squat, choose a manageable weight—a kettlebell or dumbbell—that allows you to perform 3 to 5 reps with control. The load should feel comfortable yet provide enough resistance to encourage proper form without excessive strain.

If you're a powerlifter, you might think, "If my 1RM is 400 pounds, I could probably manage 180 pounds for 5 reps easily." However, the goal in phase 5 is to make light weight feel heavy, so you should select a weight that's 10 to 30 percent of your body weight. More weight is not better. Less weight with better form and pillar engagement is what you're after.

1. Stance: Begin by setting up in your authentic squat stance (see the squat assessment on page 240). Hold a kettlebell or dumbbell close to your chest with both hands, positioning it under your chin. Keep your elbows tucked in close to your body while co-contracting your pecs and lats to stabilize the weight.

2. Bracing: Go through the bracing sequence (pages 34–35) to stabilize your pillar.

3. Execution: Perform 3 to 5 reps, focusing on controlled movement through each phase of the squat. Begin by bending at the knees and hips simultaneously, lowering yourself in a smooth, balanced motion. You should feel tension in your hips and quads. Keep the weight close to your chest and your core engaged to stabilize your torso as you descend. Aim to reach a depth where your thighs are at least parallel to the ground or go as

low as feels comfortable without compromising your form. Press evenly through your feet to return to standing, engaging your glutes and quads as you rise. Throughout each rep, ensure you meet each standard in the optimization checklist:

✓ **Neutral Spine:** Stay within your neutral spine throughout the squat, avoiding excessive rounding or arching.

✓ **No Unwanted Rotation:** Keep your shoulders, hips, knees, and ankles symmetrical.

✓ **Strong Foot and Ankle Position:** Distribute your weight in front of your ankles and press your feet firmly into the ground, creating stability through the arches and maintaining control of your ankle alignment.

✓ **Knees Tracking Toes:** Guide your knees in line with your toes to promote proper joint alignment and protect against inward collapse.

✓ **Shin Angle Roughly Matches Torso Angle:** Aim for your shin angle to match your torso angle for balanced alignment and weight distribution.

To learn more about the goblet squat and how to optimize the squat movement pattern, see the dedicated Squat chapter. This chapter provides essential assessments, exercise regressions, and optimization strategies—detailed cues and guidelines for mobility, stability, and skill—to help you build a strong foundation and address any compensations identified during your squat screen.

HINGE

ROMANIAN DEADLIFT (RDL)

PURPOSE: The RDL is an ideal exercise for screening the hinge pattern and promoting posterior chain mobility. Starting with the weight in front at the top of the movement allows you to set your pillar and establish stability more easily than having to brace from the bottom position as in a traditional deadlift, making it especially effective for the focus of phase 5.

SETUP AND EXECUTION: Select a manageable weight (typically between 10 and 30 percent of your

body weight). The load should feel comfortable yet provide enough resistance to reinforce proper form without strain, allowing you to perform 3 to 5 reps with control. You can use either a kettlebell or a dumbbell, but the kettlebell has a slight advantage due to its handle design, which allows you to generate torque and irradiation. Gripping the handle firmly and applying a slight rotational force helps activate your forearms and shoulders, creating greater stability and reinforcing shoulder engagement throughout the movement.

1. Stance: Stand with your feet hip-width apart, toes pointing straight forward. Hold a kettlebell or dumbbell in front of your thighs with straight arms. Engage your pecs and lats to stabilize the weight.

2. Bracing: Follow the bracing sequence (pages 34–35) to stabilize your core and maintain a strong pillar throughout the movement.

3. Execution: Perform 3 to 5 reps with controlled movement through the full range of motion. Initiate the movement by pushing your hips back, creating tension in your core and a stretch along your hamstrings. Keep the weight close to your thighs and shins as you descend, stabilizing your torso with core engagement. Aim to lower the weight just below your knees or as far as you can without compromising form (especially avoiding any rounding in the lumbar spine). Press evenly through your feet and drive your hips forward to return to standing, engaging your glutes and hamstrings as you rise. Focus on the following standards in each rep to meet the optimization checklist:

✓ **Neutral Spine:** Maintain a neutral spine throughout, avoiding arching or lumbar rounding.

✓ **No Unwanted Rotation:** Keep your shoulders, hips, knees, and ankles aligned.

✓ **Strong Foot and Ankle Position:** Distribute your weight across your entire foot, ensuring big toe contact with the ground as you hinge back.

✓ **Vertical Shins:** Allow a slight bend in your knees but aim to keep your shins vertical to minimize forward knee movement.

KETTLEBELL

DUMBBELL

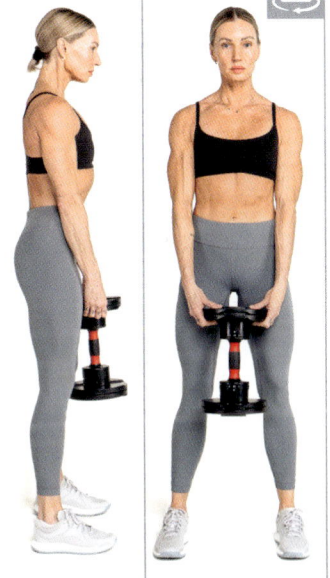

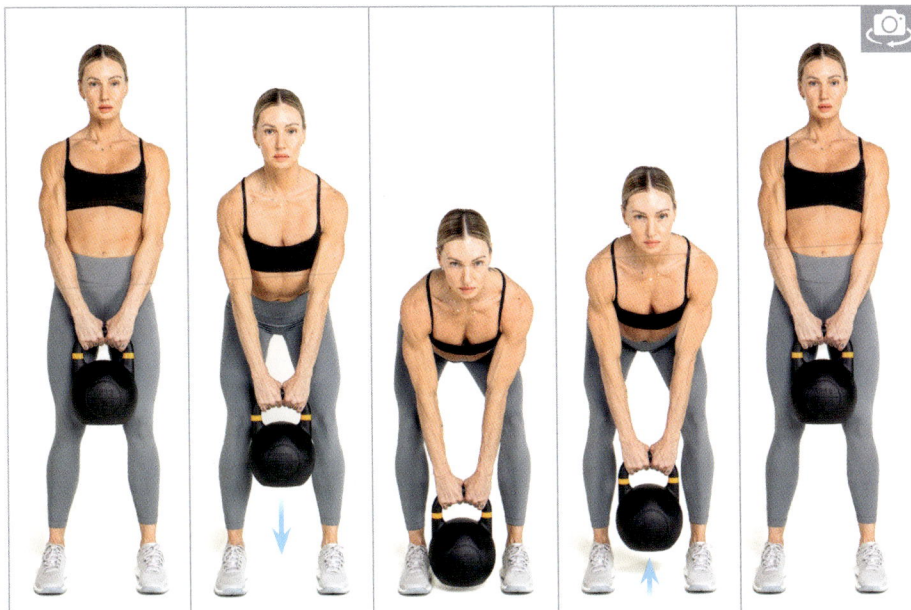

To learn more about the RDL and how to optimize the hinge pattern, see the dedicated Hinge chapter. This chapter offers essential assessments, regressions, and optimization strategies, providing detailed cues and guidelines for enhancing mobility, stability, and skill to build a strong foundation and address any compensations identified in your hinge screen.

LUNGE

The lunge pattern captures aspects of both the squat and the hinge patterns in split-stance and single-leg contexts, dynamically engaging the lower body while challenging the core, hips, and legs to promote pillar stability and functional movement.

With three options to choose from—the split squat, reverse lunge, and single-leg RDL—your choice ultimately depends on two factors: what you can perform successfully and what best complements the workout ahead.

The split squat is an excellent choice if you're new to exercise, focusing on building stability and balance, or aiming to reduce knee or back discomfort.

The reverse lunge is a great alternative if your workout will incorporate more dynamic movements, such as a loaded lunge variation. The added movement of stepping back and forward prepares you for more explosive or athletic activities later in the session.

The single-leg RDL is an ideal choice when you want to prepare for hinging movements in your workout, such as deadlifts or dynamic kettlebell exercises. This option also helps balance your overall movement pattern selections, which is particularly beneficial if you're training three or more times per week.

SPLIT SQUAT

PURPOSE: In phase 5 of the warm-up, the split squat combines stability and mobility in a functional lower body movement, reinforcing balance, pillar engagement, and control split-stance exercises.

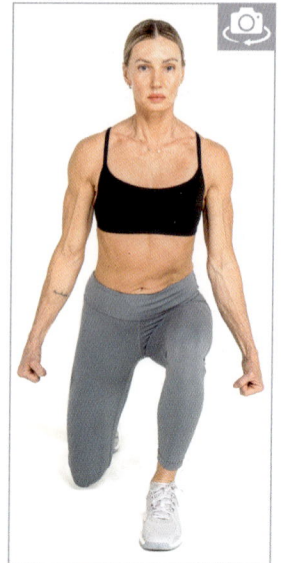
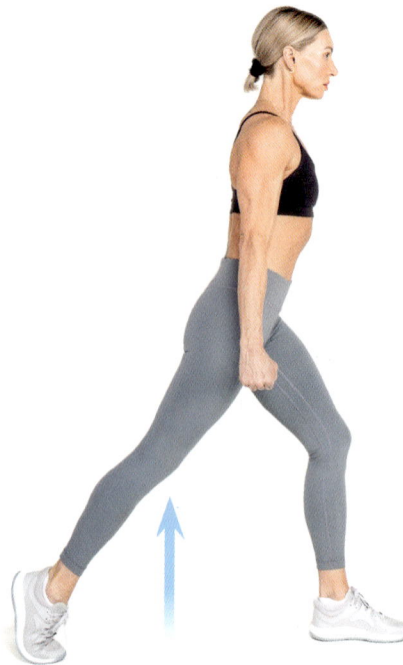
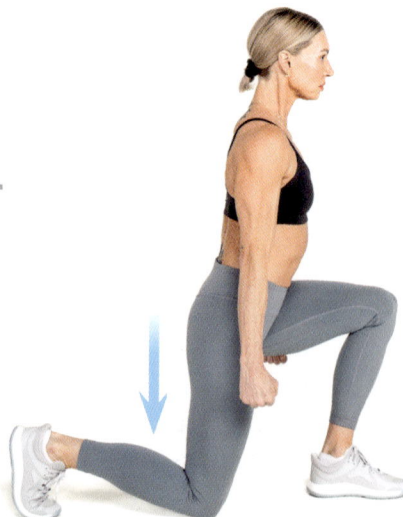
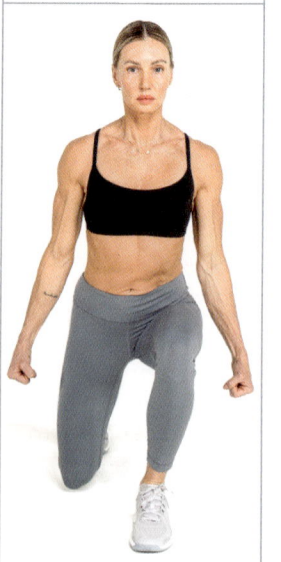

SETUP AND EXECUTION: The split squat can be performed as a bodyweight exercise, which is ideal for focusing on positioning, form, range of motion, and control—all essential for phase 5. For added challenge, you can hold a light dumbbell in each hand, but keep the load manageable to prioritize stability and controlled movement.

1. Stance: Start in a half-kneeling position with all joints at 90 degrees. Position your back knee directly under your hip with your back toes tucked under. Place your front foot so that your front shin is vertical and the knee of that leg is directly over the ankle.

2. Bracing: Go through the bracing sequence (pages 34–35) to stabilize your pillar. For split squats, it's important to dig your back toes into the ground and create torque and tension at the hips by pushing your back leg forward and pulling your front leg back (without moving your feet). This action brings your pelvis into a neutral, forward-facing position that enhances stability in the split stance.

3. Execution: Perform 3 to 5 reps on each leg, focusing on controlled movement throughout each repetition.

- **Ascending:** Push the floor away with both feet to stand up fully, maintaining your center of mass over your base of support. Your weight should be fairly evenly distributed between your feet—approximately 60 percent on the front foot and 40 percent on the back foot.

- **Descending:** Lower back down with stability and control. If you're using a pad or mat, lightly touch your back knee down. Otherwise, stop when your back knee is hovering just above the floor.

Throughout each rep, ensure you meet each standard in the optimization checklist:

✓ **Neutral Spine:** Maintain a neutral spine, specifically avoiding arching your back (which is common if you lack hip mobility or core stability).

✓ **No Unwanted Rotation:** Keep your shoulders, hips, knees, and ankles aligned symmetrically.

✓ **Strong Foot and Ankle Position:**
- *Front Foot:* Distribute your weight evenly and press your foot firmly into the ground, creating stability through the arch and maintaining control of your ankle alignment.
- *Back Foot:* Keep your foot active by pushing up onto the ball of your foot so your heel is stacked above your toes.

✓ **Knees Tracking Toes:** Guide your knees in line with your toes to promote proper joint alignment and prevent inward collapse.

✓ **Shin and Torso Angle:** While there's a range of acceptable angles, understand that different positions target muscles differently:
- *Vertical Shin and Forward Torso Lean:* Targets more glute involvement. Be cautious if your quads are weaker—you might unintentionally push your hips back to compensate.
- *Knee Traveling Forward Over Toes:* Emphasizes the quads. If you lack posterior chain stability and strength, this might be the only way you can perform the movement initially.
- *Shin and Torso Relatively Parallel:* The optimal position. This alignment helps you build strength across multiple positions and serves you well when progressing to the loaded Bulgarian split squat— one of the most functional single-leg exercises.

REVERSE LUNGE

PURPOSE: The reverse lunge is an ideal first "stepping" exercise to reinforce stability and control in the lunge pattern. With most of your body weight on the front leg throughout each rep, the reverse lunge allows you to establish bracing, tension, and stability around the hips, supporting effective screening and optimizing alignment, balance, and movement quality before progressing to more dynamic variations.

SETUP AND EXECUTION: Performing the reverse lunge as a bodyweight exercise is ideal for phase 5. However, you can hold a light dumbbell in each hand to amplify tension and stability through your pillar.

1. Stance: Stand with the majority of your body weight shifted into the leg that will remain static throughout the set.

2. Bracing: Go through the bracing sequence (pages 34–35) to stabilize your pillar. Focus on stabilizing around the leg and hip that stay static during the set.

3. Execution: Perform 3 to 5 reps on each leg, concentrating on controlled movement through each rep. Step back into a hip-width stance and position your back leg far enough back so that when you lower into the lunge, both knees bend to approximately 90 degrees. You may feel a stretch sensation in your rear quad. That's fine. Allow your torso to hinge forward slightly to keep your center of mass aligned as you step back. This will place about 75 percent of your body weight on the front leg. For the back leg, keep your toes tucked under and your foot active, stacking your heel over your toes. Push off the back foot to return to the starting position. To maintain stability with repeated reps, keep most of your weight on the static leg, tapping the moving foot down gently rather than shifting weight evenly between both feet. Just be sure to fully extend your working leg and stand tall as you complete each rep.

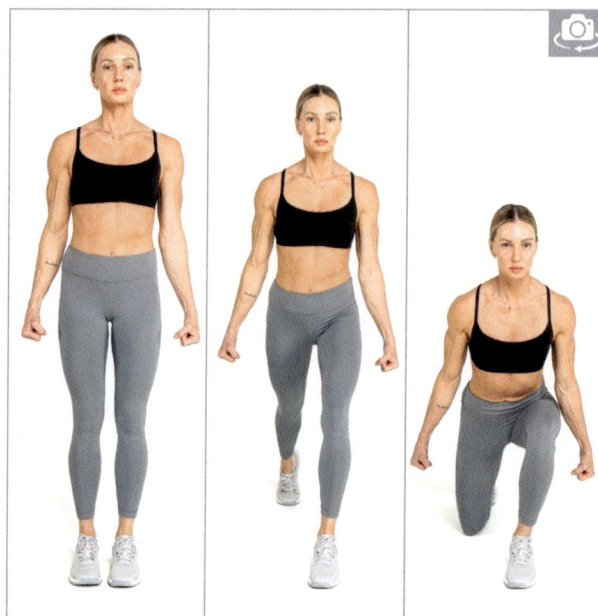

REVERSE LUNGE

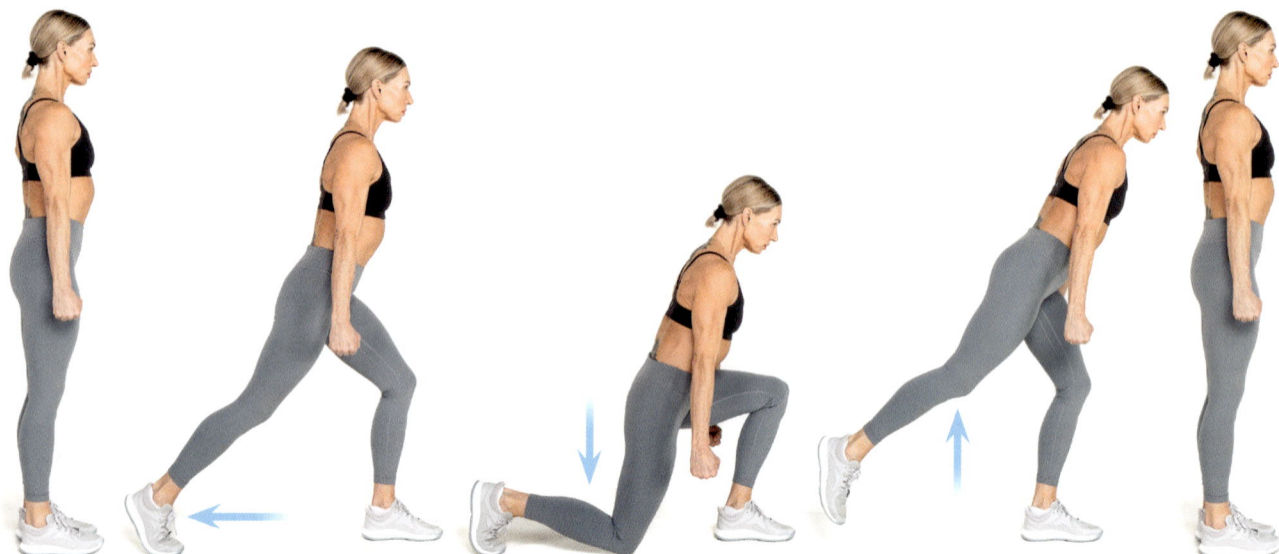

Throughout each rep, meet the standards in the optimization checklist:

✓ **Neutral Spine:** Maintain a neutral spine, avoiding arching or rounding.

✓ **No Unwanted Rotation:** Keep shoulders, hips, knees, and ankles symmetrical.

✓ **Strong Foot and Ankle Position:**

• *Front Foot:* Distribute your weight across the front of your ankle, pressing firmly into the ground to stabilize through the arch and maintain ankle alignment.

• *Back Foot:* Tuck your toes under, staying active by pressing onto the ball of your foot and stacking your heel above your toes.

✓ **Knees Tracking Toes:** Guide your knees—especially your front knee—in line with your toes for proper alignment and to prevent inward collapse.

✓ **Shin Angle & Torso Angle:** In the reverse lunge, since 75 percent of your body weight remains in the front leg, a more vertical shin and a slightly forward-leaning torso is ideal.

To learn more about the split squat, reverse lunge, and RDL and how to optimize the lunge movement pattern, see the dedicated Lunge chapter. This chapter provides essential assessments and optimization strategies—detailed cues and guidelines for mobility, stability, and skill—to help you build a strong foundation and address any compensations identified during your lunge screen.

SINGLE-LEG ROMANIAN DEADLIFT (RDL)

PURPOSE: The single-leg RDL builds balance, stability, and body awareness—essential for controlled, efficient movement. By practicing this exercise in phase 5, you set the stage for smoother, more powerful hinge and single-leg movements in your workouts, unlocking greater control and confidence across all foundational patterns.

SETUP AND EXECUTION: This movement can be challenging for many. Start by placing your hand on a wall or rack for support if needed, gradually progressing to an unsupported version as you build coordination, balance, and control. Holding a very light weight can also provide added stability by giving you a focal point to help keep your shoulders

and hips square, promoting balanced alignment throughout the movement. Additionally, the slight counterbalance can help anchor your body, making it easier to control your range of motion.

1. Stance: Begin with your feet together. Shift your weight onto your working (static) leg and bend the opposite knee to 90 degrees, keeping your foot dorsiflexed (toes to shin). This positioning enhances proprioception and stability, laying the groundwork for better movement control.

2. Bracing: Use the bracing sequence (pages 34–35) to stabilize your pillar. Since you're standing on one leg, imagine squeezing your inner thighs together to create more hip stability and alignment.

3. Execution: Perform 3 to 5 controlled reps. Begin by hinging at the hips, pushing them back as your non-working leg remains bent at 90 degrees. You should feel tension in your core and a stretch in the hamstring of your grounded leg. Reach your opposite arm toward the grounded foot. Focus on stability and form over depth; reaching just below knee level is sufficient for most people. To return to the starting position, press into the floor and drive your hips forward, maintaining alignment from your back thigh to shoulder. Throughout each rep, ensure you meet each standard in the optimization checklist:

✓ **Neutral Spine:** Stay within your neutral zone, avoiding any arching or rounding in your lower back.

✓ **No Unwanted Rotation:** Keep your shoulders, hips, knees, and ankles aligned. Focus especially on keeping both hip points facing straight ahead, as the elevated leg hip often wants to rotate outward. Resist this rotation to stay square and stable.

✓ **Strong Foot and Ankle Position:** Distribute your weight evenly across your entire foot, grounding your big toe for stability as you hinge back. Keep your ankle stacked over your foot and engage your arch to maintain a strong, active stance.

✓ **Relatively Vertical Shin:** A slight bend in your standing knee is fine, but aim to keep your shin mostly vertical to limit forward knee movement.

PUSH

PUSH-UP

PURPOSE: The push-up is a fundamental exercise for developing and screening the push pattern. It requires core activation and stability in the plank position, creating a strong platform for scapular movement and shoulder stability.

SETUP AND EXECUTION: If floor push-ups exceed your current strength capacity, try an elevated push-up on a bench, box, or barbell in a squat rack. If you experience wrist discomfort, a barbell in the rack allows a more neutral wrist position. Alternatively, on the floor, you can use wedges under your palms, hold hex dumbbells for stability, or use parallettes or push-up bars to keep your wrists neutral in a stacked position.

1. Stance: Begin in a quadruped position (or with hands on a bench, feet below hips for elevated push-ups). Spread your fingers wide (or firmly grip the bar/handles), pressing down as if you're gripping or trying to spread the floor beneath you. This activation through your hands, forearms, and shoulders creates a stable base and helps prevent shoulder shrugging. Establish strong shoulder positioning by pressing the floor away and slightly drawing your head and chin back (see push assessment for ideal hand placement).

2. Bracing: Use the bracing sequence (pages 34–35) to stabilize your pillar. Step one leg back with your toes flush with the ground. Engage your quad and glute to lock in that leg, then repeat with the other leg. Position your feet about hip-width apart. Squeeze your adductors to secure your hips and pelvis, creating full-body tension from your shoulders to your feet. Draw your ribs toward your hips to reinforce core stability.

3. Execution: Perform 3 to 5 reps with a slow, controlled movement. As you lower, keep a solid plank alignment, with your feet as the hinge point and every muscle engaged. Focus on evenly distributing pressure through both hands, pressing through your entire palm—especially the bases of your thumb and pinky fingers—to create shoulder stability. Lower to a depth that maintains full-body engagement without compromising shoulder position. To press back up, keep tension in your glutes and core, and press the floor away, extending your arms fully but avoiding elbow lockout to keep continuous activation and stability in your shoulders and torso.

Throughout each rep, meet each standard in the optimization checklist:

✓ **Neutral Spine:** Stay within your neutral zone, avoiding hip lifting or sagging.

✓ **No Unwanted Rotation:** Keep shoulders and hips symmetrical. Avoid shoulder shrugging or forward rolling.

✓ **Fully Irradiated Body:** Whether your hands are on the floor, a bar, or handles, focus on spreading your fingers wide and actively pressing down, as if you're gripping or trying to spread the floor apart beneath you. This "gripping" action activates muscles in your hands, forearms, and shoulders, creating a stable, controlled base and helping prevent shoulder shrugging.

✓ **Dynamic Scapular Movement:** Allow the scapulae to retract and depress slightly on the way down, then protract to stay flush against the rib cage as you press up.

To learn more about the push-up and how to optimize the push movement pattern, see the dedicated Push chapter. This chapter provides essential assessments and optimization strategies—detailed cues and guidelines for mobility, stability, and skill—to help you build a strong foundation and address any compensations identified during your push screen.

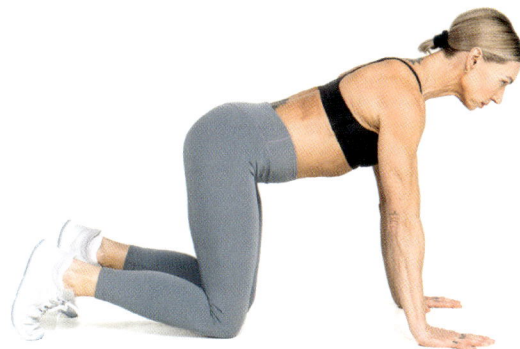

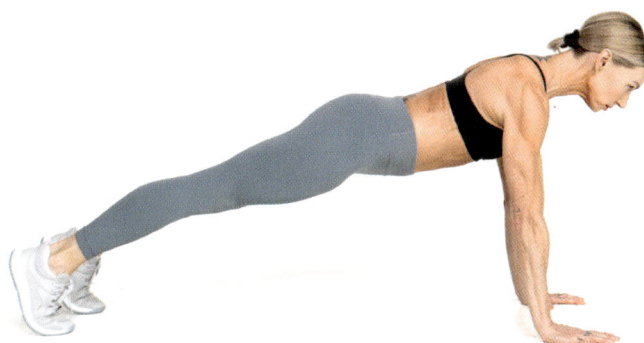

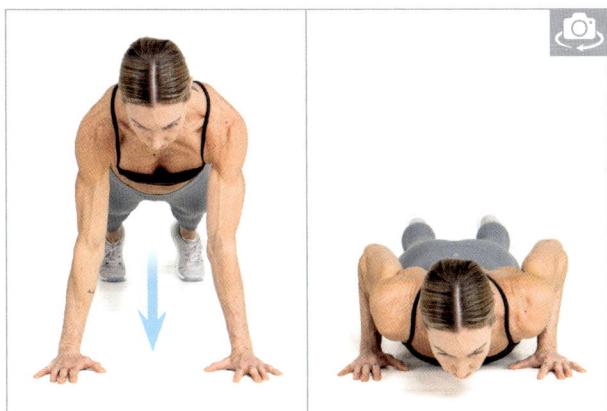

PULL

INVERTED ROW

PURPOSE: The inverted row variation is foundational for practicing and screening the pull pattern in the horizontal plane. The reverse plank position activates the posterior chain by keeping the hips extended, which engages the glutes, core, and back muscles. This full-body engagement helps maintain optimal shoulder alignment, reducing strain and promoting pain-free shoulders by distributing load evenly across stabilizing muscles.

SETUP AND EXECUTION: Before starting, ensure your suspension or ring setup is properly adjusted to allow for a full range of motion. Follow these steps to maximize alignment, stability, and control in every rep.

1. Handle Height: Adjust the handles so they're at the top of your thighs where your hip creases during a hinge. Take hold of the handles, pulling your thumbs back toward your armpits to create initial tension on the straps as you walk your feet back. Then lean back and walk your feet forward until they're directly under the anchor point. Ideally, your body should be at about a 45-degree angle; if this feels too challenging, step your feet back a few inches for a 60-degree angle.

2. Stance: Position your feet hip-width apart, with your heels, hips, shoulders, and head aligned in a straight line, forming a "reverse plank." Look toward the anchor point to keep your neck in neutral alignment. Depending on your footwear and surface, you may lift your toes to ground your heels. If sliding occurs, keep your full soles on the ground or use a bumper plate or wedge to anchor your feet.

3. Bracing: Squeeze your glutes and align your ribs with your hips to prevent arching in the lower back. Engage your lats by sliding your armpits down toward your waist, and keep your wrists and forearms aligned in a neutral position (avoid curling your wrists; palms should face each other).

4. Execution: Lower yourself down smoothly, maintaining a strong reverse plank. Brace your core, keep your glutes engaged, and maintain a firm grip. At the bottom, ensure an "active hang" by keeping your muscles engaged rather than relaxing into your connective tissues. To return to the top, drive your elbows back past your rib cage while maintaining plank alignment, using your heels as the fulcrum.

Throughout each rep, meet each standard in the optimization checklist:

✓ **Neutral Spine:** Keep a neutral spine throughout, avoiding sagging, curling, arching, or rib flaring.

✓ **No Unwanted Rotation:** Keep your shoulders and hips aligned. Avoid shoulder shrugging or rolling forward.

✓ **Fully Irradiated Body:** Maintain full-body tension from heels to head, with hips extended and posture tall.

✓ **Dynamic Scapular Movement:** Allow your scapulae to retract (draw together) and depress (move downward) on the way up, then protract (move forward) slightly to wrap around the rib cage as you lower.

To learn more about the pull and how to optimize the pull movement pattern, turn to the dedicated Pull chapter. This chapter provides essential assessment references and optimization strategies—detailed cues and guidelines for mobility, stability, and skill—to help you build a strong foundation and address any compensations identified during your pull screen.

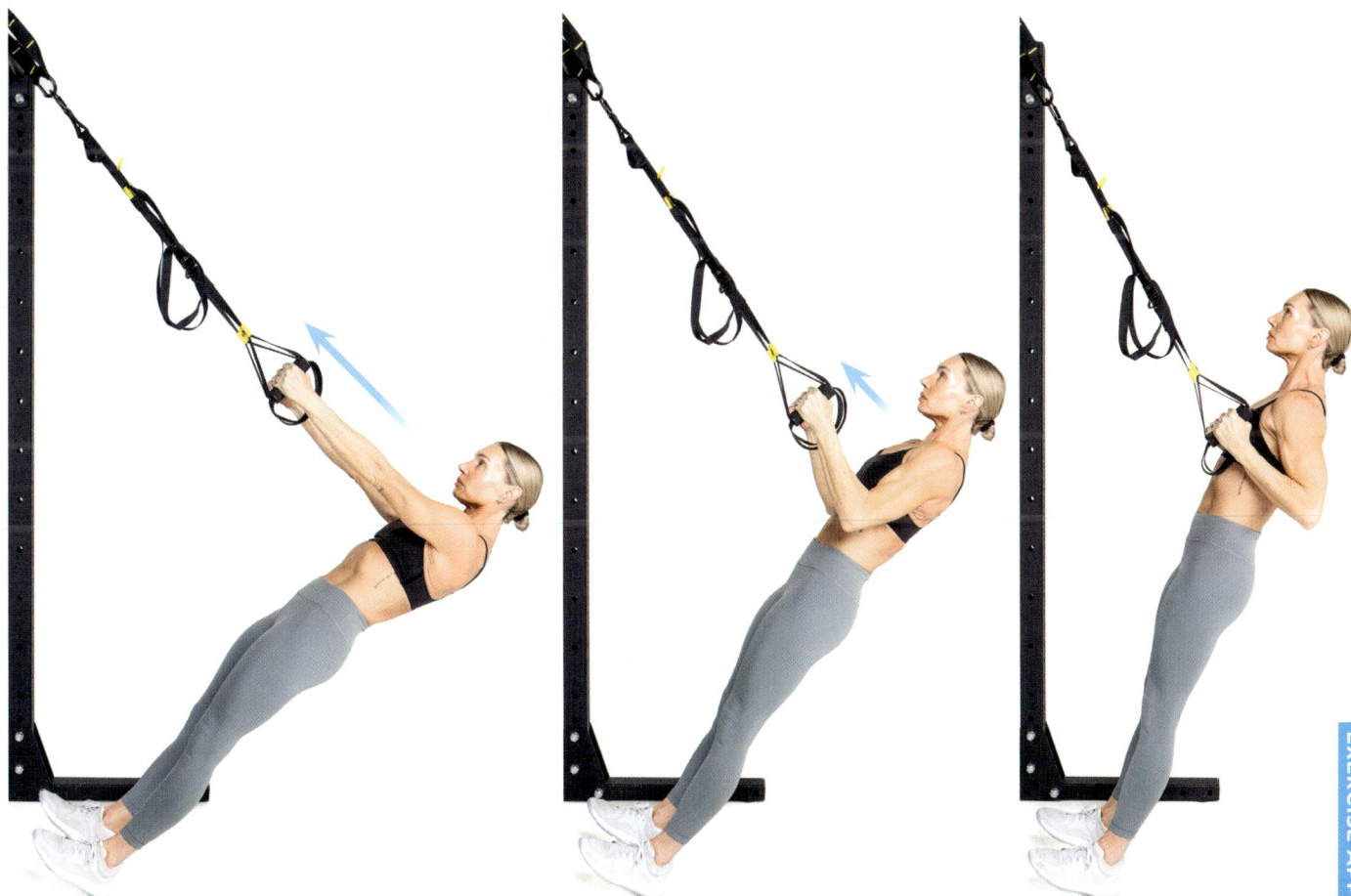

PHASE 6:
CENTRAL NERVOUS SYSTEM STIMULATION

Phase 6, central nervous system stimulation, is where you train, develop, and maintain your athletic prowess. You ramp up motor unit recruitment and ignite the CNS, locking in the benefits from the previous phases while priming the mind and body for the challenges and strain of training. Utilize two exercises, targeting different movement patterns. Move with speed and precision, placing maximal effort and focus into every rep.

For as long as I can remember, I've been obsessed with sports performance. I immersed myself in competitive sports as a youth, embracing the identity of an athlete. This meant more than just showing up for practice and games—it was a commitment that influenced every aspect of my life. I adopted the disciplined routines, focused mindset, and relentless pursuit of excellence that defined what it means to be an athlete. I learned to set goals and push through adversity, viewing each challenge as an opportunity to grow and improve. My daily choices, from how I ate and slept to how I managed my time, were all driven by my athletic aspirations, fostering a sense of purpose that revolved around competitive sports.

This dedication eventually led me to Division I baseball, where I lived and breathed the ethos of an athlete. But as fate would have it, injury struck during my sophomore year, ending any hopes of going pro. With my dreams of a professional athletic career out of reach, I turned my focus to personal training, still driven by my obsession with sports performance.

Even though I wasn't competing anymore, I still considered myself an athlete. In fact, I initially only worked with fellow athletes, applying everything I had learned from years of training, both on the field and in the weight room. My foundation had been built early, guided by my father—a high school athletic director who emphasized the importance of strength and conditioning. From an early age, he, along with other coaches, exposed me to the strategies behind building athletic attributes, which I now aimed to pass on to the athletes I trained.

As I gained more experience, working with professional athletes became a natural progression. I understood the discipline, focus, and drive it took to succeed at the highest levels, and I was determined to help them unlock their full athletic potential. Whether I was fine-tuning their programming or guiding them through proper lifting mechanics, my goal remained consistent: to optimize health and performance while keeping them pain-free.

The results spoke for themselves, and soon I found myself working with the families of the athletes— wives, mothers, even parents of some of the pros I trained. At first, I applied the same foundational principles that I used with the athletes, but without the athletic-specific components like speed and agility, as I assumed they didn't need to train at that level. However, during these sessions, I had a lightbulb moment. These individuals, although far from professional athletes, had the same core goals: to move pain-free and improve their overall functional abilities. The only difference was that they weren't aiming for peak sport performance— they were training for life performance. So why was I treating a Super Bowl champion, whose goal was health and longevity in sport, any differently than a 40-year-old mother of three with similar goals in her daily life?

That realization—that the principles of athletic performance weren't just for pros, but for everyone— became a turning point in how I approached training. I started asking myself: Why do we separate the way we think about sport and life performance? Why should attributes that define power (the ability to move fast) and athleticism (the ability to react and adapt with coordinated movement) be reserved for a select few, when they are so crucial for everyday living? And that's when the deeper truth hit me: everyone should be developing these athletic attributes, whether they realize it or not.

Even if you're not competing in sports, you should possess the ability to pivot, react, and adapt at high speeds. Whether you're navigating a crowded street, playing with your kids, or joining a spontaneous game of basketball, the physical demands of movement are universal. Just like the athletes I trained, we all need to be quick, strong, and coordinated to thrive. The stakes may not be a championship game, but the consequences of losing that ability are real.

Enter phase 6 of the warm-up where you will practice fast, dynamic movement to cultivate and maintain athletic attributes. By incorporating the exercises in this phase, you will not only fine-tune your physical capabilities and develop your athletic prowess, but you also prime your mind and body for the demands of the workout ahead. This type of training serves as a powerful catalyst, stimulating the central nervous system, which is pivotal for enhancing your overall performance. When the CNS is activated, it sharpens your mental focus, improves reaction time, and increases neural drive to the muscles, enhancing the quality of your movement and preparing you for the intensity of the exercises to follow.

Understand that this phase goes beyond preparing for a single workout. When you practice moving fast, you're not simply improving your performance for today. You're investing in your long-term physical health. This is the essence of becoming a lifelong athlete. Whether you're 18 or 80, a pro or simply someone trying to stay fit, the principles are the same. Lifelong athletes train for power, speed, and adaptability, even when they don't "need" it for sports, because these qualities protect and enhance their lives as they age.

So, while I may no longer compete on the field, I still consider myself an athlete—because I've embraced training like one. Every day, I reaffirm my commitment to moving with intention, to treating my body with the care and discipline of an athlete, and to seeing each day as an opportunity to stay agile, fast, and resilient. This is the mindset that I bring to my training and instill in everyone I coach, and it's the mindset I challenge you to adopt, too. We are all athletes in the grand game of life. And by training for life performance, you ensure that you don't just play the game—you excel in it.

THE GOALS OF CENTRAL NERVOUS SYSTEM STIMULATION

As you embarked on the 6-phase dynamic warm-up, you may have felt far from your best—your body stiff from inactivity, your mind clouded with the day's responsibilities, or perhaps you were simply grappling with the inertia of an early-morning start. This initial state, common and expected, underscores the necessity of engaging in the 6-phase dynamic warm-up, designed to transition you from this all-too-familiar starting point to a state of pain-free, peak performance.

The process started with phase 1, where soft tissue techniques effectively downregulated your central nervous system, promoting a parasympathetic response. This was akin to releasing your internal parking brake, initiating a pivotal progression that gradually alleviated the resistance shackling your body. As you unraveled knots of stress and muscular tension, you eased your mind and body into a state of relaxation and receptivity.

As you transitioned to phase 2, you engaged in dynamic stretching, further opening your body to increased ranges of motion. Each stretch, each movement, built upon the calm foundation laid by the initial phase, layering positional accessibility atop of physical readiness.

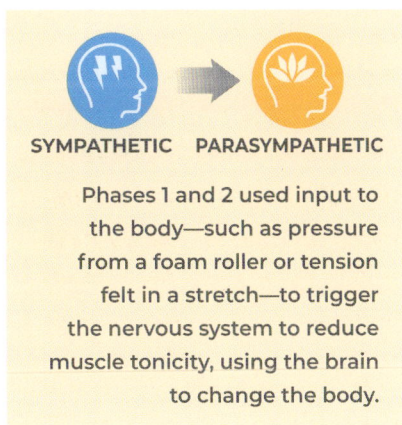

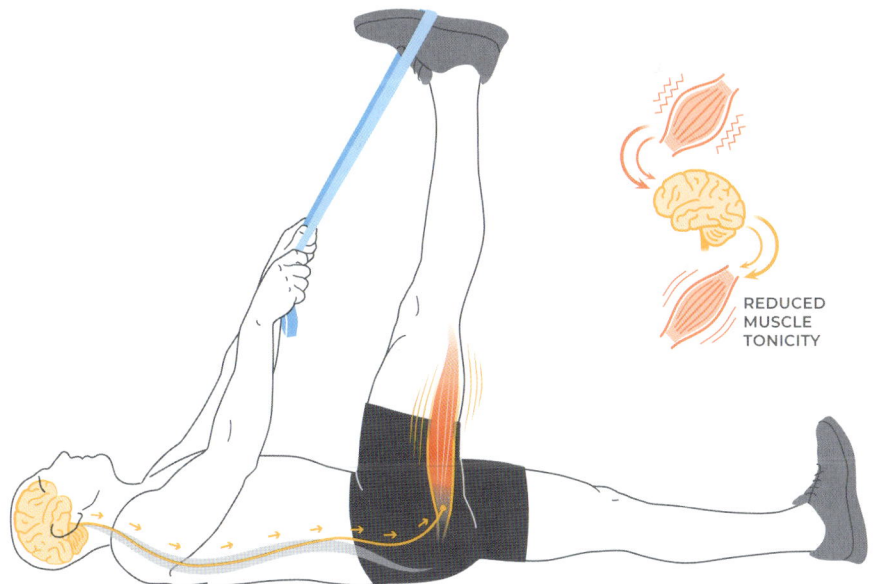

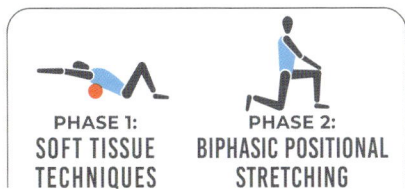

SYMPATHETIC   PARASYMPATHETIC

Phases 1 and 2 used input to the body—such as pressure from a foam roller or tension felt in a stretch—to trigger the nervous system to reduce muscle tonicity, using the brain to change the body.

REDUCED MUSCLE TONICITY

| PHASE 1: SOFT TISSUE TECHNIQUES | PHASE 2: BIPHASIC POSITIONAL STRETCHING | PHASE 3: CORRECTIVE EXERCISE | PHASE 4: ACTIVATION DRILLS | PHASE 5: MOVEMENT PATTERN DEVELOPMENT | PHASE 6: CENTRAL NERVOUS SYSTEM STIMULATION |

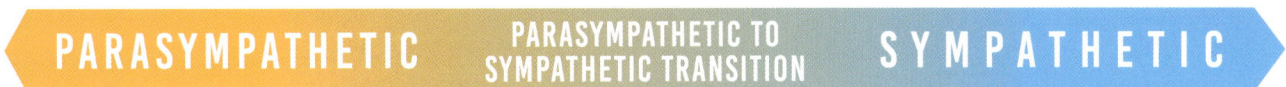

PARASYMPATHETIC — PARASYMPATHETIC TO SYMPATHETIC TRANSITION — SYMPATHETIC

With phase 3, you delved into corrective exercises. By concentrating on the sequencing, stability, and smoothness of your movement, you honed the communication between your brain and body, strengthening neural pathways that enhanced motor control, ensuring you advanced with improved symmetry and coordination.

The momentum continued to build in phase 4, where activation drills primed your muscles, igniting them with energy and purpose. The previous phases had set the stage, enabling your brain to engage muscle groups more effectively. This continuous feedback loop between brain and body consolidated the mind-muscle connection, potentiating your movement quality and muscle responsiveness. By now, the fog of lethargy had lifted, replaced by an emerging sense of focus and physical preparedness.

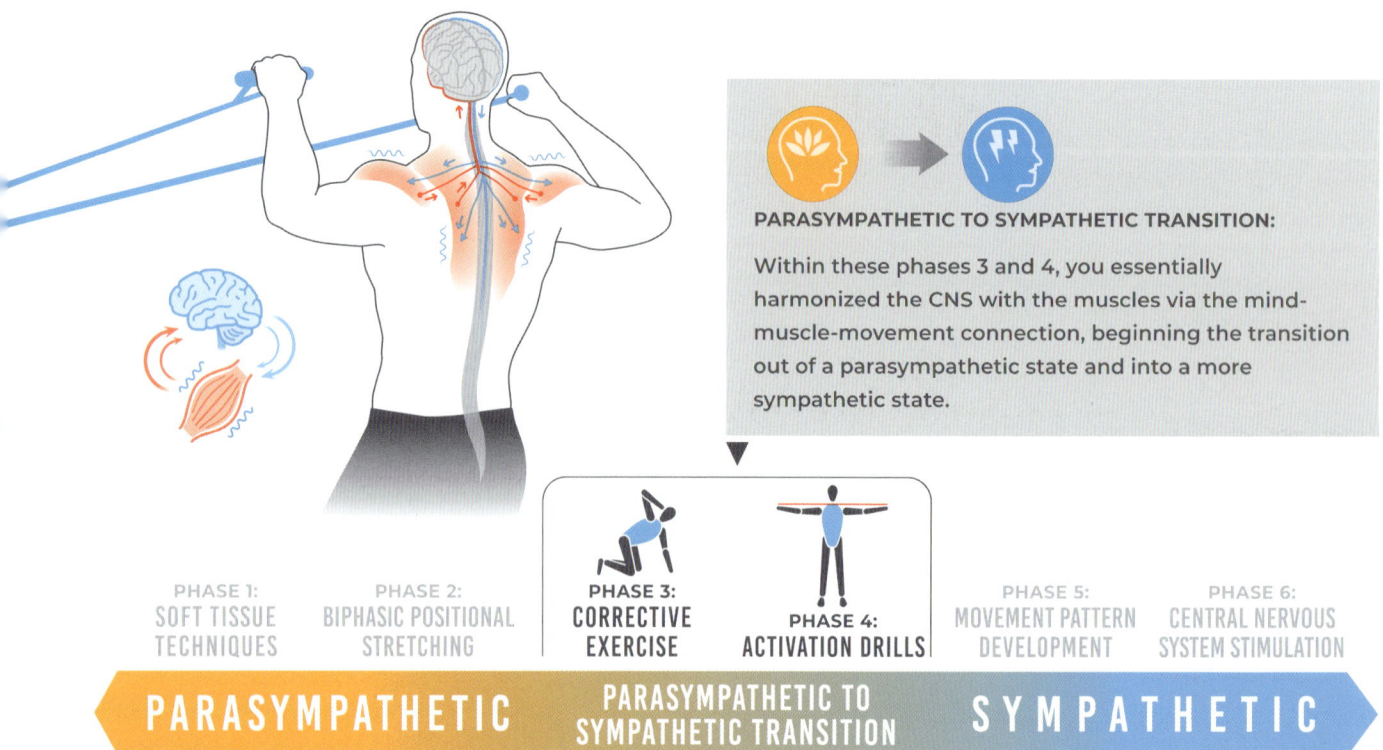

PARASYMPATHETIC TO SYMPATHETIC TRANSITION:

Within these phases 3 and 4, you essentially harmonized the CNS with the muscles via the mind-muscle-movement connection, beginning the transition out of a parasympathetic state and into a more sympathetic state.

PHASE 1:
SOFT TISSUE
TECHNIQUES

PHASE 2:
BIPHASIC POSITIONAL
STRETCHING

PHASE 3:
CORRECTIVE
EXERCISE

PHASE 4:
ACTIVATION DRILLS

PHASE 5:
MOVEMENT PATTERN
DEVELOPMENT

PHASE 6:
CENTRAL NERVOUS
SYSTEM STIMULATION

PARASYMPATHETIC

PARASYMPATHETIC TO
SYMPATHETIC TRANSITION

SYMPATHETIC

Phase 5 introduced the foundational movement patterns, where you practiced, synchronized, and refined your exercise form, consolidating the gains from the previous phases. Your body began to move with more intention and functional capacity, each improvement a testament to progress made.

As you begin phase 6, you've reached the pinnacle of the warm-up. Here, you unleash the potential cultivated through the initial five phases, channeling it into explosive, CNS-priming exercises that ignite your sympathetic nervous system.

This shift is crucial, underpinning the central goal of phase 6. The sympathetic nervous system activation helps ramp up your heart rate, increase blood flow to your muscles, and sharpen your attention, all essential for optimal performance. The prior sensations of pain, stiffness, and distraction are gone, turning the skills you perform in this phase into conduits for a surge of energy, a newfound fluidity in your movements, and an enhanced acuity in your cognitive function.

In essence, the exercises in phase 6 harness and amplify the communication between your brain and your muscles. Through this intensified neural dialogue, your brain sends rapid, precise commands to your muscles, which respond with greater speed, strength, and power. This not only prepares you physically but also mentally, as your mind enters a state of heightened awareness and alacrity. The result is a comprehensive state of preparedness, nurtured by the warm-up but now fully ignited, laying the groundwork for what comes next: enhanced performance through post-activation potentiation (PAP).

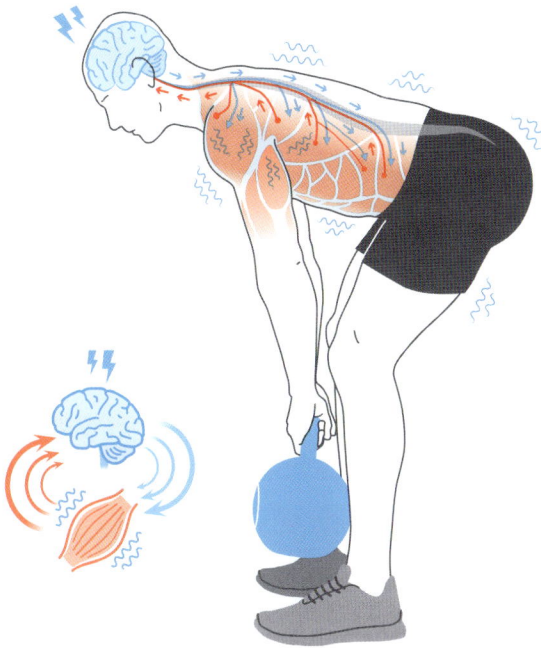

SYMPATHETIC STIMULATION:

As you transition into phase 5 and phase 6, you're amplifying the effects of the central nervous system, catalyzing the body-to-brain and brain-to-body dialogue. In phase 6, the heightened explosive focus creates more powerful performance. The fast-twitch movements (body) amplify motor neurons, sending stronger signals up the chain (brain). This improves neuromuscular coordination and efficiency, creating a constant feedback loop of potentiation.

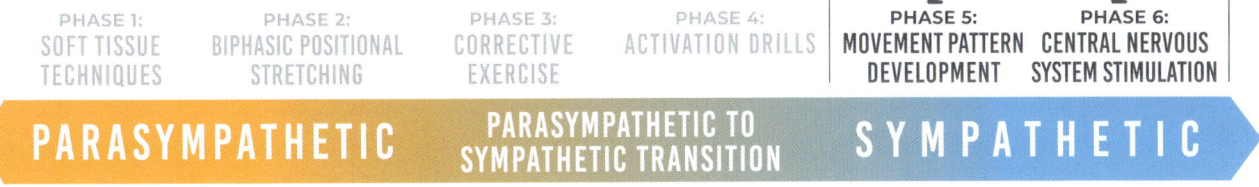

| PHASE 1: SOFT TISSUE TECHNIQUES | PHASE 2: BIPHASIC POSITIONAL STRETCHING | PHASE 3: CORRECTIVE EXERCISE | PHASE 4: ACTIVATION DRILLS | PHASE 5: MOVEMENT PATTERN DEVELOPMENT | PHASE 6: CENTRAL NERVOUS SYSTEM STIMULATION |

PARASYMPATHETIC — **PARASYMPATHETIC TO SYMPATHETIC TRANSITION** — **SYMPATHETIC**

Post-activation potentiation (PAP) isn't just a fancy training term—it's a powerhouse strategy that supercharges your muscles for peak performance shortly after a maximal effort movement, which can be either explosive, like a jump, or tension-based, like a deadlift. For example, engaging in maximal loading exercises such as a one-rep max deadlift can boost performance in a subsequent vertical jump within a short time frame, ranging from several seconds to 8 minutes (depending on the study).[1] Similarly, performing a maximal vertical jump can prime the body for improved performance in a one-rep max lift. This phenomenon illustrates the principle that "fast feeds heavy and heavy feeds fast."

In the context of a warm-up, specifically within phase 6, you stir up PAP magic through dynamic, speed-based moves like ball slams and skips. We're not max-loading someone with a compound lift here—that would be training. Instead, we're using speed-based movements to get the same neurological impact that heavy lifting provides, but from the opposite end of the spectrum. By simply moving at speed, you prime the nervous system to improve load capacity and performance. This common-sense approach maximizes efficiency without pushing the boundaries too early in a session.

In other words, speed-based exercises, such as ball slams and skips, activate and prime the muscles through rapid, explosive actions that translate directly into improved performance during the main workout. Think of it as flipping a switch in your muscles, cranking up their power output by boosting the communication lines between your brain and muscles, helping them respond more effectively and forcefully right when you need it.

Activating PAP in your warm-up isn't just about getting ready; it's about getting ahead. It sets you up for success in the immediate workout, priming your mind and body for ongoing athletic development. So, as you dive into phase 6, remember this: you're setting the stage for a training session that allows you to lift heavier, move stronger, and perform better.

USE IT OR LOSE IT

"Use it or lose it."

It's a simple but profound truth that carries a powerful message, especially as we age and particularly as it relates to our physical capabilities.

Common wisdom advises us to lift weights for strength and muscle growth, stretch and employ soft tissue techniques for mobility, and walk or engage in cardiovascular activities for general well-being. These practices are bedrock to most health-conscious fitness regimens. And for good reason: they are essential for maintaining physical health, performance, and longevity.

However, achieving pain-free performance—that sweet spot of feeling, functioning, and performing at your best—extends beyond just strength, muscle growth, mobility, and cardio. It encompasses health span, the period of life spent in good health, not just total years lived. It's about quality of life, being pain-free, and moving well at any age, no matter the demand or challenge.

To reach this pinnacle of physical wellness, it's insufficient to follow the standard fitness doctrines. You must revive the athletic attributes dulled by disuse, reclaiming the capabilities that once underpinned your youthful play and sport endeavors. Strength training alone isn't enough. As your training becomes myopic—focused solely on lifting heavier or pushing harder—you risk losing your fundamental movement skills, the very abilities that make you agile, powerful, and adaptive.

This gap in fitness routines often reveals itself in unexpected and somewhat humorous ways. In our Pain-Free Performance Specialist Certifications, for instance, a seemingly simple exercise like skipping or jumping jacks often turns into both a source of laughter and a sobering moment of self-awareness. At one particular event, we organized a light-hearted yet revealing "skip off" challenge where we incrementally introduced the skipping progressions featured in this phase. One by one seasoned trainers and fitness professionals were eliminated as they struggled with movements they had not practiced since their younger days. In the end, only two remained standing—a former track athlete and a professional dancer, experts in disciplines where such movements are daily routines.

This friendly competition wasn't merely for entertainment. It serves as a potent reminder of the consequences of neglecting basic yet essential physical skills. Those who regularly engaged in these dynamic movements excelled, while others, despite being exceptional movement experts, floundered with the simplest tasks. For many, phase 6 is the only time they will place a concentrated effort into moving with power and speed—qualities that not only improve performance in the workout but also offer protection from pain and injury.

That if you don't use, you rapidly lose.

RECOMMENDATIONS AND GUIDELINES

In phase 6, the aim is to stimulate the CNS just enough to arouse a training-effect without taxing the nervous system or inducing fatigue. The recommendations and guidelines provide a framework for achieving this balance: priming the mind and body for action while simultaneously amplifying the quality and proficiency of your movement patterns in an efficient way.

CHOOSE 2 EXERCISES

In phases 1 through 5, exercise selection is primarily guided by the specific movement pattern you're focusing on that day—such as a squat for a lower body KPI. But in phase 6, the focus shifts to fast, explosive movements that activate Post-Activation Potentiation (PAP). Here, the exact exercises matter less than your intent: move quickly and with control.

This approach makes sense when you realize that most exercises, even those categorized by body parts—like squats for the lower body or bench presses for the upper body—are actually full-body movements. A squat engages not just the legs but also the core for stability and balance. Similarly, a bench press uses leg drive and core engagement, while a pull-up requires full-body tension and control. Phase 6 capitalizes on this by emphasizing full-body integration through dynamic, athletic movements.

To get the most out of phase 6, simply choose any two fast, explosive exercises, such as skips, jacks, ball slams, or throws.

SUPERSET STIMULATION STRATEGIES

Building on the guideline of selecting two exercises, you will pair these dynamic movements into supersets. This involves performing the exercises back to back, typically with 10 to 15 seconds of rest between them. This inherent rest period, though brief, ensures that the energy and focus demanded by the first exercise does not compromise the performance and recovery of the second. With this structure, each movement can be executed with maximum intensity and effectiveness without compromising nervous system responsiveness.

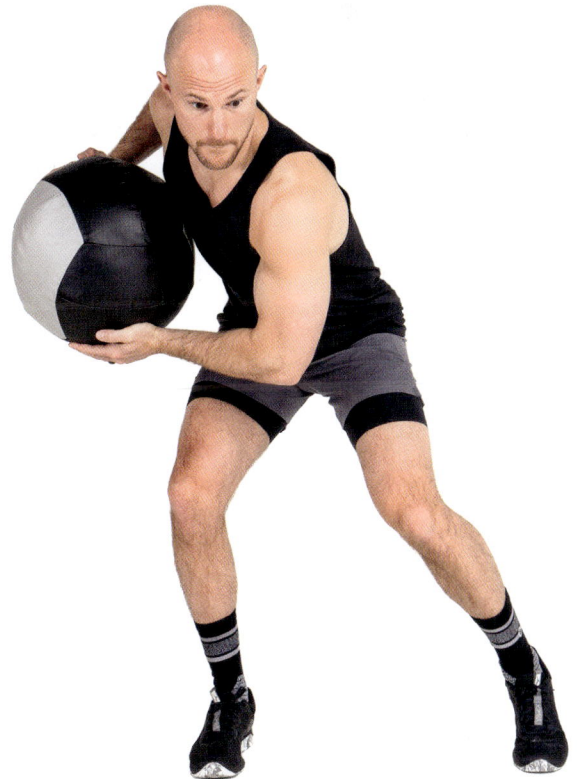

PERFORM 3 TO 5 SETS OF 3 TO 5 REPS

In phase 6, you will perform 3 to 5 supersets of 3 to 5 reps for each exercise, which might look like 5 jumping jacks immediately followed by 5 med ball slams, with 10 to 15 seconds of rest between sets. This structure ensures that you can maintain intensity and focus without overloading your CNS. Here's how it works:

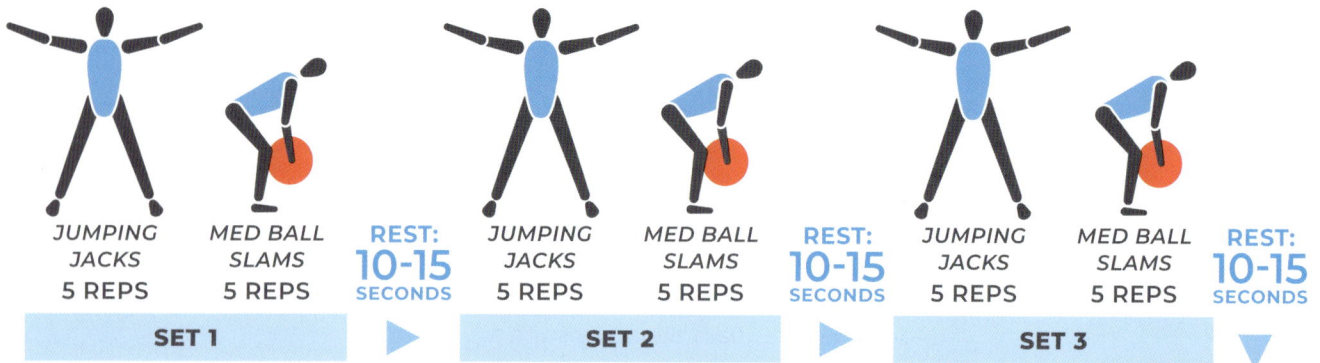

| JUMPING JACKS 5 REPS | MED BALL SLAMS 5 REPS | REST: 10-15 SECONDS | JUMPING JACKS 5 REPS | MED BALL SLAMS 5 REPS | REST: 10-15 SECONDS | JUMPING JACKS 5 REPS | MED BALL SLAMS 5 REPS | REST: 10-15 SECONDS |
| SET 1 | | | SET 2 | | | SET 3 | | |

You can finish here or repeat for another 1 or 2 sets.

As with the previous phases, you might need to fight the temptation to do more because of how great you feel. It's easy to think, "This feels incredible. I'm going to push for 10 more reps and do them as fast as I can." But here's where restraint really counts. You need to maintain a low total volume of work to avoid pre-fatiguing the CNS both centrally and peripherally. Keeping the total reps under 25 is crucial, as crossing this line of moderation can sabotage the very benefits you aim to achieve.

THE FOCUSED PROGRESSION: COORDINATION, SPEED, CHANGE OF DIRECTION

A common issue, even among seasoned athletes, is the tendency to sacrifice form for speed. They jump into their first set with the intention to "go fast" and blast off with maximal intensity, leading to sloppy execution.

Simply moving fast isn't enough—the quality, control, and intensity of each movement are what deliver the real gains. To promote movement mastery, it's helpful to follow a focused progression, prioritizing form and control and then gradually increasing speed. This is best achieved in three stages utilizing external-based cues.

STAGE 1: Coordinate your movements. If you're performing a jumping jack, for example, ensure that your arms and legs are moving in sync. In this initial stage, move slower to develop proper mechanics (i.e., move within ranges that you can control), focusing on coordination. Only increase your speed as much as you can maintain correct form.

STAGE 2: Speed up the rhythm. Once you've synchronized the pattern, begin to increase the pace of your movements. Gradually speeding up means incrementally increasing the tempo of your reps while maintaining the smooth, coordinated mechanics established in the first stage. This ensures that your form remains intact even as your speed increases. It's about finding a balance between quickness and precision so that each rep is executed with control and efficiency.

STAGE 3: Accelerate change of direction. With the jumping jack, change of direction occurs during the transition when your arms and legs come together and move apart, and vice versa. This stage comes last because it requires both coordination and speed to be firmly established. Rapid changes in direction add a layer of complexity, demanding even greater neuromuscular control, and increased ground force reaction time. Maintaining coordination and rhythm at this stage is crucial to ensure that the movements remain effective—in other words, you must be able to quickly reverse direction without losing form or control.

To incorporate each stage effectively, people familiar with the exercise and who feel primed going into phase 6 might progress through the stages quickly, sometimes within a single set. They can focus on coordination in the initial reps, then swiftly increase speed, and finally integrate rapid directional changes, all while maintaining pristine form.

Beginners, however, should take a more segmented approach. They might spend the first set solely focusing on coordination, ensuring that their movements are smooth and controlled. In the second set, they can add speed, increasing the tempo while keeping the movement quality high. By the third set, they can accelerate changes in direction, gradually moving faster and faster with every rep.

TRANSITION INTO YOUR WORKOUT WITHIN 5 TO 9 MINUTES OF FINISHING PHASE 6 (GET IN, STIMULATE, GET TO TRAINING)

Tapping into Post-Activation Potentiation (PAP) provides a temporary but powerful boost in performance, opening a window we call the "functional carryover timetable." Research suggests the ideal window is within 4 to 8 minutes after completing your last phase 6 drill.[2]

This timeline provides flexibility, but the key is reaching your main lift—the key performance indicator (KPI)—within 4 to 8 minutes after finishing the last set of your phase 6 warm-up exercise. That means you'll typically use these crucial minutes strategically, incorporating primers (lighter exercises designed to prepare you for the KPI—more on this in Part 4), targeted mobility work, or skill drills. This brief window ensures you amplify the effects of PAP right before your KPI—exactly why we rarely program the main lift first. Use this time wisely, stay off your phone, and get dialed in for peak performance.

Phase 6 exercises are designed to boost power, speed, and coordination—core attributes of athleticism—through dynamic movements like jumping jacks, skips, jumps, and med ball throws or slams. While these are the go-to pain-free performance exercises, the focus here is less about the specific exercise and more about moving quickly with control to stimulate the nervous system and activate PAP. This means any fast-twitch dynamic movement will be effective in this phase, whether it's plyometrics, jump variations, quick sprints, agility ladder drills, or cone work.

However, to stay aligned with the principles of pain-free performance, select drills that match your skill level and correlate with the training goals of your workout. What's more, it's crucial to be mindful of the equipment you use. For instance, when incorporating medicine ball slams, a 6- to 8-pound ball is ideal—heavy enough to challenge your power output but light enough to move explosively, without excessive bounce that could cause unpredictable rebounds and disrupt your flow.

Most important, stick to the guidelines outlined in this chapter, no matter which exercise or drill you choose to implement. They're your ticket to transforming all the prep work from earlier phases into real-deal performance power, ensuring you step into your workout not just ready, but fully revved up to excel.

EXERCISE APPENDIX

PHASE 6:
CENTRAL NERVOUS SYSTEM STIMULATION

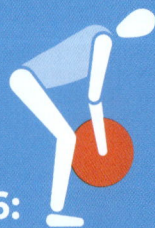

BENT-OVER MED BALL PRESS

SETUP: Stand with your feet wider than shoulder-width. Find your pillar position by engaging your pecs and lats and screwing your feet into the ground. Take a breath, brace your core, then push your hips back, lowering into an athletic hinge position. Pull the med ball to your chest with shoulders down and elbows back. Keep your neck aligned with your spine; if needed, draw your chin back slightly and focus your gaze 3 to 6 feet in front of your feet.

EXECUTION: There are two variations for this exercise. Start with the single rep variation to build a strong foundation of power and stability.

- **Single Rep Variation:** With a sharp exhale, press the ball straight down explosively, fully extending your arms. Hold the end position briefly to maximize output while maintaining body position, stability, and tension. Imagine your workout partner trying to move your knees, legs, hips, trunk, and arms—you should feel immovable. After each rep, pick up the ball, inhale, and reset it at your chest while staying in the hinged position.

VARIATION: Once you've mastered this movement with full control, progress to the repeater variation for a more advanced, continuous sequence that enhances explosive output and performance over multiple reps.

- **Repeater Variation:** As the ball hits the ground or bounces slightly, catch it immediately and pull it back to your chest. Keep your arms fully extended as you press the ball down, catching it low to the ground each time. To optimize post-activation potentiation (PAP) and improve key performance indicator (KPI) outcomes, aim to complete 3 to 5 reps increasingly faster over time, maintaining excellent form and quality in each rep.

Scan the QR code to access demos of each exercise.

BENT-OVER MED BALL PRESS

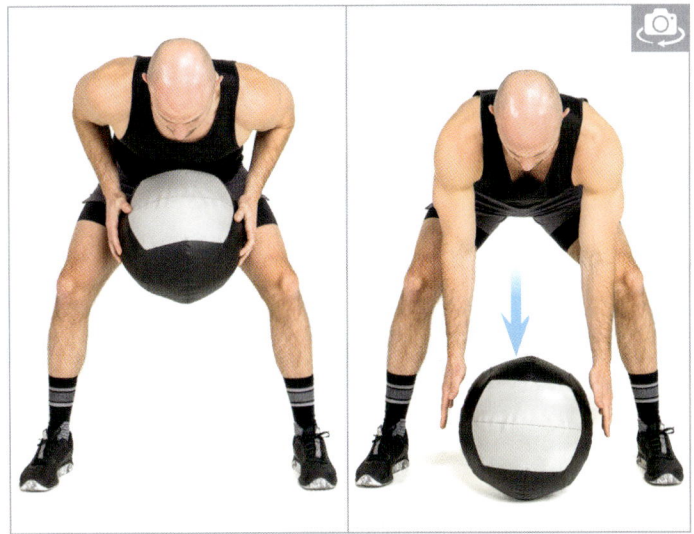

MED BALL SLAM

SETUP: Stand with your feet hip-width to shoulder-width apart. Establish your pillar position. Inhale as you then press the ball straight overhead, coming up onto the balls of your feet. If balance is challenging, keep your feet flat on the ground. Ideally, your biceps should align with your ears, placing the ball directly over your center of mass. If you experience shoulder pain, adjust the arm angle to a comfortable, pain-free position.

EXECUTION: With a sharp exhale, pull the ball down explosively while simultaneously pulling yourself into an athletic hinge position. Sweep your arms back until they align with your torso, maintaining stability and tension as if resisting pressure on your limbs and body. Hold briefly in this strong, grounded position, then pick up the ball, inhale, and reset in the standing position while reaching overhead for the next rep.

VARIATION: If you experience back discomfort in the hinge position or are focusing on stabilizing your pillar position, keep your body fully upright throughout the entire movement:

- **Anti-Flexion Variation:** Set up as above, but as you slam the ball down, keep your hips extended and torso tall. Sweep your arms down until they are just behind you, extending your fingers and engaging your triceps to hold the position tightly.

MED BALL ROTATIONAL THROW

SETUP: Stand with your feet wider than shoulder-width apart. Lift the med ball to your chest, keeping shoulders down and elbows back. Establish your pillar position by screwing your feet into the ground and engaging your pecs and lats. Take a deep breath, brace, then shift your weight to one side (e.g., the right), bringing the ball down toward your right hip as you lower into an athletic position.

EXECUTION: Rotational power in this throw begins from the ground up. As you initiate the throw to the opposite side (right in this example), shift your weight right while pivoting on your left foot. Your left knee and femur will rotate inward, allowing your hip to rotate effectively. With your weight now mostly on the right leg, your pelvis begins to rotate right, followed by your trunk and rib cage, creating a coiling effect. Use this built-up tension to powerfully throw the ball straight out to the right.

At the end of the throw, extend your arms to "push" the ball toward the target. Your right foot should be fully planted on the ground, possibly rotated slightly outward compared to the starting position, with your body weight and pillar aligned over your right leg.

Incorporating rotation into this exercise is a progression that requires strong pillar control and the ability to resist unwanted compensations: titling the torso laterally, ribs flaring up (arching), or pushing with the arms instead of properly initiating rotation through the foot and hip. Watching a recording of your throw can help you evaluate and correct this.

VARIATION: If training with a partner, try a throw-and-catch variation.

- **Partner Variation:** Set up and execute the throw as usual, but after releasing the ball, keep your body in the extended position, arms out as a target for your partner's return throw.

To catch, reverse the rotation of the throw: bend your elbows and pull the ball back toward your chest, rotating your torso back to center. As you do, rotate your pelvis back through neutral, lower the heel of your back foot, and shift your weight back into the starting leg (e.g., right). The ball returns to your starting position by your hip, ready for the next throw.

Once you have mastered the movement, find a rhythm with your partner, gradually increasing the tempo while maintaining focus and coordination.

MED BALL ROTATIONAL TOSS

SETUP: Stand with feet wider than shoulder-width apart. Hold the ball against your stomach with both hands, shoulders down and elbows back. Establish your pillar position by screwing your feet into the ground and engaging your pecs and lats. Take a deep breath, brace, then shift your weight to one side (e.g., the right), bringing the ball down toward your right hip as you lower into an athletic position.

MED BALL ROTATIONAL TOSS

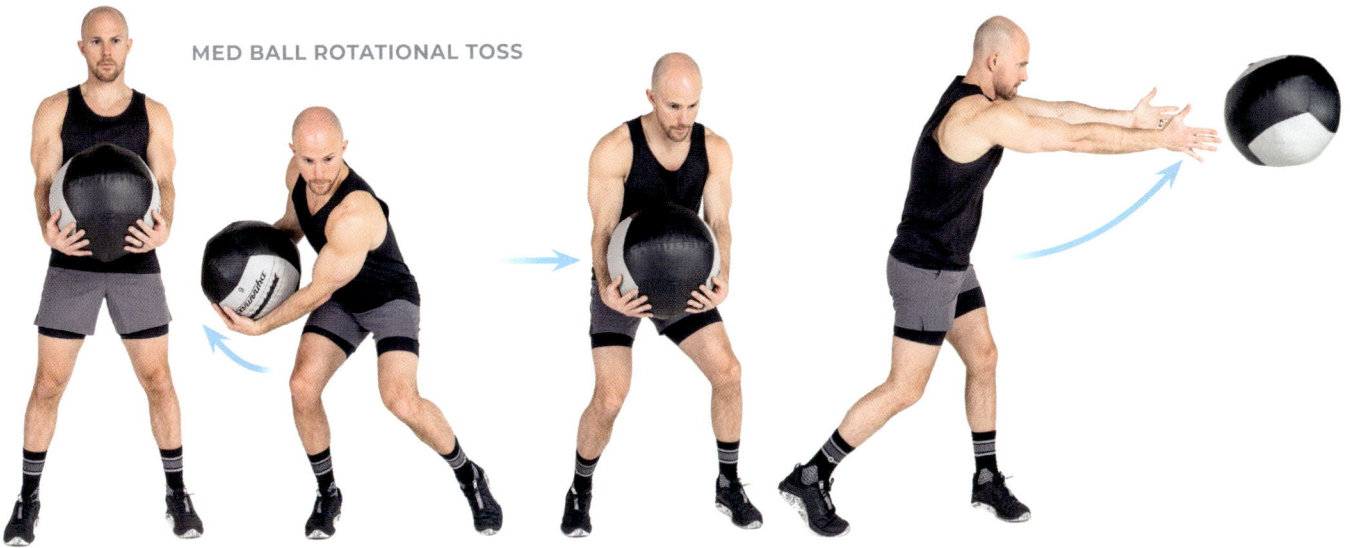

EXECUTION: The movement is similar to the rotational ball throw, but instead of pushing the ball away with bent elbows, your arms act more like ropes attached to the ball. As you rotate, let the momentum and force generated by your body propel the ball. Begin by rotating your body and letting the ball swing from your back hip, scooping it up to mid-chest height. Your lower body generates the majority of the force, while your arms simply guide the ball's path. Release at chest height to send the ball in the intended direction.

VARIATION: You can also perform this exercise as a partner variation. Hold your arms together in a basket shape to catch the ball. Your partner will toss the ball with a bit more arc, so you'll catch it on its downward path. As you catch, bend your knees to absorb the momentum, then smoothly transition into a coiled athletic position before tossing the ball back to your partner.

MED BALL ROTATIONAL CHEST PASS

SETUP: Stand with your feet wider than shoulder-width apart. For this pass, position your hands a bit wider on the ball, with each hand on either side of the midline (rather than slightly behind the ball as in the med ball throw). Lift the med ball to your chest, keeping shoulders down and elbows back. Screw your feet into the ground to engage your pecs and lats, breathe, and brace. Shift your weight to one side (e.g., the right), pulling down into an athletic stance and bringing the ball up toward your right shoulder.

EXECUTION: The movement is similar to the rotational ball throw, but the ball is positioned higher, at chest height. This setup shifts the line of drive, emphasizing the chest muscles as you push the ball away. Rotate your body from the ground up, generating power from your legs and core, and finish by driving the ball straight out from your chest in a powerful pass.

VARIATION: This is another effective drill to perform with a training partner. Aim to throw the ball in a straight line at chest height. Keep your hands in a ready position near your chest to catch the ball. As you receive it, absorb the impact by stepping back and shifting your weight to one side, bending into an athletic stance. Focus on catching and immediately returning the throw with controlled power.

VERTICAL JACKS

SETUP: Stand with your feet hip-width apart, knees slightly bent, pelvis in a neutral position, ribs stacked over hips, and arms relaxed by your sides.

EXECUTION: Jump your feet open as you bring your arms up, then pull your arms back down as you jump your feet back to hip-width apart. Stay light on your feet, absorbing each landing with a slight bend in your knees.

Unlike traditional jumping jacks where you clap overhead, focus on moving quickly and precisely. Keep your pillar stable, your body engaged, and your movements controlled. Jump to just outside shoulder-width with arms stopping at a goalpost or Y-shape. This range allows for good joint alignment (centration) and muscle engagement (co-contraction), helping you reverse direction efficiently.

SEAL JACKS

SETUP: Stand with your feet hip-width apart, knees slightly bent, with your pelvis in a neutral position and ribs stacked over your hips. Extend your arms straight out in front of you at shoulder height.

EXECUTION: Jump your feet open as you open your arms out to the sides. Then bring your arms back to the front as you jump your feet back to hip-width apart. Stay light on your feet, absorbing each landing with a slight bend in your knees.

Maintain control through your pillar, keeping your core stable, body engaged, and movements precise, just as in vertical jacks.

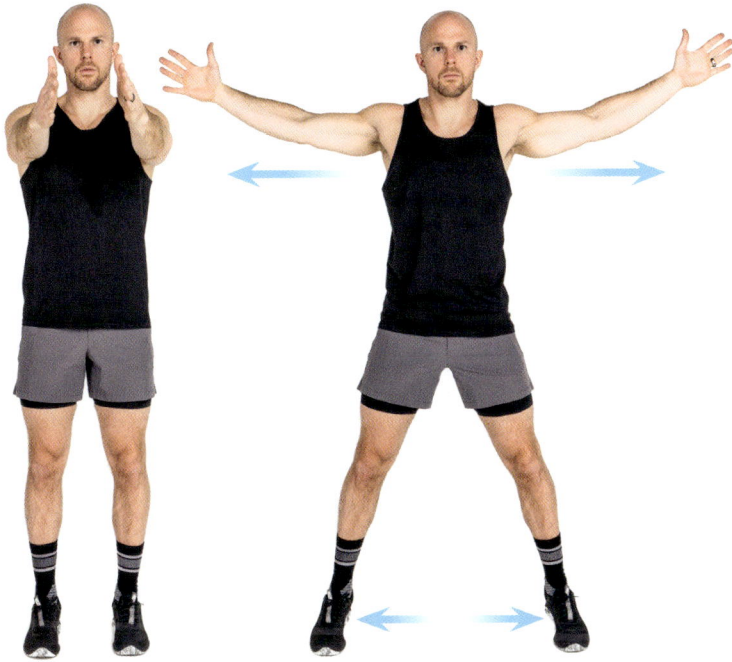

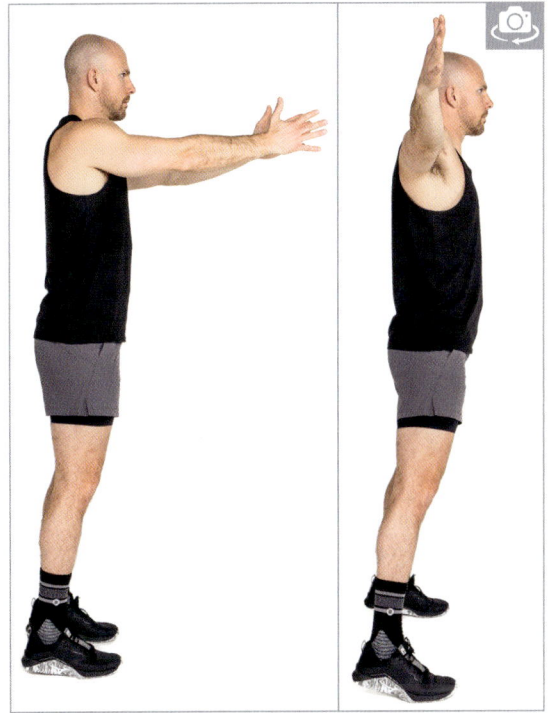

VERTICAL JUMP

SETUP: Stand with your feet hip-width apart, pelvis in a neutral position, ribs stacked over hips, and arms relaxed by your sides. Then pull yourself down into an athletic hinge, reaching your arms back so they stay in line with your torso. Lower with intention—you're actively loading the muscles in your legs, preparing for an explosive jump.

EXECUTION: To jump, push the floor away, swinging your arms up as you drive yourself straight up. Reach as high as possible, pressing through your toes and fully extending your arms to maximize power.

As you descend, pull your arms back down and land softly, touching down with your toes and then the rest of your foot. Absorb the landing by bending your ankles, knees, and hips. A "soft" landing engages your muscles to control the descent, reducing impact on your joints and preparing you to rebound into the next jump if performing repeated reps.

VARIATIONS: There are two ways to perform the vertical jump:

- **Single Jumps:** Start with single jumps to focus on smooth, controlled landings. After each jump, pause briefly to ensure balance and stability, imagining resistance against your knees, legs, torso, and arms.

- **Repeater Jumps:** Once you've mastered single jumps, progress to repeater jumps. As you land, quickly push off again, creating upward power from a high "catch" position (hips above knees). This technique maximizes jump height and power by minimizing joint range, reducing fatigue, and allowing for a quicker rebound compared to "catching low" into a deeper squat.

For individuals with limitations or prior injuries affecting the feet, ankles, knees, hips, or lower back, full jumps may feel challenging or even prohibitive. This stepwise progression offers a safe way to build the coordination, control, and muscular engagement needed for a full vertical jump by training each phase of the movement in isolation. Begin with the first drill and focus on mastering each step before moving on to the next. Progress to the subsequent variation when you can perform the current one with control, stability, and proper alignment.

- **Snap-Down:** Start here to practice the deceleration phase and develop your ability to hold a strong athletic stance. Begin standing with your feet hip-width apart, pelvis in a neutral position, ribs stacked over hips, and arms relaxed by your sides. Quickly pull yourself down into an athletic hinge, reaching your arms back in line with your torso. Hold this position with full-body tension for one second. This drill trains the deceleration and loading portion of the jump without the impact of landing. Move to the next step once you can snap down quickly and hold tension in a stable position without losing alignment.

*If you feel comfortable with the vertical jump sequence and are ready for more dynamic variations, there are additional jump options you can implement. Try incorporating **depth drops to vertical jumps**, where you step off a low platform, absorb the landing, and immediately jump upward. **Box jumps** allow you to focus on height without the impact of a full landing, while **broad jumps** emphasize horizontal distance and require strong forward propulsion. Scan the QR code next to the title to see these variations in action.*

- **Triple Extension to Snap-Down:** This adds the component of upward extension, mimicking the start of a jump without leaving the ground. Stand with feet hip-width apart, pelvis neutral, ribs stacked over hips, and arms by your sides. Reach your arms up toward the ceiling as you rise onto the balls of your feet, engaging your calves, quads, glutes, and core to help you balance for 1 second. Then quickly pull yourself down into an athletic hinge, keeping your arms in line with your torso. Hold this position with high tension for 1 second. This variation trains the transition from upward extension to deceleration. Progress to the next step once you can smoothly move from triple extension into the snap-down with control and proper form.

- **Paused Jump:** This drill incorporates the full jump movement but with a controlled pause at the loading phase. Stand with feet hip-width apart, pelvis neutral, and ribs stacked over hips. Pull yourself down into an athletic hinge, reaching your arms back as you actively load the muscles in your legs. Hold this position with high tension for 1 to 2 seconds. To jump, push the floor away as you swing your arms up and drive yourself straight up. Reach as high as possible, pressing through your toes and fully extending your arms. As you descend, pull your arms down and land softly, touching down with your toes before the rest of your foot. Absorb the landing by bending through your ankles, knees, and hips for a soft, controlled descent. Once you can perform the jump with a stable, soft landing, you're ready to move to the final progression.

- **Counter Movement Jump:** This final step combines the components of triple extension, snap-down, and jump in one fluid movement. Stand with feet hip-width apart, pelvis neutral, and ribs stacked over hips. Reach your arms up as you rise onto the balls of your feet, engaging your calves, quads, glutes, and core. Quickly pull yourself down into an athletic hinge, keeping your arms aligned with your torso. Immediately push the floor away to jump, swinging your arms up as you drive yourself straight up. At the peak, reach as high as possible, fully extending through your arms and legs. As you land, pull your arms down and absorb the impact by bending through your ankles, knees, and hips. Practice this step to refine your power, coordination, and control, ensuring you can absorb impact with a soft, stable landing.

SKIPS

Skips are a rhythmic, coordinated exercise that enhances athleticism, making them ideal for athletes, runners, and clients incorporating dynamic exercises, split stances, or agility drills in their workouts. While skipping may seem like a playground activity, it's often undertrained in adults and is essential for improving rhythm, coordination, and stability in dynamic movement patterns.

At its core, a skip is a combination of a hop (a small jump off one foot, landing on the same foot) and a step (pushing off one foot and landing on the other). A basic forward skip pattern goes hop, step-hop, step-hop, alternating as you move. Over time, you can adjust the direction, height, and distance of each hop to progress the exercise.

SKIPS PROGRESSION: To build a solid foundation for skipping, it's helpful to break down the movement into smaller progressions. By practicing each step individually, you'll develop the rhythm, coordination, and control needed for fluid, effective skips. Start with supported single skips and gradually progress as you gain stability and confidence. Each variation builds on the last, leading to a fully coordinated skip with increased height and distance.

1. **Single Supported Skips:** Hold onto a wall, rack, or suspension trainer to support balance and reduce body weight. Start with your feet together and weight on your left foot. Swing your right knee up, using the support to hop in place on your left foot. As you land, bring your right foot back down beside your left. Repeat multiple hops to practice the movement, with your right leg moving in a backward "cycling" motion, like pedaling a bike.

2. **Alternating Supported Skips:** With support for balance, start with feet together and weight on your left foot. Swing your right knee up and hop on your left foot. As your right leg lowers, step down and shift weight onto it. Then lift your left knee and hop on your right foot. This repeats the basic skip pattern slowly. As you get more comfortable, increase the rhythm and add a slight bounce.

3. **Skips in Place:** Once you are confident with supported skips, perform unsupported skips in place. Start with the same alternating pattern but without holding onto anything, allowing you to develop rhythm, coordination, and balance in the movement.

4. **Low Forward Skips:** To add forward movement, start with your weight on your left foot. Lift your right knee and perform a small forward hop on your left foot, then step forward with your right foot as it lowers. Continue by lifting your left knee and performing a small hop forward on your right foot. Practice this for about 10 yards if space allows.

5. **Forward Skips:** This variation increases both height and distance. With improved strength and coordination, aim to hop higher and move farther forward with each skip. You can measure progress by reducing foot touches over the same distance or by covering a greater distance with the same number of skips.

03

THE 6 FOUNDATIONAL MOVEMENT PATTERNS

THE SIX FOUNDATIONAL MOVEMENT PATTERNS

Squat.
Hinge.
Lunge.
Push.
Pull.
Carry.

If you aren't training these six foundational movement patterns, you're leaving both your results and your health to chance.

From the day we are born, our bodies are hardwired for movement. This inherent ability to move—and the way it manifests—is deeply rooted in our physiology. As we progress from infancy through childhood, six distinct patterns of movement emerge, each serving a foundational purpose in our lives. These movement patterns reflect our daily activities and physical interactions with the world, synergistically engage every major muscle group, and form the building blocks for the full range of human motion and capabilities.

KEY MUSCLE GROUPS UTILIZED IN THE FOUNDATIONAL MOVEMENT PATTERNS

UPPER BODY:
- BICEPS
- CORE
- DELTOIDS
- FOREARMS
- LATS
- PECTORALIS
- TRICEPS
- UPPER BACK

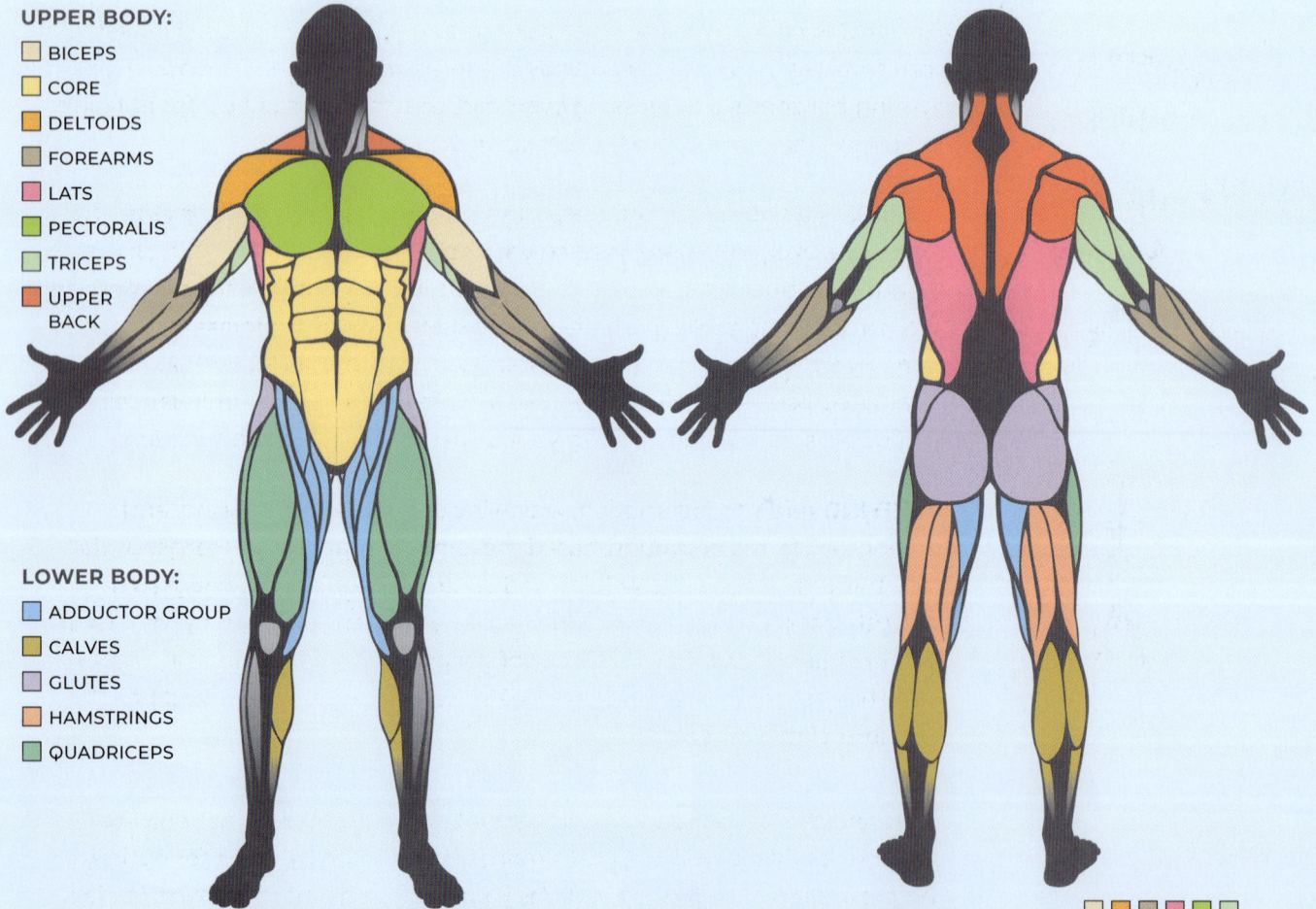

LOWER BODY:
- ADDUCTOR GROUP
- CALVES
- GLUTES
- HAMSTRINGS
- QUADRICEPS

SQUAT
1. Quadriceps
2. Glutes
3. Hamstrings

HINGE
1. Hamstrings
2. Glutes
3. Adductor group

LUNGE
1. Quadriceps
2. Glutes
3. Adductor group

PUSH
1. Pectoralis
2. Deltoids
3. Triceps

PULL
1. Upper back
2. Lats
3. Biceps

CARRY
All muscle regions + core

SQUAT

SQUATTING is the basis of everyday actions that involve lowering and raising your body with a tilted or upright posture, such as sitting down and standing up. It is essential for building lower body stability and strength, engaging the quadriceps, glutes, and hamstrings. A strong squat ensures that you can move through life's daily demands and maintain mobility as you age with less pain and limitations.

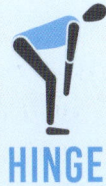

HINGE

HINGING is rooted in the motion of bending at the hips. Every time you bend over to pick something up, reach for an object on the ground, or stand upright from a bent posture, you're using the hinge. Training this movement pattern is key to protecting your back and strengthening the often neglected posterior chain (the muscles running along the back of your body).

LUNGE

LUNGING encompasses split-stance and single-leg movements like kneeling and leaning forward on one leg. It acts as the bridge between squatting and hinging in a staggered stance, challenging balance, coordination, and unilateral strength in asymmetrical positions. Strengthening your lunge enhances your ability to move confidently and safely in any direction, whether navigating uneven terrain, stepping, or performing in sports.

PUSH

PUSHING is how you move objects away from your body or push yourself away from surfaces, covering a wide array of everyday tasks and demands. From pushing horizontally to pressing overhead, this pattern is critical for building and maintaining the shoulders, chest, and triceps.

PULL

PULLING is the essential counterpart to pushing, involving movements that bring objects closer to you or bring your body closer to objects. This pattern engages the muscles of the back, shoulders, biceps, and forearms—improving grip, posture, and pulling power—vital for both athletic performance and everyday activities. In a world of forward-slumped shoulders and push-dominated patterns, pulling exercises are vital for correcting imbalances, enhancing stability, and keeping your upper body strong and functional.

CARRY

CARRYING refers to locomotion, which includes walking, crawling, and running—all forms of ground-based movements that involve "carrying" the body through space with stability and control. It requires the integration of strength, coordination, balance, and agility across the entire body. Whether it's an athletic endeavor or activities of daily living, training the carry improves your ability to move efficiently and safely, keeping you resilient and healthy for a lifetime of movement.

Mastering the six foundational movement patterns is crucial not only for meeting your aesthetic and performance goals in the gym but for optimizing and preserving the natural functions your body is meant to perform in life.

In this section, we will delve deep into each of these six movement patterns. You'll learn how to set up for each movement, how to optimize your form, and how to customize the patterns to fit your unique anatomy.

MOVEMENT TENETS

The six foundational movement patterns are at the core of human movement. To achieve peak, pain-free performance, you need to learn these patterns and refine and adapt them to suit your unique body and goals. This chapter distills the essential principles and strategies to guide you, offering a practical road map for true movement mastery.

In a world dominated by technology and convenience, a harsh reality is reshaping the way we move—or, more accurately, the way we don't move.

During our developmental years, movement is our natural language, with our bodies instinctively utilizing the full spectrum of motion. We squat deeply, hinge with ease, push ourselves up from the ground, pull ourselves to stand, and seamlessly transition from crawling to lunging to walking. In these early years, we explore, play, and engage with the world around us, testing our limits and refining our motor skills without the burden of pain or restriction.

But then something changes. As we grow older, the demands of modern life take hold. We spend more time sitting—at desks, in cars, in front of screens— and less time engaging with the dynamic, full-range movements our bodies are built for. Gradually, our natural movement patterns start to fade. What was once effortless becomes difficult, and over time, we lose the ability to move freely and confidently. By the time we reach early adulthood, many of us are already facing a troubling decline in our physical capabilities. Strength diminishes, muscles weaken, and stiffness becomes a constant companion. What's worse, chronic pain and injuries start to feel like an inevitable part of life.

This cycle of deactivation and failing health only deepens the sedentary rut we find ourselves in, leaving us vulnerable when faced with physical challenges—ones that our ancestors navigated daily but that we encounter far less frequently, if ever.

But there's good news: It's never too late to change this trajectory. Now more than ever, we must re-engage with the foundational movement patterns that our bodies were designed for. The ultimate goal?

- *To overcome and counteract the limitations imposed by our sedentary environment*
- *To reclaim the movement potential eroded and stifled by the pressures of modern life and shortsighted training practices*
- *To move pain-free, reduce vulnerability to preventable injuries, and perform at our highest level*

With this aim, training is more than just exercising to lose weight or achieve some arbitrary fitness goal. It becomes a process of building the most robust and resilient movement system possible. Yes, you want to increase strength and build muscle. Yes, you should constantly strive for better mobility, power, athleticism, and endurance. And of course, you want to improve your physique and feel great doing it. But you can never achieve these objectives unless you train in alignment with your body's natural mechanics.

Think of your body as a chain, with each movement pattern representing a critical link. No matter how strong some links may be, the chain is only as strong as its weakest one. If any link—whether it's your ability to squat, hinge, lunge, push, pull, or carry—is compromised by pain, neglect, or poor movement quality, the entire system becomes vulnerable. This weakness becomes especially evident when you face new demands, such as performing a movement you rarely practice, entering a position you can't fully control, or advancing to an exercise beyond your current abilities. When you add load or speed to these situations, the risk of pain and injury skyrockets. But by gradually exposing yourself to these challenges in a controlled environment, you can strengthen those weak links and safeguard the integrity of the entire system.

For many of us, the gym is the only place where we can actively test our body's full range of motion under load and speed. It's a space to practice, hone, and improve—experimenting with new variations while steadily advancing skill. This is how we replace pain with gains, develop the physical characteristics of health and longevity (strength, hypertrophy, mobility, power, athleticism, and conditioning), and avoid the chronic issues that arise when we neglect our basic needs.

But with this opportunity comes the challenge of knowing where to begin. To truly move, feel, and perform better—forever—you must not only train all six movement patterns but also identify your appropriate starting point and understand the principles and strategies underpinning the process. This includes the implementation of screens to optimize the patterns, assessments to individualize them, and strategies to safely progress over time. This is where the movement tenets come into play.

By systematically and thoughtfully following the guidelines in this chapter, you will gain the ability to train hard, move confidently, and, most importantly, stay healthy—capturing the true power of the pain-free performance training system.

PATTERNS VS. EXERCISES

A **movement pattern** is a general category of movements that share similar biomechanical properties, including joint angulations, structural and muscular stress, and the balance between dynamically moving and statically stabilizing muscle groups. Additionally, movement patterns involve specific neurological linkages that coordinate the body for executing a particular style of movement. Essentially, a movement pattern provides a broad framework that encompasses all the exercises and variations that can be executed within that category of movement. Together, you can think of the six foundational movement patterns as a complete blueprint for human movement.

An **exercise**, on the other hand, is a specific manifestation within a movement pattern. It involves a particular setup, uses certain tools, or adopts a unique execution style aimed at achieving a more targeted or acute goal within the broader movement pattern. Exercises allow for precision in training by enabling the manipulation of variables such as muscular emphasis, skill focus, range of motion, and load placement. Each exercise is designed to place targeted stress on the body and tailored to enhance certain aspects of the movement pattern based on individual goals or to address particular weaknesses.

In summary, a **movement pattern** provides the overarching category under which movements are classified based on shared biomechanical and neurological characteristics, and an **exercise** is a movement performed within a pattern, personalized to achieve distinct objectives. This distinction allows for a systematized approach to training—a structured, multi-tiered hierarchy—where broad movement skills are honed through exercise selection and variation, each designed to improve crucial facets of the overall pattern.

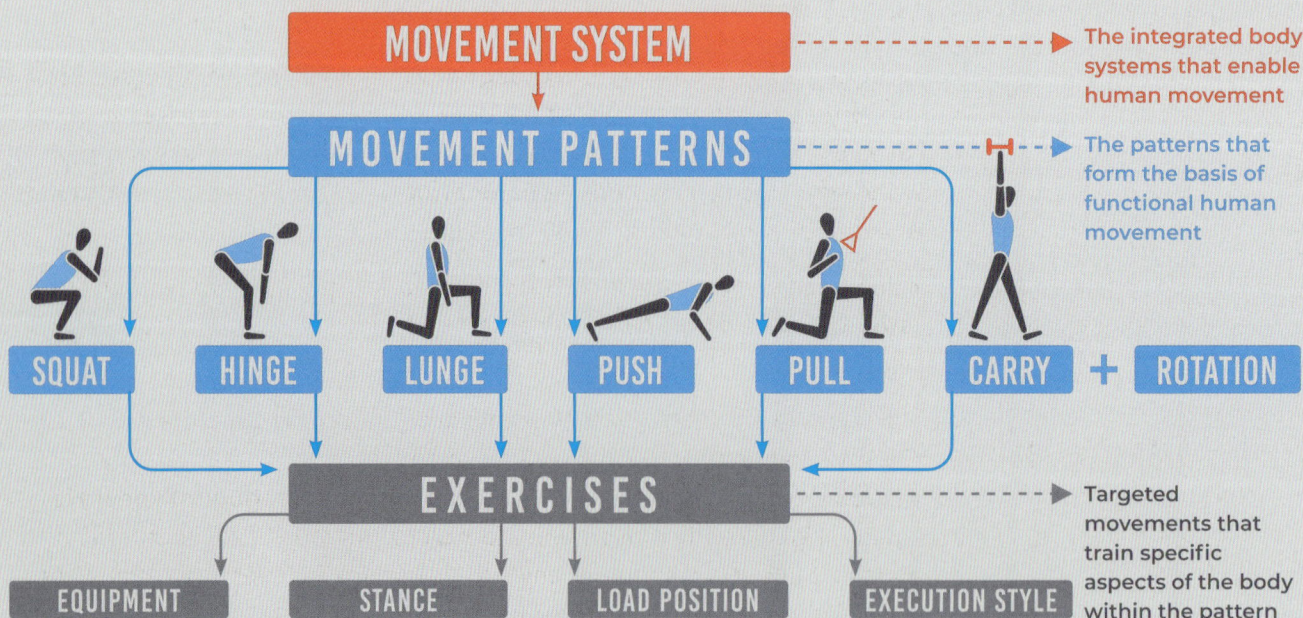

MOVEMENT SYSTEM — The integrated body systems that enable human movement

MOVEMENT PATTERNS — The patterns that form the basis of functional human movement

SQUAT · HINGE · LUNGE · PUSH · PULL · CARRY + ROTATION

EXERCISES — Targeted movements that train specific aspects of the body within the pattern

EQUIPMENT · STANCE · LOAD POSITION · EXECUTION STYLE

TRAIN ALL SIX PATTERNS—
NO PROGRAM IS COMPLETE WITHOUT THEM

I was at American Family Field in Milwaukee, Wisconsin, home of the Brewers. It was three and a half hours before game time, and I was working with one of the team's players. It was that quiet pregame lull—no fans in the stadium, just players going through warm-ups and staff hanging around, getting ready for the night ahead. When you're down there with the team, everyone's loose and relaxed, and it feels like this insider's moment where you can actually talk without the pressure of the game looming.

But I wasn't there to hang out. I was there because my client had fallen into the same trap I'd seen with so many athletes—years of overspecialization, constantly battling injuries, never fully feeling right. He'd fallen through the cracks, and I was running the pain-free performance training system to help him climb out.

While on the field, I ran into one of his teammates. We already had a connection because he'd been working with a coach certified in the system I teach. So, naturally, we started talking about his training and how he'd managed to stay healthy. I knew parts of his story, but as we talked more, he began opening up about the struggles he'd faced and the changes he'd made. The way he described his frustration and eventual breakthrough made me curious to dig deeper.

"So how'd you turn it around?" I asked, wanting to hear it all in his own words.

"I got cut," he said without hesitation. "Twice. First from one college team, then another. I spent three years in independent ball. I was about to quit, man. I was done."

It's a familiar path—athletes who were stars in high school, maybe had a shot in college, but eventually fall off the radar. Most don't find their way back. But here he was, a pitcher in the majors, throwing 100 miles per hour.

He shrugged, still processing it. "I thought I was doing everything right. For most of my career, it was all about shoulder work—isolated exercises, over and over. Every program I followed focused on that one thing: keeping my throwing arm strong. I figured the harder I worked, the better I'd get. But it never worked. I was stuck at 87, 88 miles per hour."

I nodded because it's a story I've heard too many times. Athletes zero in on one area, convinced that pushing harder will lead to breakthroughs. But it rarely does.

"When I got cut," he continued, "I knew I had to do something drastic. So I found a trainer who wasn't just focused on my arm. That's how I got connected with your system. He threw out everything I thought I knew. He had me doing full-body movements—deadlifts, Bulgarian split squats, all of it. It wasn't just about my shoulder anymore. I was linking everything together, and that's when things started to change."

He paused, thinking back. "I gained 13 miles an hour on my fastball. From 87 to hitting 100. And that happened between age 27 and 30. I thought I was done at 27. But now I'm throwing harder than ever."

His story, as remarkable as it is, didn't surprise me. Throughout my career, I've seen it play out countless times. My background in physical therapy, biomechanics, and sports performance often brings me in when athletes hit a wall—pain, burnout, or a frustrating plateau.

Though each athlete's situation was different, one recurring theme stood out: Most were neglecting or underutilizing the six foundational movement patterns. Whether it was a powerlifter ignoring three of the six, a marathon runner who trained only two, or a bodybuilder hyper-focused on four, the problem generally boiled down to overspecialization at the expense of overall physical preparedness. As a result, they developed weak links that held them back or left them vulnerable to injury.

The solution was always the same—a return to the basics by addressing the entire body as an interconnected system. That's what the pitcher figured out,

ROTATION: THE INTERCONNECTED PATTERN

Whenever I present the six foundational movement patterns—whether I'm speaking to a group of trainers or sharing on social media—someone inevitably asks, "What about rotation?"

It's a fair question because rotation is undeniably a key element of human movement. In fact, most dynamic activities involve some element of rotation. The problem is that on its own, rotation doesn't fit the criteria for a foundational movement pattern because it never occurs in isolation during full-body, multi-joint actions.

So, when someone asks me about rotation, I like to turn the question around: "Rotation of what, exactly?" This reframing helps people think critically about where rotation truly fits. If you're rotating from your shoulders, hips, or trunk, what's really happening? Which pattern is the rotation stemming from? That's when the realization hits—no matter where rotation occurs, it's always integrated within one or more of the foundational patterns.

Take throwing, for example: It's a blend of a lunge, pull, and push. Or consider a golf swing: It's a hinge paired with a rotational pull and push. Even walking incorporates rotation, as the hips and shoulders twist in opposite directions to propel you forward. In all and it's the lesson for anyone who's stuck, in pain, or chasing the next level of performance.

This can't be overstated. If you're human, training and progressing all six foundational movement patterns is non-negotiable. They are ingrained in our DNA, forming the bedrock of human movement. To overlook even one is to ignore the essence of what it means to move as a human. Yet today's fitness industry often dismisses these patterns in favor of overly specialized programs. The result? A concentrated focus on isolated body parts or specific patterns, which may yield short-term gains but ultimately leaves the body unbalanced, less connected, and more prone to injury.

Take a close look at your own training. Are you covering all six foundational patterns, or are you stuck in a loop of focusing on one area at the expense of the others? Without a solid foundation of pain-free movement across all six patterns, everything you do is built on shaky ground.

If you're human, training and progressing all six foundational movement patterns is non-negotiable.

three examples, rotation acts as the glue, binding multiple foundational patterns together. It's the plus sign in the equation, linking the movements through rotational planes of motion.

While trainers use different labels, there's a universal consensus that the squat, hinge, lunge, push, pull, and carry make up the core movement patterns because they encompass all the ways the body is designed to move. But there's more to it. To be classified as a foundational pattern, a movement must allow for progressive overload, something difficult to achieve with rotational movements alone.

For instance, you wouldn't progress from throwing a 4-pound medicine ball to a 250-pound one. Rotation is less about raw strength and more about power and synergy—how well your body can coordinate and generate force across multiple joints. The foundational patterns, on the other hand, are versatile. You can load them to build strength, increase effort to promote muscle growth, and refine them to close motor control gaps—essentially all the aspects of progressive overload that help you move better and improve over time. So, it is not just about how the body is designed to move, but also the ability to adapt the movement to a wide range

of physical characteristics. That is the basis of a foundational pattern.

Now, just because rotation is not classified as a foundational pattern doesn't mean you will neglect rotational training. Rotation is built into the pain-free performance system, and you're training it throughout the entire process. It's integrated into both the warm-ups and the exercises themselves, embedded within the six foundational patterns. As you progressively overload those core movements, you're simultaneously enhancing your rotational capabilities. Think about a baseball pitcher: There's nothing more rotational than throwing a 100-mph fastball, but that power doesn't come from practicing rotation in isolation. It's developed through the foundational patterns paired with coordination across the entire kinetic chain.

Here's the key takeaway: Rotation is a crucial element of dynamic movement, but it doesn't function as a foundational pattern on its own. Instead, it's seamlessly woven into the squat, hinge, lunge, push, pull, and carry patterns—acting as a force multiplier within each one.

SCREEN THE PATTERN—
HOW TO OPTIMIZE YOUR FORM

The pain-free performance training system might seem straightforward at first. People often assume it's as simple as performing the six foundational patterns—squat, hinge, lunge, push, pull, and carry. "It's just about doing the movements, right? Easy." But that is an oversimplification. Training these patterns is just the beginning.

Engaging in these movements means you're aware of the patterns and incorporating them into your training to some extent, but awareness alone doesn't equate to mastery. It's like receiving a textbook on the first day of graduate school and assuming you've mastered the material without ever opening the book. You have the tools, but the real journey begins when you start digging deeper.

True movement pattern mastery requires more than just going through the motions. It's a process of screening, assessing, and knowing when to progress or regress. Once you've established these patterns as the foundation of your training, the next step is to apply universal form principles to each one. This is where the screen comes in. Think of the screen as your optimization checklist—a guide to ensure you're starting with safe, effective movement while laying the groundwork for progress.

The screen evaluates five key markers of movement quality:

▼
NEUTRALITY:
Can you maintain a neutral pillar throughout the movement?

▼
SYMMETRY:
Are both sides of your body moving evenly, without unwanted rotation?

▼
STABILITY:
Are your joints stable and maintaining alignment?

▼
RANGE OF MOTION:
How deep can you move while keeping your pillar intact?

▼
CONTROL:
Are you able to manage every phase of the movement smoothly?

Going through the optimization checklist allows you to break down the movement and assess its components. Is your spine neutral? Check. Are your hips and shoulders stable? Check. Do you look symmetrical? Check. Each "yes" brings you closer to the green light for training.

If you don't meet all the standards, that's where the screen's value shines. Where are you struggling? Are you losing stability at a specific range? Is there unwanted rotation or imbalance at a joint? Are the issues rooted in mobility, stability, or skill? The screen gives you the data to pinpoint the source of these problems and make strategic adjustments to your setup and execution.

SCREENING WITH PURPOSE AND PRACTICALITY

As a personal trainer or group class instructor, your time is limited, and your clients' needs are varied. That's why the goal of the screening protocol in the Pain-Free Performance Specialization Certification (PPSC) is to get clients training as quickly and effectively as possible. The focus is practicality—ensuring clients can move safely and see progress immediately.

Keep It Simple, Keep It Safe

Most trainers only have an hour per session. The screen helps you zero in on the essentials: Can your client meet the standards of the optimization checklist and train safely today? If they can, that's "good enough" to start. Perfection isn't required—functional, safe, and effective movement is the priority.

Adapt in Real Time

The screen also allows for real-time adjustments during the session. Start your client with a standardized setup, like those outlined in Phase 5 of the warm-up. From there, adjust based on what you see or what the client reports. For example, if they feel discomfort at a specific range or struggle to meet the checklist standards, you can modify their stance, alignment, or execution on the spot. These small, strategic tweaks help refine their movement without the need for a full assessment.

Know When to Assess

A detailed assessment is only necessary if the screen reveals unresolved issues, such as difficulty maintaining a neutral pillar, noticeable asymmetry, or pain that can't be resolved with simple cues. Assessments give deeper insights into these challenges, enabling you to tailor solutions. However, the key is knowing how to interpret the screen, improve form, and select the right exercise from the movement pattern pyramid to ensure safe training that day.

Start Where They Succeed

Most clients begin with foundational progressions—the easier exercises at the base of the pyramid—to build confidence and proficiency. As they master these, you can consider running an assessment to uncover opportunities for further refinement. The pyramid ensures that progression is scalable and appropriate for every individual.

Empower Your Clients

If you're working in a group setting or don't have time for a detailed assessment, encourage clients to film their movement screens. This allows them to review their form against the optimization checklist provided in this book. Even with a trainer, seeing their movement firsthand fosters deeper understanding and empowers them to take ownership of their progress.

Train the muscles while sparing the joints.

The principle behind the optimization checklist is simple but profound: Train the muscles while sparing the joints. The screen identifies when your form is placing unnecessary strain on your joints instead of properly activating your muscles. This insight gives you the opportunity to make meaningful corrections that will enhance performance and prevent injuries.

In the movement pattern chapters, you'll find clear examples of how to apply the optimization checklist to foundational progressions. These baseline exercises are designed to help you evaluate your form while providing a practical way to develop and improve your movement. The same exercises are incorporated into Phase 5 of the warm-up, turning your daily warm-up routine into a built-in movement screen. This means that every time you warm up, you're not just preparing your body for the session ahead—you're actively practicing and refining the key standards outlined in the optimization checklist.

ASSESS THE PATTERN—
HOW TO INDIVIDUALIZE AND ENHANCE YOUR EXECUTION

Meeting the standards in the optimization checklist through the screen lays a solid foundation for progress. It highlights key principles for safe and effective movement, pinpoints weak links or sources of discomfort, and establishes a baseline for improvement. But the real power of the process comes from building on this foundation with the assessment—a deeper dive into understanding how your body moves and identifying the specific adjustments you need to make to perform at your best.

The assessment isn't just about meeting general standards; it's about uncovering the unique mechanics of your setup, stance, range of motion, and execution style. It ensures that your movement patterns are customized to your individual anatomy rather than forcing you into a generalized mold. You've likely heard the phrase, "Everyone is different." If that's true, how can everyone move the same way? They can't—and they shouldn't.

Some assume there's a "perfect" position or alignment that works for everyone, but the reality is that no two bodies are identical. Variations in limb length, joint structure, and muscular development mean that what's optimal for one person may be uncomfortable—or even harmful—for another. The assessment helps you move beyond one-size-fits-all thinking and find what works for your body.

This emphasis on individuality is crucial. The right stance, range of motion, and execution style may not look "textbook," but it will feel stable, controlled, and pain-free. This approach avoids the common trap of mimicking external cues or positions that might not suit your anatomy, which can lead to inefficiency, discomfort, or even injury. Instead, the assessment helps you refine your movement in a way that respects the way your body was designed to function.

While some trainers use general adjustments based on body type—like recommending specific setups for long limbs or short torsos—this method only scratches the surface. The assessment digs deeper, examining the unique characteristics of your joints, skeletal alignment, and movement tendencies. Tailoring your setup and execution to these factors doesn't just improve how effectively you move; it reduces strain on your joints, lowering the risk of pain or dysfunction.

This understanding is vital because many people mistakenly believe that improving movement is about stretching or foam rolling. While these techniques can help, they can't change fixed factors like the depth of your hip socket or the angle of your femur. A more effective approach is to embrace the structural realities that influence your movement and focus on optimizing what you can control: mobility, stability, and skill.

Assessments don't have to be time-consuming or repeated frequently. When done correctly, they're efficient, insightful, and provide lasting benefits, as your bone structure doesn't change (barring significant surgery like a hip replacement). You also don't need to assess everything at once. Instead, focus on identifying and prioritizing the weakest link in your movement chain. For instance, if your

OPTIMIZING MOVEMENT: SCREEN VS. ASSESSMENT

A **screen** is a broad evaluation tool used to check your form against universal standards (referred to as the "optimization checklist"). It provides a quick and effective way to identify fundamental movement faults, compensations, or imbalances that could be holding you back or leading to pain. Think of the screen as a baseline test of your movement quality, focusing on key markers like joint neutrality, symmetry, stability, range of motion, and control.

In traditional approaches, screens are often more rigid and can feel disempowering—as if the focus is on pointing out everything you're doing wrong. However, in the pain-free performance approach, the screen is seamlessly integrated into your training session, specifically in phase 5 of the warm-up. If you meet the standards in the optimization checklist, you're ready to train. If compensations or weaknesses appear, you can use the optimization strategies provided in each chapter to improve your form and address your weak links.

What's more, the screen serves as a dynamic tool to guide your training. It allows you to make informed decisions—whether that means regressing an exercise, homing in on a specific weakness, or modifying your training program to better suit your needs.

An **assessment** takes the screening process further by personalizing the movement to your unique body. While the screen provides a general overview of how you're moving, an assessment dives deeper into the specifics of your anatomy and biomechanics—revealing your optimal stance, setup, and execution style. This is where the movement is tailored to your bone structure, limb lengths, and mobility.

Traditional methods often treat assessments as standalone protocols, which can make people feel "broken" or as though they're failing some arbitrary standard. In contrast, pain-free performance uses the data from the assessment to refine and adjust your movement so that you can better meet the standards outlined in the optimization checklist.

Unlike a screen, which is utilized in phase 5 before every training session, an assessment is only done once since your bone structure won't change. However, it's especially useful when you need to fine-tune your form, break through a plateau, or resolve ongoing pain or mobility limitations.

In essence, screens offer a quick, standardized check to ensure you're moving safely, while assessments allow you to customize the movement for your unique anatomy.

Together, they help you train smarter, addressing weak links before they lead to injury and fine-tuning your movements for long-term, pain-free progress. With both the screen and assessment, the goal isn't to judge or label, but to gather data that you or your coach can use to make performance enhancing adjustments.

squat feels off, start there. Addressing one limitation often has a ripple effect, improving other patterns like lunging or hinging. This interconnected nature of the body means progress in one area can unlock potential across the entire system, making assessments a strategic investment in overall performance.

This interconnected approach is why assessments are valuable for everyone, not just beginners. Even advanced trainers and seasoned athletes benefit from the process. In PPSC courses, trainers often uncover subtle adjustments during their own assessments that unlock pain-free ranges or improve efficiency. These breakthroughs reinforce that assessments are a critical tool for continuous refinement and optimal performance at every level.

Together with the screen, the assessment provides a comprehensive view of your movement. This combination allows you to train smarter, push harder, and stay consistent without setbacks. By personalizing your setup and execution, you're not only improving how you move; you're building a foundation that supports lifelong performance.

IDENTIFY AND CORRECT COMPENSATIONS—
OPTIMIZATION STRATEGIES TO ENHANCE MOBILITY, STABILITY, AND SKILL

In the chapters that follow, you'll notice a deliberate structure designed to guide you step-by-step toward better movement. Each movement pattern begins with a screen, followed by an assessment, and culminates with optimization strategies. This sequence ensures a comprehensive approach to improving your form and performance.

The screen provides a starting point by using the optimization checklist to evaluate your current movement capabilities. It identifies areas where your form meets the standards and highlights any compensations or weak links that may need attention. This is where you begin to build awareness of your movement quality and establish a baseline for progress.

The assessment takes the process further, diving into the unique variables that shape how your body moves. Factors like hip structure, limb length, and joint mobility are examined to uncover the adjustments you need for a setup, stance, and execution style tailored to your anatomy.

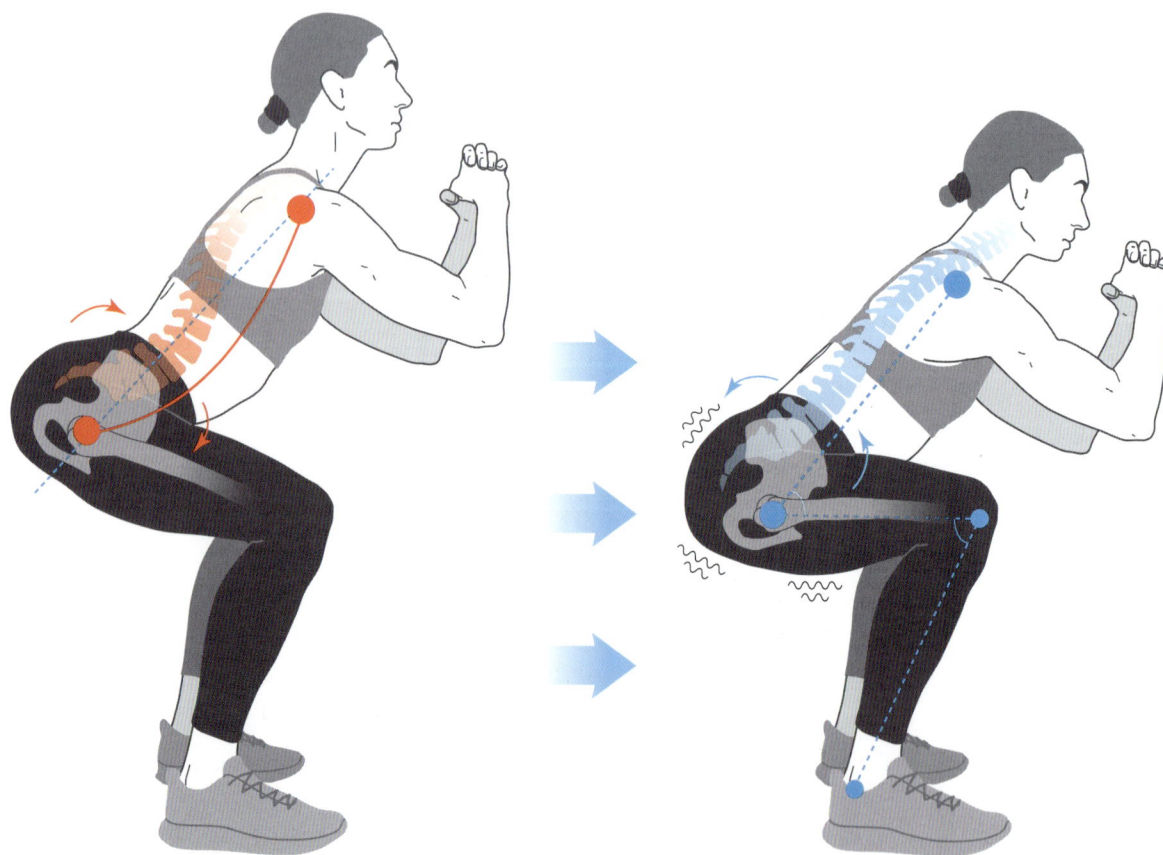

After completing the assessment, it's crucial to retest your form using the optimization checklist. This step ensures that the adjustments made during the assessment have addressed any compensations identified in the screen. By following this test-and-retest model, you gain measurable feedback and actionable insights about your progress, confirming whether your movement now aligns with the standards set by the screen.

Once you've fine-tuned your setup and execution to fit your body, the next step is to address any lingering compensations that may still impact your movement. This is where the optimization strategies become essential— because compensations might not stop you from training now, but left unchecked, they can lead to discomfort, inefficiency, or even injury over time.

Compensations often arise from one of three key areas: mobility, stability, or skill.

MOBILITY

Mobility refers to the active range of motion your joints can control. When it's limited, your body compensates in ways that shift strain to other areas. For example, stiff hips or ankles might cause your knees to collapse inward or your lower back to round during a squat. These adaptations reduce efficiency and increase the likelihood of pain.

STABILITY

Stability is the ability to maintain control of a joint throughout its range of motion. When stability is lacking, your movements lose alignment, and faults like unwanted rotation, a collapsing spine, or buckling knees can occur. Stability is the foundation of strong, efficient movement—when it's compromised, everything else becomes more difficult.

SKILL

Skill is the coordination and control required to execute a movement with precision. If your form feels unsteady or jerky, it often points to gaps in motor control, a lack of practice, or unfamiliarity with the movement. Skill is what ties everything together, ensuring movements are smooth, efficient, and repeatable.

The good news is that every compensation has a solution. By pinpointing weak links and applying targeted optimization strategies, you can improve mobility, enhance stability, and develop skill that not only refine your form but also build a stronger, more adaptable body.

In the coming chapters, we'll take a closer look at these strategies, breaking them down for each movement pattern. Whether you're working to unlock hip mobility for deeper squats, stabilize your core for better lunges, or fine-tune your hinge mechanics, you'll find clear, actionable steps to address the challenges holding you back.

THE PRINCIPAL STAGE PROGRESSIONS—
PROGRESS OR REGRESS BASED ON HOW YOU FEEL, FUNCTION, AND PERFORM

When it comes to mastering the six foundational movement patterns, it's not just about optimizing the exercises within the patterns; it's about understanding the progression of those exercises to achieve continual, pain-free gains. The principal stage progressions are designed to help you build a solid foundation from the ground up, stacking motor skills from easiest to hardest layer by layer so you can develop and maintain a movement system that is both strong and adaptable.

To help you conceptualize this process, imagine each progression as a building block in a pyramid. The foundational exercises form the wide, stable base, where motor control and movement quality are developed with minimal load and complexity. As you move up the pyramid, the exercises increase in difficulty, allowing you to expand your movement quality and skill through more advanced variations. In other words, each layer of the pyramid supports the next, ensuring that as you progress to more challenging exercises, you're well prepared to maintain form, avoid injury, and effectively handle increased loads or more complex movements.

I'll be the first to admit that there are countless ways to progress and endless exercise variations you could implement. If I included every possible variation, there would be thousands of exercises for each pattern. The progressions featured within the movement pattern pyramids are the "big hitters." They represent the principal options that effectively illustrate how to progress from easier to more advanced movements based on factors like motor control demands, load position, stance, and execution.

I set them up this way to provide a clear, adaptable pathway for everyone—from beginners to experienced movers. They offer structure but also flexibility, allowing you to customize and individualize your training based on your goals, training style, and background. No matter where you start on the movement pattern pyramid, the aim is to implement the progression near the edge of your ability—enough to stimulate progress, but not so much that you risk pain or injury.

This is tricky because everyone has a different starting point. Someone who is brand-new to exercising should obviously start at the base of the pyramid with the first stage progression. But I'm guessing that most of you are not beginners. In fact, many of you are, for better or worse, already performing exercises at or near the top of the pyramid. Does that mean that the principal-stage progressions do not apply to you? Absolutely not, and here's why.

Let's take the example of an experienced lifter who can handle massive loads with complex variations like the barbell back squat or deadlift. On the surface, this might seem like the pinnacle of strength training, but what if these movements are causing frequent injuries or chronic pain? In that case, the pattern itself needs to be rebuilt and the exercise regressed.

This is where stage progressions become crucial, even for seasoned lifters. By running the screen and assessment, you can quickly identify any linchpins in your movement. From there, working your way back up the pyramid—starting with simpler variations—allows you to rebuild the pattern with a stronger, more stable foundation. This process doesn't take long and can make all the difference in helping you determine not only the right exercises for your situation, but also the modifications that you may need to make to those exercises to stay pain-free.

Another scenario where the stage progressions come into play is when you run the assessment and modify your body position or execution. For instance, if you've always performed a squat or deadlift with a particular stance, a sudden change fundamentally alters how your body performs the exercise. Your neural sequencing and motor control are wired for the old stance, so when you adjust it, you may need to regress—either by moving lower on the pyramid or reducing the load or range of motion—to adapt to the new position. In these situations, regression isn't a setback but rather a strategic move to build a stronger base. This ensures that when you progress again, you do so safely and effectively, setting yourself up for long-term success.

As you advance through the stage progressions, your strength, skill, and confidence will naturally grow. However, remember that progress is rarely linear. It's essential to regularly assess your readiness—not only to move to more advanced exercises but also to determine when you might need to regress to an easier variation. This means continuously evaluating where you are in your journey and being mindful of how your body is responding. Several factors come into play, such as your current physical state (including sleep quality, muscle soreness, stress levels, and any pain), how well you've mastered the previous stage, and whether you can maintain proper form under more challenging conditions.

So, how do you know when it's time to move on to a more advanced exercise or regress to an easier variation? The answer lies in how you feel, function, and perform.

FEEL

Does the exercise feel right? When everything is firing correctly, the correct muscles should engage, and the movement should feel strong, stable, and smooth. You should experience a sense of control and coordination, with no awkwardness or apprehension. If the movement flows naturally and you feel in sync with your body, it's a good indication that you're ready to progress to the next stage. However, if you notice any pain, discomfort, or any other red flags during the screen, you may need to regress to an easier variation.

Can you perform the exercise with proper form? If your technique breaks down, it's a sign that the exercise is too advanced, and you should consider regressing to a movement where you can maintain control and stability. However, if you can consistently perform the exercise with excellent form—you can pass the screen for that exercise, for example—it may be time to advance up the pyramid to continue building strength and motor control.

PERFORM

Can you execute the exercise under challenging conditions—such as with added load, increased speed, or greater effort—without compromising form? If you can, it's a sign that you're ready to progress up the pyramid. But if the added challenge causes your form to falter, regressing to a simpler variation is necessary to ensure safe and effective training while you build the capacity to handle more demanding exercises.

One of the biggest mistakes people make in training is jumping straight into the most advanced, high-risk exercises—those at the top of the pyramid that demand high skill and heavy loads—before they're truly ready. It's like trying to leap up a flight of stairs only to come crashing down, leading to a cycle of injury, reinjury, and disuse. The principal stage progressions are your road map for avoiding that cycle. They guide you in building a strong, pain-free body by ensuring your training is always aligned with your current capabilities. This approach helps you steer clear of the pitfalls of overreaching and undertraining, keeping your progress steady and sustainable.

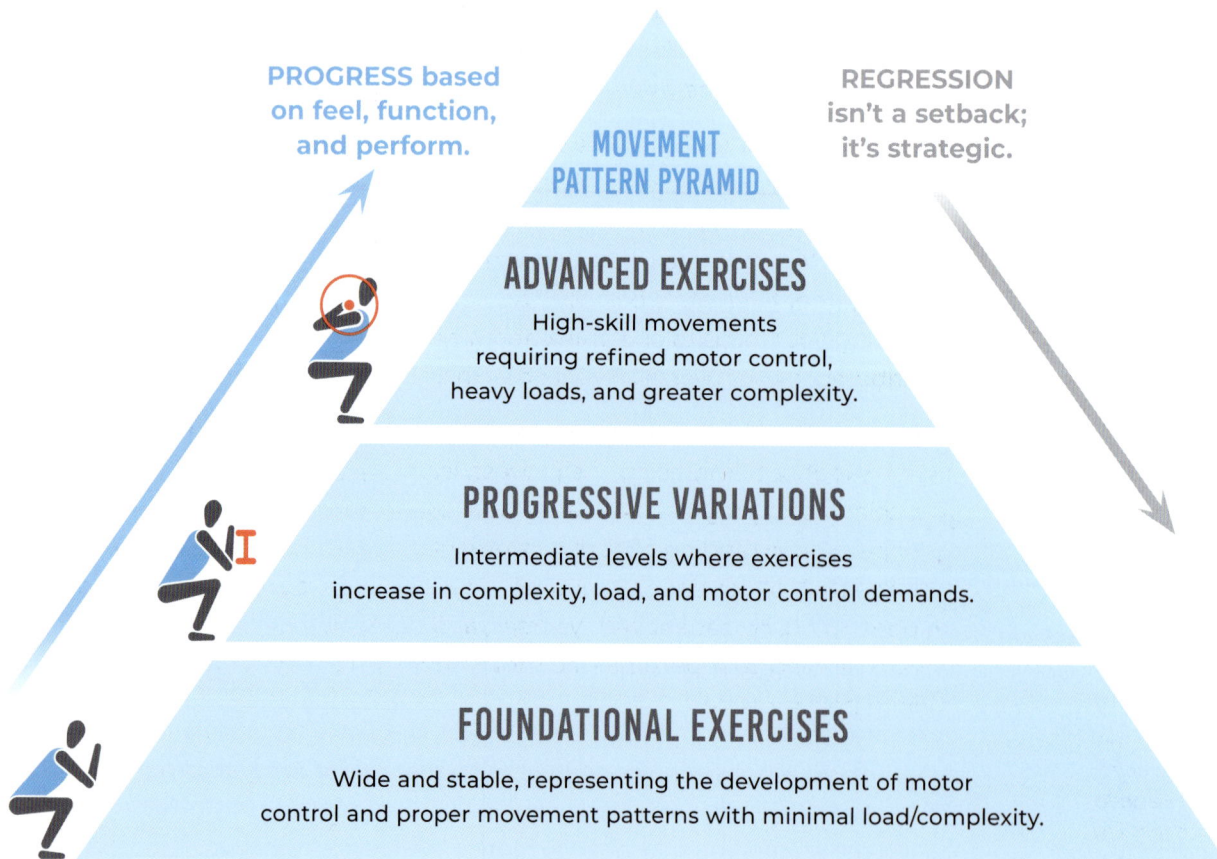

PROGRESS based on feel, function, and perform.

REGRESSION isn't a setback; it's strategic.

MOVEMENT PATTERN PYRAMID

ADVANCED EXERCISES
High-skill movements requiring refined motor control, heavy loads, and greater complexity.

PROGRESSIVE VARIATIONS
Intermediate levels where exercises increase in complexity, load, and motor control demands.

FOUNDATIONAL EXERCISES
Wide and stable, representing the development of motor control and proper movement patterns with minimal load/complexity.

TRAIN
THE PATTERNS

Train six patterns: push, pull, hinge, squat, lunge, and carry

Evaluate program balance regularly

SCREEN
THE PATTERNS

Screen the optimization checklist

Film yourself or get coaching feedback

If you meet the standards, that's "good enough" to train

ASSESS
THE PATTERNS

Personalize movement to your body

Retest and screen the patterns from your authentic setup and execution

CORRECT
THE PATTERNS

Identify your linchpins

Address mobility, stability, and skill issues

Utilize optimization strategies to fix form

PROGRESS
THE PATTERNS

Progress or regress based on feel, function, and performance

Build from foundational to advanced movements

ADOPT THE MOVEMENT MASTERY MINDSET—
DON'T CHASE PERFECTION

Having read all the movement tenets, you might be thinking, "How can I possibly keep all of this in mind? What if I can't get it exactly right?" This concern often stems from several factors: the challenge of executing movements correctly, the psychological and emotional scars of past injuries, and the seemingly daunting task of rebuilding foundational movement patterns from scratch. It's a lot to take in, and the fear of not getting it perfect can quickly take hold, leading to destructive thinking patterns that can hinder your progress.

This can manifest in thoughts like, "If I can't do the most advanced exercise, I might as well not do it at all," or believing that a movement is either wholly safe or always harmful. You might even think, "If my form isn't perfect, the entire exercise is a failure." This type of all-or-nothing, black or white mindset is common yet counterproductive. It can create unnecessary pressure and prevent you from making the consistent, meaningful progress that truly defines movement mastery.

As you might recall from Part 1, adopting the movement mastery mindset means seeing improvement as a continuous journey rather than a destination. Your progress should be measured against your own potential—what you're truly capable of—rather than some unattainable ideal. Ultimately, this mindset leads to a healthier, more sustainable relationship with exercise, one that allows you to grow and evolve without the pressure of being perfect.

It's also crucial not to fixate on a single exercise or pattern, believing that mastering it will solve all your physical challenges. Human movement is far more complex than that. No single movement or exercise can address everything. What's more important is how different movements and patterns work together to create a balanced and effective training routine. Instead of narrowing your focus to one, think about how each movement you perform contributes to your overall physical health and functional abilities.

As you dive into the next chapters, remember that the path to movement mastery is about embracing the process, learning from each experience, and celebrating progress, no matter how small. Along the way, you'll gain a deeper understanding of both movement and your body, equipping you with the tools to continue this journey with confidence and optimism. Keep an open mind, be patient with yourself, and trust that every step you take toward refining your personalized movement will bring you closer to pain-free, lifelong performance.

SQUAT

The squat is one of the most butchered movement patterns. Years of poor habits, misguided training practices, and everyday environmental pressures have turned what should be a fundamental human movement into a source of pain for many. But it doesn't have to be that way. By learning how to squat correctly and practicing it in a way that aligns with your body's natural mechanics and anatomy, you can regain lost function, experience less pain, build more strength, and protect yourself from injury in the long run.

It was my first night on the job with the Chinese Olympic Committee, and I was about to experience a cultural initiation I'll never forget. As is customary for new Western coaches, they took me out for dinner and drinks. Now, I've never been much of a drinker—I'm more of a "glass of water, early bedtime" kind of guy—but I didn't want to seem disrespectful. I figured I'd have a drink or two, be polite, and call it a night. But, as I was about to find out, that's not how the night was going to unfold.

When we walked in, I immediately noticed crates of baijiu—a clear liquor I'd heard whispers about—stacked in the corner. Twelve people sat at a table, and each person had their own bottle. I quickly realized this wasn't going to be the kind of casual "have a beer and chat" night I was hoping for. But hey, new country, new job. "When in Rome," I thought.

What followed was 90 minutes of nonstop toasting, standing, and downing baijiu like it was a competitive sport. We'd stand up, say something nice to each other—complimenting everything from watches to haircuts—clink glasses, and down a full cup of this throat-burning jet fuel. Each toast seemed to escalate, and before long, I was hammered. Desperate for a break, I stumbled to the restroom and noticed something odd: One of the urinals was chest height. "Who on Earth is using this?" I thought, squinting at it as if my impaired vision would somehow give me an answer.

Then I saw the toilets—or rather, the holes in the floor. Pretty standard in China, but at the time, I was too drunk to fully grasp the situation. I shrugged, did what I'd gone there to do, and stumbled back to the table, none the wiser.

The next morning, I woke up with a hangover that could knock out a horse. My head was pounding, and as I tried to piece together the night, I remembered the chest-high "urinal." It dawned on me with painful clarity: That wasn't a urinal—it was the designated puke station, where everyone else had been discreetly throwing up to keep the party

going. Meanwhile, I had missed the memo and suffered through, leaving me to endure a full day of athlete assessments while barely functioning.

Back then, I was using a popular movement screen to assess athletes' movement patterns and identify issues. My first test was the overhead deep squat, and on that miserable, hungover day, I ran it on hundreds of China's elite and upcoming athletes. I fully expected to see the usual flaws I often encountered in the U.S.—compensations, imbalances, all the stuff I was used to coaching.

But to my surprise, nearly every one of them performed flawless squats—deep, symmetrical, and pain-free.

At first, I thought I'd messed up the assessments. My head was throbbing, and I couldn't believe what I was seeing. I even suggested we rescreen everyone. But via some translation, they told me, "No, we squat well in China." That's when it clicked: The squat toilets I'd encountered the night before weren't just bathroom fixtures, but represented a fundamental difference in daily movement patterns. Throughout my travels in China, I began to notice that squatting was a way of life—people squatted to rest, to work, to socialize. The deep squat wasn't just an exercise; it was an everyday movement pattern ingrained from childhood.

Meanwhile, in the West, we've engineered the full-range squat out of our daily lives. Elevated toilets, squatty potties to unkink our bowels, and sitting with our hips locked at 90-degree angles for most jobs and activities have eliminated the need for deep hip flexion. This sedentary lifestyle directly impacts how most people squat in the gym. Accustomed to stopping at 90 degrees, many perceive a shallow, parallel squat as "full depth." Over time, this limited range of motion not only reinforces poor movement patterns but also increases stress on the knees. By stopping abruptly at parallel with added load, the knees absorb forces that would otherwise be distributed through the hips and glutes in a deeper squat.

In cultures where deep squatting is part of everyday life, the movement is a natural part of the body's routine. Squatting to full depth not only maintains range of motion but also helps people instinctively adopt a squat stance and style that suits their unique body structure. The more you squat pain-free, the more your body finds the most efficient way to perform the movement, adapting to your individual hip, ankle, and leg anatomy. This is just one reason why, in these cultures, deep, unrestricted squats are second nature.

In the West, however, we lose this ability. Then, when people try to push beyond their limited range in the gym—whether adding weight or aiming for a deeper squat—it often gets butchered. The hips tuck under, the lower back rounds, and compensations kick in to make up for the lack of mobility, stability, and skill. And while many think they know what a squat is, their idea is often limited to the gym version—feet shoulder-width apart, knees bent, hips back. For some, this works, but it's only a shadow of the full, unrestricted squat pattern we're naturally capable of. The gym squat often prioritizes lifting heavy loads, while the deeper, innate squat pattern deteriorates over time—not just due to our sedentary lifestyles but because we continually practice this limited version and ingrain poor habits.

It's a classic example of how years of poor movement patterns directly impact gym performance. Without a solid foundation, people force their bodies into positions they're not prepared for, thinking that simply adding weight or going lower is the answer. But it's not. To squat well—whether in the gym or in daily life—you have to reclaim the full, natural movement your body was designed for. Most importantly, you should be able to do it pain-free, without compensations or unnecessary strain that could lead to chronic discomfort or long-term injury. This requires a willingness to approach the squat with a mindset of exploration and adjustment, recognizing that an ideal squat looks different for everyone and depends on your unique structure, mobility, and movement history.

Take, for example, a 23-year-old strength coach I recently worked with. He told me, "Squats kill my knees and back. But I just tough it out." And that's where he—and so many others—get it wrong. Rather than adjusting the movement to suit their own anatomy, they try to force their bodies into a one-size-fits-all squat, which only compounds the pain. They don't consider that their bodies may need adjustments—perhaps a different stance, foot position, or squat depth—to make the movement work for them. By sticking rigidly to a "universal" squat technique, they unknowingly butcher their form and cause issues that could have been avoided with simple modifications.

There's a better way. The first step is to reassess how you're squatting in the first place, making sure your form suits your body's needs. Just as important is knowing the difference between the typical discomfort that comes with lifting and the kind of pain that signals something is wrong.

Matt Wenning, one of the greatest squatters of all time, put it best when he told me: "A squat shouldn't feel comfortable when you're braced properly. But it shouldn't hurt, either." The message is simple: Squatting should feel tight, controlled, and stable, with every muscle working together to support the movement.

Too often, people confuse pain with progress, believing that pushing through will lead to gains. But forcing through pain is a recipe for injury and setbacks. A truly effective squat means moving well first before adding load. It starts with mastering the fundamentals: proper setup, bracing, and smooth, controlled movement. Nail those basics, and the strength will naturally follow as your body becomes more stable, more efficient, and more powerful.

But to get there, you need more than just effort; you need to screen and assess the pattern to identify where your form is breaking down, where you might be compensating, and where you need to improve. By running a movement screen, you'll see if you're maintaining a neutral pillar, achieving symmetry, and controlling the full range of motion. These are your markers—your baseline for safe, pain-free squatting. If you're experiencing pain or limitations during the screen, the assessment will point you toward the adjustments you need to make, whether it's altering your range of motion or tweaking your stance.

Once you've identified your ideal squat setup and execution, it's time to move through the progressions. Start with the exercises at the base of the squat pyramid and gradually build up to more advanced variations as your mobility, stability, and skill improve. Don't rush it—mastery takes time. Focus on the subtleties of each stage and allow your body to adapt as you build a solid, pain-free foundation. By following these progressions and addressing any weak links, you'll unlock the full potential of your squat, transforming it from a butchered movement into the natural, powerful pattern it is meant to be.

A truly effective squat means moving well first before adding load.

SQUAT SCREEN

The screen is your first opportunity to apply key cues that ensure you're moving with the best form possible. This isn't about perfection, but rather a starting point to guide the process.

There are a couple of ways to approach the squat screen, depending on your experience. If you already squat regularly, start with the stance that feels most natural to you, while avoiding a stance that is excessively wide or narrow. If you're new to squatting—or if you feel your squat pattern needs a reset—I recommend following the setup and execution steps outlined below. This generalized setup works for most people, but keep in mind that it may not align with your unique hip anatomy.

The goal of the screen is to test your squat against the standards covered in the optimization checklist and to identify any potential weak links that could be compromising your form. In other words, it introduces the correct way to squat, giving you a framework to measure your current squat pattern and highlight any areas that need improvement.

By using this baseline, you'll have a better sense of what adjustments to make. Then the assessment will lock it in, helping you fine-tune a setup, depth, and foot position that is more specific to your body.

SETUP: STANCE and BODY POSITION

1. **Stance:** Stand with your feet about shoulder-width apart, toes slightly turned out. Bring your hands to your neckline. Make a fist with one hand and cup the other hand around your knuckles.

2. **Stabilize the Pillar:** Begin the cueing sequence to stabilize your pillar. Co-contract your pecs and lats by pressing your hands together and squeezing your arms toward your ribs. Then engage your glutes and adductors while pressing your big toes into the floor to create an arch in your feet. Simultaneously, rotate your knees outward without moving your feet.

3. **Breathing and Bracing:** Inhale deeply through your nose, expanding your diaphragm in all directions (360-degree expansion). Once you've reached maximal inhalation, hold your breath and brace your core by contracting the muscles around your torso.

For a more detailed explanation of how to stabilize and brace the pillar, see pages 34–35.

EXECUTION: PERFORMING THE SQUAT

Eccentric Phase: With your body stabilized and maximally tensioned, begin the squat by pushing your hips back and bending your knees simultaneously. As you lower, allow your torso to tilt slightly forward to maintain balance, keeping your spine neutral, your pelvis stable, and your weight evenly distributed across your heel, big toe, and little toe (referred to as the tripod foot position).

Continue descending with your knees tracking over your toes while keeping a strong foot and ankle position. Your shins should angle forward in a way that roughly matches the forward tilt of your torso as you approach the bottom of the squat. Lower your hips as far as you can while maintaining a neutral spine and avoiding compensations or unwanted rotation at your ankles, knees, hips, or shoulders.

Change of Direction (Amortization Phase):

The transition between the eccentric (lowering) and concentric (rising) phases—known as the amortization phase—is a critical point in the movement where faults often occur. Move slowly enough during the eccentric phase to maintain position and stability as you reach the bottom. Avoid bouncing or collapsing into the change of direction, which can exacerbate instabilities. Keep full-body tension through this phase, ensuring smooth control as you reverse the movement.

Concentric Phase:
As you begin the ascent (concentric phase), drive through your entire tripod foot, actively pushing the ground away while keeping your knees tracking over your toes and your hips and shoulders rising together at the same rate. Maintain full-body tension, focusing on engaging your glutes, hamstrings, and core to drive the movement.

Avoid losing foot pressure, allowing your knees to cave in, or shifting your weight excessively toward your toes or heels. Keep your rib cage stacked over your pelvis, and ensure your spine and pelvis remain neutral throughout the upward motion.

Key Considerations:

Smooth Tempo: During the eccentric phase, move at a pace that maintains stability and alignment without sacrificing the fluidity of the movement. Avoid going so slowly that it disrupts your natural mechanics or reduces full-body tension.

Control Throughout: Ensure tension is never lost, even during the change of direction at the bottom of the squat. This consistency helps prevent joint stress and enhances movement efficiency.

Alignment and Balance: Keep your spine neutral, your pelvis stable, and your weight evenly distributed across your tripod foot throughout the entire movement.

By maintaining **stability, control, and tension** in every phase of the squat, you can reduce the risk of compensatory patterns, improve joint health, and build a strong foundation for safely handling increased loads over time.

Utilizing the squat setup and execution strategy, the next step is to film yourself performing the movement from both front and side angles. This provides a clear visual baseline and allows you to compare your pre-assessment form with your post-assessment results. Ideally, have someone measure how deep you can squat while adhering to the standards outlined in the optimization checklist. If that's not possible, take photos to capture your squat depth and positioning. Once you've gone through the assessment and retested with your personalized squat stance, you'll be able to see how much deeper and more controlled your squat becomes, providing a clear picture of the progress you've made.

HIP VARIATION AND SQUATTING—
THE ENDLESS HIP ANTHROPOMETRICAL DIFFERENCES

To optimize your squat stance, it's essential to appreciate the vast differences in hip anatomy among individuals. Variations in the shape and alignment of the hip joint and femur significantly influence which stance will feel most natural, effective, and pain-free for you.

- **Femur Neck Length and Angle:** The femur's neck can lean forward (anteversion) or backward (retroversion), affecting how your feet and hips should be positioned. For instance, Caucasian men typically average around 7 degrees of anteversion, while Chinese men average about 14 degrees. Retroversion also varies, with Caucasian men experiencing it in about 24.1 percent of cases, African American men at 15.1 percent, and women across all ethnicities at 14.3 percent.[1] This variability means some people feel better with a more "toes-out" stance, while others prefer "toes-forward."

- **Hip Socket (Acetabular) Orientation and Depth:** The tilt and depth of your hip socket also vary. A deeper or more angled socket might require a wider stance or more hip hinge to squat comfortably, while a shallow or forward-tilted socket might make a narrower, upright squat easier.

THE IMPORTANCE OF A PERSONALIZED APPROACH

It's the combination of variables—femoral length/angle, hip socket depth/orientation—that gives each person a unique range of motion and squat stance. This is why a one-size-fits-all approach to squatting doesn't work.

Even common recommendations based on body type tend to oversimplify things. For example, it's often said that people with longer torsos and shorter legs should squat more upright, while those with shorter torsos and longer legs should lean forward. But that's not always the case. Some people with short torsos and long femurs still squat upright and vice versa—likely due to the aforementioned factors.

The key takeaway is that your anatomy affects how you squat. Fortunately, you don't need to know every detail of your hip structure to squat correctly. That's the purpose of the assessment: It helps identify your optimal squat stance and depth without the need for in-depth knowledge of your internal anatomy.

DIFFERENCES IN FEMORAL NECK LENGTHS AND ANGLES

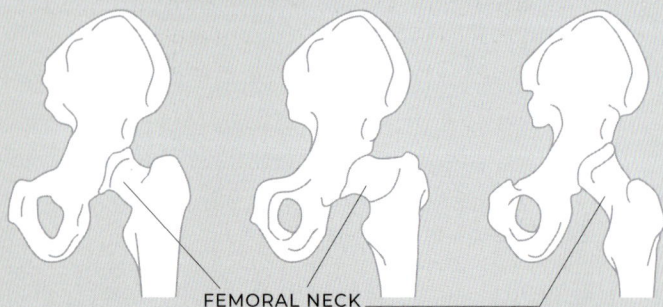

DIFFERENCES IN HIP SOCKET ORIENTATION AND DEPTH

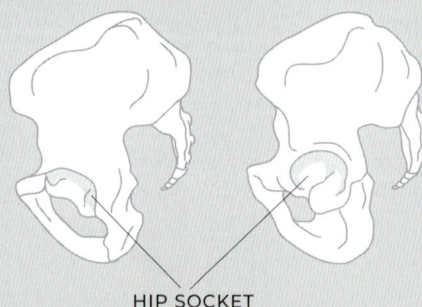

FEMORAL NECK

HIP SOCKET

✓ NEUTRAL SPINE

Maintaining a neutral spine while squatting means keeping your spine stable and aligned, though some movement is natural. The goal is to stay within a zone of neutrality—a range in which your spine remains stable and safe under load.

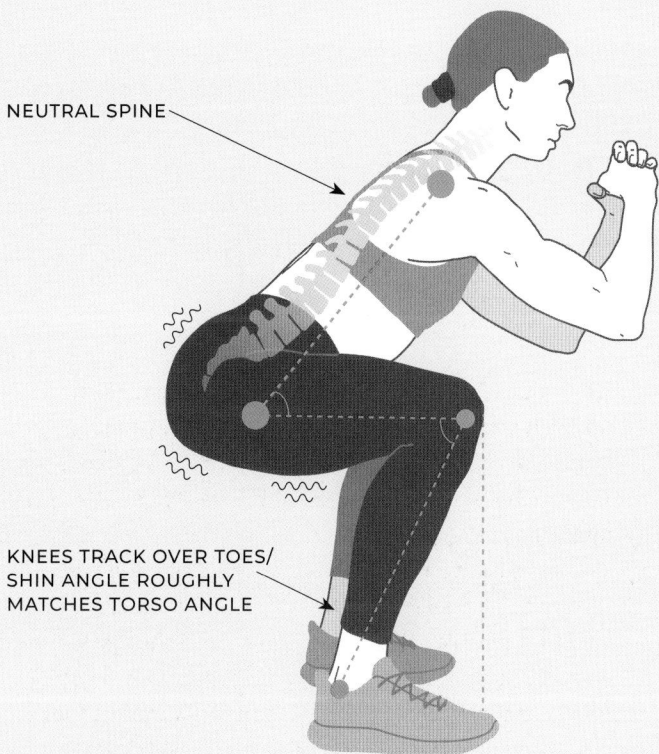

✓ NO UNWANTED ROTATION

Resisting unwanted rotation during the squat means preventing asymmetrical or uncontrolled rotational movements. While some degree of rotation is natural due to the way human anatomy is structured—our muscles, ligaments, and tendons are organized in layers, slings, and oblique patterns—unwanted rotation refers to imbalances or compensations that occur during the movement, leading to instability and inefficiency.

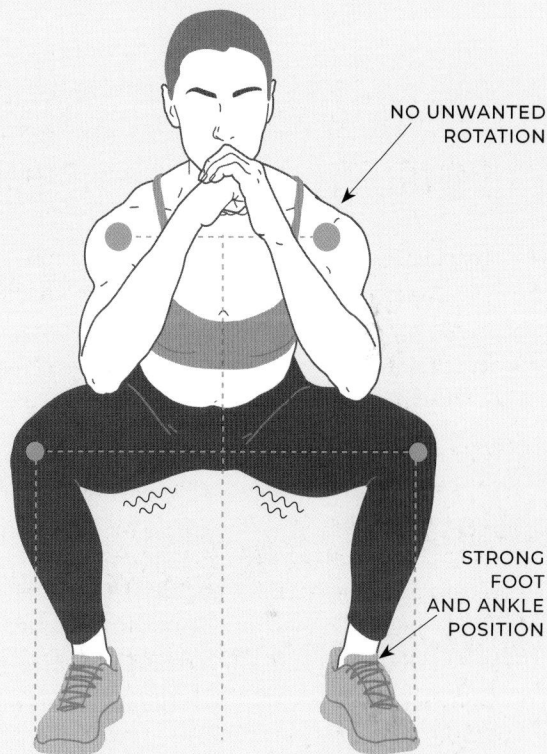

NEUTRAL SPINE

NO UNWANTED ROTATION

KNEES TRACK OVER TOES/ SHIN ANGLE ROUGHLY MATCHES TORSO ANGLE

STRONG FOOT AND ANKLE POSITION

✓ KNEES TRACK OVER TOES/ SHIN ANGLE ROUGHLY MATCHES TORSO ANGLE

A key element of proper squat mechanics is ensuring two things. First, the midline of your kneecap (patella) should track over the fifth digit (pinky toe). This ensures your knees move forward in line with your feet, preventing them from caving inward or flaring outward excessively.

Second, the angle of your shins should match the angle of your torso as you move through the squat. This alignment creates better force angles, reduces stress on your joints, and promotes a stable, powerful squat from start to finish.

By maintaining proper knee tracking and shin/torso alignment, you not only protect your knees and ankles but also keep your hips and spine in a stacked, stable position. This allows you to engage the right muscles, maintain balance, and enhance both performance and safety.

✓ STRONG FOOT AND ANKLE POSITION

A strong ankle and foot position is fundamental to executing a proper squat. Your feet are the only point of contact with the ground, and how they engage with the surface has a direct impact on your stability and movement efficiency. Similarly, your ankles play a crucial role in transferring power up through your legs and hips. By maintaining a stacked joint position, where your ankle is aligned over your foot, and keeping your feet actively engaged, you can create stability and torque from the ground up, reducing compensations up the chain (in your knees, hips, and lower back).

SQUAT ASSESSMENT

The squat has long been one of the most debated topics in fitness, sparking discussions across all levels of the industry—from bodybuilding to powerlifting, Olympic-style lifting, and CrossFit. As barbell sports have gained influence, the way we view the squat has shifted, often reducing it to a sport-specific exercise. But in focusing too heavily on performance within the confines of the gym, many have lost sight of the squat as a fundamental human movement—one that serves us in everyday life, not just under a loaded bar.

As the fitness industry continues to evolve, we've gained new insights into the unique anatomical, biomechanical, and neuromuscular differences between individuals. Specifically, the structure of the hips can vary widely from person to person, making it clear that no two people should squat exactly the same way. The one-size-fits-all approach doesn't work. It's time to embrace a more personalized strategy that aligns with each individual's anatomy and movement capabilities.

This is where the squat assessment plays a crucial role. If your initial screen felt good, you're ready to train. But for many, small adjustments in stance width, foot orientation, or squat depth can make a significant difference in how the movement feels and performs. The upcoming assessment is designed to help pinpoint these subtle refinements, giving you the ability to fine-tune your squat for greater comfort, safety, and strength.

In practice, these tweaks can lead to breakthrough moments. It's not uncommon to see someone struggle with their squat, only to gain an extra 10 inches of authentic range of motion after making a few strategic changes. These refinements often unlock a squat pattern they didn't know they had.

SQUATTING FROM YOUR NON-AUTHENTIC SQUAT STANCE

Your "authentic" squat stance is the one best suited to your body's mechanics—optimized for strength, movement efficiency, and long-term health. But that doesn't mean you can't or shouldn't train other stances. In fact, working from a "non-authentic" stance—like wider or narrower than usual—can help target weak links, boost muscular recruitment, and strengthen different ranges of motion. Just remember, regardless of stance, the rules remain the same: Maintain spine neutrality and manage rotation to avoid pain and injury.

Take powerlifters, for example. Their competition stance is designed to hit parallel depth with maximum load—often not their authentic stance, but one that helps them achieve specific performance goals. They prioritize a stance that gets them just to parallel, which may not allow for full range of motion but is necessary for their sport. However, this doesn't mean they should ignore their authentic stance in training. By focusing on their optimal stance outside of competition, they can build better long-term movement health and strength capacity, while still using non-authentic stances to meet specific performance objectives.

In summary, prioritizing your authentic stance is essential for building and maintaining a solid, pain-free squat pattern. Non-authentic stances, on the other hand, are valuable tools to work on targeted goals—whether it's building strength in specific ranges of motion, emphasizing certain muscle groups, strengthening weak links, or preparing for a competition.

And that's exactly what you're aiming for with this assessment. By customizing your squat to fit your individual hip structure and movement profile, you'll move smarter, safer, and more efficiently—not just for barbell lifts, but every squat you do.

THE HIP QUADRANT TEST— DETERMINING YOUR AUTHENTIC SQUAT STANCE

To find your ideal squat stance and depth—and understand how your hip joint functions during a squat—you can use a simple orthopedic assessment known as the Hip Quadrant Test (or Hip Scour Test). Traditionally, this test has been used by medical professionals to evaluate hip function and identify the presence and location of issues such as labral tears or joint degeneration. However, in this context, the focus is on understanding how your femur and hip socket (acetabulum) naturally move together, free from soft tissue restrictions, to help you discover the most comfortable and effective squat stance and depth for your body.

1. STARTING POSITION

▶ **Action:** Lie on your back with a neutral spine, keeping your legs straight and heels touching the ground.

▶ **Goal:** Keep your pelvis stable throughout the test, avoiding any compensatory movement (like the opposite leg or tailbone lifting off the ground).

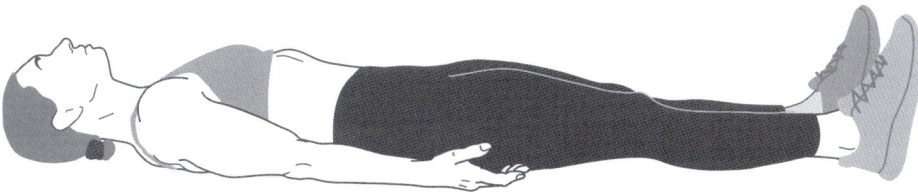

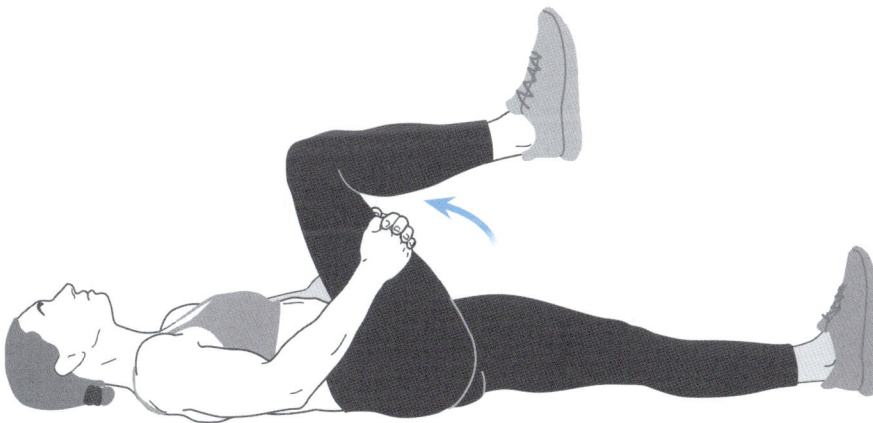

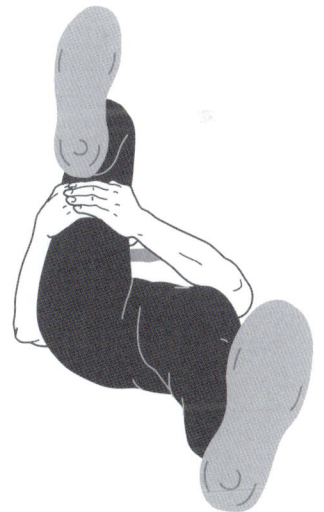

2. KNEE-TO-CHEST FLEXION

▶ **Action:** Slowly bring one knee toward your chest. Then grip your hamstrings with both hands to guide your knee farther toward your chest. Keep the movement controlled, aiming to bring your knee directly upward without allowing it to move outward. Stop when you feel resistance and hit the natural block.

▶ **Goal:** Maximize hip flexion while keeping your pelvis stable (no rounding of the lower back or lifting of the opposite leg). You're assessing how close you can bring your knee to your chest without compensations.

▶ **Observation:** Note how close your knee comes to your chest without forcing the movement or causing any other part of your body to shift. This knee-to-chest position provides an initial marker for assessing your hip flexion and, ultimately, your potential squat depth when standing upright as you continue with the assessment.

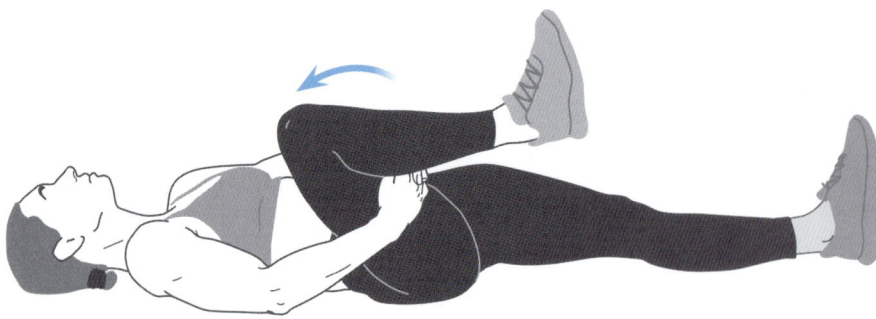

3. HIP EXTERNAL ROTATION AND ABDUCTION

▶ **Action:** After reaching the flexion limit, gently move your knee outward (external rotation), allowing your femur to move away from your midline (abduction). Continue to guide your knee closer to your chest/shoulder, seeing how much additional range of motion you can achieve.

▶ **Goal:** Minimize the distance between your knee and chest by adding external rotation and abduction. You're assessing how much closer your knee can come to **your** chest with this adjustment. The closer **your** knee comes, the more squat depth you'll achieve when standing on your feet.

▶ **Observation:** Watch for any compensations like the opposite leg lifting off the ground, rotation through the torso or shoulders, and pelvis rounding with tailbone coming off the floor. Only the hip you're testing should be moving. Reset back to the previous step if you notice any compensations.

4. REPEAT WITH OPPOSITE LEG (TEST BOTH LEGS SIMULTANEOUSLY)

▶ **Action:** Hold the leg you assessed in the previous step (e.g., your right leg) in the relative end range testing position. Once stabilized, slowly and under control, perform the test on the opposite leg (e.g., the left leg) while maintaining the position of the first leg. This process allows you to evaluate both sides together and yields the most accurate measurements. Take note of differences in range of motion, comfort, and symmetry between the sides. For precision, measure key variables such as heel-to-heel distance, knee-to-knee distance, butt-to-heel distance, and both toe angles (refer to images for clarity).

▶ **Goal:** Determine your authentic squat depth and stance. Pay attention to four key variables:

- **Heel Position:** The width between your heels, which will help determine your ideal squat width.

- **Toe Angle:** The degree to which your toes are turned out (foot abduction). If your test required more external rotation, you'll likely need a more toed-out stance for squatting.

- **Knee Position:** Check the distance between your knees to ensure they align properly in your squat stance.

- **Hip Flexion:** Roughly determine the distance between your hips and heels to roughly determine your squat depth.

▶ **Observation:** If you don't have someone available to take measurements, mentally note the four key variables or capture a photo or video for reference. Use this information to replicate your optimal stance when transitioning into a standing position.

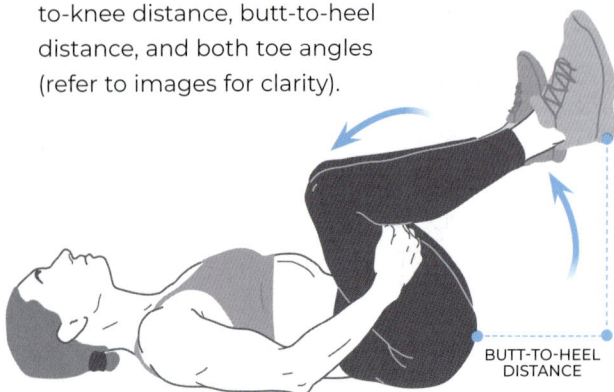

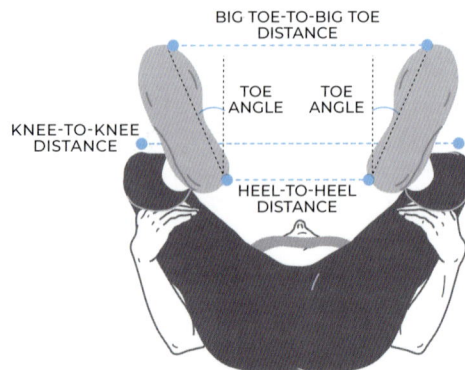

5. TRANSFER TO STANDING POSITION

▶ **Action:** Stand up and try to replicate the position you found in the test.

▶ **Goal:** Try your best to replicate the result from the assessment into the standing position.

▶ **Observation:** If it feels different from how you usually squat, that's okay—you're getting closer to your authentic squat stance.

6. ADJUST AND RETEST

▶ **Self-Assessment:** After standing in the position that mirrors the results of your test, try squatting. Focus on replicating the foot width, toe angle, and knee distance from the test. Based on how the squat feels, make slight adjustments to the width of your feet or the angle of your toes.

▶ **Goal:** Follow the optimization checklist. If your new stance feels more comfortable and stable, you've found a better starting position and execution for your squat. If it still feels off, continue tweaking these variables to match what felt most natural during the assessment. It's worth noting that other factors can come into play when standing—such as limited ankle mobility, knee pain, and insufficient muscle activation or motor control. If you're new to exercise, practice this stance only to a depth that feels comfortable, paying attention to each item on the optimization checklist. As you accumulate more reps, you'll improve your movement, build strength, and eventually be able to go deeper.

▶ **Observation:** When you perform squat screen and retest using the optimization checklist from your authentic stance, take note of how you feel, function, and perform. Do you have less pain, more range of motion, and control? If you still have glaring compensations—you don't meet one or more of the standards outlined in the optimization checklist due to mobility, stability, or skill—address those utilizing the strategies covered below.

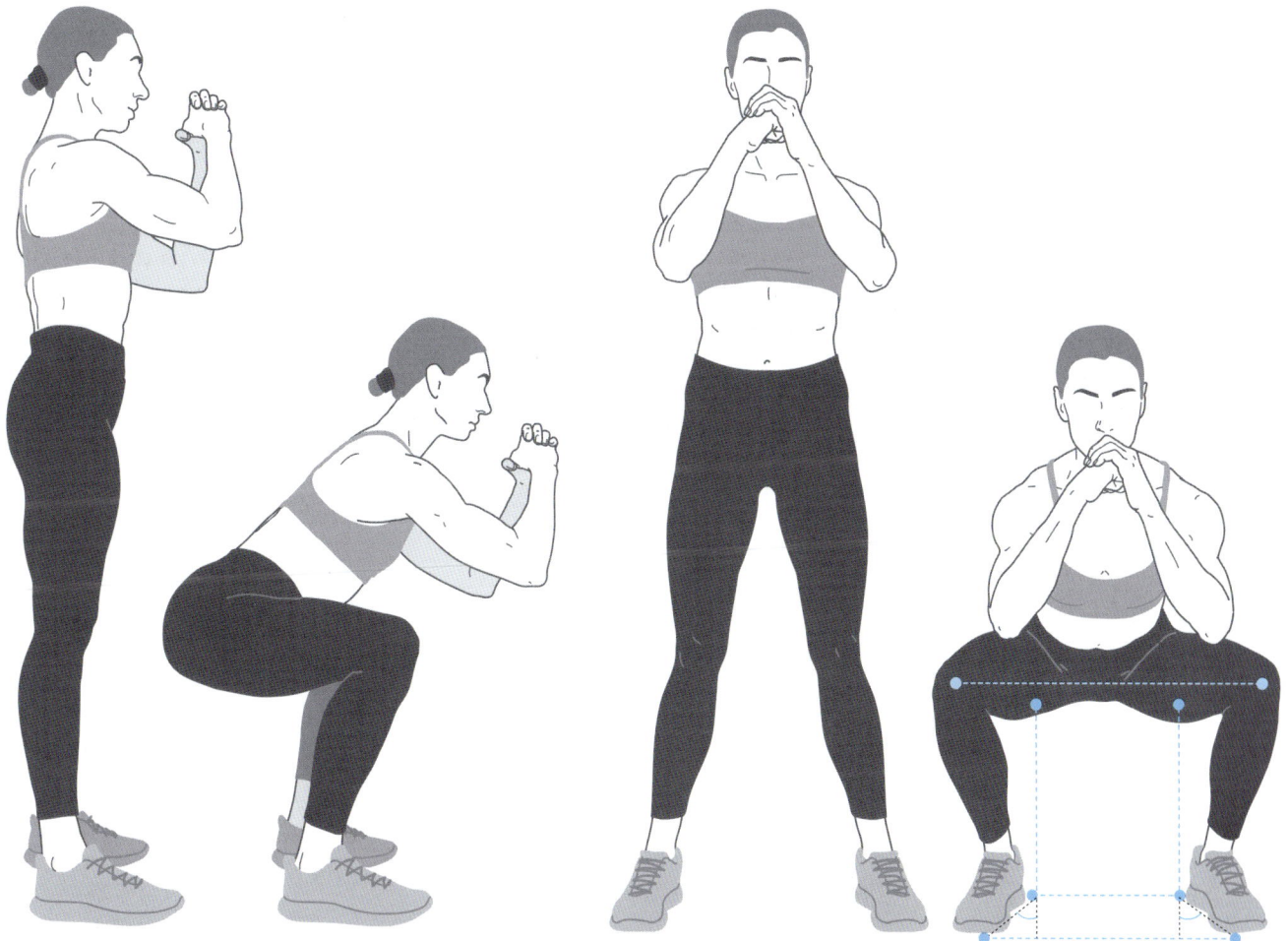

OPTIMIZATION STRATEGIES

Now that you've completed the screen and retested your squat using the optimization checklist from your authentic stance (see Step 6: Adjust and Retest in the assessment protocol), you may still notice some compensations that place unnecessary strain on your knees, hips, or lower back. If these compensations cause pain flare-ups or limit your performance, they should be addressed with strategies tailored to your individual needs. It's important to understand, however, that not every compensation leads to pain or injury, nor does it mean you're fragile or incapable of training effectively. In fact, some individuals may feel stronger or move better in positions that would traditionally be considered "faults." The key is finding what works best for your body and goals.

Not every compensation leads to pain or injury, nor does it mean you're fragile or incapable of training effectively.

Fortunately, the squat pattern is highly adaptable, and every compensation has a targeted mobility, stability, or skill-based solution. With the right optimization strategies, you can refine your mechanics, address weak links, and build a stronger, more resilient squat—no matter your starting point, unique anatomy, or movement history.

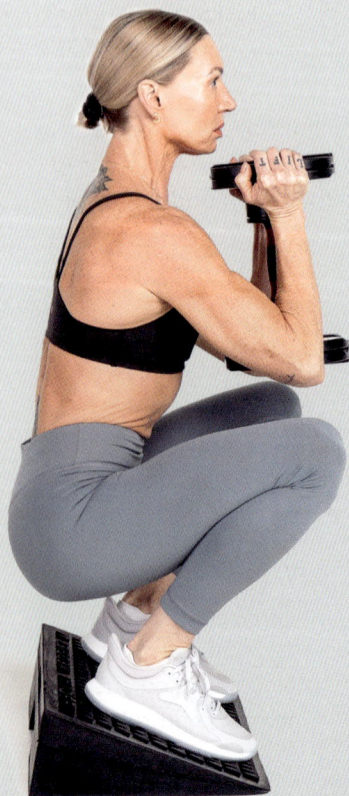

THE ROLE OF THE SQUAT WEDGE: TOOL OR CRUTCH?

You should be able to perform a high-quality squat on flat ground without relying on external aids.

A squat wedge can instantly improve nearly every movement fault—ankle mobility, knee positioning, hip alignment, lumbopelvic stability, core control, and even upper body positioning. It's an incredibly effective tool for accessing better ranges of motion and cleaner squat mechanics. However, it's just that—a tool, not a long-term solution.

When the goal is to rebuild and optimize your squat pattern, relying on a wedge as a permanent fixture creates a dependency rather than addressing the root cause of your movement faults. Instead, think of the wedge as a temporary aid to help you learn, refine, and reinforce proper mechanics.

That said, wedges have a valid place in your training toolbox. They can adjust muscular targeting, modify load capacity, and increase the trainability of certain squat variations. But when it comes to movement optimization, the ultimate goal is clear: You should be able to perform a high-quality squat on flat ground without relying on external aids.

COMPENSATION: LUMBAR HYPEREXTENSION WITH ANTERIOR PELVIC TILT

MOBILITY: Tight hip flexors and quads, often caused by prolonged sitting or specific postures (e.g., standing with locked knees and an arched back), pull the pelvis into an anterior tilt. This is typically paired with a poorly braced pillar. You can identify this issue if

▼ Your pelvis tilts forward (anterior pelvic tilt), causing an exaggerated curve in your lower back.

▼ Standing upright often feels tight in your lower back, hip flexors, and hamstrings, making it uncomfortable to stand for long periods and causing compensations into anterior pelvic tilt and lumbar extension.

OPTIMIZATION STRATEGIES:

▶ Refer to the **Hip Mobility A Linchpin Blueprint** (page 469) for targeted mobility exercises.

▶ Perform goblet squats, split squats, and reverse lunges to balance hip mobility and stability.

▶ Strengthen glutes and hamstrings with supine hip hinges (glute bridges, hip thrusts) and anterior-loaded good mornings, emphasizing neutral spine alignment.

▶ Add recovery stretches like the prone quad stretch to lengthen tight hip flexors and quads.

STABILITY: Insufficient pillar stability often leads to compensations like anterior pelvic tilt. This typically occurs when initiating the squat and when rising out of the bottom position. A lack of diaphragmatic breathing and bracing results in over-reliance on the lower back for support, which can contribute to low back pain. Indicators of poor pillar stability include

▼ Difficulty maintaining a neutral spine and pelvis when standing, sitting, or squatting

▼ A tendency to "break" at the lower back, especially when moving at higher speeds or under load

OPTIMIZATION STRATEGIES:

▶ Refer to the **Core Stability A (Supine) Linchpin Blueprint** (page 472).

▶ Practice the **Prone Breath Corrective** (page 46) to establish proper diaphragmatic breathing.

▶ Incorporate goblet squats using a box to control depth and prevent compensations.

▶ Add stability-focused exercises like glute bridges, hip thrusts, and anterior-loaded good mornings to reinforce a stable and neutral spine.

SKILL: A lack of motor control or proper sequencing often shows up as an inability to brace effectively or maintain a neutral spine throughout the movement. You might notice:

▼ Excessive arching (lumbar extension) at the top of a squat, often followed by rounding (lumbar flexion) during the descent, indicates poor core control and pelvic stability

▼ A lack of smooth, controlled motion—often seen as jerky or inconsistent movement, particularly during the squat descent—tends to worsen under load or with fatigue

OPTIMIZATION STRATEGIES:

▶ Ensure proper setup: Keep your pelvis neutral, ribs stacked over hips, and breathe 360 degrees into your torso (hands on your waist can help with feedback).

▶ Perform goblet box squats to support proper alignment while building skill.

▶ Practice RNT (Reactive Neuromuscular Training) by placing a band around your knees to reinforce abduction.

▶ Refer to the squat screen, the optimization checklist, and the Pillar chapter for detailed cueing techniques to establish and maintain neutral spinal alignment.

ANKLE MOBILITY: THE MISUNDERSTOOD LIMITER OF SQUAT PERFORMANCE

Ankle mobility has become the go-to scapegoat for nearly every squat-related issue in the weight room. Lifters and athletes often assume their inability to hit proper depth, maintain stability, or move without pain stems from restricted ankle dorsiflexion (the ability to flex your ankle upward). This belief has led to countless hours of foam rolling, extreme mobility drills, and elaborate prehab rituals—often without meaningful results.

While proper ankle mobility is essential for maintaining balance, alignment, and depth in your squat, it's crucial to screen for limitations before jumping to conclusions—because what might appear to be an ankle mobility issue often turns out to be something else entirely.

After screening thousands of coaches and athletes, we've found that in over 90 percent of cases, ankle mobility isn't actually the root cause of poor squat performance. Instead, the ankle becomes functionally restricted due to other weak links in the kinetic chain, including

- Core stability deficits
- Lumbopelvic instability
- Skill and motor control gaps
- Stance mismatches or setup errors

If your ankle mobility drills haven't been delivering results, it's time to stop chasing mobility myths and start screening effectively. A proper screen will help you determine whether you're dealing with a true ankle mobility limitation and, if so, whether it's caused by a soft tissue restriction or a joint-related issue. This clarity ensures you're not wasting time on ineffective strategies and allows you to target the root cause directly for more meaningful and lasting progress.

HALF-KNEELING DORSIFLEXION SCREEN

When it comes to ankle mobility, many lifters mistakenly self-diagnose dorsiflexion restrictions when, in reality, their limitations stem from poor movement patterns rather than true soft tissue or joint restrictions. If your foundational squat mechanics are flawed, your ankle complex will often act as a neurological parking brake, limiting mobility to protect your body from potential harm. This is your body's built-in protective adaptation—a safety mechanism designed to prevent injury. The challenge lies in overcoming this adaptation and retraining your body to move efficiently.

Before jumping into self-treatment for ankle mobility, it's essential to objectively measure your dorsiflexion range of motion to establish a clear baseline. Think of this baseline as both your functional starting point and a pass-or-fail screen. This screen will reveal whether ankle mobility is a true red flag, impacting your movement mechanics from the ground up, or if your ankles are actually functioning within a normal range of motion and the issue lies elsewhere.

Because everyone has unique anthropometrics—differences in body types, joint structures, and functional skill sets—you'll use a universal screening method to measure dorsiflexion accurately. Using the width of your fist (approximately 4 inches for men and 3.5 inches for women) as a reference point, you can establish a baseline range of motion and determine a pass-or-fail result to determine whether you should prioritize ankle mobility drills or shift your focus to other areas of movement optimization.

SETUP:

- Get into a half-kneeling position with one knee down and your front foot flat on the floor. (You can remove your shoes for a more accurate assessment.)
- Place your fist perpendicular to your longest toe to establish a measurable range of motion reference point.
- Use a vertical marker, such as a foam roller or a wall.

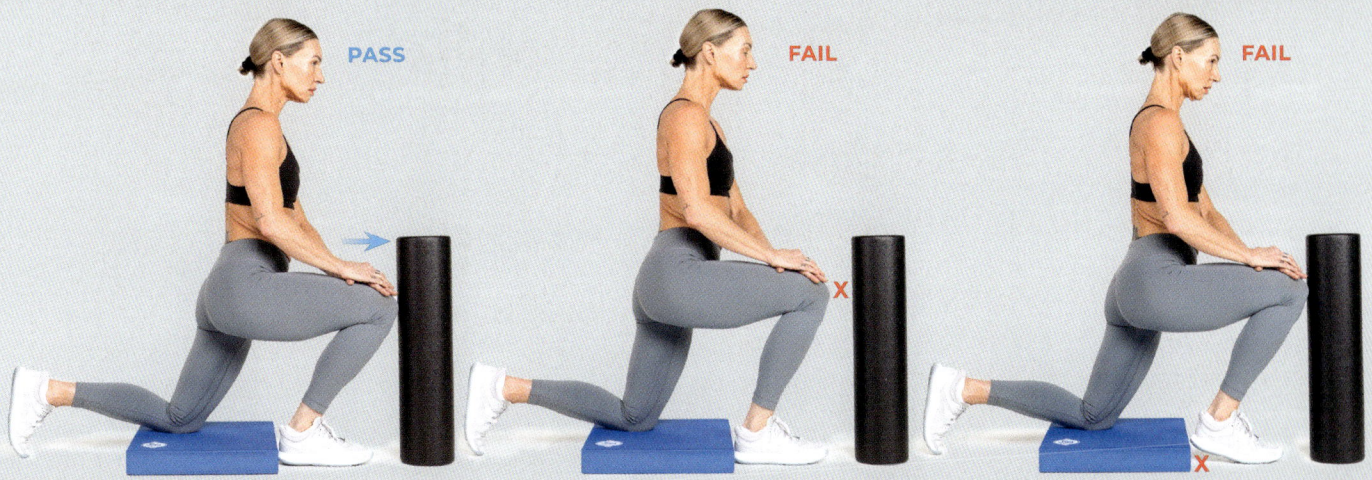

PASS FAIL FAIL

SCREEN:

· Drive your front knee forward over your toes as far as possible without your heel lifting off the ground. Maintain a neutral pillar with an upright posture.

· Observe the relationship between your kneecap and the marker (foam roller, wall, or fist distance) during the forward knee drive.

RESULTS:

✓ **PASS:** If your kneecap passes the marker while you keep your heel down and foot flat, you have a functionally normal range of motion and do not need to prioritize ankle mobility drills.

✗ **FAIL:** If your kneecap does not pass the marker or you can't reach it without your heel lifting off the ground, this indicates a restriction in ankle dorsiflexion and establishes a baseline for mobility work. Failed screens qualify you for ankle mobility drills—like the ones covered in the Ankle Mobility Linchpin Blueprint (page 468) to address the limitation effectively.

HEEL DROP SCREEN

The ankle is one of the most biomechanically complex regions of the body, often referred to as the ankle complex for good reason. It consists of five synergistic joints surrounded by both contractile (muscles and tendons) and non-contractile (ligaments and fascia) tissues that allow movement in all three cardinal planes of motion, as well as multi-angled oblique planes. With such a high degree of movement variability, accurately identifying the type of ankle mobility restriction—whether it's soft tissue based or joint based—is essential. This differentiation determines the most effective corrective strategy for restoring functional ankle mobility.

Simply put, an ankle (or any other articulating joint) can be restricted in two primary ways: soft tissue tone and tightness, or joint restriction. If you feel a stretch through the back side of your lower leg during both straight- and bent-knee testing positions, the restriction is likely soft tissue related. If there's a blocking sensation on the front side of

your ankle in both positions, the restriction is likely joint based. In rare cases, if you feel a difference in the restriction between straight- and bent-knee positions, it indicates a combination of soft tissue and joint mobility limitations.

The distinction matters because while soft tissue restrictions typically can be addressed with techniques like foam rolling, stretching, and targeted soft tissue mobilization, these same methods cannot improve joint restrictions. In fact, attempting to force soft tissue techniques into a joint restriction can potentially exacerbate the issue and worsen range-of-motion limitations.

This is why screening is nonnegotiable—it eliminates guesswork and provides a clear pathway forward. By identifying whether your limitation is soft tissue or joint related, you'll avoid wasting time on ineffective strategies and focus your efforts where they'll deliver meaningful progress.

Option 1: Squat Wedge

- Place one foot on a squat wedge, ideally barefoot, with your toes elevated and your heel firmly planted at the lowest point of the wedge.

- Ensure your toes are pointing straight forward.

Option 2: Elevated Surface (e.g., step or weight plate)

- Step onto an elevated surface, such as a step or weight plate.

- Place the ball of your foot on the edge of the surface with your toes pointing straight forward and your heel hanging off the edge.

Perform the screen one ankle at a time.

SCREEN:

Straight Knee Position:

- Shift your weight onto the testing ankle.

- With a straight knee, drive your heel down toward the lowest point of the wedge (or toward the floor if using an elevated surface) while keeping your toes in contact with the surface.

- Slightly lean your body forward to accentuate the stretch.

- Hold the position for 5 to 10 seconds and assess the sensation:
  Do you feel a stretch at the back of the lower leg (Achilles region) or a blocking sensation at the front of the ankle joint?

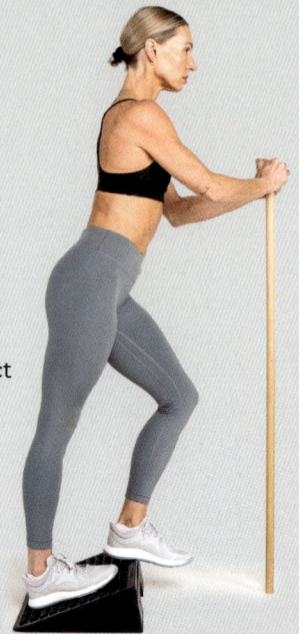

HOW TO ADDRESS SOFT TISSUE RESTRICTIONS

Soft tissue restrictions are often caused by excessive muscle tone or tightness in the lower leg, particularly in the calf and Achilles region. To address these effectively, refer to the **Ankle Mobility Linchpin Blueprint** (page 468), focusing your efforts on these three exercises.

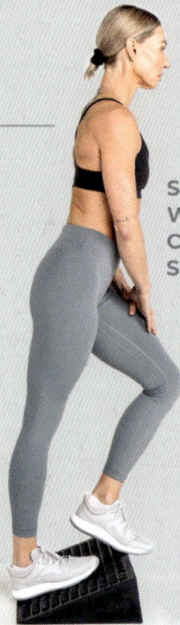

STANDING WEDGE CALF STRETCH

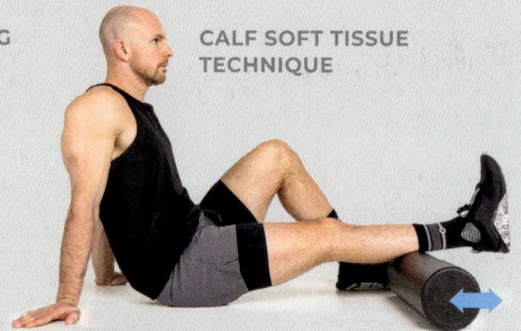

CALF SOFT TISSUE TECHNIQUE

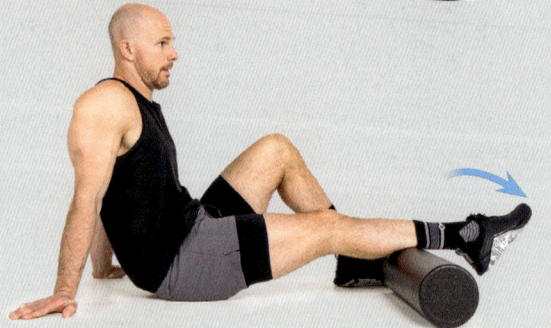

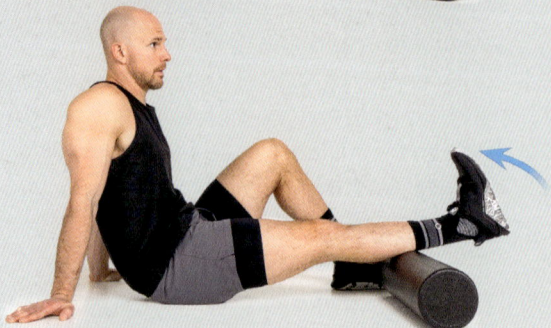

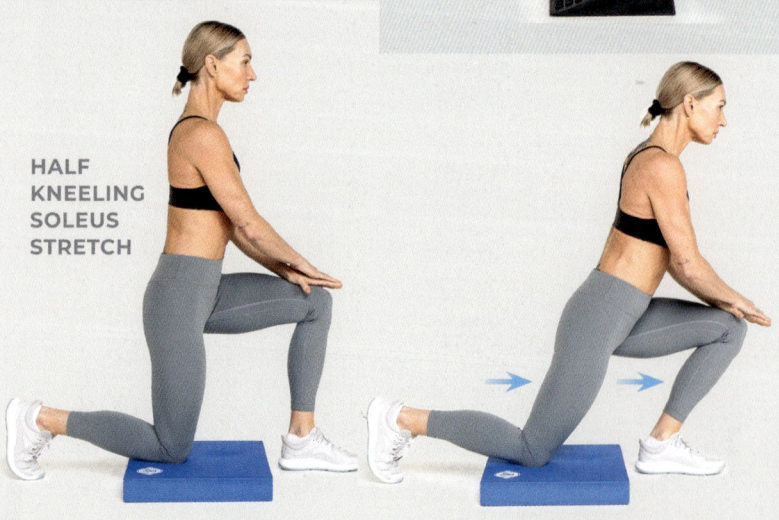

HALF KNEELING SOLEUS STRETCH

Bent Knee Position:

- Repeat the same test, but this time bend your knee slightly while maintaining the same foot position.

- Hold for 5 to 10 seconds and reassess the sensation:
  Do you feel a stretch at the back of the lower leg (Achilles region) or a blocking sensation at the front of the ankle joint?

RESULTS:

- ✓ **PASS:** If you feel no significant restriction or discomfort in either position and your range of motion appears normal, you do not need focused ankle mobility work.

- **Soft Tissue Restriction:** If you feel a stretching sensation at the back of the lower leg in both positions, you are likely dealing with a soft tissue limitation.

- **Joint Restriction:** If you feel a blocking sensation at the front of the ankle in both positions, you are likely dealing with a joint restriction.

- **Mixed Restriction:** If the restriction sensation differs between the straight and bent knee positions, you may need to address both soft tissue and joint mobility limitations (a rare but possible scenario).

HOW TO ADDRESS JOINT RESTRICTIONS

Joint restrictions are typically the result of structural limitations or stiffness within the joint capsule, leading to a blocking sensation at the front of the ankle. To address joint restrictions, follow the **Ankle Mobility Linchpin Blueprint** (page 468), with an emphasis on the three-way ankle mobility drill.

KEY TAKEAWAY:

Don't spend endless hours on ankle mobility drills unless the screen shows a legitimate restriction. Instead, focus on other linchpins like core stability, hip mobility, and skill-based refinements, which often yield far greater improvements in your squat mechanics, efficiency, and load capacity.

For those individuals who do have a true ankle mobility issue, it can often be resolved within 1 to 2 minutes of targeted soft tissue and/or joint mobilization drills.

THREE-WAY KNEE-OVER-TOES ANKLE MOBILITY DRILL

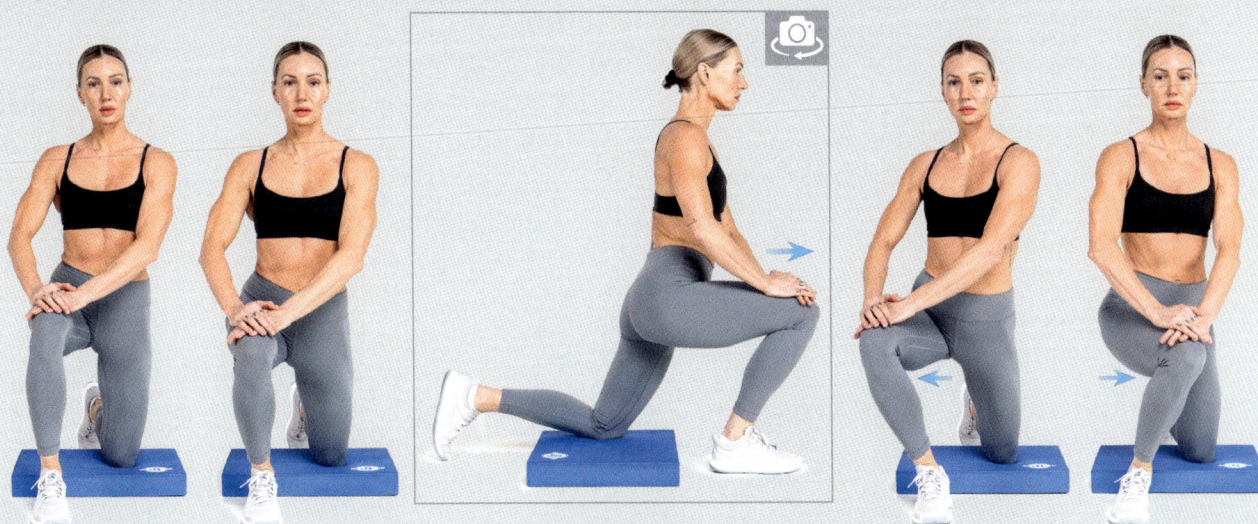

COMPENSATION: FORWARD ROUNDING OF THE UPPER BACK

MOBILITY: Tight pecs and upper traps are common culprits behind forward rounding of the upper back. This issue can be exacerbated by poor posture or overemphasis on pushing exercises without balancing pulling movements. Signs of limited mobility include

▼ Difficulty maintaining an upright torso and "tall chest" during a squat, often paired with an inability to fully extend the mid-back

▼ Persistent tightness in the neck, shoulders, and chest, along with a sensation of feeling "stuck" when attempting to extend the upper back

OPTIMIZATION STRATEGIES:

▶ Refer to the **T-Spine Mobility Linchpin Blueprint** (page 471) for solutions to improve thoracic extension and shoulder mobility.

▶ Use goblet or front rack positions to encourage an upright posture—avoid holding dumbbells at your sides, as this can reinforce forward rounding.

▶ Incorporate pulling exercises (e.g., rows, face pulls) into your programming.

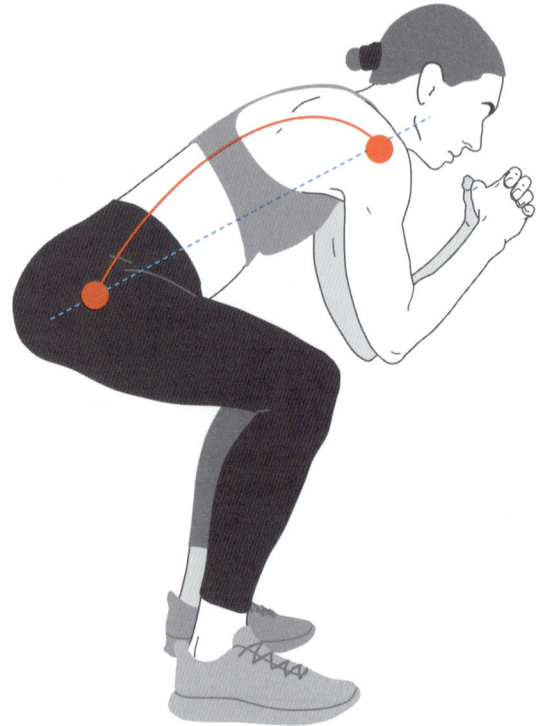

STABILITY: Poor scapular stability often stems from prolonged seated, rounded-forward postures or insufficient training of the muscles responsible for extension and external rotation. Indicators include

▼ Unstable shoulders and shoulder blades often lead to flared elbows, elevated shoulders, internal shoulder rotation, and scapular winging during movement or under load

▼ Difficulty generating tension in the lats during co-contraction, along with an inability to engage the upper back for stability

OPTIMIZATION STRATEGIES:

▶ Start at the bottom of the squat progression pyramid, only adding variations as you meet the standards in the optimization checklist.

▶ Refer to the cueing sequence in the Pillar chapter (page 34) to improve bracing setup and execution.

SKILL: Rounding in the upper back during squats often results from a lack of body awareness or insufficient training. When mobility and stability are not limiting factors, this compensation is likely due to poor movement patterns. Signs of a skill gap include

▼ Losing an upright posture during the descent of a squat, with difficulty regaining a neutral position

▼ A tendency to look down at the floor during a squat, paired with a flexed upper back and neck, indicates poor head and thoracic positioning

▼ Difficulty maintaining neutral shoulders and spinal alignment under increased load or fatigue

OPTIMIZATION STRATEGIES:

▶ See the **Scapular Stability Linchpin Blueprint** (page 473) for targeted exercises to improve scapular control.

▶ Prioritize pulling variations in your program to restore balance between the chest and back. Include face pulls, band pull-aparts, and scapular retraction drills.

▶ For recovery, use stretches like the 90/90 chest stretch (page 122) to release tight pecs, and practice 90/90 Supine Parasympathetic Positional Breathing (page 54) to relax tight neck and upper back muscles caused by forward head posture.

COMPENSATION: ROUNDING THE LOWER BACK; POSTERIOR PELVIC TILT (AKA "BUTT WINK")

MOBILITY: Limited hip and/or ankle mobility are often a contributing factor to the butt wink. However, anatomical differences, such as femur and hip socket alignment, can play a significant role, meaning mobility drills alone may not fully address the issue. Signs that mobility could be the limiting factor include

▼ A rapid posterior pelvic tilt ("butt wink") near the end range of the squat

▼ Inability to maintain lumbo-pelvic stability in the bottom quarter of the squat, even with an optimal stance and bracing

▼ A fast, uncontrolled descent (eccentric drop) amplifies compensations, exposing mobility limitations in the ankles, hips, or knees, and often results in a posterior-to-anterior pelvic shift when bouncing out of the bottom

OPTIMIZATION STRATEGIES:

► Perform the **Ankle Mobility Screens** (page 246) to assess ankle mobility and determine if it's a limiting factor.

► Use the **Ankle Mobility Linchpin Blueprint** (page 468) and/or the **Hip Mobility B Linchpin Blueprint** (page 469), depending on the results of the screen.

► Assess your squat (see **Hip Quadrant Test** on page 241) to determine your natural ROM.

► Use a box to manage depth if needed.

► Incorporate exercises like split squats, reverse lunges, RDLs, and side lunges to promote functional ROM.

► Include recovery stretches, such as the supine hamstring stretch with strap, prone quad stretch, adductor rock-back, and dynamic pigeon stretch.

STABILITY: The "butt wink" often occurs when pillar stability is sacrificed to achieve deeper squat depth. This can happen as core tension loosens at the bottom, leading to posterior pelvic tilt and lower back rounding. Signs of instability include

▼ Losing spinal and pelvic neutrality at the bottom of the squat

▼ Difficulty maintaining a strong brace in the hips and core at the bottom position of the squat

OPTIMIZATION STRATEGIES:

► Refer to the **Core Stability B (Prone) Linchpin Blueprint** (page 473) for exercises and cues to build a strong, stable pillar.

► Perform the squat assessment (see **Hip Quadrant Test** on page 241) to optimize range of motion while preserving stability.

► Use a box to manage squat depth and ensure pillar engagement is maintained throughout.

► Add anterior-loaded exercises like goblet squats to emphasize bracing and core control.

► Strengthen abductors to support proper hip positioning, which can improve ROM over time without sacrificing stability.

SKILL: The "butt wink" can stem from insufficient body awareness or poor motor control during the squat. This is often seen in beginners or individuals who lack experience in managing proper form throughout the movement. Indicators of a skill gap include

▼ Descending too far into the squat, beyond the ability to maintain a neutral spine and pelvis with proper bracing

▼ Relying on a fast, uncontrolled eccentric drop and "bouncing" out of the bottom of the squat

OPTIMIZATION STRATEGIES:

► Perform the squat assessment to determine the ideal stance and depth for your anatomy.

► Prioritize movement mastery by following the optimization checklist, progressing through the squat progression pyramid, and sticking to a controlled depth you can manage.

► Cue proper bracing and focus on maintaining alignment throughout, emphasizing form over depth or speed.

COMPENSATION: KNEES ROTATING INWARD (VALGUS COLLAPSE)

MOBILITY: Tight calves or adductors can contribute to inward knee rotation by limiting ankle dorsiflexion or inhibiting abduction (knees out position). These restrictions often stem from improper footwear (such as high heels), undertraining, or unresolved injuries. You can identify mobility issues if

▼ You feel tightness in your calves or inner thighs when attempting to push your knees outward as you approach squat depth.

OPTIMIZATION STRATEGIES:

▶ Perform the **Ankle Mobility Screens** (page 246) to assess ankle mobility and determine if it's a limiting factor.

▶ Use the **Ankle Mobility Linchpin Blueprint** (page 468) or the adductor-focused **Hip Mobility B Linchpin Blueprint** (page 469), depending on the results of the screen.

▶ Elevate your heels using a slant board, wedges, or small weight plates if ankle mobility is restricted.

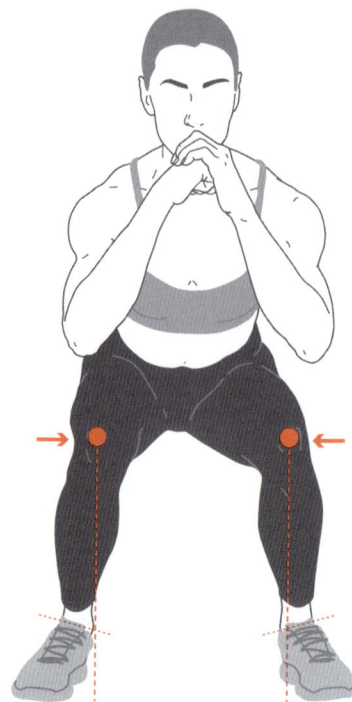

STABILITY: Poor stability in the foot, ankle, or hip often contributes to valgus collapse. This instability can stem from poor footwear, undertraining, or previous injuries, and it may cause a chain reaction affecting the knees, hips, spine, and shoulders. Indicators of poor stability include

▼ Inward rotation or collapsing of the foot and ankle during the concentric phase of the squat

▼ Difficulty maintaining proper "knees tracking over toes" alignment, especially under load during the upward phase of the squat

OPTIMIZATION STRATEGIES:

▶ Perform squats from your authentic or a modified stance that allows for better ankle and foot stability. For some, this might involve a slightly wider stance with reduced depth until stability improves.

▶ Use RNT (Reactive Neuromuscular Training) with a miniband:

· Place the band above the knees to encourage abduction and prevent inward collapse.

· Place the band above the ankles to strengthen foot and ankle positioning.

▶ Incorporate single-leg exercises like split squats, reverse lunges, and single-leg glute bridges.

▶ Focus on strengthening the abductors, glutes, and lower limbs to enhance alignment and stability.

SKILL: Knee valgus often results from poor body awareness and a lack of coordination during the squat. In some cases, lifters overemphasize depth or speed, sacrificing stability for range of motion. Other contributing factors include failing to engage the pillar or improperly sequencing movement patterns. Signs of a skill gap include

▼ Difficulty feeling activation of the glutes and hamstrings during the eccentric phase of the squat

▼ A tendency to default into an anterior knee-dominant squat, leading to internal rotation and inward knee collapse during the concentric phase

OPTIMIZATION STRATEGIES:

▶ Focus on actively driving the knees outward as you descend into the squat. Visualize "spreading the floor" with your feet to engage the glutes and create external rotation at the hips.

▶ Practice squats with a miniband above the knees to provide tactile feedback and reinforce abduction.

▶ Perform goblet squats or use a suspension trainer to develop better alignment and control without overloading.

▶ Slow down the movement and focus on deliberate, controlled repetitions to improve coordination and sequencing.

▶ Use a box squat to limit depth while you build strength and control through the desired range of motion.

COMPENSATION: KNEES ROTATING EXCESSIVELY OUTWARD

MOBILITY: Tight lateral tissues, such as the peroneal muscles, lateral quad, and TFL, can pull the knees outward relative to foot positioning. This is often exacerbated by suboptimal foot and hip alignment, such as attempting to squat with feet pointing straight forward when your hip structure requires a more abducted (toes out) stance. Signs that mobility is the issue include

▼ Difficulty maintaining knee alignment over the toes during the eccentric phase of the squat

▼ Tightness or discomfort around the upper quads, lateral hip, or IT band

OPTIMIZATION STRATEGIES:

► Refer to the **Hip Mobility C Linchpin Blueprint** (page 470).

► Perform the squat assessment to find the ideal foot angle for your hip structure. Gradually progress to full ROM exercises, such as split squats, and reverse lunges, focusing on proper alignment between feet, knees, and hips.

► Supplement with abductor strengthening exercises like starfish side planks or side-lying abduction leg raises to create balance and support new ranges of motion.

► Include recovery stretches such as the dynamic pigeon stretch, side-lying quad stretch (with focus on lateral line stretch), and supine hamstring stretch with a strap, slightly pulling the foot across the body to target lateral tissues.

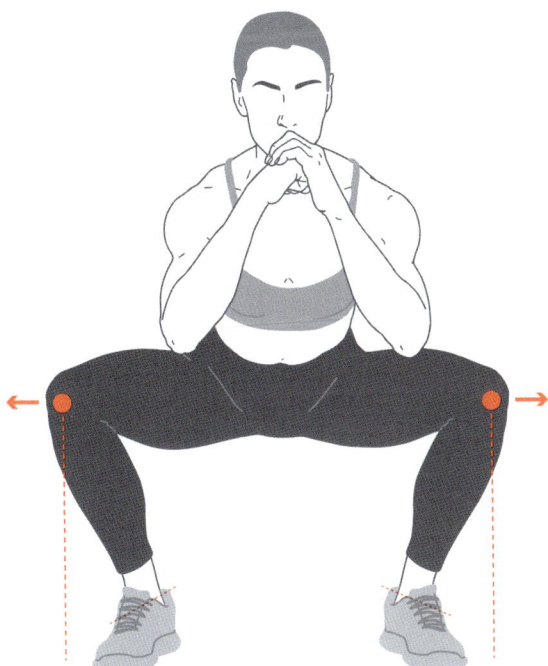

STABILITY: Excessive knee abduction can result from a lack of overall stability, often seen in hypermobile individuals who seek wider knees-out position for a sense of control or muscular engagement. Indicators of poor stability include

▼ Jerky or inconsistent knee movement, shifting between valgus (knees caving inward) and varus (knees pushing outward) during the lowering and raising phases of the squat

▼ A preference for excessively wide stances to artificially create stability, even when mismatched with one's optimal squat stance and hip anatomy

OPTIMIZATION STRATEGIES:

► Refer to the **Core Stability A (Supine) Linchpin Blueprint** (page 472) and the **Hip Stability A Linchpin Blueprint** (page 475) to build a more stable foundation.

► Use RNT (Reactive Neuromuscular Training) with a miniband under your feet, encouraging a strong arch and proper knee alignment.

► Incorporate stability-focused exercises like dead bugs, bird dogs, glute bridges (holding a light med ball or yoga block between the knees), and starfish side planks or side-lying abduction leg raises to improve hip positioning and muscle balance.

SKILL: Excessive knee abduction is often linked to misunderstandings of technique cues, such as overemphasizing "drive your knees out." This can lead to compensatory patterns, especially in group settings where cues may be generalized. Signs of a skill issue include

▼ Inconsistent or improper knee tracking, especially during the concentric (rising) phase of the squat

▼ Shifting weight to the outer edges of the feet during the squat

OPTIMIZATION STRATEGIES:

► Use the optimization checklist and squat assessment to identify your ideal setup and hone your form.

► Practice squats from your authentic stance, focusing on maintaining knees over toes alignment.

► Allow time to adapt to any stance adjustments. Rebuild your "autopilot" in this new position before progressing to higher loads or volume.

► Focus on distributing your weight evenly through your heel, big toe, and pinky toe (tripod foot position).

COMPENSATION: ASYMMETRICAL HIP SHIFT (ONE HIP DROPS OR MOVES MORE THAN THE OTHER)

MOBILITY: Limited mobility in the ankles or hips can lead to a hip shift, especially if one side is tighter or more restricted. This may become apparent during unilateral movements like lunges or split squats. Signs of mobility limitations include

▼ Difficulty achieving symmetrical depth in the squat

▼ Feeling more restricted or tight on one side during stretches or warm-up movements

OPTIMIZATION STRATEGIES:

▶ Perform the **Ankle Mobility Screens** (page 246) to assess ankle mobility and determine if it's a limiting factor.

▶ Use the **Ankle Mobility Linchpin Blueprint** (page 468) or the **Hip Mobility B Linchpin Blueprint** (page 469), depending on the results of the screen.

▶ Strengthen within the symmetrical range you can control and gradually increase depth over time.

▶ Use exercises like split squats, reverse lunges, and lateral lunges to address imbalances and improve mobility.

▶ Add supplemental stretches such as the half-kneeling hip flexor stretch, adductor rock-back, dynamic pigeon, prone quad, and supine hamstring stretches with a strap.

STABILITY: A hip shift can occur when the body compensates for poor hip centration or lack of overall pillar stability. This can result from mismatched squat stances, excessive load, or squat variations that aren't suited to your body. Indicators of instability include

▼ A noticeable shift, tilt, or rotation of the hips during the lowering or raising phases of the squat

▼ Difficulty maintaining a neutral spine and pelvis throughout the squat

OPTIMIZATION STRATEGIES:

▶ Refer to the **Hip Stability A Linchpin Blueprint** (page 475) to prepare for squats.

▶ Perform a squat from your authentic stance (see **Hip Quadrant Test**, page 241) and manage depth with a box or bench. Videoing your squat from behind can help ensure your setup prevents shifting.

▶ Apply RNT (Reactive Neuromuscular Training) by using a miniband around the knees to focus on abduction or a light pull-up band around the hips, pulling in the same direction as the shift to provide feedback and encourage correction.

▶ Add supplemental unilateral exercises like split squats, lunges, 1.5 stance hinge variations, side plank variations, glute drills, and lateral lunges (curtsy lunges).

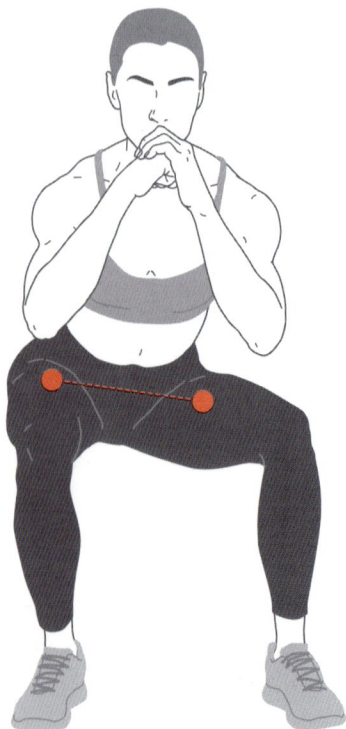

SKILL: Asymmetry can stem from repetitive patterns in life, work, or sport (e.g., always throwing, lunging, or sitting in a specific position). These habits carry over into gym movements, reinforcing imbalances. Signs of a skill gap include

▼ Difficulty maintaining a symmetrical squat pattern

▼ Habitual compensations or movement biases become more apparent under increased load or speed

OPTIMIZATION STRATEGIES:

▶ Start your session with the **Hip Stability A Linchpin Blueprint** (page 475) to address imbalances.

▶ Program an authentic or modified stance that promotes stable and symmetrical squats.

▶ Regress to a squat variation that prioritizes movement quality and symmetry, controlling depth with a box if needed.

▶ Focus on setup: align stance, stabilize the pelvis by co-contracting glutes and adductors, breathe 360 degrees, and brace to maximize intra-abdominal pressure. Maintain full-body irradiation throughout the squat to support stability and control.

COMPENSATION: ANKLES ROLL INWARD (PRONATION) OR OUTWARD (SUPINATION)

MOBILITY: A lack of ankle dorsiflexion can lead to compensatory pronation as the body attempts to achieve depth. Alternatively, tight lateral tissues can cause supination. Signs of limited mobility include

▼ Difficulty keeping the foot tripod (heel, big toe, pinky toe) grounded during the squat

▼ A noticeable collapse inward or outward of the ankle joint when squatting

OPTIMIZATION STRATEGIES:

▶ Perform the **Ankle Mobility Screens** (page 246) to assess ankle mobility and determine if it's a limiting factor.

▶ Refer to the **Ankle Mobility Linchpin Blueprint** (page 468) for targeted solutions.

▶ Incorporate lower-limb soft tissue work and dynamic stretches during the 6-phase warm-up.

▶ Train the lower limb through a full ROM with exercises like calf raises, elevated calf raises, and squat or split squat iso-soleus raises.

▶ Use recovery stretches such as the wall or wedge calf stretch and the half-kneeling knee-to-wall soleus stretch, elevating your toes on a wedge to increase effectiveness.

STABILITY: Poor footwear, lack of proprioception, or previous injuries can impair ankle stability. Indicators include

▼ Inward collapse of the ankle during the squat indicates instability or weakness in the foot and ankle complex

▼ Difficulty maintaining a stable tripod foot—equal pressure through the heel, big toe, and little toe

OPTIMIZATION STRATEGIES:

▶ Refer to the **Ankle Stability Linchpin Blueprint** (page 468) to build ankle strength and proprioception.

▶ Focus on creating a strong foot tripod and maintaining good alignment during squats. Perform bodyweight or light/moderately loaded squats barefoot to improve engagement.

▶ Add balance and strengthening drills like balance holds, low step-downs/step-ups, and split squats or reverse lunges.

▶ Include calf raises, soleus raises, and tib raises between exercises or at the end of workouts to increase volume and build endurance.

▶ Progress stability demands by performing squats, hinges, and lunges in a proprioceptively rich environment, such as standing on a foam pad to challenge balance.

Gradually introduce barefoot or minimalist walking for foot strength. Start with 20 minutes per session, increasing volume gradually.

SKILL: Foot and ankle compensations may result from poor awareness, ingrained movement habits, or lack of endurance. Sudden increases in activity, such as transitioning from a sedentary lifestyle to high walking volume, can also strain the feet and lead to compensatory patterns. Signs of a skill issue include

▼ Inconsistent foot and ankle alignment under the knees during the squat, which indicates poor stability or control in the lower limbs

▼ Difficulty maintaining an active foot arch and proper tripod stance—balanced pressure through the heel, big toe, and little toe

OPTIMIZATION STRATEGIES:

▶ Perform phases 1–4 of the **Ankle Stability Linchpin Blueprint** (page 468) three to seven times per week as part of your warm-up or as standalone secondary or off-day recovery sessions.

▶ Focus on maintaining a strong foot tripod, engaging the arch, and ensuring proper alignment during squats. Use bodyweight or light/moderate loads to refine technique.

▶ Practice balance drills, step-downs, and step-ups to improve coordination and foot control.

▶ Add volume to lower limb strengthening with calf raises, soleus raises, and tib raises between sets or at the end of workouts.

▶ Gradually increase barefoot or minimalist walking to rebuild proprioception and strengthen the feet, starting with short sessions and progressing slowly.

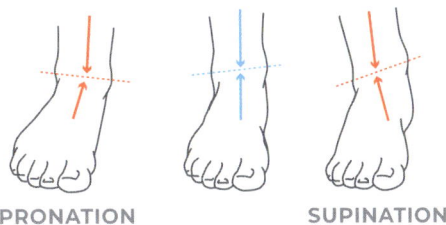

PRONATION   SUPINATION

COMPENSATION: SHOULDER ROTATION (UNEVEN BAR PATH OR TORSO TWIST)

MOBILITY: Postural habits from desk work, driving, or texting can create upper body tightness or asymmetry that affects squat mechanics. Tightness in the thoracic spine, pecs, or lats may limit your ability to maintain symmetry under the barbell. Signs of mobility issues include

▼ Stiffness in the upper back, making it difficult to extend the thoracic spine and maintain an upright torso, often causing the shoulders to round forward

▼ A pulling or tight sensation across the chest when positioning the barbell, especially in front or back rack setups, leading to uneven alignment

▼ Tightness along the sides of the torso or under the armpits, making it challenging to grip or stabilize the barbell symmetrically and maintain proper shoulder positioning

OPTIMIZATION STRATEGIES:

▶ Perform the **T-Spine Mobility Linchpin Blueprint** (page 471) with a pec emphasis if thoracic rotation is restricted, or the **Shoulder Mobility B (Vertical) Linchpin Blueprint** (page 472) with a lats emphasis if overhead restrictions are observed in the pull assessment.

▶ Use an alternative squat variation, such as the safety bar squat, landmine squat, Zercher squat, or goblet squat, to maintain a strong pillar while addressing mobility limitations.

▶ Incorporate full-ROM exercises like lat pulldowns, DB or cable pullovers, chest fly variations, and single-arm push and pull variations that include rotational components.

▶ Include recovery stretches such as the 90/90 chest stretch, prone chest stretch, supine twist with the back arm extended in a T-shape, suspension trainer T-spine and posterior shoulder stretches, and child's pose.

STABILITY: Shoulder rotation during squats can stem from instability in the shoulder complex or poor scapular control, leading to a breakdown in pillar alignment. Indicators of instability include

▼ Difficulty securing the barbell in a stable position without relying on an excessively wide hand placement or high bar position

▼ Discomfort in the shoulders, neck, or upper back during squats

▼ Inability to fully grip the barbell with an appropriate hand width and position

OPTIMIZATION STRATEGIES:

▶ Refer to the **Overhead Stability Linchpin Blueprint** (page 474) to strengthen the shoulder complex and improve shoulder stability.

▶ Select a squat tool or load position that promotes symmetry, such as the safety bar squat, Zercher squat, or landmine squat, if shoulder rotation is observed during barbell squats.

▶ Incorporate stability-focused push and pull exercises like DB and cable presses and rows (prioritize single-arm variations), face pulls, rear delt flies, KB arm bars, and high plank shoulder taps.

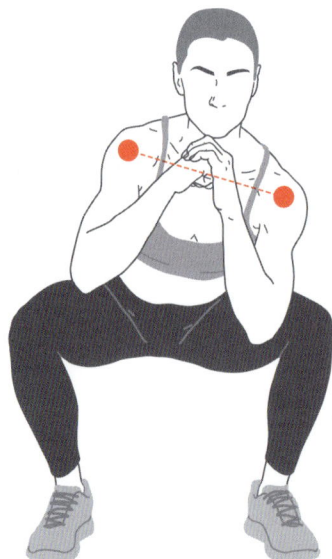

SKILL: Maintaining good posture and a strong brace throughout a squat is a learned skill that requires practice. Shoulder rotation can result from poor setup, insufficient bracing, or a lack of awareness about upper body alignment. Signs of a skill gap include

▼ An inconsistent bar path, including twisting, dipping, or uneven movement from right to left during squats

▼ Difficulty maintaining full-body tension, irradiation, and stable hand placement

OPTIMIZATION STRATEGIES:

▶ Review the Pillar chapter to refine your setup and bracing technique. Focus on aligning the pelvis and rib cage, breathing 360 degrees, and bracing to maximize intra-abdominal pressure.

▶ Follow the exercise recommendations in the stability section above to build strength and control in the feet and ankles.

▶ Ensure the bar is centered and gripped evenly before unracking. Actively pull the bar into your traps to create tension in the upper back.

▶ Focus on applying equal force through both feet, keeping the bar path straight during the descent and ascent.

▶ Use a fixed point in front of you to maintain alignment and reduce unnecessary torso rotation.

▶ Practice with lighter loads to focus on symmetry, and video your squat to identify any visible rotation or imbalances.

COMPENSATION: HEELS LIFTING OFF THE GROUND

MOBILITY: Restricted ankle mobility, particularly in dorsiflexion, is a common cause of the heels lifting during squats. Tightness in the gastrocnemius or soleus may force the weight onto the toes, compromising stability. Signs of mobility limitations include

▼ Heels lifting off the ground during the descent

▼ A tendency to shift weight forward, making it difficult to maintain balance

OPTIMIZATION STRATEGIES:

▶ Perform the **Ankle Mobility Screens** (page 246) to identify restrictions and determine whether they stem from the gastrocnemius, soleus, or joint structures.

▶ Refer to the **Ankle Mobility Linchpin Blueprint** (page 468) for targeted drills to improve dorsiflexion.

▶ Focus on maintaining full foot contact (big toe, little toe, and heel) during squats, even if it requires pulling the hips back and lowering the torso slightly.

▶ Use wedges or plates to elevate the heels for a quick improvement in foot position and a more upright torso during squats. *Note:* This is a temporary solution and should not be used as a long-term crutch.

▶ Train the lower limb through a full ROM with exercises such as calf raises, elevated calf raises, and squat or split-squat iso-soleus raises.

▶ Incorporate recovery stretches like the wall or wedge calf stretch and the half-kneeling knee-to-wall soleus stretch, enhancing them with a wedge under the foot to elevate the toes.

STABILITY: Balancing on the balls of the feet during a squat is inherently less stable than maintaining full foot contact. Developing a strong, stable squat pattern requires prioritizing proper foot alignment and contact. Indicators of stability issues include

▼ Difficulty maintaining a balanced, upright posture during squats

▼ Feeling unstable or wobbly while descending

▼ Difficulty maintaining a stable tripod foot position—balanced pressure through the heel, big toe, and little toe

OPTIMIZATION STRATEGIES:

▶ Begin your session with the **Core Stability B (Prone) Linchpin Blueprint** (page 473) to establish a stable base and prepare the body for squatting.

▶ Use a suspension trainer–assisted squat to unload body weight and lean back slightly, helping to maintain full foot contact and an upright torso.

▶ Use wedges or plates to elevate your heels, facilitating better alignment and balance during squats.

▶ Train lower limb stability with exercises such as balance holds, elevated calf raises, and squat or split-squat iso-soleus raises. These exercises improve both proprioception and foot strength.

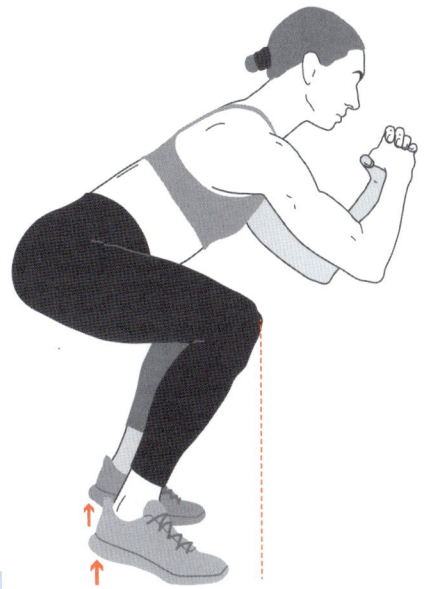

SKILL: For beginners or those returning to exercise, learning to manage the center of mass over the base of support takes time. The center of gravity (around the belly button) should remain stacked over the base of support (the feet) to maintain balance and effectively recruit major muscle groups. Signs of a skill gap include

▼ Heels lifting due to a forward shift of the center of mass

▼ Difficulty coordinating the descent and ascent of the squat

OPTIMIZATION STRATEGIES:

▶ Warm up with the **Core Stability B (Prone) Linchpin Blueprint** (page 473) to build awareness of proper alignment and bracing.

▶ Focus on weight distribution— see the optimization checklist for strong foot and ankle and knee tracking over toes.

▶ Use a suspension trainer–assisted squat to offload body weight and practice keeping your center of mass over the base of support.

▶ Focus on setup, including proper stance, pelvis and rib cage alignment, and co-contraction of the glutes and adductors to stabilize your pelvis. Practice breathing 360 degrees, bracing to maximize intra-abdominal pressure, and maintaining full-body irradiation during squats.

COMPENSATION: FEET TURNED OUT EXCESSIVELY OR ROTATING OUTWARD

MOBILITY: When ankle dorsiflexion is limited, the feet may turn out as a compensation to allow the body to lower into the squat. Tightness in the gastrocnemius, soleus, or joint structures can also restrict movement. Signs of mobility limitations include

▼ Feet turning out excessively during the descent of the squat

▼ Difficulty maintaining full foot contact or an active arch

OPTIMIZATION STRATEGIES:

▶ Perform the **Ankle Mobility Screens** (page 246) to assess mobility restrictions and identify whether they stem from soft tissue or joint limitations.

▶ Use the **Ankle Mobility Linchpin Blueprint** (page 468) to address any mobility deficits.

▶ Program an authentic or modified stance with an appropriate foot abduction angle for your hip structure. Gradually increase ROM while improving motor control.

▶ Focus on maintaining full foot contact through the big toe, little toe, and heel, with the ankle stacked and an active arch throughout the movement.

▶ Train the lower limb through full ROM exercises like calf raises, elevated calf raises, and squat or split squat iso-soleus raises.

▶ Incorporate recovery stretches such as wall or wedge calf stretch variations and the half kneeling knee-to-wall soleus stretch, elevating the toes on a wedge to increase intensity.

STABILITY: Poor foot positioning or outward foot rotation may indicate that your squat stance doesn't match your hip anatomy. Performing the squat assessment to find your authentic stance will help address this. Adjusting to a new stance may require time and practice to sync improved foot positioning with hip centration. Indicators of stability issues include

▼ Feet rotating outward during the descent and ascent of a squat

▼ Inconsistent foot contact and alignment with the ground, especially at end-range squat depth

OPTIMIZATION STRATEGIES:

▶ Use the **Hip Stability B Linchpin Blueprint** (page 475) to solidify your new foot position and improve motor control.

▶ Program an authentic or modified stance that aligns with your hip structure and improves knee tracking. Adjust depth as needed while building stability in the new position.

▶ Focus on maintaining full foot contact with an active arch and stacked ankle throughout the squat.

▶ Incorporate balance and lower limb strengthening exercises such as balance holds, low step-downs/step-ups, and suspension trainer–assisted split squats and reverse lunges, ensuring proper foot and ankle positioning.

▶ Add calf raises, soleus raises, and tib raises to improve stability and endurance, either during rest periods or at the end of workouts.

SKILL: Improving motor control in a new squat stance takes practice and patience. Once your stance is optimized, you'll need time to develop comfort and precision in your new positioning. Signs of a skill gap include

▼ Struggling to maintain proper alignment in your new stance during loaded or fatigued squats

▼ Difficulty syncing the new foot position with improved hip centration

OPTIMIZATION STRATEGIES:

▶ Refer to the **Hip Stability B Linchpin Blueprint** (page 475) to refine motor control and strengthen the connection between foot position and hip alignment.

▶ Program an authentic or modified stance tailored to your anatomy, focusing on proper alignment and gradually increasing ROM and depth.

▶ Maintain full foot contact with an active arch and stacked ankle, paying attention to consistent knee tracking.

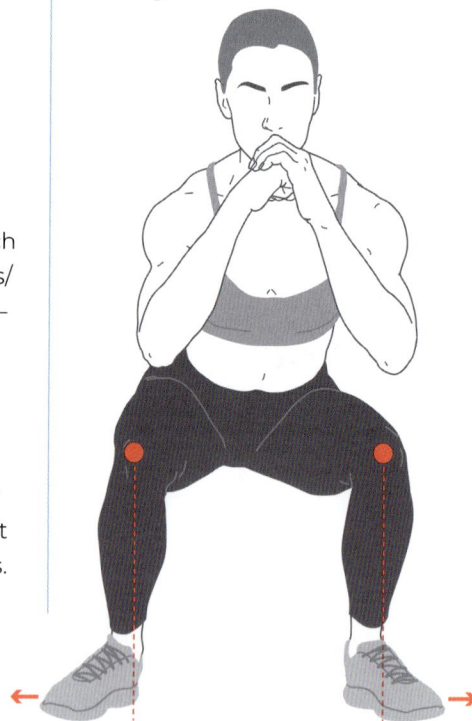

COMPENSATION: EXCESSIVE FORWARD LEAN (SHIN ANGLE DOESN'T MATCH TORSO ANGLE)

MOBILITY: Limited ankle dorsiflexion forces the hips to shift back, increasing the torso lean to maintain balance. Signs of restricted mobility include

▼ Difficulty allowing the knees to move forward over the toes during squats

▼ A feeling of tightness or restriction in the back of the lower leg when attempting to keep the heels down while squatting

OPTIMIZATION STRATEGIES:

▶ Perform the **Ankle Mobility Screens** (page 246) to assess mobility restrictions and identify whether they stem from soft tissue or joint limitations.

▶ Use the **Ankle Mobility Linchpin Blueprint** (page 468) to address any mobility deficits.

▶ Elevate heels with a slant board, wedges, or weight plates to improve foot positioning and maintain a more upright torso. *Note:* This should be used as a temporary intervention to correct form, not as a long-term solution.

▶ Train through full ROM with exercises like calf raises, elevated calf raises, and squat or split squat iso-soleus raises.

▶ Incorporate recovery stretches such as the wall calf stretch, toe-elevated calf stretch, quadruped single-leg adductor stretch, or bilateral frog stretch to enhance ankle mobility.

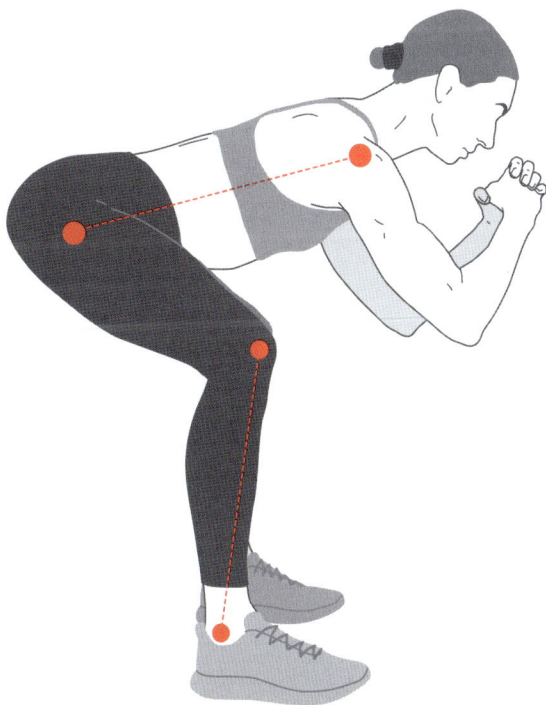

STABILITY: If ankle mobility is sufficient, weak pillar engagement or underdeveloped spinal erectors can cause excessive forward lean. Signs of instability include

▼ Struggling to maintain an upright torso and neutral spine at the bottom of a squat

▼ Jerky motions, wobbling, shaking, and inconsistent tension during the eccentric phase of the squat, especially under load

OPTIMIZATION STRATEGIES:

▶ Use the **Core Stability B (Prone) Linchpin Blueprint** (page 473) to address core strength.

▶ Perform suspension trainer–assisted squats to unload body weight and maintain a more upright torso by engaging the arms and upper back.

▶ Strengthen the posterior chain with exercises like glute bridges, hip thrusts, low cobras, Supermans, flutter kicks, reverse hypers, and back extensions.

▶ Add recovery stretches to open the front side of the body, such as the half-kneeling hip flexor stretch, prone quad stretch, sphinx stretch, or lying supine over a stability ball. Stretch the lower back with supine knees-to-chest and supine twists to reduce post-workout tension.

SKILL: Learning to stack your center of gravity over your base of support and maintain alignment during squats requires practice. This often involves retraining movement patterns to reduce excessive forward lean. Signs of a skill gap include

▼ Displaying inconsistent movement patterns with unpredictable forward torso lean

▼ Having difficulty coordinating the descent and ascent, resulting in a loss of balance or uneven control

OPTIMIZATION STRATEGIES:

▶ Follow the recommendations in the stability section above to build strength and coordination.

▶ Gradually progress to heavier loads and greater ROM as stability improves, unlocking more optimal movement patterns over time.

SQUAT PROGRESSION PYRAMID

The squat progression pyramid is all about building from the ground up. Each stage builds upon the last, allowing you to develop a squat pattern while training safely and pain-free.

Bodyweight squats form the foundation, locking in the movement pattern without the added complexity of external load. Once you meet the standards covered in the optimization checklist, you will progress to **goblet box squats**. This progression introduces a light anterior load, which helps you learn how to create pillar tension, irradiation, and bracing while providing the safety and feedback of the box to refine your depth and form.

From there, **goblet squats** remove the box, challenging your range in free space. This prepares you for the **front squat**, where the anterior load increases, demanding even more mobility, stability, and skill to maintain proper form under increased load.

Finally, the **back squat** represents the highest load capacity and motor control of any squat variation. With the weight on your back, you must lean forward, creating a more hip-dominant squat that challenges your ability to maintain full-body tension and precise coordination under heavier loads.

In this section, I break down each exercise in the squat progression pyramid, highlighting the unique aspects that set each variation apart. While the movements progress in complexity, they all share the same foundational mechanics. These mechanics, outlined in the optimization checklist, serve as your reliable guide. From bodyweight squats to heavily loaded variations, the principles remain consistent, ensuring your form stays solid as you advance up the pyramid.

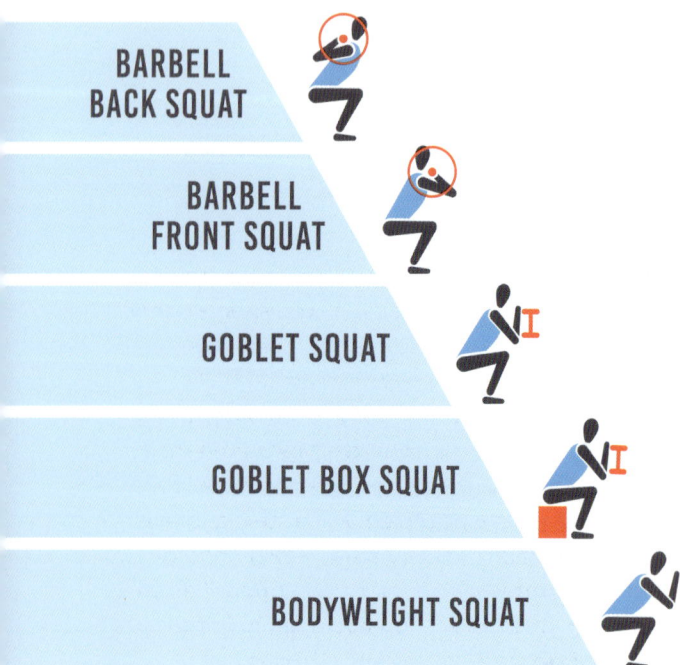

BARBELL BACK SQUAT

BARBELL FRONT SQUAT

GOBLET SQUAT

GOBLET BOX SQUAT

BODYWEIGHT SQUAT

BODYWEIGHT SQUAT

The bodyweight squat forms the base of the pyramid and is the key to building a strong squat pattern. This is crucial because, without mastering the pattern first, you're more likely to hit walls and experience setbacks when progressing to more advanced variations.

The transition from bodyweight to the first stage progression happens quickly, especially if you've followed the screen and assessment protocol. Once you meet the standards in the screen, you're ready to advance to the next stage (goblet box squat).

While the bodyweight squat may seem simple, it's the foundation for all future squat variations. Getting it right here will set you up for long-term success, eventually leading to more advanced squat exercises with load.

For guidance on mastering the bodyweight squat, refer to the squat screen and optimization checklist covered earlier in the chapter.

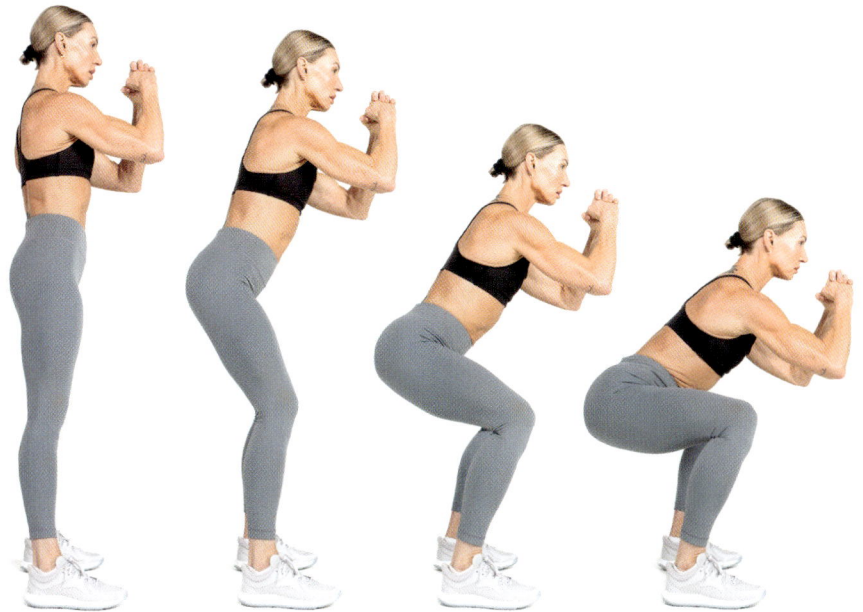

ECCENTRIC PHASE

CONCENTRIC PHASE

GOBLET BOX SQUAT

The goblet box squat is the perfect bridge between bodyweight squats and loaded variations, providing the structure and feedback needed to refine your movement. The box serves as a guide to ensure you're squatting within the range of motion identified in your assessment. For example, if your assessment shows you can squat to 10 inches, the box should be set to that height. This helps you meet the standards outlined in the optimization checklist while avoiding compensations caused by exceeding your available range.

What sets the goblet box squat apart is its ability to provide instant feedback on your movement. By focusing on controlled deceleration and a stable base of support, the box eliminates the guesswork of depth and encourages intentional, repeatable movement.

This variation also reinforces proper biomechanical principles. The box provides a target for the hips to "sit," reinforcing a hip-dominant squat pattern, while the goblet position's anterior load encourages an upright torso and a strong, braced core. These mechanics reduce the likelihood of common compensations, such as lumbar flexion (butt wink) or excessive forward lean, helping you build confidence and control with load.

SETUP: Begin by selecting a stable platform such as a box, bench, risers, or a stack of bumper plates. Ensure the box matches the depth identified during your squat assessment and is secure enough to remain steady under you without shifting or tipping.

ECCENTRIC PHASE

CONCENTRIC PHASE

LOAD POSITION: The choice of load is important for performance and comfort. While both dumbbells and kettlebells are effective, **dumbbells are often preferred due to their versatility and ease of handling.** A dumbbell offers a neutral hand position, meaning your palms face each other while gripping the weight. This position allows for better alignment of the wrists, forearms, and shoulders, reducing strain and awkwardness compared to the supinated grip typically required for a kettlebell. The neutral grip also enables the dumbbell to be stacked closer to your sternum, improving balance and control during the movement.

Using a dumbbell also lets you pull your elbows in tighter against the bottom of the weight, which increases irradiation—tension radiating through the arms and shoulders—and enhances overall stability. This setup creates a secure, compact position that supports proper form and reinforces pillar strength.

For a kettlebell, hold it by the horn to ensure a strong grip and proper irradiation back into your shoulders. Many flip the kettlebell upside down and hold the bell itself. While this mimics the position of the dumbbell, getting into the position requires a clean and catch motion—a skill not suited for most lifters and difficult with higher loads.

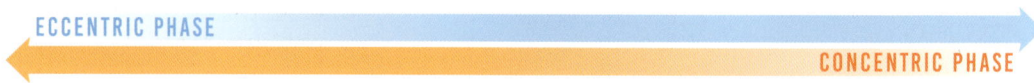

Once you've selected your load, pick it up using a neutral and stable pillar to avoid unnecessary strain on your lower back. Ideally, lift the weight from a bench or box around thigh or waist height. Hold the weight close to your chest, gripping it firmly with both hands. Your palms should press into the sides of the load, creating tension through your forearms and shoulders. This tension stabilizes the shoulder girdle and enhances total-body engagement. Keep your elbows slightly angled downward to ensure the weight feels secure while maintaining a strong brace throughout your core.

EXECUTION: Take a few small steps to position yourself in front of the box and adjust your feet into your authentic squat stance.

Lower yourself with control, keeping your spine neutral and distributing your weight evenly across your tripod foot (heel, big toe, and little toe).

As you reach the box, deload about 50 percent of your body weight onto it. This partial deload allows you to engage the posterior chain more effectively while maintaining core tension.

AVOID TWO COMMON MISTAKES:

1. Fully relaxing, which releases tension in the hip flexors and collapses the spine against the box.

2. Staying overly tense, which negates the purpose of using the box (also known as "touch and go").

Instead, find balance by partially deloading while maintaining a slight rocking motion. **Shift 3 to 5 degrees back and forth on the box to emphasize posterior chain dominance.** This interaction breaks the stretch-shortening cycle, creating a distinct eccentric phase, a brief pause, and a powerful concentric drive.

It's this slight rocking mechanism—**sit, shift, shift, raise**—that allows you to catapult out of the bottom position with sound biomechanics. The anterior load from the goblet position keeps your torso upright, while the box interaction maximizes hip engagement.

Drive through your feet with steady force to ascend, keeping your core braced and knees tracking over your toes. Maintain full-body tension to ensure stability, alignment, and smooth, controlled reps.

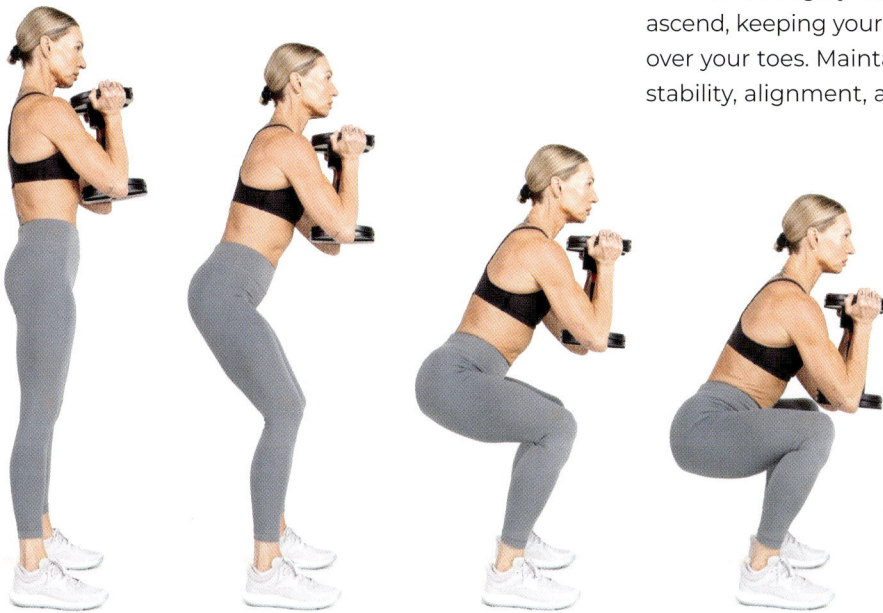

ECCENTRIC PHASE

CONCENTRIC PHASE

GOBLET SQUAT

The goblet squat is the natural progression from the goblet box squat, where you remove the box and the external cue it provides. With the box gone, the goal is to maintain the same squat pattern and depth you've already established, moving smoothly from the eccentric (lowering phase) to the concentric (rising phase) in free space—a key step that prepares you for the more advanced stages of the progression pyramid.

SETUP: Begin in your authentic squat stance.

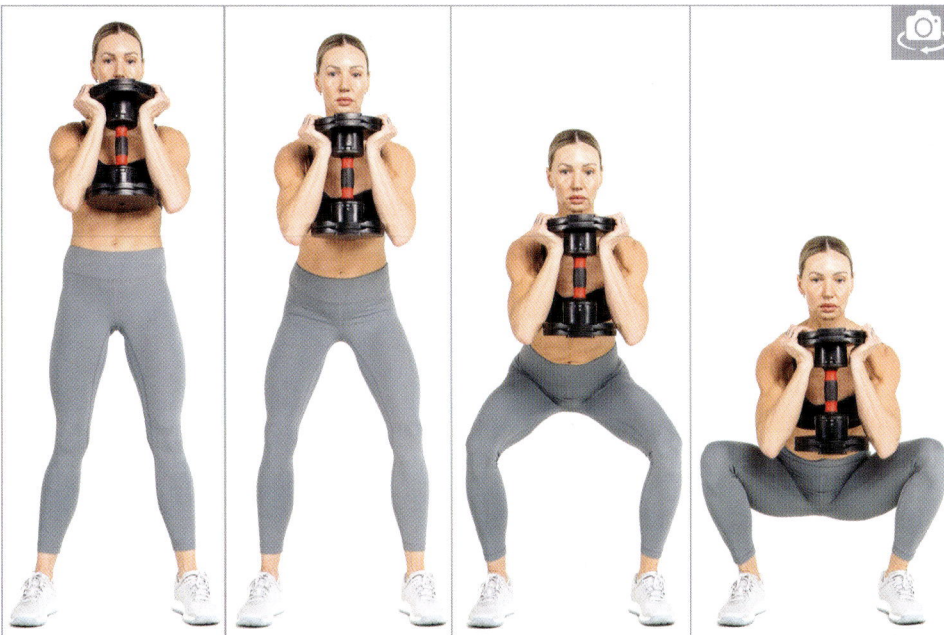

LOAD POSITION: The load position remains consistent with the goblet box squat:

- **Hold a dumbbell or kettlebell close to your chest with both hands.** If using a dumbbell, press your palms firmly into the sides of the weight, creating tension that radiates through your forearms and shoulders. If using a kettlebell, hold it by the horns to ensure proper grip engagement and irradiation back into the shoulders.

- **Keep your elbows slightly angled downward to secure the weight and maintain stability.**

EXECUTION: **Lower yourself in a controlled manner, maintaining a neutral spine and braced core.** Without the box as a target, focus on transitioning smoothly through your authentic range of motion. Expect a slightly knee-forward, quad-dominant movement compared to the hip-dominant mechanics of the goblet box squat.

Descend until you reach the depth established during your assessment, keeping your hips and knees aligned over your foot tripod (heel, big toe, and little toe).

At the bottom of the squat, you no longer have the support of a box to gauge depth. This requires a quick and controlled change of direction from the eccentric to the concentric phase. This is where most movement faults occur. Watch for issues such as ankle instability, knee valgus, pelvic tilt, or excessive flexion in the lower or upper back. Maintaining a neutral pelvis and spinal alignment throughout this transition (amortization phase) is critical.

On the ascent, drive through your feet with controlled force. Keep your pillar braced and ensure your knees track directly over your toes. Emphasize full-body tension as you rise, stabilizing your pelvis and preserving a neutral spine for optimal alignment and power.

FRONT SQUAT

The front squat is a pivotal step up the squat progression pyramid, bridging the gap between foundational exercises like the goblet squat and advanced, heavy back squats by introducing increased loading potential in a front-loaded position.

While the barbell is the most commonly used tool for this exercise, it's not the only option. The front squat encompasses a variety of variations—including safety bar squats, dumbbell front squats, and kettlebell front squats—that all adhere to the same movement principles. What matters most is the load position: The weight must stay close to your center of mass— the point where your body's weight is evenly distributed— and directly over your base of support, which is the area between your feet providing stability during the movement.

ECCENTRIC PHASE

CONCENTRIC PHASE

This alignment ensures balance and control, allowing you to maintain an upright torso, which reduces stress on the lower back, promotes proper alignment of the spine and hips, and encourages better activation of the core. These elements not only reinforce pillar stability but also prepare you for heavier, pain-free back squatting by teaching you to manage load efficiently while maintaining safe and effective mechanics.

Whether you're using a barbell, safety bar, or another implement, the front squat challenges you to stabilize, control, and resist forward flexion under the heavier anterior load, making it an essential progression in the squat hierarchy.

SETUP: Success with the front squat begins with proper setup. **Start by setting the barbell on J-hooks at mid-sternum height (around your chest or "nipple line").** This height allows you to unrack the bar without going onto your toes and ensures smooth reracking.

LOAD POSITION: Take a grip on the bar just outside shoulder width, ensuring your wrists are in line with your forearms for proper alignment.

Step under the bar with your feet in a hip-width power stance, with the bar positioned across the front shelf of your shoulders. **The bar should rest securely in the groove between your anterior deltoids and collarbone, creating a stable platform.**

Next, raise your elbows so they point forward and remain parallel to the ground. **Then retract your shoulders and pull them slightly down and back to lock the bar in place.** This upper body stability is crucial for maintaining balance and control throughout the lift.

If wrist, elbow, or shoulder mobility limits your ability to achieve a full grip, the lifting strap modification can provide a more accessible and pain-free alternative. To use straps:

1. Attach the straps securely to the barbell, positioning them evenly at shoulder width.

2. Wrap the straps around your hands, allowing you to maintain a neutral grip with your thumbs pointing down.

3. Drive your elbows up in front of your shoulders to create the front rack shelf.

4. Externally rotate your shoulders to enhance torque and stability.

5. Maintain a neutral thoracic spine by actively stabilizing your shoulder blades down and together.

This strap modification reduces stress on the wrists and elbows while improving shoulder and thoracic spine positioning. It allows for cleaner movement patterns, enhanced stability, and better motor control.

Avoid the cross-arm hold, as it compromises stability and increases the risk of bar movement, especially with heavier loads. More specifically, this position forces the shoulders into deep internal rotation and protraction, making it difficult to achieve proper centration in the front rack, which is essential for maintaining a strong pillar.

Before unracking, perform a breathe-and-brace protocol. Inhale deeply through your nose, expand your core 360 degrees, and engage your diaphragm to create intra-abdominal pressure. This stabilizes your spine and prepares you to manage the load effectively.

EXECUTION: With your setup and load position secure, it's time to move. **Lift the bar straight up by extending your legs and step back in three small, deliberate movements: one step with your dominant foot, one with your non-dominant foot, and a final adjustment to set your squat stance.** Keep these steps efficient to minimize unnecessary time under tension.

Begin the squat by unlocking your hips and knees simultaneously. The front-loaded position naturally shifts the emphasis to a more knee-dominant pattern, challenging your ability to maintain an upright torso and strong core engagement.

Lower yourself with control, ensuring your elbows stay lifted and your chest remains tall. Descend to your full range of motion, keeping your feet firmly grounded in a balanced tripod position (heel, big toe, and little toe). Focus on staying braced and aligned throughout the eccentric phase.

The transition between lowering (eccentric) and rising (concentric) is where most movement faults occur. **Maintain tightness through your core and shoulders to avoid issues like dropping elbows, rounding your upper back, or allowing your knees to collapse inward.**

To stand back up, drive through your feet while keeping your elbows high and your core engaged. **Think about pushing your body into the bar and maintaining full-body tension as you return to the starting position.** This ensures a controlled and powerful ascent while keeping pillar alignment intact.

BACK SQUAT

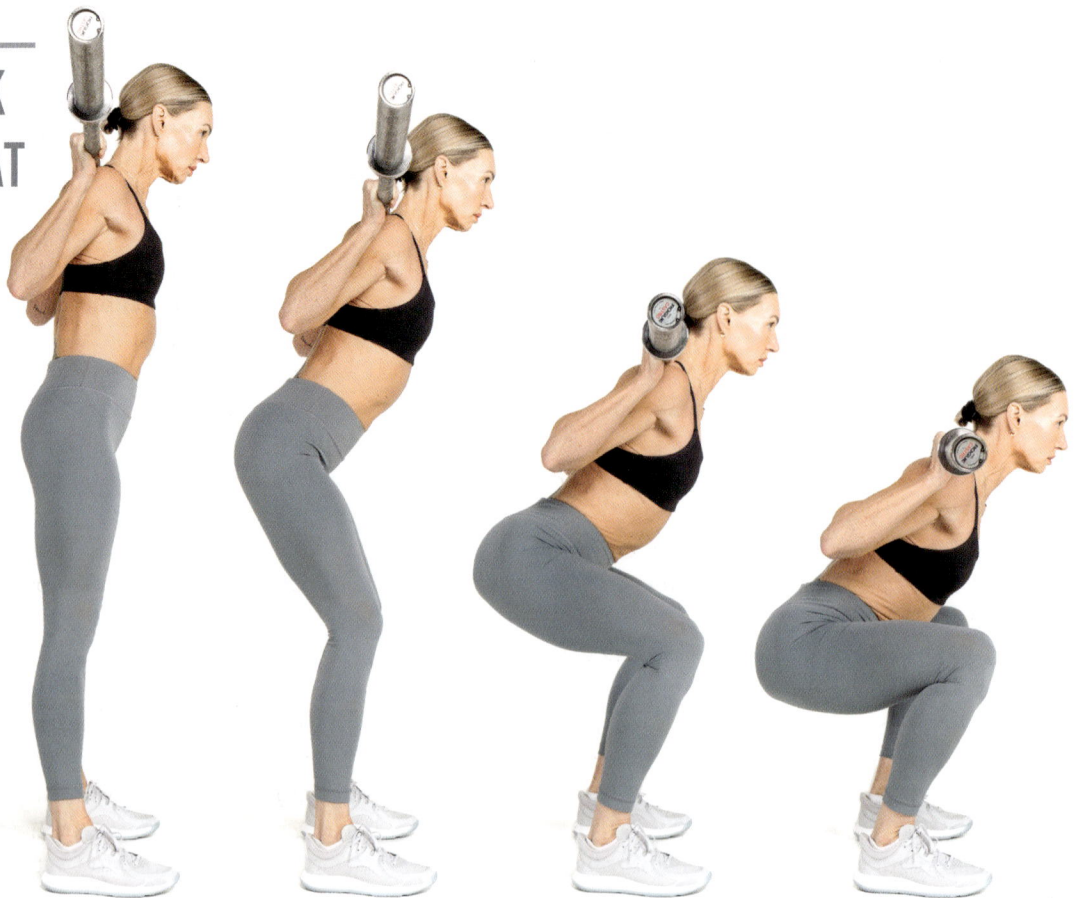

ECCENTRIC PHASE

CONCENTRIC PHASE

The back squat represents the pinnacle of the squat progression pyramid. It's the ultimate expression of strength, coordination, and control, but it's also one of the most butchered and misapplied movements in training. Defined by its posteriorly loaded position, the back squat emphasizes the glutes, hamstrings, and lower back while engaging the quads and core. Its unique load distribution allows for greater weight capacity than anteriorly loaded squats, but with that increased potential comes greater complexity. Managing the heavier load requires a perfect balance of mobility, stability, and skill—qualities that elevate the back squat to its rightful place at the top of the pyramid.

Yet, for all its benefits, the back squat isn't for everyone—and that's okay. One of the biggest mistakes coaches, athletes, and rehab pros make is force-feeding the barbell squat to lifters who aren't suited for it. Pain, mobility restrictions, training history, and even personal goals all play a role in determining whether the back squat is the right fit. And the idea that every lifter must conform to a specific bar placement, like high-bar or low-bar, is outdated and often counterproductive. Long-term success—whether in performance, injury resilience,

or overall strength—comes from individualizing the movement to meet your unique needs, not forcing a one-size-fits-all setup.

For example, bar placement and torso angle should be dictated by the position where you can generate the most tension and stability while maintaining proper alignment. For most people, this will fall somewhere in the middle of the torso angle and bar position continuum.

The back squat's complexity is also its strength. It exposes weaknesses and demands integration across the entire kinetic chain. A lack of stability in the upper back, scapula, or thoracic spine can lead to compensations in the lower back and pelvis, capping your performance and increasing the risk of injury. Customizing the setup based on your ability to generate torque and maintain tension through these areas is critical for both safety and success.

Unless you're a competitive powerlifter, your back squat setup doesn't need to adhere to rigid sport-specific standards. Instead, the focus should be on creating a setup that allows you to squat pain-free, build strength, and maintain longevity in your training. This might involve experimenting with tools like the safety bar or adjusting your bar position to suit your body's needs, not forcing yourself into a position that feels awkward or painful.

At its core, the back squat isn't just about loading up the heaviest barbell; it's about building resilient strength that carries over to all aspects of training and life. Its position at the top of the squat progression pyramid reflects its demand for mastery, but also its reward: When approached with intention and tailored to individual needs, the back squat becomes an unparalleled tool for developing full-body strength, coordination, and control.

SETUP: Begin by setting the barbell on J-hooks at mid-sternum or nipple height. This allows you to unrack the bar smoothly without standing on your toes and ensures easy reracking after your set.

Grip the bar, choosing a grip width that suits your shoulder mobility. A closer grip increases upper back stability but should remain comfortable and pain-free. Many lifters prefer a false grip, with the thumbs resting over the bar alongside the fingers. This grip reduces wrist strain and allows you to focus on retracting and externally rotating your shoulders, creating a secure "shelf" for the bar.

LOAD POSITION: Step under the bar with your feet in a power stance—hip-width apart with toes slightly angled outward. Position the bar across your upper back based on your anatomy and mobility. Most lifters will find the strongest position somewhere between the high-bar placement (just below the base of the neck) and the low-bar placement (slightly lower, across the rear deltoids). The goal is to find a placement that allows for maximum stability and comfort while minimizing strain on your shoulders.

Once the bar is in position, retract your shoulder blades and pull them slightly down. Co-contract your pecs and lats to lock the bar in place.

EXECUTION: With your grip set, upper back tight, and bar in position, brace your core by taking a deep breath and creating intra-abdominal pressure. **Extend your legs to lift the bar straight up off the hooks and step back into position with three deliberate movements: one step with your dominant foot, one with your non-dominant foot, and a final adjustment to set your squat stance.** Pause briefly to let the bar settle securely onto your body, ensuring stable contact before continuing.

Begin the squat by simultaneously unlocking your hips and knees. As the barbell is posteriorly loaded, your torso will naturally lean forward more than in a front squat. This is normal and necessary for proper alignment in a back squat. Focus on maintaining a neutral spine and braced core as you descend.

A helpful cue is to "pull yourself down" using your hamstrings. This keeps tension throughout your posterior chain and ensures a controlled descent. **Allow your knees to move slightly forward while keeping your hips moving down and back.** The exact angle of your torso and hip position will depend on your individual anatomy, limb lengths, and squat style.

At the bottom of the squat, maintain tension in your core and lumbopelvic region. Avoid collapsing or losing stability. This phase is where movement faults often occur, such as hips rising too quickly or the torso folding forward.

Drive upward by pressing through your feet, ensuring your knees and hips extend simultaneously. **A key cue here is to "drive your back into the bar," which keeps the bar path straight and engages the entire posterior chain.** Avoid letting your hips shoot up faster than your shoulders, as this can compromise stability and shift the load unevenly.

Maintain control and full-body tension throughout the ascent, finishing in a strong, upright position.

SAFETY AND BEST PRACTICES

Use spotter arms: Failing safely is just as important as lifting safely. Always set up spotter arms in the rack at a height just below your full squat depth. This ensures that if you fail a lift, the bar can be safely set down without risking injury.

Rack the bar properly: At the end of your set, step forward deliberately, matching the same controlled steps you used to unrack. Ensure the bar contacts the J-hooks, then lower it into place. Avoid rushing or "dumping" the bar back into the rack.

Respect your limits: Use proper progressions, pay attention to form, and prioritize safety over ego. This ensures long-term success and progression without unnecessary setbacks.

Face the right direction: I get it—you want that perfect, unobstructed Instagram shot. But facing out of the rack for a better camera angle is a serious safety risk. Imagine trying to rerack the bar backward while fatigued after a heavy, taxing set. Without clear visibility, you're one misstep away from disaster. Prioritize your safety over social media—face into the rack, focus on your lift, and use spotter arms to ensure you can train smart and stay safe.

HINGE

The hinge has become the forgotten movement pattern. Despite it being one of the most essential movements for overall strength and function, many people have lost the ability to hinge correctly. The consequences of this shift are significant, as the hinge isn't just another movement—it's the foundation for every other pattern. If you want to move well, get stronger, and avoid injury, you must reclaim the ability to hinge with proper form. This chapter will show you how.

You step up to the barbell, take a deep breath, and pull. Everything feels fine—until halfway through the lift, your back rounds. Suddenly, all the pressure shifts to your spine, sending a sharp pain through your lower back. You drop the weight, knowing something went wrong. But it's too late. The damage is done. You tweaked your back deadlifting.

It's an all-too-common scenario—one that has given the deadlift a bad rap. From commercial gyms to university weight rooms, many lifters, athletes, and even trainers have written off the deadlift as an inherently dangerous exercise, branding it as a high-risk movement that's not worth the potential injury. The reputation is understandable—after all, stories of tweaked backs and strained muscles seem to follow the deadlift wherever it goes.

But is the deadlift really to blame? Or is the problem that most people aren't executing it in a way that aligns with their mobility and movement capabilities? I'll be the first to admit: Jumping straight into heavy deadlifts without mastering the basics is a recipe for disaster.

Take my own experience, for example. When I was 22, I was interning at the University of Buffalo, immersed in a Westside Barbell–inspired training system. For the first time, I was pulling heavy weights from the floor in a conventional deadlift stance with little regard for my mechanics. My numbers climbed fast—four plates on the bar, personal records every few weeks. But those gains came at a cost. Every Tuesday after my Monday deadlift sessions, my lower back would ache. I convinced myself that pain was just part of the process, the cost of getting stronger.

Until the day everything snapped—literally.

I hadn't even touched the barbell yet. As I bent down to set up for my lift, before my hands even reached the bar, a sharp pop shot through my lower back. I was instantly locked in flexion, unable to move, stand, or straighten up. In that moment, I wasn't a strong, young athlete. I was a 22-year-old, bent over at 90 degrees, helpless and terrified.

That injury didn't just change my workouts—it reshaped my entire life. Sitting through graduate school lectures became unbearable. Sleeping was painful. Training, even just my upper body, felt impossible.

What made it worse was the cycle that followed. Every time I felt a little better, I'd return to deadlifting without addressing the root problem. And every time, I'd re-injure myself. For years, I was stuck in this vicious cycle of pain, frustration, and self-doubt. It wasn't until I finally started from scratch—rebuilding the hinge pattern, addressing my range of motion, and creating a resilient movement system—that I truly broke free.

On my 37th birthday, I pulled a lifetime PR: pain-free, beltless, and with the kind of confidence I'd been chasing for over a decade. But the story doesn't end there. That same night, I went straight to the baseball field to coach, throwing over 200 pitches and hitting balls for two hours. The next morning, I felt 100 percent—no aches, no setbacks, just ready to crush my next session. For me, that was the ultimate breakthrough. It wasn't just about hitting big numbers in the gym—it was about being strong, functional, and fully capable of living the life I wanted. It's one thing to deadlift a PR, but it's another to follow it up with real life activities and not being sidelined by pain.

So, yes, the deadlift can be harmful if you don't respect your own range of motion and have the right mechanics in place. But that doesn't mean the deadlift itself is inherently dangerous. The real issue is that most people don't differentiate between the deadlift as an exercise and the hinge as a foundational movement pattern. They go straight to the top of the pyramid without understanding the mechanics of the hinge itself—the art of loading the hips while keeping the spine stable and pillar engaged.

Without mastering that foundation, you're setting yourself up for failure. And failure, especially when it comes with pain, creates a cycle of fear and avoidance that only worsens the problem. You've likely seen it yourself: People experience pain or injury with deadlifts and then steer clear of the hinge pattern altogether. But avoiding it doesn't address the underlying issue; it only limits your potential and weakens nearly every movement you do in the gym.

To break this cycle, it's crucial to understand that the hinge is more than just the deadlift—it's the backbone of functional movement. It teaches you how to generate power from the hips and stabilize the pillar, a skill that carries over to almost every activity: lifting, swinging, running, jumping, and even maintaining better posture in daily life. If your hips are the engine driving your body's power, the hinge is the mechanism that fuels and develops it, tapping into some of the biggest and strongest muscle groups: your glutes, hamstrings, and the entire posterior chain. When you master the hinge

pattern, you gain access to one of your body's most powerful and efficient movements—one that enhances mobility, stability, and skill across all other patterns.

Don't wait for another strained back to learn how to hinge properly. There's a simple solution that can rewrite the outcome. Before you even touch a barbell again, you need to establish your range of motion, learn how to control your hips, and maintain stability through your pillar. Once that foundation is in place, the hinge won't be a movement you fear—it will become your most powerful tool for protecting your spine and building long-term strength and power.

In this chapter, you'll learn exactly how to reclaim and refine your hinge pattern. By breaking it down into manageable steps, you'll build a strong base that prepares you for more advanced lifts like the deadlift—all while keeping you safe and pain-free.

If your hips are the engine driving your body's power, the hinge is the mechanism that fuels and develops it.

HINGE SCREEN

The hinge is one of the most fundamental movement patterns—and yet it's often forgotten, buried beneath years of habits and exercises that fail to engage its full potential. In a world where squats and presses dominate gym routines, the hinge is sometimes overshadowed, despite being bedrock to many powerful and efficient movements. The hinge screen is your chance to reclaim this essential pattern, ensuring your movement is both safe and effective while uncovering any limitations that may be holding you back.

Whether you've been hinging for years through exercises like deadlifts and kettlebell swings or you're unsure where to start, this screen will meet you where you are. If you're experienced, begin with your usual setup and evaluate how well your movement aligns with the standards in the optimization checklist. If the hinge feels unfamiliar—or if past injuries or poor habits have caused you to avoid it—follow the setup and execution steps outlined here to rediscover this powerful movement pattern.

The goal of the screen isn't just to test your hinge against a set of benchmarks but to reconnect with the mechanics that unlock your body's potential. A proper hinge teaches you how to load your hips, stabilize your spine, and tap into the strength of your posterior chain—your body's engine for generating power and stability. When this pattern is forgotten, it's not just your lifts that suffer; you lose the foundation for nearly every athletic movement and risk exposing your lower back to unnecessary strain.

By starting here, you'll establish a baseline for your hinge, identifying your strengths as well as any areas needing attention. From there, the assessment will help you refine your positioning, range of motion, and mechanics in a way that's specific to your body. This process not only helps you rediscover the hinge but also ensures it becomes a cornerstone of your training, empowering you to work up the movement pattern pyramid with confidence.

SETUP: STANCE and BODY POSITION

1. **Stance:** Stand with your feet hip-width apart, toes pointing straight forward. This position represents the most authentic setup for a hinge, allowing you to maximize posterior chain engagement while minimizing unnecessary knee bend or hip rotation. Distribute your weight evenly across a balanced tripod foot position: 50 percent on your heels, 25 percent on your big toe, and 25 percent on your little toe. This ensures stability and prevents excessive backward or forward shifting during the movement.

   Place your hands in a hand-over-hand position for added stability and tension. Cup one hand over the knuckles of the other, pressing your hands together to create active engagement through your pecs and lats. This positioning helps reinforce pillar stabilization and encourages proper alignment throughout the hinge.

2. **Stabilize the Pillar:** Begin by creating tension throughout your body. Co-contract your pecs and lats along with your glutes and adductors.

For a detailed explanation of breathing and bracing, refer to pages 34–35.

3. Breathing and Bracing: Take a deep 360-degree breath through your nose, expanding your diaphragm in all directions. Hold your breath at maximal inhalation and brace your core by contracting the muscles around your torso. This step locks in spinal stability for the movement.

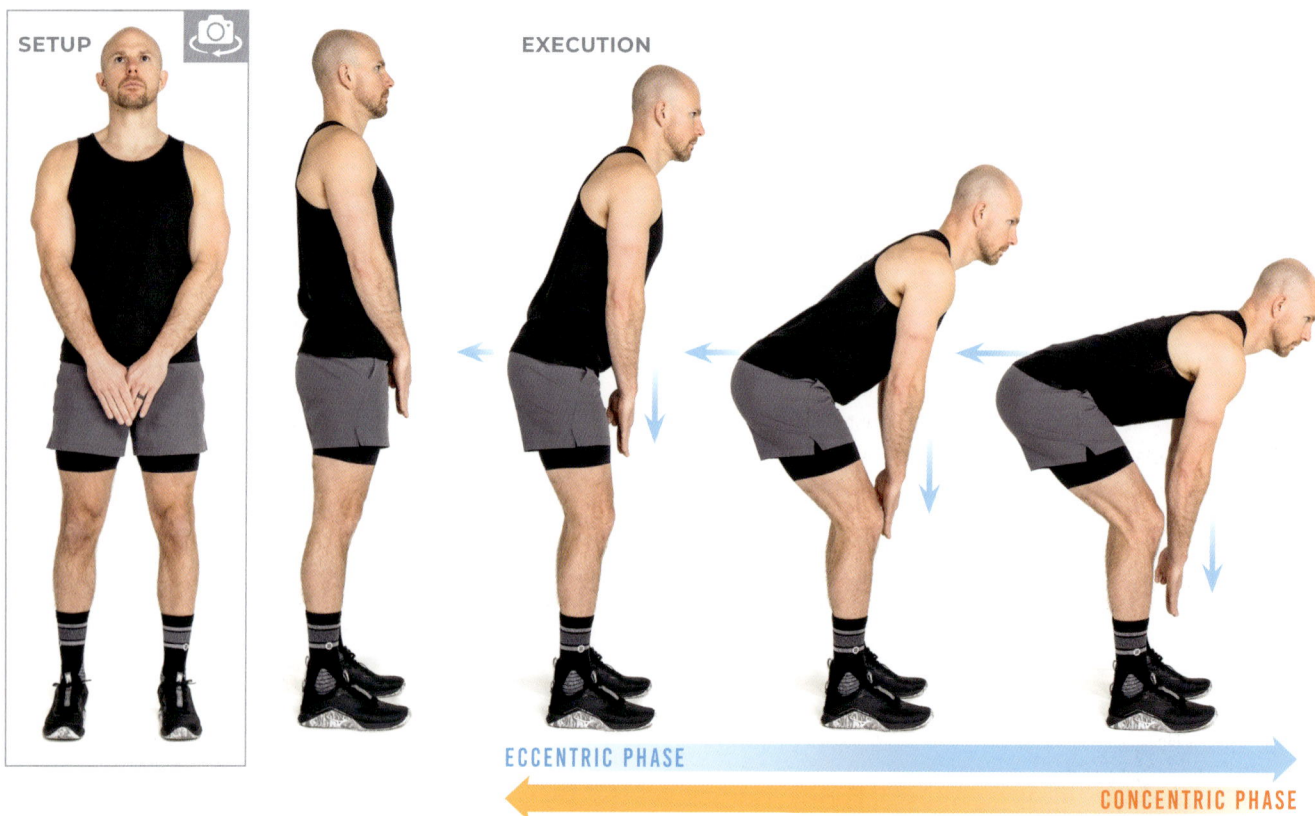

SETUP

EXECUTION

ECCENTRIC PHASE

CONCENTRIC PHASE

EXECUTION: PERFORMING THE HINGE

With your body stabilized and tensioned, initiate the hinge by sending your hips back rather than bending at the waist, ensuring the movement is driven by the posterior chain—glutes, hamstrings, and lower back—while maintaining a neutral spine and stable pelvis. Your shins should remain vertical, and your knees should avoid forward movement to keep the pattern purely hip dominant.

As you descend, direct your hands toward your heels, keeping your arms close to your body. This cue prevents your hands from drifting forward, which could shift the movement away from the hips and into the lower back.

Lower your torso as far as you can without compensating—your knees bending forward or your back rounding. Your palms should pass below your knees, but the exact depth will depend on your range of motion and ability to maintain proper form.

Avoid collapsing or shifting your weight backward onto your heels. Instead, maintain equal weight distribution across your tripod foot, with pressure balanced between your heels, big toes, and little toes.

Throughout the movement, keep your entire body controlled and stable. Whether lowering into the hinge (eccentric phase) or returning to standing (concentric phase), ensure that your spine remains neutral, your hips drive the motion, and your pillar stays engaged. This precision helps reinforce proper mechanics, making the hinge both safe and effective as a foundational movement.

OPTIMIZATION CHECKLIST

The next step is to record yourself performing the hinge from both a front and side perspective. This gives you a visual reference point to evaluate your initial form and identify areas for improvement. By analyzing your alignment and depth against the standards in the optimization checklist, you'll gain valuable insights to guide the adjustments needed for better mechanics and movement efficiency.

✓ NEUTRAL SPINE

Maintaining a neutral spine during the hinge means keeping your back stable and aligned as you move. While some natural curvature in the spine is expected, the goal is to avoid lumbar flexion and extension (rounding and arching of the lower back), which shifts the load from the hips to the spine. A neutral spine ensures the posterior chain—glutes, hamstrings, and lower back—remains the primary driver of the movement, reducing strain and enhancing power.

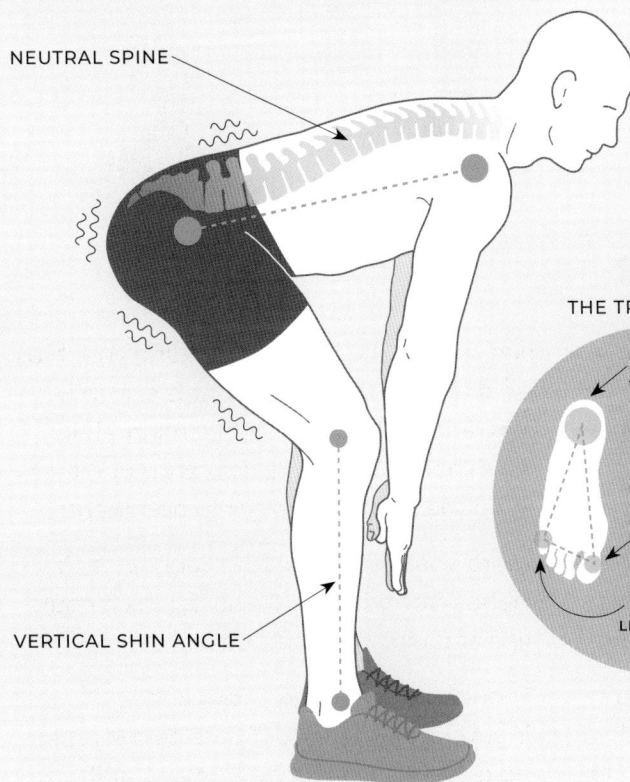

✓ NO UNWANTED ROTATION

Resisting unwanted rotation during the hinge requires maintaining symmetry and stability throughout the body. Unwanted rotation occurs when one side compensates for the other, leading to inefficient movement and potential injury risk. For the hinge, this means keeping the ankles, knees, hips, and shoulders symmetrical as you descend and rise, ensuring better force transfer and stability across the posterior chain.

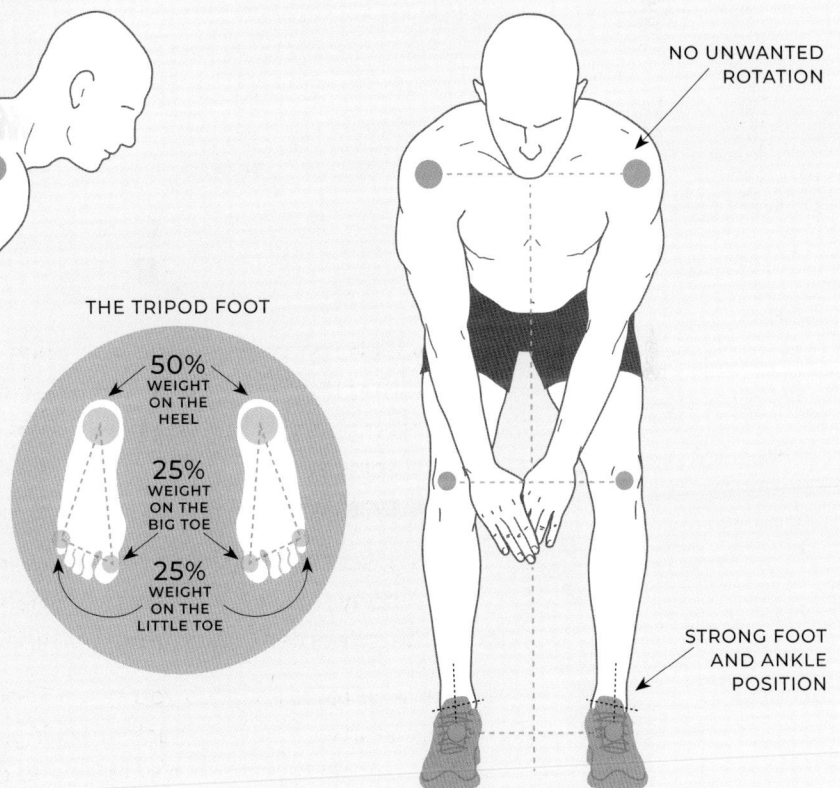

NEUTRAL SPINE

THE TRIPOD FOOT

50% WEIGHT ON THE HEEL

25% WEIGHT ON THE BIG TOE

25% WEIGHT ON THE LITTLE TOE

NO UNWANTED ROTATION

VERTICAL SHIN ANGLE

STRONG FOOT AND ANKLE POSITION

✓ VERTICAL SHIN ANGLE

A proper hinge relies on a vertical shin angle to maintain a hip-dominant pattern. Forward knee movement shifts the load away from the hips and onto the quads, altering the movement mechanics. By keeping your shins vertical, you ensure the hinge is driven by the posterior chain. This positioning not only reinforces proper mechanics but also protects the knees and encourages optimal engagement of the glutes and hamstrings.

✓ STRONG FOOT AND ANKLE POSITION

Your foot and ankle position provide the foundation for a strong hinge. The tripod foot—50 percent weight on the heel, 25 percent on the big toe, and 25 percent on the little toe—ensures stability and even weight distribution. Similarly, a stable ankle position prevents unnecessary movement, enabling you to load the hips effectively. Maintaining active engagement through the feet reduces compensations higher up the chain, particularly in the knees and lower back.

HINGE ASSESSMENT

The hinge assessment goes beyond the basics, offering a deep dive into your movement mechanics to reveal your true range of motion and ability to hinge without placing undue stress on your spine or other joints. At its core, this test addresses a fundamental question in strength training: **Should you be pulling from the standard barbell height of 8.75 inches off the ground?**

This height, rooted in the history of lifting rather than individual biomechanics, has become an arbitrary benchmark for the deadlift. The 8.75-inch standard originated in the early days of Olympic lifting, when barbell heights were set to prevent lifters' heads from being crushed against the ground during failed overhead lifts. While this rationale made sense in its historical context, it now forces modern lifters—regardless of their limb length, mobility, or skill level—to conform to a standard that often fails to align with their unique anatomy or range of motion.

Our data, gathered from over 20,000 certified coaches and athletes of all skill levels, reveals a striking statistic: 93 percent of individuals cannot maintain optimal mechanics while pulling from this height. Yet, despite these findings, the fitness world continues to prioritize this arbitrary standard over personalized approaches. The result? Many lifters unknowingly hybridize their movement patterns, turning their hinge into a squat-hinge hybrid and breaking key biomechanical principles. This leads to inefficiency, compensation, and the very injuries that give the deadlift its notorious reputation.

The hinge assessment is designed to cut through this confusion and focus solely on your body's available range of motion in a **pure hip hinge pattern**. By evaluating your mobility, stability, and skill, this test provides a clear answer to whether you should be lifting from the ground—or if adjustments, such as elevating the barbell, are necessary to accommodate your movement capabilities.

The goal of this assessment is not to rule out lifting from the ground but to confirm that you can do so with proper mechanics and without unnecessary risk. With your baseline established, you'll have the clarity needed to advance your lifts strategically and adapt your patterns to suit your individual range of motion when necessary.

WHAT IS A PURE HIP HINGE PATTERN?

A pure hip hinge pattern starts with the hips moving backward (posterior translation) to initiate the movement. The knees bend slightly—around 20 to 45 degrees—as the hips push back. However, unlike a squat, the knees remain at this fixed angle while the hips continue to bend further (hip flexion), allowing the torso to hinge forward. Throughout the movement, the spine and pelvis stay neutral, meaning they maintain proper alignment without rounding or arching.

The end result is maximum hip movement with minimal knee bending (20 to 45 degrees). This differs from a squat, where the hips and knees bend fully and simultaneously as the body lowers and rises. Put simply, the hinge isolates hip movement, while the squat involves both joints working together.

THE HINGE BACK TEST—
DETERMINING YOUR AUTHENTIC HINGE STANCE and ROM

This assessment evaluates your ability to perform a pure hip hinge by identifying the maximum range of motion you can maintain while adhering to proper mechanics outlined in the optimization checklist. For example, in a Romanian deadlift (RDL), this test determines the lowest position you can reach while maintaining pure hinge mechanics. Similarly, for conventional deadlifts from the floor, it identifies the highest position you can start from while preserving those same mechanics. This ensures your movement capacity is optimized for all hinge variations, allowing for safe and effective performance tailored to your unique range of motion.

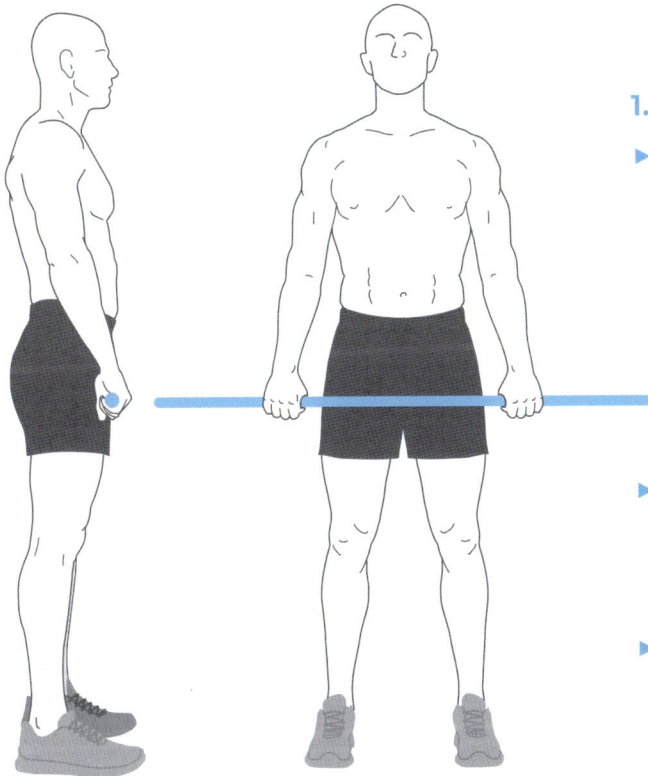

1. STARTING POSITION

▶ **Action:** Stand with your feet hip-width apart, toes pointing forward, and a dowel in your hands. Place your thumbs on your hips and grip the dowel firmly with both hands, keeping it aligned horizontally across your thighs. This grip mimics the position your hands will take when gripping a barbell, helping you build familiarity with proper hand placement and tension needed for effective hinge mechanics.

▶ **Goal:** Maintain a stable stance with your weight distributed evenly across the tripod foot (heel, big toe, and little toe) while setting up for the assessment.

▶ **Observation:** Ensure your pelvis is neutral, and the dowel remains in contact with your thighs as you initiate the test.

2. INITIATING THE HINGE

▶ **Action:** Begin by pushing your hips back as you guide the dowel down the front of your thighs. Keep your spine neutral and your shins vertical, avoiding forward knee movement. Focus on maximizing the backward motion of your hips while maintaining control.

▶ **Goal:** Evaluate how far your hips can move backward without breaking your neutral zone or compensating with forward knee movement.

▶ **Observation:** Watch for any rounding and arching of the lower back (lumbar flexion and hyperextension) or excessive knee bend.

3. DETERMINING YOUR MAXIMUM DEPTH

▶ **Action:** Lower the dowel down your legs as far as you can, sticking to the standards outlined in the optimization checklist. Stop at the point where you feel you are about to compensate, such as losing spinal neutrality or allowing forward knee movement. Avoid pushing past this range to prevent breaking form.

▶ **Goal:** Identify the precise depth where you can maintain a pure hip hinge without sacrificing form for additional range of motion (rounding your back or excessive knee bend, for example).

▶ **Observation:** Note the dowel's position on your leg. This is your maximum hinge depth representing your authentic hinge range of motion and serves as a reference for end-range RDL exercises and your start position for the barbell deadlift.

HINGING FROM YOUR NON-AUTHENTIC HINGE STANCE

Your "pure hinge" stance is the foundation for safe, effective movement—a hip-width position with toes pointing forward that maximizes posterior chain engagement and establishes your most authentic hip hinge mechanics. Mastering this stance is essential for building strength, maintaining long-term movement health, and enhancing performance in all other hinge variations.

While the pure hinge remains the cornerstone of training, adopting different stances—such as hybrid or sumo—can be valuable tools for targeting specific muscles, meeting sport-specific demands, or addressing individual goals. Regardless of stance, the mechanics learned in your pure hinge—loading the hips effectively, maintaining a neutral spine, and avoiding compensatory patterns—should always guide your movement.

Here's a breakdown of the primary hinge stances, their purposes, and when to use them:

PURE HINGE STANCE

• **Stance:** Feet hip-width apart, toes pointed straight forward.

• **Purpose:** This stance represents the authentic hinge pattern, focusing on isolating the posterior chain. It's the most biomechanically efficient position for loading the hips and maintaining a neutral spine, often referred to as the "power position." By aligning the glutes and hamstrings in an optimal biomechanical setup, this stance allows for maximum force generation. To find this position, hop up and down a few times and "catch" your landing—nearly every time, your feet will land naturally in this hip-width, toes-forward alignment.

• **When to Use:** Use the pure hinge stance to rebuild movement patterns, prevent compensations, and establish a baseline for pain-free hinging. This stance not only strengthens your posterior chain but also enhances all other stances, forming the foundation for long-term training and movement health.

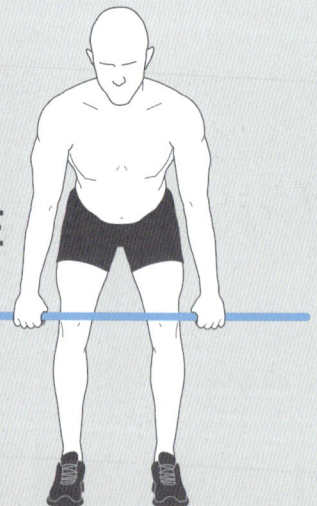

4. ADJUST AND RETEST

▶ **Action:** Perform 3–5 repetitions of the hinge. Each repetition should aim to reach your maximum depth while maintaining proper mechanics, such as a neutral spine, vertical shins, and strong foot positioning. Afterward, screen your movement against the optimization checklist to confirm adherence to the standards for a proper hinge.

▶ **Goal:** Refine your hinge pattern through practice while ensuring your form adheres to key criteria and avoiding any compensations. Use the baseline measurement to guide your training, ensuring that all loaded hinges stay within your authentic range of motion. Recognize that your hinge depth is not static and can improve with consistent practice and the integration of mobility, stability, and skill work.

▶ **Observation:** Retest periodically to confirm adherence to the optimization checklist and note progress in range of motion and stability over time. If the dowel stops significantly above the ground, consider elevating the barbell or implementing corrective strategies to address your most glaring linchpins.

HYBRID STANCE

• **Stance:** Feet shoulder-width apart with toes angled outward (15–20 degrees).

• **Purpose:** A blend of a hinge and a squat pattern, the hybrid stance (also known as "squat stance") allows for more knee flexion and greater depth, making it a useful option for improving range of motion closer to the floor. It emphasizes both posterior and anterior chain muscles.

• **When to Use:** Great for lifters with limited mobility or for developing strength in ranges of motion that mimic deeper barbell pulls. This stance can also help bridge the gap between pure hinge mechanics and competition-specific patterns.

SUMO STANCE

• **Stance:** Feet positioned wider than shoulder width with toes angled out (30–50 degrees).

• **Purpose:** This stance is a hinge-squat hybrid that emphasizes mobility, knee flexion, and external rotation. The sumo stance involves increased quad activation and promotes a more upright torso, reducing lower back demands while still engaging the hips. While effective for certain goals, it introduces more knee bend, external rotation torque, and vertical torso positioning compared to a pure hinge.

• **When to Use:** Ideal for powerlifters or athletes aiming to maximize strength in specific ranges of motion. However, it should only be incorporated alongside a pure hinge—such as Romanian deadlift (RDL) variations—to maintain balanced development and mechanics. The sumo stance complements, but does not replace, the biomechanical benefits of a pure hinge.

OPTIMIZATION STRATEGIES

After completing the hinge assessment and retesting your movement against the optimization checklist (see Step 4: Adjust and Retest in the assessment protocol), you may still notice subtle compensations—minor deviations that shift the workload away from your muscles and onto your joints. These compensations are often influenced by factors such as limited range of motion (mobility), difficulty maintaining alignment (stability), or challenges in coordinating the movement (skill).

It's important to recognize that these compensations are not inherently harmful or indicative of fragility. While they may contribute to discomfort or limit performance for some individuals, others might move comfortably and effectively despite them. The key is understanding how these patterns impact your unique movement and addressing them when they hinder your goals or create unnecessary strain.

The good news is that the hinge pattern is highly trainable, and every compensation has a targeted solution. By identifying and addressing weak links through tailored optimization strategies, you can refine your mechanics, build strength in your posterior chain, and set yourself up for long-term success.

With that in mind, let's explore the most common compensations and the practical steps you can take to overcome them.

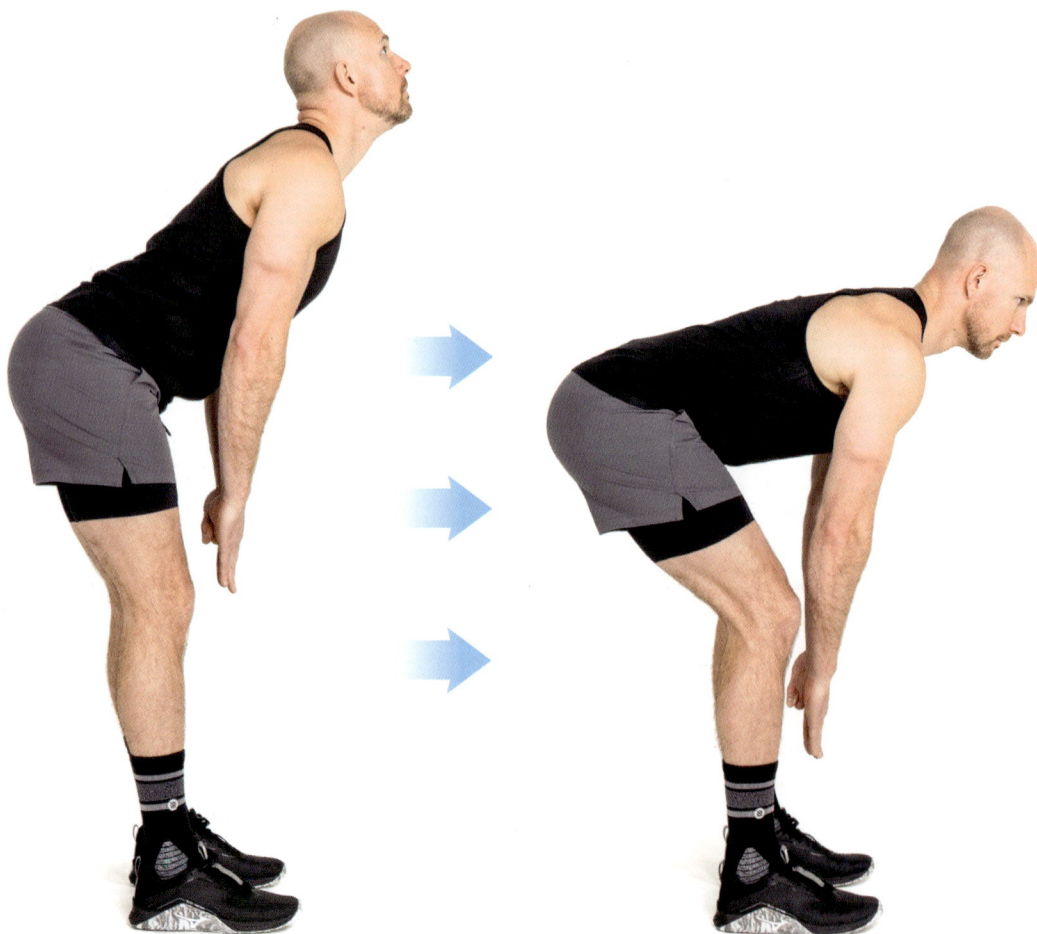

COMPENSATION: LUMBAR HYPEREXTENSION with ANTERIOR PELVIC TILT

MOBILITY: Tight hip flexors and quads, often caused by prolonged sitting or specific postures (e.g., standing with locked knees and an arched back), pull the pelvis into an anterior tilt. This is typically paired with a poorly braced pillar. You can identify this issue if

▼ Your pelvis tilts forward, causing an overly extended lower back curve

▼ Standing upright feels "tight" in your lower back, hip flexors, and hamstrings

▼ Prolonged standing becomes uncomfortable, leading to compensation into anterior pelvic tilt (APT) and lumbar extension

OPTIMIZATION STRATEGIES:

▶ Refer to the **Hip Mobility A Linchpin Blueprint** (page 469) for targeted mobility exercises.

▶ Perform hands-banded bodyweight hinges, anterior-loaded good mornings, split squats, and reverse lunges to balance hip mobility and stability.

▶ Strengthen glutes and hamstrings with supine hip hinges (e.g., glute bridges, hip thrusts) and core exercises like dead bugs and front planks, emphasizing neutral spinal alignment.

▶ Add recovery stretches, such as the prone quad stretch to lengthen tight hip flexors and quads, and child's pose to stretch the lower back muscles.

STABILITY: Insufficient pillar stability often leads to compensations like anterior pelvic tilt. A lack of diaphragmatic breathing and bracing results in over-reliance on the lower back for support, which can contribute to low back pain. Indicators of poor pillar stability include

▼ Difficulty maintaining a neutral pelvis when standing, sitting, or hinging

▼ Increased spinal extension and flexion during movement, especially when moving quickly or under load

OPTIMIZATION STRATEGIES:

▶ Refer to the **Core Stability A (Supine) Linchpin Blueprint** (page 472).

▶ Practice the **Prone Breath Corrective** (page 46) to establish proper diaphragmatic breathing.

▶ Incorporate pull-throughs with a band or cable to engage anterior core muscles that stabilize the pillar.

▶ Add stability-focused exercises such as glute bridges, hip thrusts, and goblet squats to reinforce a stable and neutral spine.

SKILL: A lack of motor control or proper sequencing often exacerbates compensations. This manifests as an inability to brace effectively or maintain a neutral spine throughout movement. Signs of this include

▼ Overcompensation into lumbar extension at the top of the hinge or lumbar flexion toward the bottom

▼ A lack of smooth motion during the descent or shifting between hips pushing back and knees bending, often worsening under load or fatigue

OPTIMIZATION STRATEGIES:

▶ Ensure proper setup: Maintain a neutral pelvis, stack ribs over hips, and breathe 360 degrees into your torso. Placing hands on your waist can help with feedback.

▶ Perform pull-throughs with a band or cable to support core activation while building skill.

▶ Practice Reactive Neuromuscular Training (RNT) by placing a band around your knees to reinforce abduction and posterior chain stability.

▶ Refer to the Pillar chapter for detailed cueing techniques to establish and maintain a neutral spinal alignment.

COMPENSATION: LUMBAR FLEXION (ROUNDING LOWER BACK)

MOBILITY: Limited hamstring mobility can contribute to lumbar flexion during hinges. However, a lack of pelvis or core stability can result in the hamstrings being used as a "backup" for stability. Signs that mobility may be a limiting factor include

▼ Comparing a standing toe touch to a seated toe touch. If both are limited, improving posterior chain mobility will enhance performance in pure hinge movements. (If the seated toe touch shows increased range of motion, stability work may also be beneficial.)

▼ Difficulty pushing the hips back during the hinge, leading to the spine curling or rounding

▼ Feeling significant resistance in the hamstrings, with knees bending or moving forward to compensate

OPTIMIZATION STRATEGIES:

▶ Refer to the **Posterior Chain (Hinge) Mobility Linchpin Blueprint** (page 470) for targeted mobility exercises.

▶ Practice Reactive Neuromuscular Training (RNT) by placing a band around your hips (anchored behind you) to encourage better spinal extension and proper hip movement.

▶ Incorporate exercises like the kneeling banded hip thrust to establish proper hinge mechanics and glute contribution, reducing reliance on the hamstrings as the primary extensor. Include supine hinge exercises like glute bridges and hip thrusts.

▶ Add recovery stretches such as the supine hamstring stretch with a strap, child's pose, or dynamic pigeon stretch, and the supine twist.

STABILITY: Rounding of the lower back often occurs due to weak pillar stability and/or insufficient ability to create and maintain a brace under load. Indicators of instability include

▼ Loss of spinal and pelvic neutrality during the hinge

▼ Difficulty maintaining a brace through the hips, core, and shoulders

OPTIMIZATION STRATEGIES:

▶ Refer to the **Core Stability B (Prone) Linchpin Blueprint** (page 473) for exercises and cues to build a strong, stable pillar.

▶ Practice Reactive Neuromuscular Training (RNT) with a band around your hips (anchored behind you) to promote better spinal extension and hip engagement.

▶ Perform non-vertical hinge variations, such as pull-throughs, to ensure pillar engagement is maintained throughout the movement.

▶ Incorporate exercises like glute bridges, hip thrusts, and side planks to improve hip stability.

SKILL: A lack of motor control or insufficient body awareness is often seen in beginners or individuals guarding against pain or previous injuries. Signs of a skill gap include

▼ Descending beyond the range you can control with a neutral spine and proper bracing

▼ Focusing more on "lowering" the chest or weight rather than pushing the hips back

OPTIMIZATION STRATEGIES:

▶ Beginners or individuals returning after an injury may benefit from performing supplemental hinge exercises like glute bridges and hip thrusts for 4 to 12 weeks before progressing to standing hinge variations.

▶ Prioritize movement mastery by following the optimization checklist and progressing through the hinge progression pyramid using non-vertical hinge variations to build competence and confidence.

▶ Cue proper bracing and focus on maintaining alignment throughout, emphasizing form over depth or load.

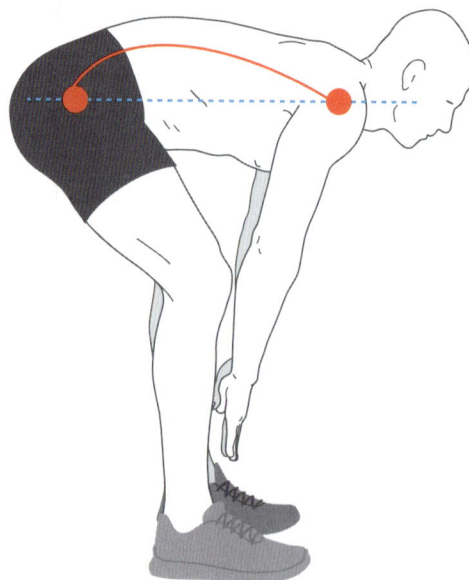

COMPENSATION: UPPER BACK ROUNDING with T-SPINE FLEXION

NOTE: *For older clients, the observed curvature in the upper back may reflect a remodeled spinal position, which is different from temporary spine flexion and shoulder movement on the rib cage. In such cases, the spine in this position cannot extend. Improvements in soft tissue mobility will not change the curvature of the spine. Instead, the focus should be on empowering the client, training what is available, and preventing further forward rounding.*

MOBILITY: Tight pecs and upper traps are common culprits behind the forward rounding of the upper back and shoulders. This issue can be exacerbated by poor posture or an overemphasis on pushing exercises without balancing pulling movements.

Signs of limited mobility include

▼ Difficulty maintaining a "tall chest" in a standing position and/or a lengthened upper torso during the hinge

▼ Tightness in the neck, shoulders, and chest

▼ Feeling "stuck" when extending the upper back or opening the arms wide to a T-shape

OPTIMIZATION STRATEGIES:

▶ Refer to the **T-Spine Mobility Linchpin Blueprint** (page 471) for exercises to improve thoracic extension and shoulder mobility.

▶ Use glute bridges, hip thrusts, or non-vertical load variations like pull-throughs to encourage better posture.

▶ Incorporate pulling exercises (e.g., rows, face pulls) into your programming to restore proper posture.

▶ Prioritize the 90/90 chest stretch to open the pecs and improve upper body alignment.

STABILITY: Poor scapular stability often stems from prolonged seated or rounded-forward postures, as well as insufficient training of the muscles responsible for extension and external rotation. Indicators include

▼ Shoulders and shoulder blades feel unstable, causing elbow flaring, internal rotation, elevated shoulders, and scapular winging

▼ Difficulty creating tension in the lats during co-contraction, leading to an inability to utilize the upper back effectively under load

OPTIMIZATION STRATEGIES:

▶ Refer to the **Scapular Stability Linchpin Blueprint** (page 473) for targeted exercises to improve scapular control.

▶ Practice Reactive Neuromuscular Training (RNT) by placing a band around a dowel, barbell, or your wrists and facing the anchor point. Pulling the weight toward you will engage the lats and improve posture and pillar stability.

▶ Prioritize pulling variations to restore balance between the chest and back. Include exercises like face pulls, band pull-aparts, and scapular retraction drills.

▶ For recovery, use stretches such as the 90/90 chest stretch (page 122) to release tight pecs, and practice 90/90 Supine Parasympathetic Positional Breathing (page 54) to relax tight neck and upper back muscles caused by forward head posture.

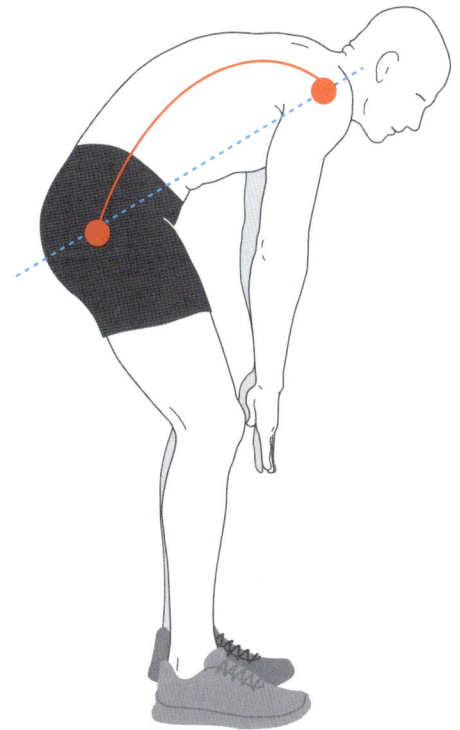

SKILL: Rounding in the upper back during hinges often results from a lack of body awareness or insufficient training. When mobility and stability are not limiting factors, this compensation likely stems from poor movement patterns. Signs of a skill gap include

▼ Losing upper body posture as you descend, with difficulty regaining neutral alignment

▼ Struggling to maintain a neutral pillar, especially under load or when fatigued

OPTIMIZATION STRATEGIES:

▶ Start with supplemental hinge movements like glute bridges and hip thrusts, progressing through the hinge progression pyramid only after meeting the standards in the optimization checklist.

▶ Refer to the cueing sequence in the Pillar chapter (page 34) to refine bracing setup and execution.

COMPENSATION: ASYMMETRICAL HIP SHIFT (ONE HIP TILTS, SHIFTS or ROTATES)

MOBILITY: Muscular imbalances often result in reciprocal inhibition over time, where one muscle becomes short, dominant, or tight while the opposing muscle is lengthened, weak, or inhibited. Since the hip is the second most mobile joint in the body as a ball-and-socket joint, it involves numerous muscles and allows movement in multiple directions. However, prolonged sitting and sedentary habits can lead to restricted hip mobility, making it a common linchpin for dysfunction. Indicators include

▼ Feeling more restricted or tight on one side during stretches or warm-up movements

▼ Favoring one side when sitting down or getting up from the floor, or difficulty getting up and down altogether

OPTIMIZATION STRATEGIES:

▶ Refer to the **Hip Mobility B Linchpin Blueprint** (page 469) to address tight or short muscles around the hip joint.

▶ Strengthen within the symmetrical range you can control, gradually increasing depth over time (e.g., using a rack or blocks to control depth).

▶ Incorporate exercises such as 1.5 stance glute bridges, hip thrusts, RDLs, split squats, reverse lunges, and lateral lunges to address imbalances and improve mobility.

▶ Add supplemental stretches like the half-kneeling hip flexor stretch, adductor rock-back, dynamic pigeon stretch, prone quad stretch, and supine hamstring stretch with a strap.

STABILITY: Where reciprocal inhibition is present, there are also lengthened, weak, or under-trained muscles. This can lead to a lack of stability, especially in those with limited exercise experience or a sedentary lifestyle with low daily activity levels. (Walking, which is reciprocal in nature, is an excellent way to establish baseline hip stability and function!) Lacking hip stability can be identified by

▼ A noticeable shift or rotation in the hips during the descent or ascent in a hinge

▼ Difficulty maintaining a neutral pelvis and spine and/or balance during activities such as walking, changing directions, walking up or down stairs, or performing split squats and lunges

OPTIMIZATION STRATEGIES:

▶ Refer to the **Hip Stability B Linchpin Blueprint** (page 475) to prepare for hinges.

▶ Use a modified stance to promote better stability and manage depth with a rack or blocks. Recording your hinge from behind can help ensure your setup minimizes shifting.

▶ Apply Reactive Neuromuscular Training (RNT) by using a miniband around the knees to encourage abduction or a long resistance band around the hips, pulling in the same direction as the shift to provide feedback and promote correction.

▶ Include supplemental unilateral exercises like split squats, lunges, 1.5 stance hinge variations, side planks, glute drills, lateral lunges, and possibly curtsy lunges.

▶ Finish workouts with additional hip stability work, such as phase 3 and phase 4 drills or similar movements, as a burnout finisher.

SKILL: Asymmetry often stems from repetitive patterns in daily life, work, or sports (e.g., consistently throwing, lunging, or sitting in a specific position). These habits carry over into gym movements, reinforcing imbalances. Signs of a skill gap include

▼ Struggling to control movement patterns in symmetrical hinge exercises

▼ Biases or ingrained habits during setup or execution (e.g., foot placement, stance width, or how you "pick up" the load)

OPTIMIZATION STRATEGIES:

▶ Start your session with the **Hip Stability B Linchpin Blueprint** (page 475) to address imbalances.

▶ Program a stance or modification that promotes stable and symmetrical hinges.

▶ Regress to a non-vertical hinge variation that prioritizes movement quality and symmetry, using a box, bench, rack, or blocks to control depth as needed.

▶ Focus on setup: align your stance, stabilize the pelvis by co-contracting the glutes and adductors, breathe 360 degrees, and brace to maximize intra-abdominal pressure. Maintain full-body irradiation throughout the hinge, including lat engagement, to support stability and control.

COMPENSATION: KNEES ROTATE INWARD

MOBILITY: Tight muscles can "pull" bones out of alignment, especially when they are lengthened during movement. In the case of a pure hinge, this often involves the hamstrings, particularly the laterally connected attachments, or the adductors. Indicators include

▼ Difficulty touching your toes from a standing or seated position

▼ Feeling tight or restricted when attempting a wide stance hinge (sumo) or performing split squats or lunges

OPTIMIZATION STRATEGIES:

▶ Refer to the **Posterior Chain (Hinge) Mobility Linchpin Blueprint** (page 470) for hamstring-focused work or the **Hip Mobility B Linchpin Blueprint** (page 469) for adductor-focused work.

▶ Use Reactive Neuromuscular Training (RNT) by placing a band around your legs just above your knees to promote abduction and better leg alignment.

▶ Incorporate single-leg exercises such as split squats, reverse lunges, and single-leg glute bridges.

▶ Perform recovery stretches like the quadruped adductor stretch, frog stretch, and supine hamstring stretch with a strap, slightly drawing the leg across the body to target the lateral hamstring.

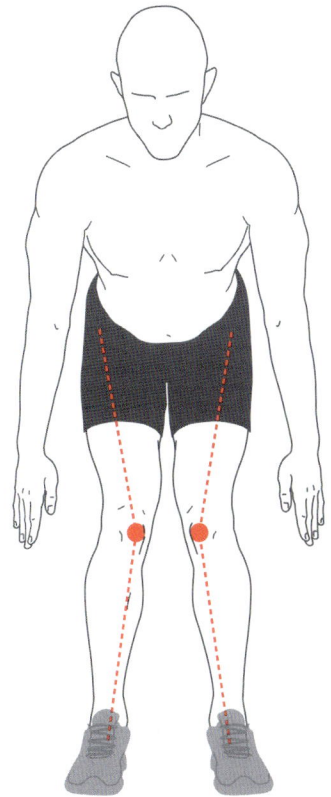

STABILITY: Poor stability in the foot, ankle, or hip often contributes to valgus collapse. This instability may result from poor footwear, undertraining, or previous injuries, creating a chain reaction that affects the knees. Indicators of poor stability include

▼ Wobbling or collapsing at the foot and ankle, causing the knee to fall inward

▼ Difficulty maintaining proper "knees tracking over toes" alignment, particularly under load when pulling the weight up

OPTIMIZATION STRATEGIES:

▶ Begin your session with the **Hip Stability B Linchpin Blueprint** (page 475).

▶ Adjust your stance to improve ankle and foot stability. For some, this may involve a slightly wider stance with reduced depth until stability improves.

▶ Use RNT with a miniband to address alignment:

· Place the band above the knees to encourage abduction and prevent inward collapse.

· Place the band above the ankles to strengthen foot and ankle positioning.

▶ Incorporate single-leg exercises such as split squats, reverse lunges, and single-leg glute bridges.

▶ Focus on strengthening the adductors, glutes, and lower limbs to improve alignment and stability.

SKILL: Knee valgus often results from poor body awareness and a lack of coordination during the hinge. Lifters may overemphasize depth or load, sacrificing stability for range of motion or an ego lift. Additional factors include failure to engage the pillar or improper sequencing of movement patterns. Signs of a skill gap include

▼ Difficulty "feeling" the activation of glutes and external rotators to drive the knees outward

▼ Inability to set and maintain a strong pillar and brace, resulting in forward knee movement and internal rotation, causing the knees to collapse inward during the upward phase of the hinge

OPTIMIZATION STRATEGIES:

▶ Actively drive the knees outward as you set up and push your hips back into the hinge. Visualize "spreading the floor" with your feet to engage the glutes and create external rotation at the hips.

▶ Practice hinges with a miniband above the knees to provide tactile feedback and reinforce abduction.

▶ Slow down the movement and focus on deliberate, controlled repetitions to improve coordination and sequencing.

▶ Use a non-vertical hinge, emphasizing horizontal hip movement backward, or limit depth with a rack or blocks while building strength and control through the desired range of motion.

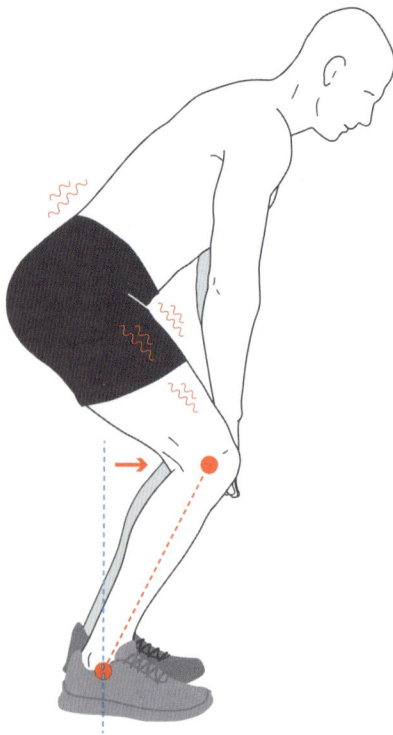

COMPENSATION: FORWARD KNEE MOVEMENT

If you struggle to push your hips back, another way to lower yourself is by bending the knees, sending them forward past the ankle, and employing more of a squat pattern. While this isn't inherently wrong, it doesn't align with a pure hinge pattern. With increased knee bend during a hinge, the load shifts to the quadriceps and compensates by overloading the lower back. Over time, this can lead to weakness, imbalance, reduced performance, and an increased risk of injury or pain.

MOBILITY: Tight hamstrings or a restricted posterior chain are the most common causes of forward knee movement, as the descent of a pure hinge lengthens the hamstrings. Indicators include

▼ Difficulty keeping relatively straight legs while descending in a pure hinge

▼ Tightness in the hamstrings and possibly the lower back during seated or standing folds

OPTIMIZATION STRATEGIES:

► Perform the **Posterior Chain (Hinge) Mobility Linchpin Blueprint** (page 470) to increase range of motion for hinge patterns.

► Focus on the eccentric (lowering) portion of the hinge movement, moving slowly and with control to maximize the loaded stretch. Work within a range of motion where you can maintain minimal forward knee bend, improving mobility over time.

► Incorporate recovery stretches, such as the supine hamstring stretch with a strap or legs-up-the-wall pose. Static stretching for 10 minutes per week per muscle group has been shown to improve mobility.

STABILITY: Maintaining a strong pillar and neutral spine is a common challenge in hinge patterns. A lack of stability can lead to compensations such as forward knee movement. If you struggle to pressurize your pillar, it becomes harder to create tension and stability in the posterior chain, leading to knee-bending instead of the desired "hips pushing back" movement. Indicators of poor stability include

▼ Lagging glute/adductor co-contraction and bracing, making it difficult to stabilize the posterior chain before movement begins

▼ Difficulty maintaining a strong brace when driving the hips back

▼ Difficulty "feeling" the hamstrings and glutes during hinge exercises (a common challenge for very flexible individuals)

OPTIMIZATION STRATEGIES:

► Perform the **Core Stability B (Prone) Linchpin Blueprint** (page 473) to improve pillar control and overall stability.

► Prioritize pull-through variations with a band or cable to encourage posterior chain recruitment and reduce knee bending.

► Incorporate posterior chain strengthening exercises such as glute bridges, hip thrusts, hamstring curls, reverse hypers, and back extensions.

SKILL: Your body naturally defaults to the easiest or strongest movement patterns unless you intentionally train for balanced, functional strength. Because daily life often involves squat and lunge-like movements, the hinge pattern is often undertrained. Forward knee movement during a hinge may indicate a lack of experience or body awareness. Signs of a skill gap include

▼ Defaulting to knee-bending in hinge variations

▼ Difficulty "feeling" the hamstrings and glutes during hinge exercises

OPTIMIZATION STRATEGIES:

► Focus on maintaining a strong foot tripod by engaging the arch and co-contracting the glutes and adductors to stabilize the pelvis. This creates more torque and tension around the hips. Use body weight or light/moderate loads to refine your technique.

► Prioritize pull-through variations with a band or cable to promote proper hip hinge mechanics.

► Incorporate posterior chain strengthening exercises such as glute bridges, hip thrusts, hamstring curls, reverse hypers, and back extensions.

HINGE PROGRESSION PYRAMID

The hinge progression pyramid is your road map to building a strong, pain-free hinge pattern. At the foundation of the pyramid is the **bodyweight hinge**. This simple, unloaded movement teaches you the basics of how to hinge at your hips—moving your pelvis back while keeping your spine neutral. It's all about learning the pattern and setting the stage for everything that comes next. Once you meet the standards covered in the optimization checklist, you're ready to move up the pyramid.

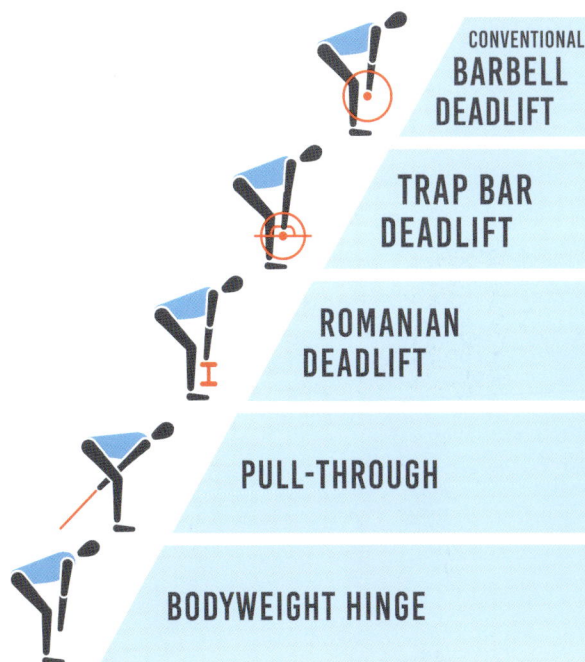

CONVENTIONAL BARBELL DEADLIFT

TRAP BAR DEADLIFT

ROMANIAN DEADLIFT

PULL-THROUGH

BODYWEIGHT HINGE

The **pull-through** refines the hinge by helping you feel how your hips should move. A cable or band applies tension in a horizontal direction, gently pulling your hips back. This helps you practice shifting your weight into your hips (instead of your lower back) and guides you through the correct movement. It's like having a coach physically cueing your hips to move the right way—safe, effective, and easy to learn.

Next comes the **Romanian deadlift (RDL)**, where you start adding vertical resistance to the pattern using dumbbells, kettlebells, or a barbell. This introduces load to your hinge, making it more challenging while still giving you control over the movement. The RDL also focuses on lowering the weight slowly (the eccentric phase), which improves your ability to stabilize your body as you move.

The **trap bar deadlift** steps things up by adding more load and slightly adjusting the setup to make the movement more accessible. The trap bar's handles are elevated, so you don't have to reach as far down as with a barbell, and the weight sits directly in line with your body. This setup is easier on your back and lets you lift heavier while keeping your form in check. The neutral grip also makes it easier to stabilize your shoulders and core, helping you maintain and develop pillar strength and control.

Finally, at the top of the pyramid is the **conventional barbell deadlift**, the most advanced hinge variation due to the significant demands it places on the hips and the high level of motor control required. Here, you'll be lifting from a pure hinge posture, which puts more strain on your back, hips, and core. It's a test of everything you've built so far—your ability to brace, maintain alignment, and generate force. For many people, adjusting the height of the bar with blocks or plates can make the movement safer and better aligned with their natural range of motion.

Each stage of the hinge progression pyramid builds on the last, ensuring you develop mobility, stability, and skill every step of the way. In forthcoming pages, you'll find specific tips for honing each movement, helping you progress with purpose and achieve your strongest, safest hinge.

BODYWEIGHT HINGE

The bodyweight hinge lays the groundwork for the entire hinge progression pyramid, forming the basis of a movement pattern you perform every day.

Whether you're recovering from an injury, starting fresh, or honing your technique, the bodyweight hinge allows you to fine-tune your movement in its simplest form.

For guidance on mastering the bodyweight hinge, refer to the hinge screen and optimization checklist covered earlier in the chapter.

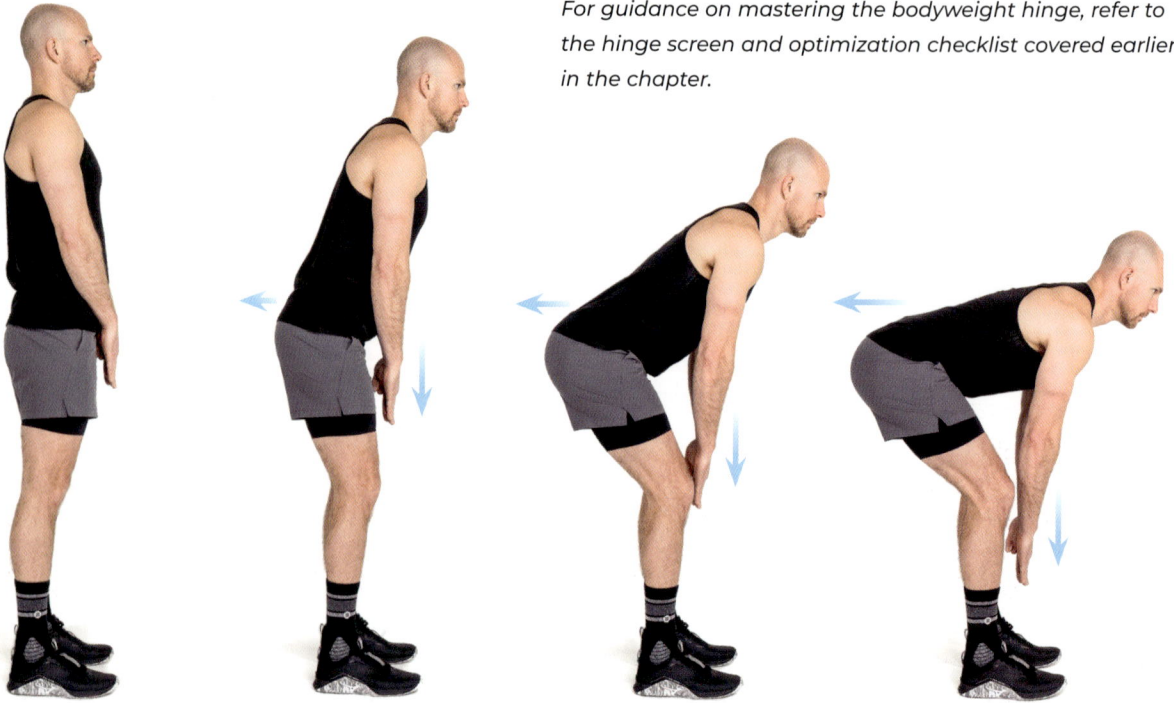

ECCENTRIC PHASE

CONCENTRIC PHASE

PULL-THROUGH

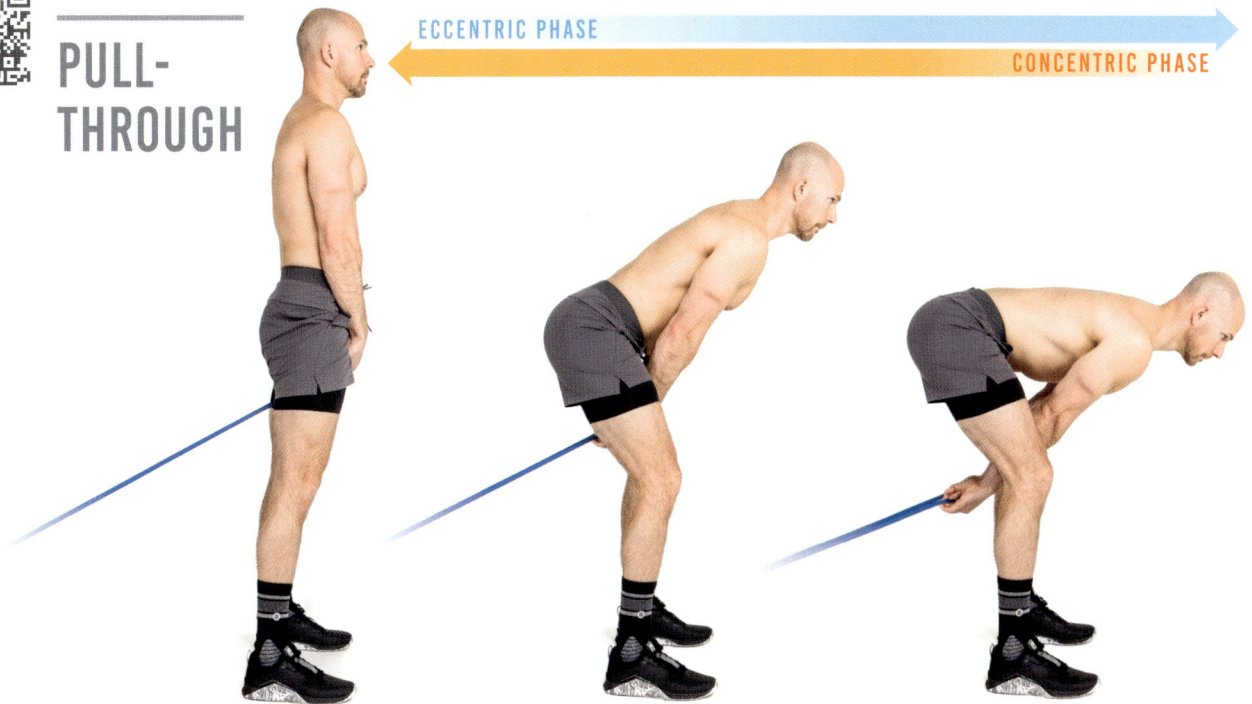

The pull-through is a key step in mastering the hinge pattern. By adding horizontal resistance with a band or cable, this exercise helps you lock in the hip movement that defines a proper hinge—pushing your hips back and driving them forward—without the common mistake of squatting the movement. That gentle pull from the resistance gives you immediate feedback, so you know when your hips are doing the right work, all while keeping your spine neutral and safe.

Think of the pull-through as your "aha" moment for understanding how your glutes, hamstrings, and lower back work together. It strips away the pressure of heavy loading and focuses entirely on hinging mechanics with minimal strain on your spine. If you're just starting out, managing lower back pain, or rebuilding your hinge, this exercise lays the foundation for success as you progress to heavier, more advanced variations.

SETUP: Start by selecting your implement: either a long resistance band or a cable machine with a rope attachment.

- **The band** provides accommodating resistance, meaning the tension increases as you extend your hips and transition into an upright posture. This feature helps guide your hips into a neutral position at full extension, locking in proper alignment and emphasizing the role of the glutes at the top of the movement. The band's forgiving nature and tactile feedback make it ideal for beginners or those rebuilding their hinge pattern, as it provides constant guidance to reinforce clean mechanics.

- **The cable** provides consistent tension throughout the entire movement, making it a great choice for more advanced lifters looking to increase load. What's more, the weight stack allows for incremental progressions, enabling you to fine-tune resistance as your strength improves. While the cable offers excellent control, it is generally better suited as an accessory movement once you've mastered the basic mechanics with a band.

Anchor the band or cable low to the ground—6 to 12 inches off the floor is ideal. A low anchor ensures the resistance follows the proper angle, facilitating a pure hip hinge motion without impeding mechanics or risking awkward contact with the body.

Face away from the anchor point and position yourself directly above it, with the band or cable on slack positioned between your legs. Grab the handles (or the band itself) with a neutral grip—palms facing each other.

From there, take three full steps forward to create tension in the band or cable. This ensures the resistance is constant throughout the movement and that the cable doesn't rack the weight stack prematurely. Once tension is set, adjust into your authentic hinge stance.

LOAD POSITION: As you establish your starting position, engage your lats and pull your shoulders back and down. This creates tension through your upper body and ensures your pillar is stable. A neutral spine and braced core are non-negotiable, setting the foundation for a clean hinge.

EXECUTION: Begin by hinging your hips back, allowing the band or cable to guide your hips into a pure posterior shift. Your shins should remain vertical throughout, with the knees stacked directly over the ankles. Avoid excessive forward knee movement or hyperextension of the legs. Keep your spine neutral and avoid rounding or overextending through the back.

Lower into the hinge slowly and with control, focusing on an eccentric stretch through the hamstrings. Stop once you reach your full range of motion, as determined by your hinge assessment—this is typically where your spine begins to round or where tension shifts to compensatory patterns.

To return to the starting position, reverse the motion by driving your hips forward in a controlled yet dynamic concentric phase. Think about leading the movement with your glutes while maintaining alignment through your torso. Lock your hips into a neutral position at the top by contracting your glutes and stabilizing your lumbopelvic region.

Repeat for the prescribed number of reps, maintaining consistent tension and control throughout. Each repetition should reinforce the hip-dominant movement, training the hips to move smoothly from a backward to forward position without compensations.

ROMANIAN DEADLIFT (RDL)

ECCENTRIC PHASE

CONCENTRIC PHASE

DUMBBELL RDL

The Romanian deadlift (RDL) marks the first introduction of axial loading to the hinge pattern. Unlike earlier stages like the bodyweight hinge or pull-through, the RDL challenges your ability to stabilize under a vertical load while moving through a controlled, full range of motion. It emphasizes the eccentric (lowering) phase of the movement, allowing for maximum recruitment of the hamstrings and glutes while reinforcing proper alignment and pillar stability.

The top-down approach of the RDL offers unique advantages. Starting from a neutral standing position allows you to brace and stabilize effectively. This method also enables you to customize the range of motion based on your hinge assessment findings, ensuring that your movement stays within your authentic limits.

When it comes to implements, the RDL provides flexibility. Beginners should start with a single kettlebell or dumbbell positioned over the mid-foot for ease of control and proximity to the center of mass. From there, progressions include double kettlebells, dumbbells, or even barbell variations, with each step introducing more complexity and loading potential. As the load shifts farther away from the body, the demands on your motor control, stability, and strength increase, making this a scalable movement for lifters at all levels.

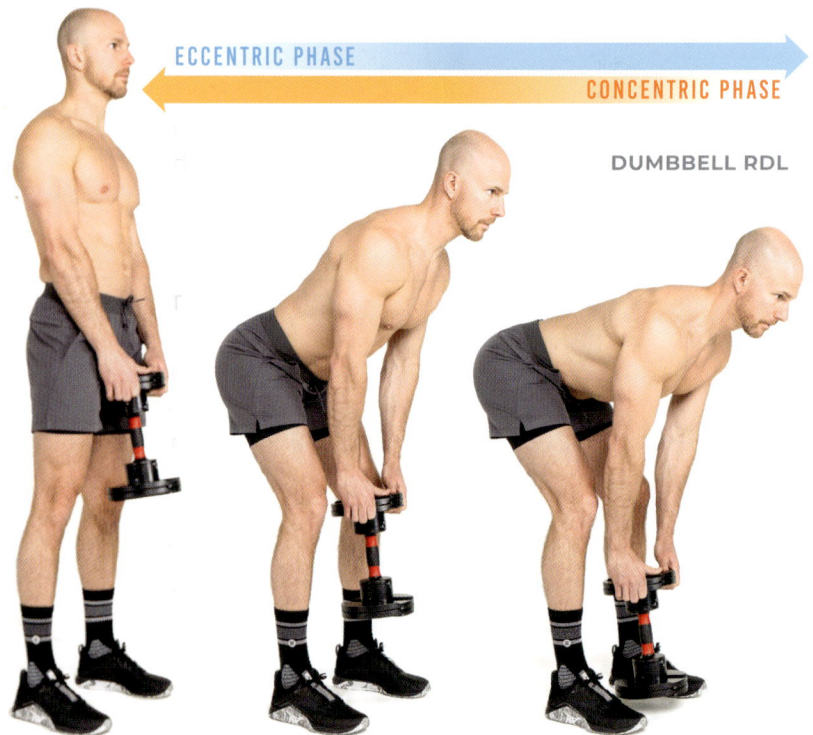

The RDL is the go-to exercise for building foundational strength and function. It trains the pure hip hinge pattern through a full range of motion while integrating the upper and lower body, making it one of the most valuable exercises in the hinge hierarchy. If you had to choose one loaded hinge exercise to master, the RDL should be at the top of your list.

SETUP: If you're working with a light load to refine your movement, such as an 8 kg kettlebell in a phase five warm-up training scenario, you can start by standing directly over the weight. Use a squat position with a neutral spine to grab the kettlebell, bring it into position, and establish your brace before initiating your first rep.

However, as the weight increases to something more challenging—beyond what you can comfortably lift for 10 reps—it's important to elevate the starting position. For kettlebells or dumbbells, place them on a bench or box at about knee height to simplify the lift-off. For barbell use, rack the barbell in J-hooks set just below hip height to create a similar starting position. This minimizes strain, allows you to start in a strong, neutral position, and mirrors the setup for other loaded hinge patterns. Once the weight is in position, take three deliberate steps back: one with your dominant foot, one with your non-dominant foot, and a final adjustment step into your authentic hinge stance.

LOAD POSITION: **Regardless of the implement—a single kettlebell, double kettlebells, dumbbells, or a barbell—the weight should remain close to your body throughout the movement.** Your arms hang straight down, with the weight aligned over your center of mass. The key is maintaining a packed shoulder position, co-contracting your pecs and lats, and maximizing grip tension through irradiation. This creates a stable and controlled movement, ensuring that the load doesn't swing or deviate from its vertical path.

For kettlebells or dumbbells, the weight should glide up and down the front of your legs, acting as a tactile guide to maintain the proper hinge pattern. Keeping the load tight to your body not only reinforces pure hip-dominant mechanics but also prevents unwanted lumbar rounding or compensatory squatting.

EXECUTION: The RDL follows the optimization checklist covered in the hinge screen. Begin by taking a deep diaphragmatic breath and bracing your core to stabilize your spine. **Push your hips back to initiate the hinge, allowing the weight to travel down while maintaining a neutral spine.** Your knees should remain slightly bent and your shins vertical, ensuring that the movement stays hip-dominant.

The eccentric phase should be slow and deliberate, stretching and lengthening the hamstrings as your hips move into full flexion. Once you reach your maximum range of motion without compensating through your spine or pelvis, reverse the movement by driving your feet into the ground and hips forward.

The concentric phase—the rising portion—should be smooth and dynamic, with a hard flex at the top of the rep. Think about driving your hips forward into the kettlebell, dumbbell, or barbell to emphasize the horizontal displacement of your hips. This ensures full engagement of the glutes and locks in the lumbopelvic structure at the top.

KETTLEBELL RDL

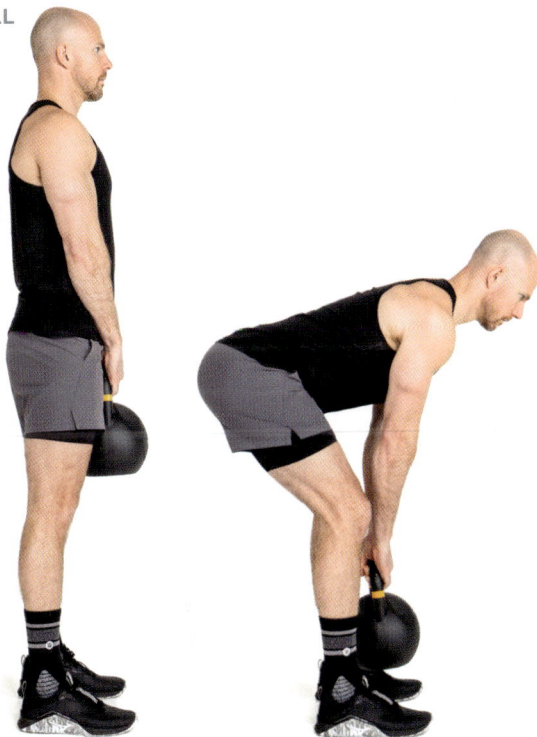

ECCENTRIC PHASE

CONCENTRIC PHASE

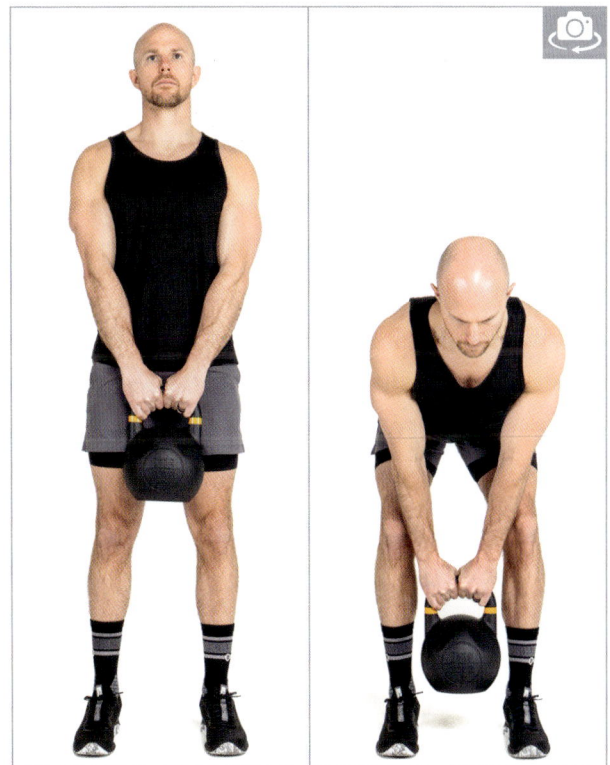

ECCENTRIC PHASE

CONCENTRIC PHASE

TRAP BAR DEADLIFT

The trap bar deadlift is one of the most practical and beginner-friendly ways to build strength and improve your hinge mechanics. It's the next logical step in the hinge progression pyramid, giving you the ability to handle heavier loads without the steep learning curve or strain that can come with a conventional barbell deadlift. By stepping inside the bar and aligning the handles over your center of mass, the trap bar deadlift feels natural and balanced, making it accessible for anyone—whether you're new to lifting or an experienced lifter.

One key advantage of the trap bar is its adjustable pulling height. The high handles, typically 3 to 5 inches above a standard barbell height, make it easier to set up in a strong position while reducing excessive strain. However, many lifters don't realize that the trap bar also offers customizable deadlift heights beyond just "high handle" or "low handle" variations. By flipping the bar to the low handles (8.75 inches off the ground—the same as a standard barbell) or elevating the bar on blocks to match your authentic hinge range, you can fine-tune the setup to better suit your mobility and mechanics. Instead of being locked into a fixed range of motion, this approach allows you to train at the depth that best aligns with the result of your hinge assessment results.

If you're looking for a deadlift variation that balances accessibility with progression, the trap bar deadlift is an essential tool. Its versatility and setup not only make it safer and easier to learn but also provide a strategic way to load your hinge that minimizes strain on your lower back.

SETUP: **Start by selecting a trap bar with elevated handles to allow for easier access to the bar.** Stand inside the bar with your feet hip-width apart and your toes pointing straight ahead or slightly outward. Position the middle of your feet directly in line with the bar collars to align the load with your center of mass.

Begin in a standing position to establish tension through your body. Progress through the pillar cueing sequence (page 34), creating stability across your shoulders, hips, and core. Only after this full-body engagement should you hinge your hips back and lower yourself to the bar. Keep your shins vertical, your spine neutral, and your chest slightly elevated as you descend. Grip the handles with a firm, neutral grip (palms facing your body), ensuring your hands are positioned evenly on both sides.

LOAD POSITION: With the bar positioned directly over your center of mass, the load is distributed evenly, minimizing unnecessary strain on your back. Maintain a neutral shoulder position by retracting and slightly depressing your shoulder blades, engaging your lats to lock in stability.

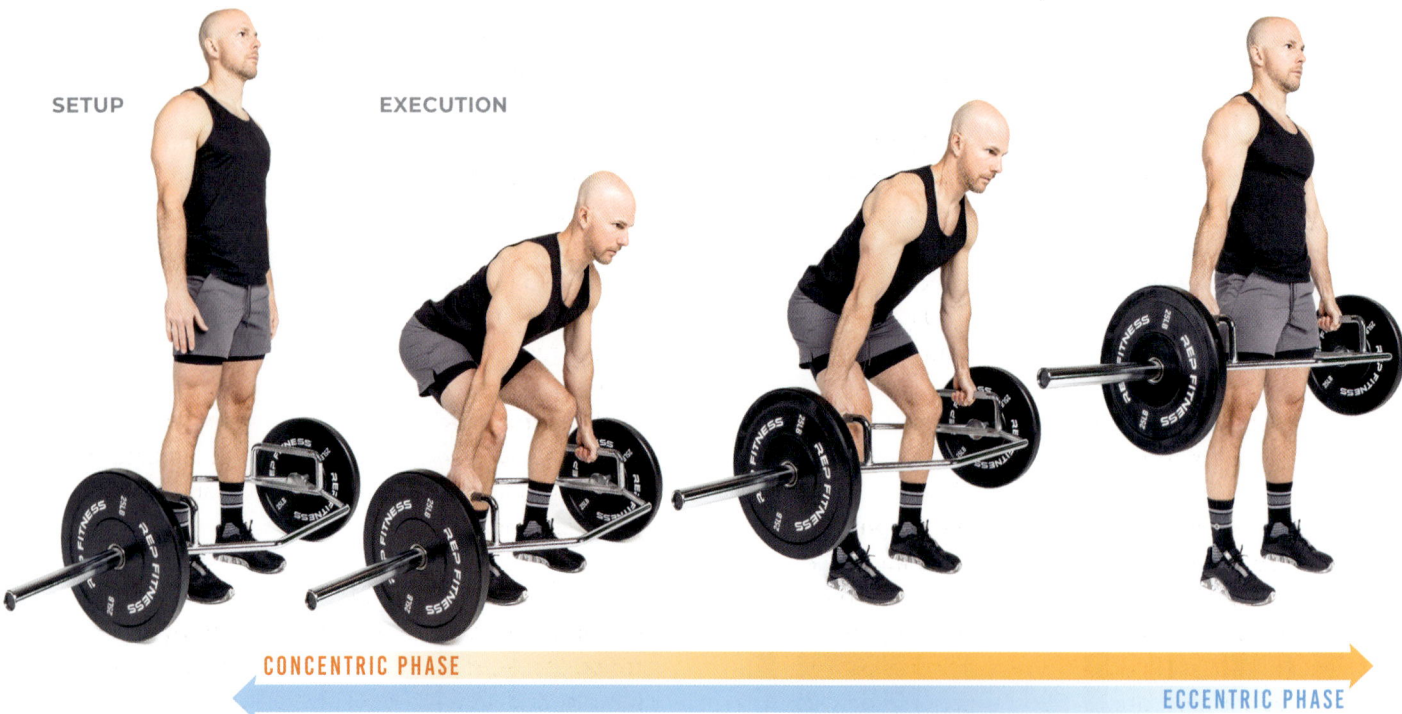

SETUP

EXECUTION

CONCENTRIC PHASE

ECCENTRIC PHASE

Before initiating the lift, take a deep diaphragmatic breath and brace your core. The slack in the bar should be minimal due to the lack of ball bearings in most trap bars, but you should still focus on maintaining tension through your body.

EXECUTION: Begin the lift by driving your hips up and forward, keeping your shins vertical and your knees stacked over your ankles. Focus on generating force through your hips while maintaining a neutral spine. The initial pull should be dynamic, transitioning into a strong, controlled lockout as your hips reach full extension. At the top, ensure your glutes are fully engaged, and avoid leaning back or hyperextending your spine.

On the descent, mirror the mechanics of an RDL by pushing your hips back and maintaining a neutral spine. Lower the bar in a controlled manner. Bring the bar to a complete stop on the ground, allowing for a momentary reset while maintaining full-body tension. Avoid bouncing the bar or sacrificing your brace at the bottom.

Between reps, re-engage your breath and brace before initiating the next pull. This ensures consistency in form and prevents unnecessary strain or loss of tension. Repeat for the desired number of reps, focusing on precise execution and maintaining alignment throughout.

CONVENTIONAL BARBELL DEADLIFT

The conventional barbell deadlift stands at the peak of the hinge progression pyramid, representing the most advanced and demanding variation in the hinge pattern. Its position at the top is earned by the complexity it introduces—requiring precision in bracing, exceptional motor control, and the ability to lift heavy loads from a pure hinge position. Unlike the trap bar deadlift, which centers the load over your base of support, the barbell deadlift places the weight anteriorly (in front of your center of mass). This creates significantly more torque on the spine and increases the demand on your posterior chain, including the hamstrings, glutes, and lower back.

This anterior loading, combined with the need to brace from a flexed position, makes the conventional deadlift a true test of strength, stability, and technical skill. For many lifters, adjustments such as elevating the bar with blocks or plates are necessary to align the lift with their authentic range of motion, as determined by the hinge assessment. When performed correctly, the barbell deadlift builds unparalleled strength and power, but its complexity demands attention to setup, load position, and execution to maximize performance and minimize the risk of potentially harmful compensations.

SETUP: Begin by adjusting the bar height to match your authentic range of motion, as determined in your hinge assessment. This might mean elevating the bar on blocks, plates, or power rack pins if the standard starting position feels inaccessible or causes compensations. Your feet should be placed in a power stance—hip-width apart, with toes pointed forward or slightly out, depending on your individual mechanics.

Position the barbell over your mid-foot, keeping your shins 2 to 3 inches away from the bar. This setup ensures a proper starting position where your hips, shoulders, and core can brace effectively.

Hinge down to the bar with a neutral spine, maintaining co-contraction of the shoulders, and hips as you lower yourself. Grip the bar with a double overhand grip or use lifting straps if grip strength is a limiting factor. Avoid a mixed grip, as it introduces asymmetries that can lead to biceps tears or imbalances.

LOAD POSITION: With the barbell in hand, create tension through your entire body by packing your shoulders, engaging your lats, and gripping the bar tightly. Your hands should be positioned just outside your knees at about a thumbs distance from your shins.

Your hips should drop slightly as you "wedge" into position, taking any slack out of the bar while maintaining alignment between your torso and shin angles. At this point, take a deep breath through your mouth, brace your core, and lock in your pillar for maximal stability.

EXECUTION: Begin the lift with an explosive concentric movement by driving through your tripod foot—pressing evenly through your heel, big toe, and little toe to create a stable base. This ensures balanced force production and prevents shifting weight excessively onto the heels or toes, which can compromise alignment and control. **As you drive upward, extend your hips while maintaining a neutral spine, keeping tension throughout your posterior chain.**

Focus on synchronizing your torso and shin angles to prevent your hips from rising too **quickly**—a common fault that shifts strain onto the lower back instead of distributing the load across your hips.

At the top, achieve full hip extension without overextending your lower back. Slightly squeeze your glutes to lock in the finish while keeping your rib cage stacked over your pelvis.

For the eccentric phase, lower the bar in a **controlled manner, keeping it close to your body to maintain tension and stability. Descend by hinging at the hips first, allowing your knees to bend naturally as needed.** Let the bar return to the ground with a slight reset between reps to reinforce proper bracing before initiating the next rep.

SETUP

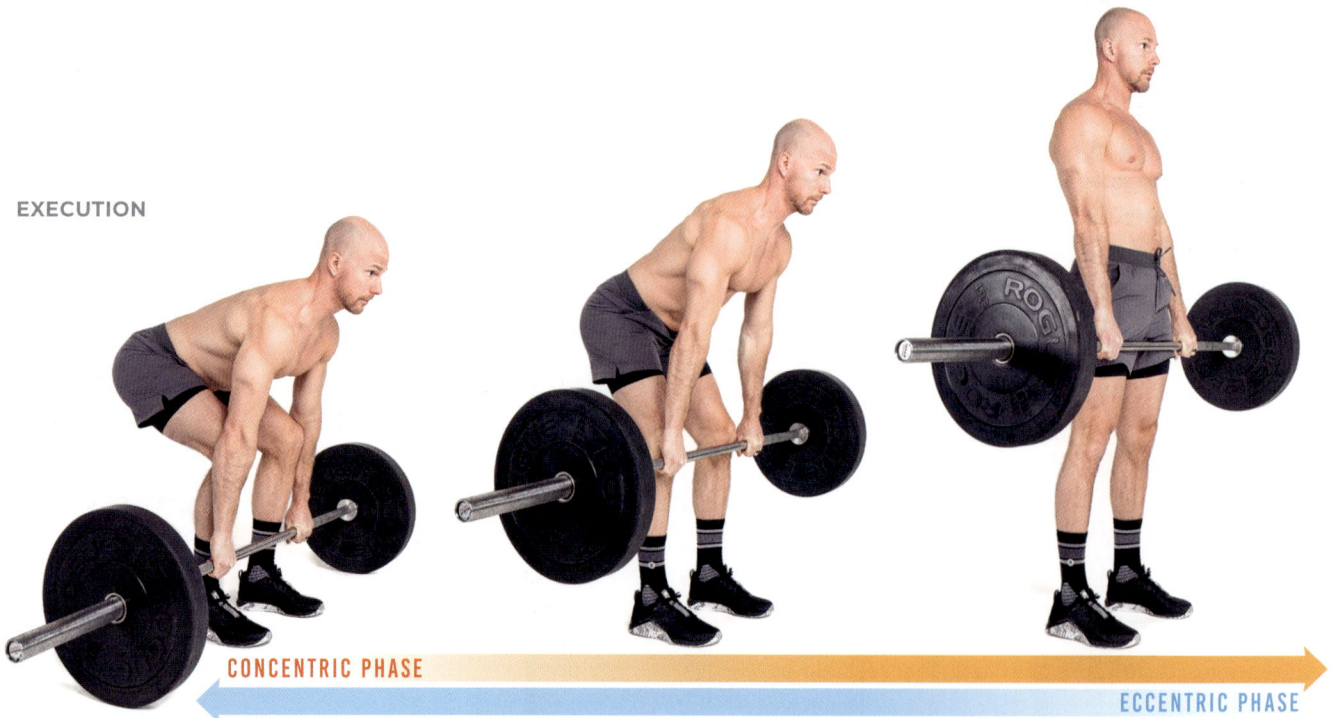

EXECUTION

CONCENTRIC PHASE

ECCENTRIC PHASE

GRIP CONSIDERATIONS

When performing the conventional barbell deadlift, grip considerations are vital for safety and performance. Lifting straps offer a practical and effective solution for grip fatigue, allowing you to focus on the movement pattern and maximize strength development. Avoid the mixed grip, as the risks far outweigh the benefits, especially if you're not a competitive power lifter. Instead, prioritize symmetrical grip options like the double overhand grip, hook grip, or straps to ensure proper mechanics and long-term success in your training.

LIFTING STRAPS

Lifting straps are a valuable tool for the conventional barbell deadlift, especially when grip strength becomes the limiting factor. The goal of the deadlift is to strengthen the hinge movement pattern and target the posterior chain, not to let grip fatigue dictate your performance. By using lifting straps, you remove grip as a limiting variable, allowing you to focus on maintaining proper form, building strength, and safely managing heavier loads.

When to Use Lifting Straps:

- **Grip Strength Limitation:** If your grip fails before your muscles do, straps help you continue training effectively.

- **Higher Volume or Maximal Lifts:** They're particularly useful in high-rep sets or when approaching maximal loads where grip fatigue becomes a significant factor.

- **Preventing Compensations:** Without straps, lifters may unintentionally alter their technique or adopt risky grip strategies, like a mixed grip, to compensate for grip limitations.

Caveats: While straps are excellent for prioritizing the hinge pattern, they should be used selectively. Grip strength is still an important aspect of overall performance and should not be ignored. Incorporate grip-focused exercises, like farmer's carries or double overhand deadlifts with lighter loads, into your training to ensure balanced development.

MIXED GRIP

A mixed grip involves placing one hand in an overhand position and the other in an underhand position while gripping the bar. While this technique can help lifters manage heavier loads by stabilizing the bar and preventing it from rolling, it comes with significant drawbacks and risks.

Drawbacks of the Mixed Grip:

- **Asymmetrical Forces:** The mixed grip inherently creates uneven tension in the shoulders, torso, and spine. This asymmetry can lead to imbalances, compensations, and increased risk of injury over time.

- **Biceps Tear Risk:** The underhand grip places the biceps tendon under significant strain, especially during maximal lifts. This increases the likelihood of biceps tears, which are a devastating and preventable injury.

- **Compromised Alignment:** Mixed grip often leads to subtle shifts in shoulder and hip positioning, compromising the lumbopelvic alignment needed for a strong, safe lift.

Alternatives to Mixed Grip:

- **Double Overhand Grip:** This grip promotes symmetry and is ideal for moderate weights or as a way to build grip strength.

- **Hook Grip:** Used by many competitive lifters, the hook grip locks the bar in place by trapping the thumb under the fingers, providing added stability without introducing asymmetry.

- **Lifting Straps:** As discussed, straps are a safer and more effective alternative for managing grip fatigue while maintaining alignment and reducing injury risk.

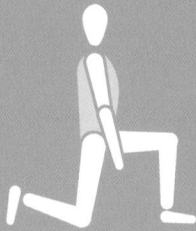

LUNGE

The lunge is one of the most overlooked and undertrained movement patterns. Despite its essential role in building strength and stability, many lifters neglect it—or avoid it entirely. But this oversight comes at a cost. The lunge includes nearly all single-leg and asymmetrical stance movements, making it crucial for correcting imbalances and enhancing athletic performance.
If your goal is to move better, feel stronger, and stay pain-free, training the lunge is non-negotiable.

When I arrived at the Olympic Training Center in China, I stepped into a world of raw power and precision. Around me were some of the strongest athletes on the planet—lifters who could launch hundreds of pounds overhead with effortless control, their technique refined through years of relentless practice. Their quads were the size of my torso, their strength unmatched. Watching them move the barbell with such mastery was awe-inspiring.

But that mastery was deceiving.

For all their dominance with a barbell, their training was laser-focused on perfecting a very specific set of movements. I wasn't there to teach them how to lift. That was their domain, their sport. My role was to address something they hadn't fully developed—something that, despite their extraordinary abilities, had been overlooked: functional training.

The term gets thrown around so often that its meaning can feel diluted. In this case, it meant identifying weaknesses that years of specialization had created. These lifters had mastered their sport-specific movements, but their training had left them with blind spots. To support their Olympic lifts, they needed more than just strength and power. They needed movement capacity—balance, stability, and control in novel positions.

The solution was deceptively simple: squat, hinge, lunge, push, pull, and carry. These foundational movement patterns are the backbone of all human motion, but I focused on one in particular—the lunge. More specifically, squatting and hinging from a split stance, using exercises that exposed their weaknesses in a way they weren't accustomed to.

Olympic lifters are no strangers to the split stance, particularly in the jerk, where they catch massive weights overhead. But that movement is explosive, brief, and supported by momentum. What they hadn't developed was the ability to generate and control strength through an extended range of motion in these positions—slowly, deliberately, and under sustained load.

That became clear the moment I introduced Bulgarian split squats. The protocol was straightforward—3 to 4 sets of 8 to 10 reps with 35-pound dumbbells. For athletes who had been squatting and cleaning for years, this should have been easy. It wasn't.

Their faces told the story: frustration, surprise, and the unmistakable strain of muscles being challenged in ways they hadn't experienced before. Their legs trembled, their balance wavered, and they fought for stability rep after rep.

I watched in disbelief. These were some of the strongest athletes in the world. But the moment they had to generate strength and stability from a staggered stance, everything changed. They weren't just weak in this position; they lacked the neuromuscular coordination to control it. Their strength wasn't translating. And that realization hit them just as hard as the exercise itself.

This wasn't a failure. It was an opportunity. The gap in their training had finally been exposed, and now we could do something about it.

Over the following weeks, the transformation was dramatic. Bulgarian split squats and unilateral exercises did more than build strength—they rewired movement patterns. By engaging glutes and adductors as stabilizers, they developed a new movement intelligence. Neuromuscular coordination improved, allowing them to resist knee valgus, maintain rotational control, and stabilize under asymmetrical loads.

The results went beyond traditional performance metrics. Reduced muscular strain, faster recovery, and more intentional movement became their new normal. What started as a simple intervention—introducing single-leg work—not only reconstructed their athletic foundation but also helped mitigate the risk of training injuries by addressing chronic sport-specific stress.

The experience in China stayed with me. It was a stark reminder that even at the highest level, specialization has consequences. These lifters had refined their technique to near perfection, but their reliance on symmetrical, bilateral barbell movements had created gaps in their movement capacity that single-leg training quickly brought to light—and corrected.

Years later, I saw the same issue play out in a completely different arena: powerlifting.

Olympic lifting is about explosive power and precision. Powerlifting, on the other hand, is pure brute strength—moving as much weight as possible in three lifts: the squat, the bench press, and the deadlift. The sport revolves around bilateral force production, pushing it to its absolute extreme. And while powerlifters and Olympic lifters may train differently, they often share the same blind spots.

That's how I found myself in Columbus, Ohio, working with Dave Tate—one of the most legendary figures in powerlifting. If the Olympic lifters had movement gaps, Dave's were even more entrenched. His life had been dedicated to powerlifting, and his body bore the marks of that devotion: hip replacements, back issues, shoulder pain, elbow problems.

When I started working with him, our goal wasn't to chase numbers. It was to rebuild—starting from the ground up. The first step was a movement pattern audit to assess his capacity outside the powerlifting framework.

His squatting? Still possible, but only to a box set at knee height to achieve parallel depth. Pushing? No problem—bench pressing was second nature. But pulling movements? Virtually nonexistent. Overhead work? Not even an option. And as for split-stance and single-leg training? I already knew what his response would be.

"What the fuck? I don't do that bullshit," he said, his tone a mix of disdain and disbelief.

Dave never sugarcoated anything. His bluntness and colorful language were as much a part of his persona as his superhuman strength.

"Exactly," I shot back, meeting him head-on. "That's why we're starting here. If you only train what you're good at, nothing changes."

In our first session, I introduced the simplest variation of a lunge pattern: split squats. Dave, a man who had squatted close to 1,000 pounds in competition, couldn't complete a single rep without assistance. His movements were unsteady, his coordination off, his frustration obvious.

"This fucking sucks," he muttered. "Twice as hard, half the weight, and humbling every single time."

That's the reality of single-leg training. It reveals every imbalance, every weakness, and every gap in coordination. Even as Dave progressed over the next few weeks—moving from assisted to unassisted split squats and eventually adding dumbbells— he started to grasp what I had been trying to show him. Strength isn't just about moving heavy weight. It's about mobility, stability, and skill.

And just when you think you've figured it out, single-leg training finds new ways to humble you. No matter how much you improve, these exercises continue to challenge you. And fundamentally, the movements that challenge you most are usually the ones you need most.

Whether you're chasing PRs, competing on the field, or simply trying to move better in everyday life, the payoff is undeniable. Functional training— true functional training—builds patterns and strength that align with how your body moves in the real world. This approach is critical because life rarely occurs in static, bilateral stances. Walking, running, and most dynamic athletic movements rely on split-stance or single-leg patterns. Yet many conventional training programs remain dominated by bilateral movements—a disconnect that frequently leads to chronic pain, compensatory movements, and increased injury risk.

The lunge pattern bridges this gap, offering benefits that extend far beyond the gym. Unlike heavy bilateral lifts, split-stance and single-leg exercises provide a strength and muscle-building stimulus without excessive loading, sparing your joints while still delivering impressive results.

Dave Tate said it best: "Twice as hard, half the weight, and humbling every single time."

Exactly what your body needs.

LUNGE SCREEN

The lunge pattern is divided into three progressive levels: the split squat, reverse lunge, and single-leg Romanian deadlift (RDL). Each level builds on the last, progressively reducing your base of support while increasing the demands on your mobility, stability, and motor control. These progressions are not just exercises—they're a systematic way to train the mechanics required to excel in split-stance and single-leg movements.

The lunge screen serves as a critical litmus test, offering insight into your entry point within this progression. It helps you identify weaknesses or imbalances, predict your ability to handle the demands of the lunge pattern, and assess your readiness for both starting-point strength and stimulatory load capacity. By using the screen to guide your training, you can ensure that your approach matches your current abilities, setting you up for safe and effective progress through increasingly complex movements.

LEVEL 01 SPLIT SQUAT

The split squat is the foundation of split-stance training, and it's all about control. With both feet grounded, you'll feel stable enough to focus on the basics: balancing your weight, stabilizing your hips, and keeping your pillar strong. Meeting the standards outlined in the optimization checklist at this level lays the foundation for progressing to the next stage, so don't rush it. After all, even the pros—Olympic lifters, powerlifters, and seasoned athletes—struggle here when they've neglected the lunge pattern.

SETUP: STANCE and BODY POSITION

1. **Start in Half Kneeling:** Place one knee on the ground with the opposite foot flat in front of you, forming a roughly 90-degree angle at both knees. Your front knee should align directly over your ankle, with your back knee directly beneath your hip. Maintain a vertical torso and ensure your hips are square.

2. **Foot Placement:**

- **Front Foot:** Flat on the ground, pointed straight, with weight evenly distributed across the tripod foot (heel, big toe, and little toe).

- **Back Foot:** Toes tucked under, creating tension through the big toe and arch to enhance irradiation.

3. **Stabilize the Pillar:** Create full-body tension by co-contracting your pecs and lats, locking your upper body into a stable position. Since the hands remain down by your sides, create irradiation through the fists while engaging the pecs and lats—this serves as the first line of tension in your pillar prep. Because this is a split stance, activation differs from bilateral squat and hinge patterns. Here, focus on a "scissoring" action between the glutes and adductors of both the front and back leg—squeezing inward to create stability from opposing positions. This deep co-contraction enhances lumbopelvic control and positioning, a key factor in maintaining alignment and force transfer. Root your feet into the ground by pressing down and flexing your toes, creating torque at the feet to further reinforce stability. Maintain an active, neutral spinal position throughout, ensuring your pillar remains strong and aligned.

4. Breathing and Bracing: Take a 360-degree breath to expand your diaphragm and brace your core as if preparing for a lift. This stabilizes your spine and pelvis before movement.

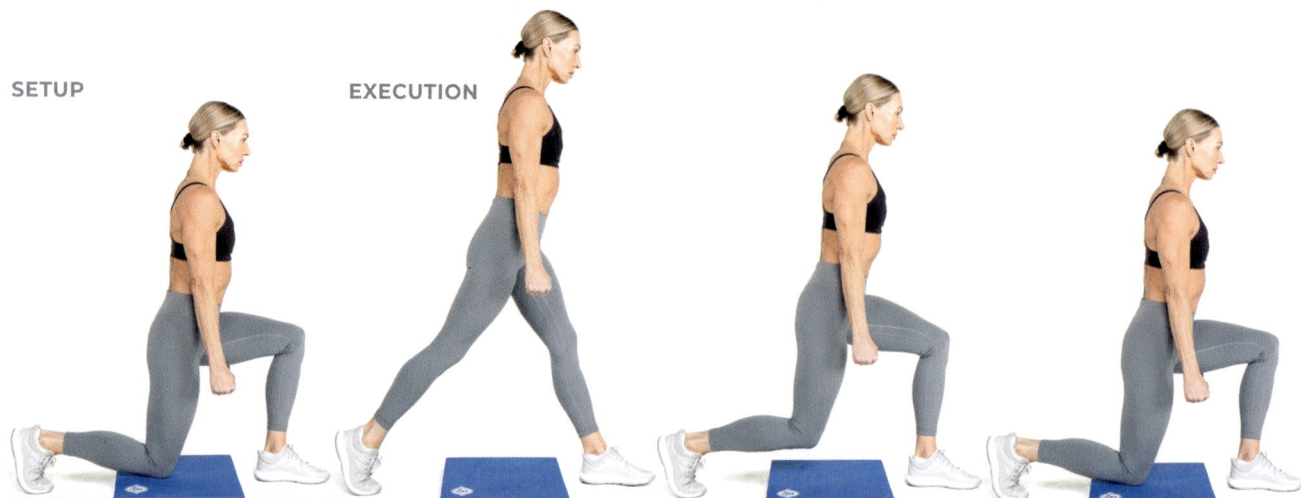

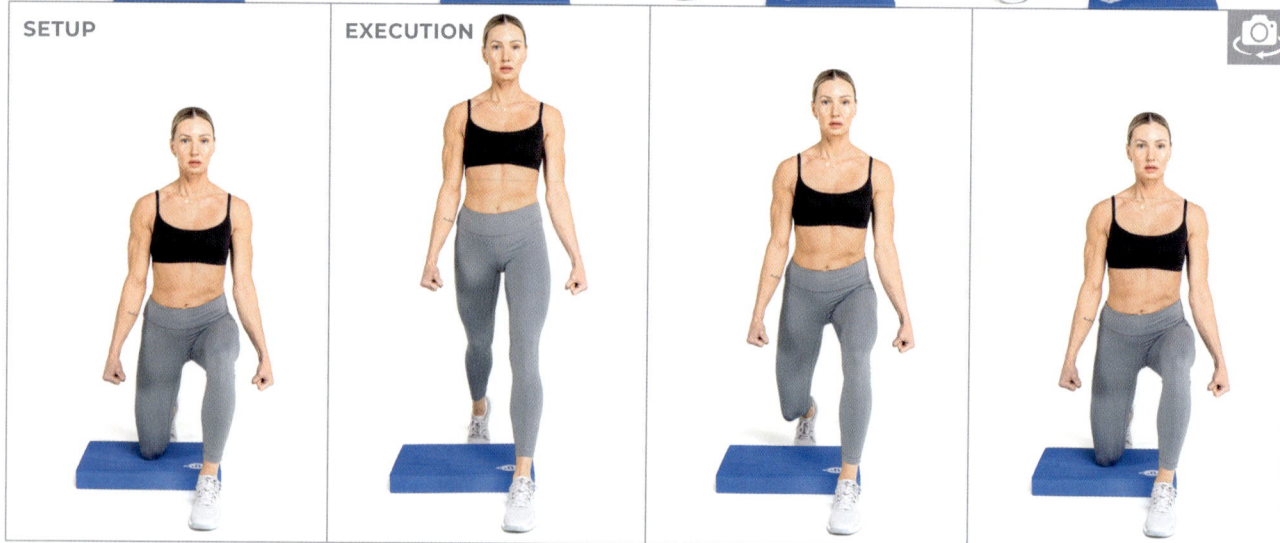

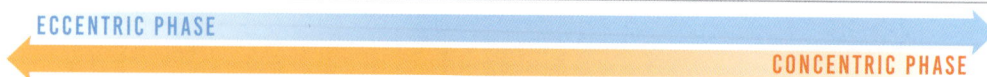

SETUP EXECUTION

SETUP EXECUTION

ECCENTRIC PHASE

CONCENTRIC PHASE

EXECUTION: PERFORMING THE SPLIT SQUAT

From the half-kneeling position, drive through your front foot to rise in the concentric phase, moving in a direct vertical line without any forward or backward deviation. Keep your torso upright, pillar engaged, and spine in a neutral position. As you extend your front leg, remember that not everyone can achieve full knee extension. Your priority should always be maintaining control and proper alignment as you transition from the ground to standing.

As you lower back into the eccentric phase, bend your front knee and allow your back knee to lightly touch the ground. Control the descent to maintain stability, avoiding any sudden shifts or loss of balance.

Focus on even weight distribution between your front and back legs, ensuring approximately 50/50 effort from both.

Throughout the exercise, maintain a strong foot and ankle position, and avoid any unwanted rotation at the ankles, knees, hips, or shoulders. Keep your torso angle consistent, and ensure your front knee tracks over your foot.

LEVEL 02 REVERSE LUNGE

The reverse lunge introduces dynamic movement into the lunge pattern, challenging your ability to decelerate with control. Your front leg bears most of the load, while the back leg contributes to balance and stability without driving the movement. This level builds on the stability developed in the split squat, paving the way for the heightened balance demands of the single-leg RDL.

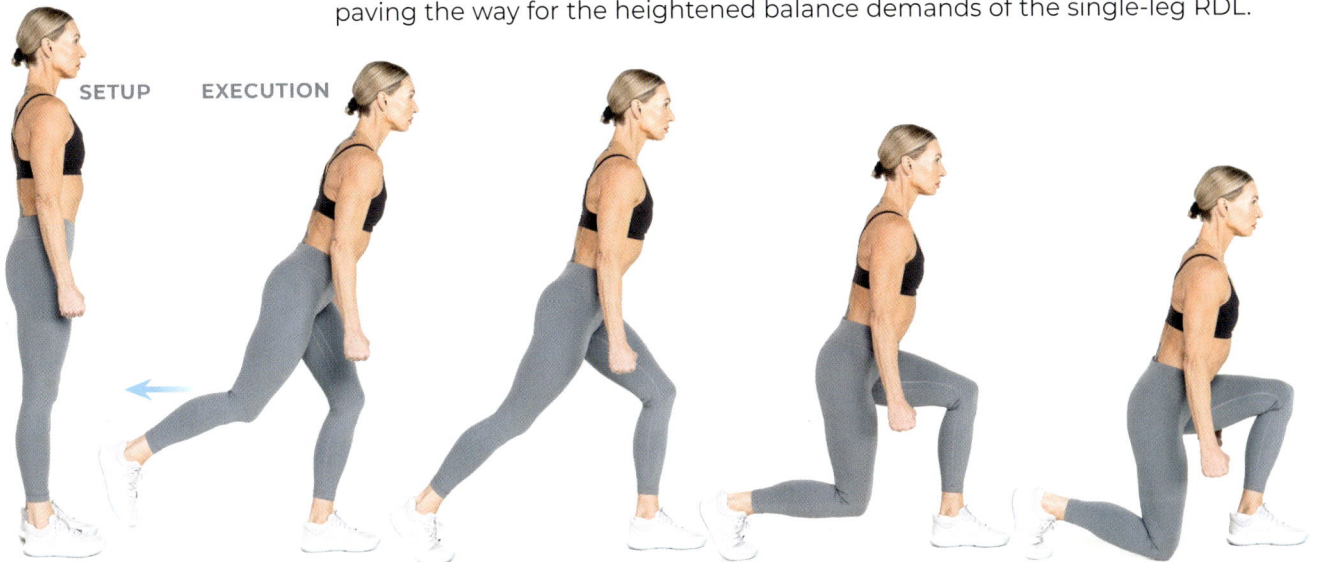

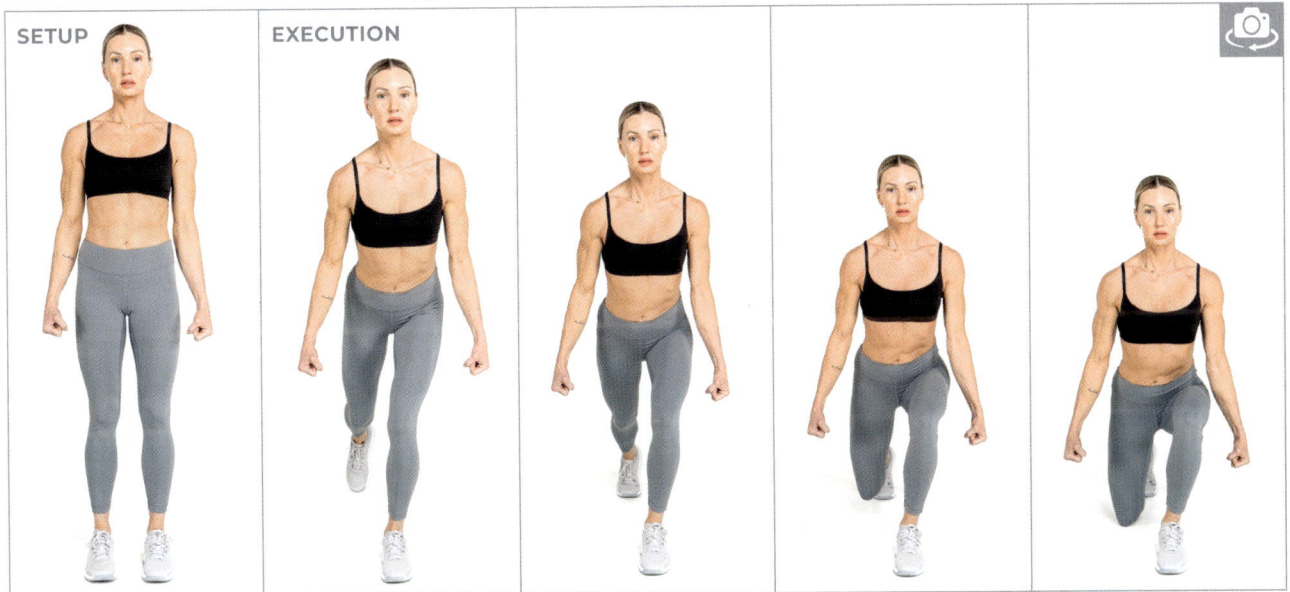

SETUP   EXECUTION

SETUP   EXECUTION

ECCENTRIC PHASE

CONCENTRIC PHASE

SETUP: STANCE and BODY POSITION

1. **Start in Standing Position:** Begin with your feet hip-width apart, toes pointing forward, and weight evenly distributed. This neutral stance sets the foundation for the movement.

2. **Stabilize the Pillar:** Brace your shoulders, hips, and core to create full-body tension while maintaining a neutral spinal position.

3. **Breathing and Bracing:** Take a deep 360-degree breath and brace your core before initiating the movement.

EXECUTION: PERFORMING THE REVERSE LUNGE

Step back with one leg while maintaining a neutral spine and avoiding any unwanted rotation at the ankles, knees, hips, or shoulders. Your back foot should land softly, ensuring your stride is neither too short nor too long.

Before lowering, take a quick moment to assess your alignment—your front foot should be firmly planted with your knee tracking over your toes, while your hips and spine remain neutral.

With control, begin descending into the lunge by bending both knees and allowing your back knee to move toward the floor in a deliberate, even motion. The front leg should bear 70 to 75 percent of the load, with the back leg offering the remaining support. Focus on stability rather than speed.

At the bottom of the movement—when your back knee hovers just above the floor or lightly taps a pad—pause momentarily. This brief moment of stillness reinforces balance and ensures full engagement of the stabilizing muscles before you initiate the ascent.

To return to the starting position, push off the ground with your back toes while driving through your front foot. This combined effort between the front and back legs promotes proper mechanics and alignment as you rise.

LEVEL 03 SINGLE-LEG RDL

The single-leg RDL represents the pinnacle of single-leg training, unlocking the highest level of single-leg strength, balance, and control—an essential foundation for efficient, pain-free movement.

However, many people struggle with this exercise, often attributing their difficulty to a "lack of balance." In reality, balance is a trainable skill, and you can build toward the single-leg RDL by strengthening the same movement pattern in a more stable position. If you aren't yet able to perform this movement with control, you can still develop a well-rounded, effective training program by focusing on split squats, lunges, and bilateral or kickstand hinge variations (you'll learn the kickstand RDL, which serves as a progression for the single-leg RDL, in the lunge pyramid on page 315).

SETUP: STANCE and BODY POSITION

1. **Start in a Kickstand Position:** Begin with your front foot firmly planted and your back foot lightly touching the ground, toes down for balance. This creates stability and prepares you for the single-leg phase.

2. **Foot Placement:** Focus on your tripod foot, actively pressing into the ground with equal pressure through the heel, big toe, and little toe. This is your primary base of support.

3. **Stabilize the Pillar:** Brace your core, engage your lats, and align your hips and spine in a neutral position.

4. **Breathing and Bracing:** Take a deep diaphragmatic breath and brace your core. This step is critical for maintaining stability during the movement.

EXECUTION: PERFORMING THE SINGLE-LEG RDL

Shift your weight fully onto your front leg, lifting the back leg into the single-leg position. Maintain a slight bend in the front knee to activate the hamstrings and stabilize the pelvis. Ensure your spine remains neutral, with no unwanted rotation at the ankles, knees, hips, or shoulders. Keep your front foot firmly grounded in a tripod position to provide stability and prevent compensations.

Initiate the movement by hinging at the hips, sending them back while keeping your shin angle somewhat vertical with minimal forward knee movement. As you hinge forward, bend your back leg to approximately 90 degrees. This engages the hamstring of the back leg, making it easier to stabilize the pelvis and maintain proper alignment.

As your back leg extends behind you with the knee bent, lower your torso while maintaining a neutral spine and square hips. Avoid twisting or compensating with your lower back.

Keep your arms close to your body and reach your palm toward your front foot as far as your mobility allows, ensuring your shoulders remain stable and do not round.

Reverse the motion by driving your hips forward, returning to the standing position while keeping your back foot off the ground between reps.

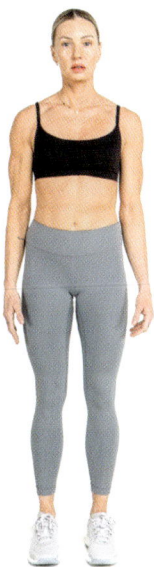

SETUP

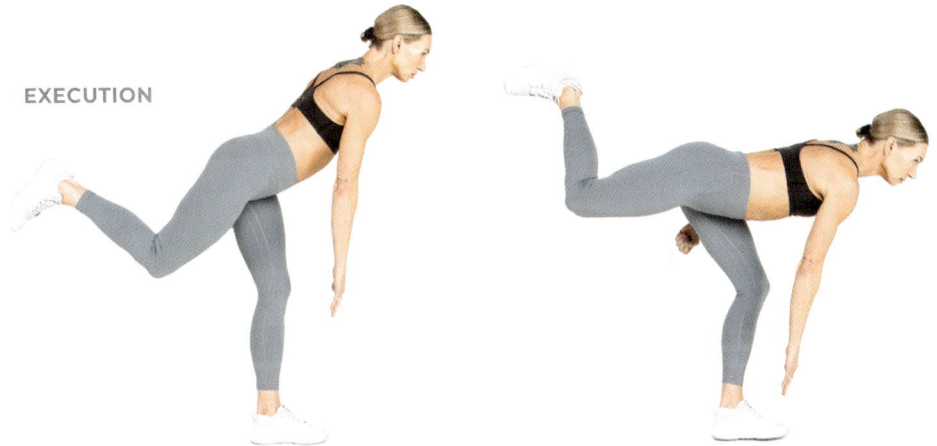

EXECUTION

SETUP

EXECUTION

ECCENTRIC PHASE

CONCENTRIC PHASE

OPTIMIZATION CHECKLIST

This checklist helps you screen your form and identify areas for improvement at every level of the lunge pattern. Start by recording yourself performing the split squat, reverse lunge, and single-leg RDL from both front and side angles. Use these recordings to evaluate your alignment, balance, and control, comparing your performance against the checklist standards.

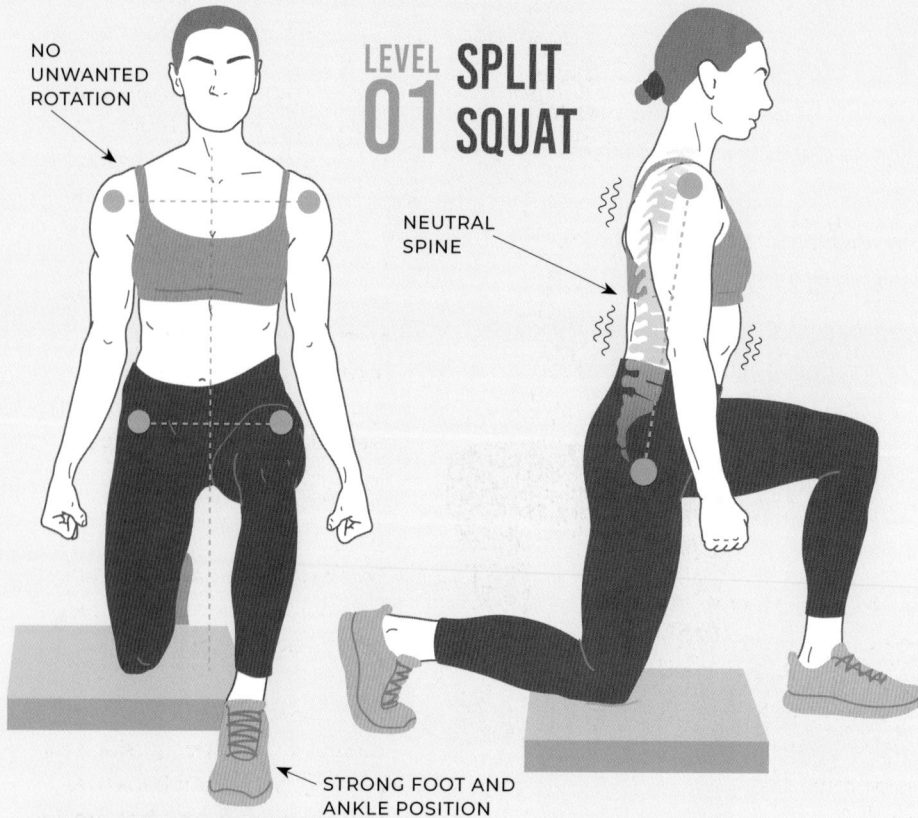

LEVEL 01 SPLIT SQUAT

NO UNWANTED ROTATION

NEUTRAL SPINE

STRONG FOOT AND ANKLE POSITION

✓ **NO UNWANTED ROTATION**

Unwanted rotation in the split squat often occurs when one leg compensates for the other, leading to misalignments through the hips or shoulders. By keeping your body symmetrical and aligned, you ensure both legs work evenly, improving stability and efficiency.

✓ **STRONG FOOT AND ANKLE POSITION**

In the split squat, a strong foot and ankle position provide the foundation for balance and control. Distribute your weight evenly across your front foot's tripod (heel, big toe, and little toe) and engage your back foot by pushing up onto the ball of your foot and to stabilize your rear leg. This balanced positioning helps you maintain alignment and stability throughout the movement.

✓ **NEUTRAL SPINE**

Maintaining a neutral spine during the split squat ensures that your torso stays upright and stable throughout the movement. The goal is to avoid excessive arching or rounding, which can compromise alignment and shift the load away from the legs. By bracing your pillar and keeping your spine neutral, you promote proper force transfer between your lower body and the ground, supporting stability and control.

LEVEL 03 SINGLE-LEG RDL

✓ **NEUTRAL SPINE**

A neutral spine is critical in the single-leg RDL to maintain balance and prevent compensations during the hinge. Any spinal rounding or excessive knee bend increases the risk of instability and shifts the load to your lower back.

✓ **NO UNWANTED ROTATION**

The single-leg RDL tests your ability to resist rotation while balancing on one leg. Any twisting through the hips or shoulders disrupts form and can lead to instability. Keeping your pelvis level and your shoulders square ensures symmetry, promoting balance and optimal force transfer.

✓ **STRONG FOOT AND ANKLE POSITION**

The single-leg RDL relies heavily on a strong foot and ankle position, as your foot is your sole point of contact with the ground. Press evenly through the tripod of your foot to create stability and prevent compensations up the chain. Maintaining active engagement through the ankle ensures balance, allowing your hips and posterior chain to drive the movement.

LEVEL 02 REVERSE LUNGE

✓ NEUTRAL SPINE

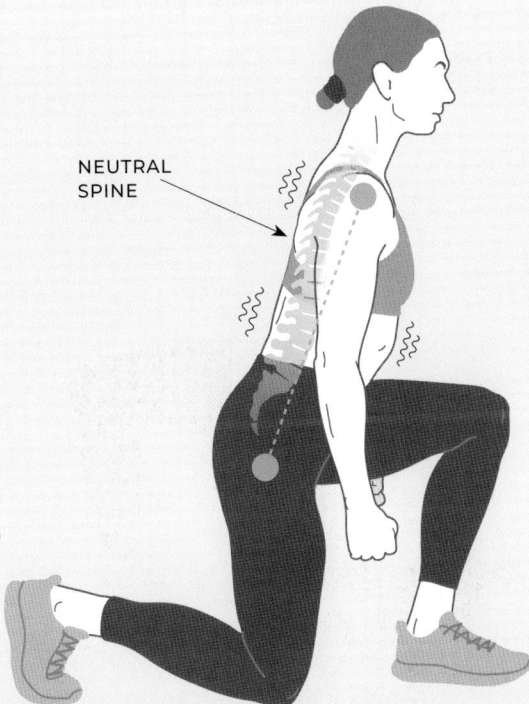

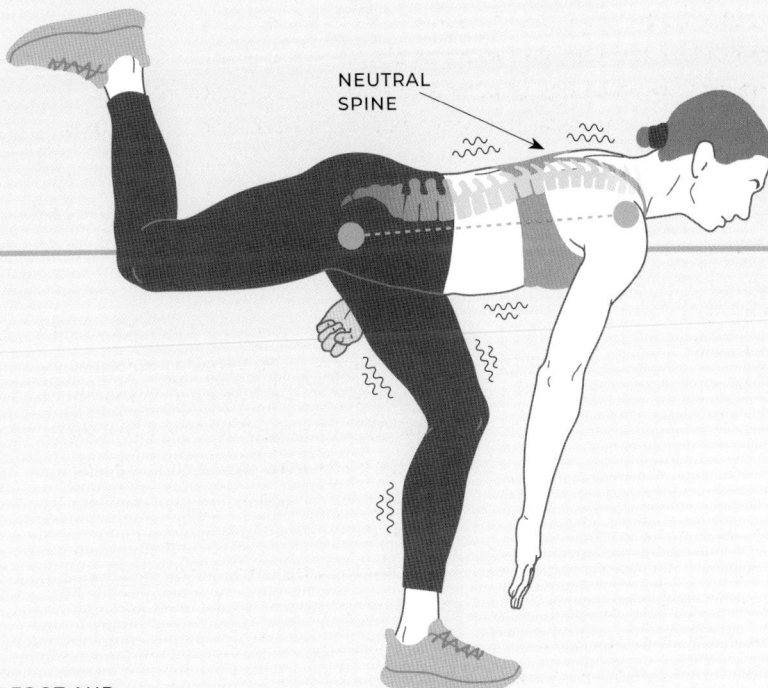

In the reverse lunge, a neutral spine helps manage the dynamic transition between standing and the lunge position. As you step back, maintaining spinal alignment within your neutral zone prevents unnecessary strain on your lower back and ensures the work stays in your legs. Proper bracing and pillar engagement are key to keeping your torso steady as you lower and rise.

NO UNWANTED ROTATION

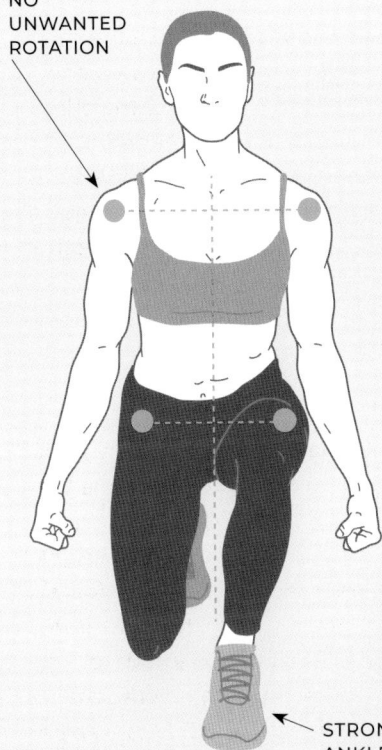

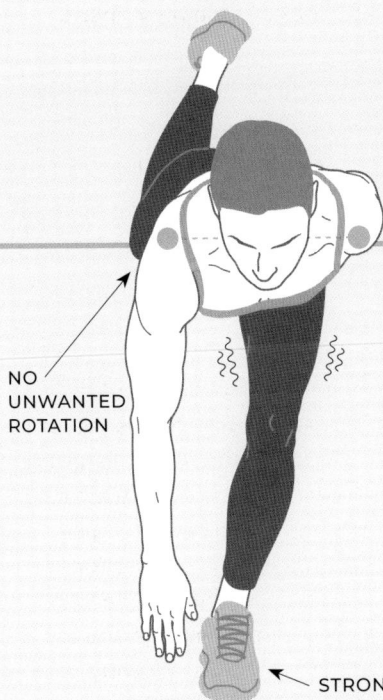

NEUTRAL SPINE

STRONG FOOT AND ANKLE POSITION

✓ NO UNWANTED ROTATION

In the reverse lunge, resisting unwanted rotation is even more important due to the added movement. As you step back, maintain alignment through your ankles, knees, hips, and shoulders to prevent one side from dominating. Proper symmetry ensures efficient movement and stability as you transition between positions.

✓ STRONG FOOT AND ANKLE POSITION

Foot and ankle positioning in the reverse lunge are crucial for managing the dynamic nature of the movement. Your front foot should remain firmly rooted in the tripod position for stability, while your back toes and ball of your rear foot provide support and balance during the lunge.

NO UNWANTED ROTATION

NEUTRAL SPINE

STRONG FOOT AND ANKLE POSITION

LUNGE ASSESSMENT

The lunge is one of the most versatile and functional movement patterns, blending the knee-dominant strength of the squat with the hip-dominant power of the hinge. It's a unique hybrid that challenges your ability to balance stability and dynamic control—all while working in split-stance or single-leg positions that mimic how we move in sport and life.

But let's be honest: lunges often get a bad rap because they're hard, humbling, and for many, downright painful—especially for the knees. Whether it's questions like "Should my knee go past my toes?" or "Why do my knees hurt when I lunge?" these concerns come up constantly. Most of the time, the problem isn't the lunge itself—it's how it's performed. Poor alignment, misunderstood mechanics, and a lack of personalization are often the culprits.

Enter the lunge assessment. It's designed to cut through the confusion and help you lunge in a way that aligns with your unique anthropometry—the individual proportions of your limbs and joints. By focusing on proper knee positioning and mechanics, the assessment addresses common pain points and ensures you're maximizing the benefits of this foundational movement pattern.

THE TF RATIO HIP FLEXION TEST— DETERMINING YOUR AUTHENTIC KNEE and TORSO ANGLE

The TF Ratio Hip Flexion Test is a cornerstone of the lunge assessment, offering an essential way to customize split-stance and single-leg patterns by analyzing the relationship between your tibia (shinbone) and femur (thighbone) lengths. These proportions are critical for tailoring lunge mechanics to your unique skeletal structure, helping to mitigate common issues such as knee pain or hip discomfort.

Why does this matter? If lunges feel awkward or leave you with sore knees, it might stem from a stance misaligned with your skeletal proportions. The TF Ratio Hip Flexion Test evaluates the relative lengths of your tibia (T) and femur (F) and compares them to a normalized ratio of 0.8—where the tibia is 20 percent shorter than the femur. While research indicates that deviations from this ratio correlate with an increased risk of knee arthritis, patellofemoral pain syndrome (front knee pain),[1] and hip impingement, it does not explain why. This is where the TF Ratio Hip Flexion Test factors in.

Your limb lengths are a fixed, unchangeable variable, but your lunge mechanics are not. By identifying your ratio and adjusting your movement patterns accordingly, you can train more intelligently to avoid discomfort and injury.

For example:

- **If your tibia is longer than your femur (ratio greater than 0.8),** lunges will naturally shift more stress onto your knee, especially when your knee moves forward excessively. Without proper alignment adjustments, you're likely to experience increased knee discomfort or pain. Reducing forward knee travel and adjusting your stance can help redistribute stress and minimize strain.

- **If your tibia is shorter than your femur (ratio less than 0.8),** you'll likely need to allow more forward knee travel and adopt a greater torso lean to maintain proper form. If you don't make these adjustments, you risk increasing strain on your hips or lower back. Balancing knee- and hip-dominant movements to match your proportions is crucial for comfort and optimal mechanics.

These real-world examples illustrate how understanding your unique TF ratio allows you to customize lunge patterns for optimal performance and pain-free movement. Rather than comparing tibia and femur lengths as equals, the focus is on how different they are and what those differences mean for your mechanics.

By combining your tibia-to-femur ratio with an isolated hip flexion range-of-motion test, this assessment creates a personalized blueprint for optimizing your lunge technique. **The tibia-to-femur ratio determines knee tracking relative to your toes, while the hip flexion test identifies the ideal angle of your torso.** Together, these tests provide a hybridized lunge pattern designed to maximize muscular recruitment, strength, and stability, tailored to your unique structure.

NOTE: *This test applies to all split-stance and single-leg movements, including split squats, reverse lunges, and single-leg RDLs, and all progressions and variations within each level.*

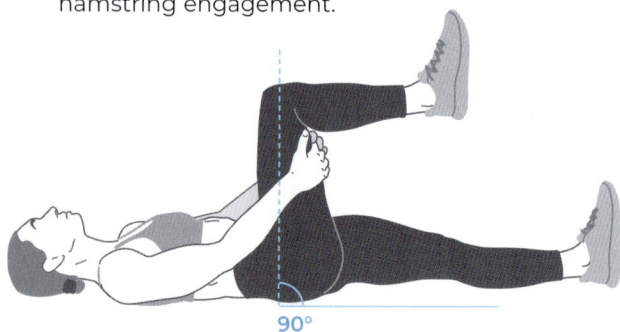

GREATER TROCHANTER

FEMUR

LATERAL CONDYLE

TIBIAL TUBEROSITY

TIBIA

ANKLE CREASE

STEP 1: MEASURE TIBIA AND FEMUR LENGTHS

▶ **Action:** Measure the length of your tibia and femur to calculate your tibia-to-femur ratio.

1. **Measure the Tibia (T):** Locate the tibial tuberosity (bony prominence below the kneecap) and measure to the ankle crease where the tibia meets the foot.

2. **Measure the Femur (F):** Identify the greater trochanter (bony prominence on the side of your hip) and measure to the lateral condyle (bony prominence on the outer side of the knee).

3. **Calculate the Ratio:** Divide the tibia length (T) by the femur length (F). For example, if the tibia measures 16 inches and the femur measures 20 inches:

TIBIA-TO-FEMUR RATIO = T ÷ F
16 ÷ 20 = 0.8

▶ **Goal:** Determine your tibia-to-femur ratio to understand how your skeletal proportions influence knee and torso angles during lunges.

▶ **Observation:**

· **A ratio of 0.8** places you in the middle of the anatomical spectrum, balancing between an upright posture with minimal knee travel and a forward knee position with pronounced torso lean.

· **Ratios above 0.8** indicate a longer tibia relative to the femur, which may require a more upright torso and limited forward knee movement.

· **Ratios below 0.8** indicate a shorter tibia relative to the femur, allowing for greater forward knee movement and more torso lean.

STEP 2: ASSESS HIP FLEXION RANGE

▶ **Action:** Lie on your back with your legs extended. Slowly bring one knee toward your chest, keeping the opposite leg straight. Continue raising your thigh toward your torso until you feel a block, pinch, discomfort, or notice compensations such as your pelvis tilting.

▶ **Goal:** Mentally and visually note your maximal hip flexion range to determine how much forward lean your torso can accommodate during lunge movements. For example, if your thigh stops at 90 degrees of flexion (perpendicular to the floor), your torso will need to remain more upright to stay aligned. In contrast, if your thigh moves closer to 140 degrees, your torso can lean forward more naturally, allowing for greater glute and hamstring engagement.

▶ **Observation:**

• **90 degrees of hip flexion:** Limited range of motion means your thigh is more vertical relative to your torso. To maintain alignment, your torso should remain upright, as leaning too far forward may cause compensation or strain in the hips and lower back.

• **140 degrees of hip flexion:** Greater range allows your thigh to approach your torso. This increased angle supports a more forward torso lean, enabling you to maximize glute and hamstring recruitment while maintaining alignment and stability.

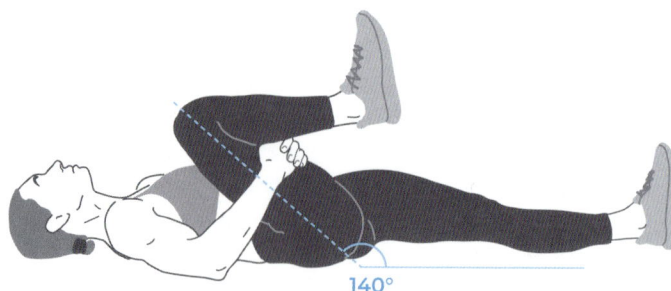

90°

140°

STEP 3: COMBINE DATA TO ESTABLISH YOUR MIDLINE POSITION

▶ **Action:** Use your tibia-to-femur ratio and hip flexion findings to establish your optimal alignment for split-stance and single-leg movements.

▶ **Goal:** Develop a personalized midline position that balances knee-dominant and hip-dominant mechanics, ensuring pain-free and efficient movement.

▶ **Observation:** Use a mirror or video to confirm your knee, shin, and torso angles align with the optimal position for your unique proportions. This combination—proper knee-over-toe tracking and torso alignment—maximizes muscular recruitment, strength, and stability, ensuring the movement feels controlled and pain-free.

Normal Ratio (0.8): Position the knee slightly over the toes with a slight forward torso lean, balancing knee and hip mechanics.

Ratios Above 0.8 (Longer Tibia): Maintain a more upright torso and limit forward knee movement to reduce stress on the knee joint.

Ratios Below 0.8 (Shorter Tibia): Allow the knees to move farther forward and the torso to lean more to avoid excessive hip and lower back strain.

STEP 4: ADJUST AND RETEST

▶ **Action:** Perform the lunge screen with the variation most appropriate for your current level: split squat, reverse lunge, or single-leg RDL. Execute several repetitions while making small adjustments to your knee and torso angles based on your personalized midline position from the assessment.

• **For the split squat and reverse lunge**, focus on maintaining the authentic biomechanical positions determined by your tibia-to-femur ratio and hip flexion test. These factors determine the ideal balance between knee tracking and torso lean, ensuring proper joint alignment and maximal muscular recruitment. This "hybrid" position—allowing for as much natural forward torso angle and knee travel as your structure permits—is key to achieving maximal stability, joint centration, and efficient force production. Simply put, **your strongest position is your most stable position**.

• **For the single-leg RDL**, expect a more knee-dominant position, with your knee naturally moving farther over your toes while maintaining a strong hinge pattern. This adjustment allows for optimal muscular recruitment and control during the more dynamic demands of this variation.

• Make these refinements gradually, ensuring each repetition feels strong, stable, and aligned with your unique structure.

▶ **Goal:** Successfully meet the standards outlined in the optimization checklist for each level. Retest the screen in phase 5 to confirm progress.

▶ **Observation:** If you struggle to meet any of the standards due to limitations in mobility, stability, or skill, incorporate targeted optimization strategies to address the issue.

OPTIMIZATION STRATEGIES

The optimization strategies are designed to help you address compensations identified in step four of the assessment. These compensations often arise from three key areas: mobility (limited range of motion or control), stability (challenges with balance or alignment), and skill (difficulty coordinating the movement).

It's important to understand that these compensations don't mean you should avoid or stop training the lunge pattern but rather highlight areas where your movement can be refined for greater efficiency and control. For some, these deviations might feel natural and pose no immediate issues, while others may find them limiting or uncomfortable. The goal is not to strive for perfection but to identify and polish the patterns that best support your individual needs and goals.

With that in mind, let's dive into the most common challenges in the lunge pattern and explore how targeted optimization strategies can help you move more efficiently and confidently.

NOTE: *Many of the compensations in the lunge pattern originate from the same underlying issues identified in the squat and hinge. If you encounter a compensation not listed here, revisit those sections for further guidance. Improving foundational squat and hinge mechanics often enhances your lunge performance, as common linchpins frequently affect multiple patterns. Recognizing these recurring limitations simplifies your corrective approach, since the strategies follow a similar framework.*

COMPENSATION: FORWARD ROUNDING OF THE UPPER BACK

MOBILITY: Tight pecs and upper traps are common culprits behind forward rounding of the upper back. This issue can be exacerbated by poor posture or an overemphasis on pushing exercises without balancing pulling movements. Indicators of limited mobility include

▼ Difficulty maintaining an upright torso in a split squat or lunge without collapsing forward

▼ Tightness or pulling sensations in the chest and shoulders when attempting to extend the upper back

OPTIMIZATION STRATEGIES:

▶ Refer to the **T-Spine Mobility Linchpin Blueprint** (page 471) for exercises to improve thoracic extension and shoulder mobility.

▶ Use goblet or front rack positions to encourage an upright posture— avoid holding dumbbells at your sides, as this can reinforce forward rounding.

▶ Incorporate pulling exercises (e.g., rows, face pulls) into your programming to counteract tightness from pushing movements.

▶ Prioritize the 90/90 chest stretch to open the pecs and improve posture.

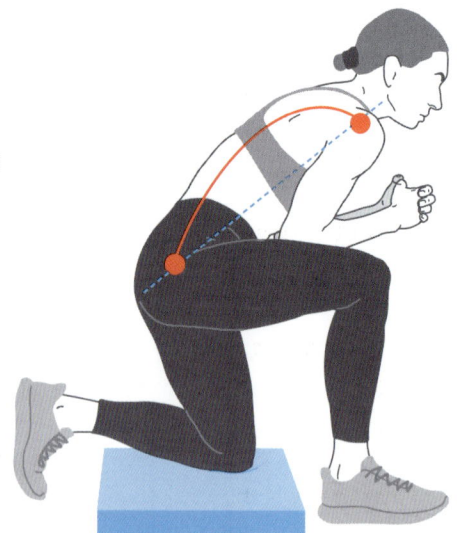

LEVEL 1

SKILL: Rounding in the upper back during lunges often results from a lack of body awareness or insufficient training. When mobility and stability are not limiting factors, this compensation is likely due to poor movement patterns. Signs of a skill gap include

▼ Losing upper body posture as you descend into a split squat or lunge

▼ Looking down at the floor during split squats and lunges, leading to a flexed upper back and neck position

▼ Struggling to maintain a neutral pillar and shoulder position, particularly under load or when fatigued

OPTIMIZATION STRATEGIES:

▶ Start at the bottom of the **Lunge Progression Pyramid** (page 315) with split squats and reverse lunges, only adding variations once you meet the standards in the optimization checklist.

▶ Refer to the cueing sequence in the Pillar chapter (page 34) to improve bracing setup and execution.

STABILITY: Poor pillar stability often stems from prolonged seated or rounded-forward postures, as well as insufficient training of the muscles responsible for deep core function, spinal extension, and shoulder external rotation. Challenges associated with poor stability may present as

▼ Discomfort in the neck or upper back when trying to extend the spine and "get tall" or pull the shoulders back

▼ Difficulty engaging the core or feeling tension in the lats

▼ Inability to establish intra-abdominal pressure to support an upright posture

OPTIMIZATION STRATEGIES:

▶ Refer to the **Core Stability A (Supine) Linchpin Blueprint** (page 472) for targeted exercises to improve core function and posture.

▶ Use a suspension trainer to allow your arms to assist in pulling you into a more upright position. Avoid holding dumbbells at your sides, as this can reinforce forward rounding.

▶ Incorporate pulling exercises into your programming to offset forward rounding.

▶ Use recovery stretches such as child's pose and 90/90 pec stretch to improve mobility and posture.

LEVEL 2

LEVEL 3

COMPENSATION: LUMBAR HYPEREXTENSION WITH ANTERIOR PELVIC TILT

MOBILITY: Tight hip flexors and quads, often caused by prolonged sitting or specific postures (e.g., standing with locked knees and an arched back), pull the pelvis into an anterior tilt. This is typically paired with a poorly braced pillar. Mobility restrictions may present as

▼ Anterior pelvic tilt, causing an overly extended lower back curve

▼ Standing upright feels tight in your lower back, or you experience an intense stretch in the back-leg hip flexor/quad when lowering into a split squat or lunge

OPTIMIZATION STRATEGIES:

▶ Refer to the **Hip Mobility A Linchpin Blueprint** (page 469) for targeted mobility exercises.

▶ Reduce the depth of lunge pattern exercises to ensure proper form:

• **Split squats & lunges:** Using pads or yoga blocks under your back knee can help manage depth.

• **Single-leg RDL:** Stop with your hands above or in line with your knee rather than chasing mid-shin or below.

▶ Strengthen the glutes and hamstrings with supine hip hinges (glute bridges, hip thrusts) and anterior-loaded good mornings, emphasizing neutral spine alignment.

▶ Add recovery stretches such as the prone quad stretch and half-kneeling hip flexor stretch to lengthen tight hip flexors and quads, and child's pose or a supine twist to alleviate lower back tightness.

LEVEL 3

LEVEL 1

LEVEL 2

SKILL: A lack of motor control or proper sequencing often exacerbates compensations, leading to difficulty maintaining a neutral spine and effective bracing throughout movement. Signs of a skill gap include

▼ Overcompensation into lumbar extension at the top of split squats or lunges

▼ Loss of balance or a lack of smooth motion (jerkiness, especially in the descent), exacerbated under load or fatigue

OPTIMIZATION STRATEGIES:

▶ Ensure proper setup: maintain a neutral pelvis, stack ribs over hips, and breathe 360 degrees into your torso. Placing your hands on your waist can provide feedback.

▶ Practice Reactive Neuromuscular Training (RNT) using a long resistance band (light):

• **Split squats & lunges:** Step your front leg into the loop so the band is positioned outside your knee. This reinforces abduction, increasing hip stability and glute activation during the movement.

• **Hinge progression:** Step both feet into the loop and face away from the anchor point to perform a hip-banded hinge. This is a great way to build the hinge pattern from a two-foot stance before progressing to a 1.5 stance hinge, moving toward a successful single-leg RDL.

▶ Refer to the Pillar chapter for detailed cueing techniques to establish and maintain neutral spinal alignment.

OPTIMIZATION STRATEGIES:

▶ Refer to the **Core Stability A (Supine) Linchpin Blueprint** (page 472).

▶ Practice the **Prone Breath Corrective** (page 46) to establish proper diaphragmatic breathing.

▶ Start with supported variations using a suspension trainer or holding onto a stable surface to focus on posture and bracing.

• **Split squats & reverse lunges:** If the suspension trainer variation feels too easy, progress to loaded variations in the goblet position to increase anterior core activation.

• **Single-leg RDL:** Use a suspension trainer while keeping your arms straight and reaching forward as you push your hips back. Alternatively, touch your hands down to a bench or box at the bottom of the rep, or use a wall or rack for support.

▶ Add stability-focused exercises such as glute bridges, hip thrusts, and anterior-loaded good mornings to reinforce a stable and neutral spine. These will help you progress toward more hinge variations, including the single-leg RDL.

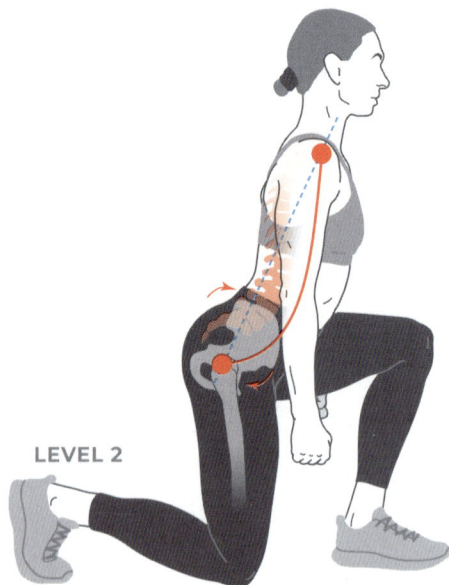

STABILITY: Insufficient pillar stability often leads to compensations like anterior pelvic tilt. A lack of diaphragmatic breathing and bracing results in over-reliance on the lower back for support, which can contribute to low back pain. Indicators of instability include

▼ Difficulty maintaining a neutral pelvis when standing, sitting, or performing lunge variations

▼ Increased spinal movement (extension and flexion), exacerbated under speed or load

COMPENSATION: FORWARD KNEE MOVEMENT / HEEL LIFT

MOBILITY: Tight, short, or restricted plantar fascial tissues and/or calves are common issues that can lead to a heel lift when the knee travels forward. This can be exacerbated by a weak arch, improper footwear, or repetitive movement without appropriate mobility and recovery. Mobility restrictions may present as

▼ Difficulty achieving adequate dorsiflexion without collapsing the arch or rotating the knee inward

▼ A feeling of tightness in the ankle or back of the lower limb when walking, bending the knees forward, or climbing stairs

OPTIMIZATION STRATEGIES:

▶ Refer to the **Ankle Mobility Linchpin Blueprint** (page 468) for solutions to improve ankle dorsiflexion and lower limb mobility.

▶ Use a suspension trainer or a supported hand position to help maintain your center of mass between both feet (rather than shifting forward over the front foot).

▶ Perform split squats and lunges with a focus on maintaining a vertical shin, ensuring the knee stays stacked over the ankle of the front leg—unless this causes pain, in which case, use the angle recommended by your TF ratio.

STABILITY: A lack of stability in the arch, hip, or core can result in unbalanced body weight and compensations while performing split squats and lunges. Signs of instability include

▼ Difficulty setting and maintaining full foot contact (tripod stance: big toe, little toe, and heel)

▼ Inability to maintain a strong foot and ankle position, knee alignment, or neutral pillar—especially during the descent of a split squat or lunge, or when moving under load

OPTIMIZATION STRATEGIES:

▶ Refer to the **Hip Stability B Linchpin Blueprint** (page 475) for lower body stability solutions.

▶ Use a suspension trainer or a supported hand position to help maintain full foot contact and keep your center of mass between both feet (instead of shifting forward over the front foot).

▶ Incorporate balance exercises and unilateral supplemental movements such as glute bridges, hamstring curls, step-ups, and calf/soleus raises.

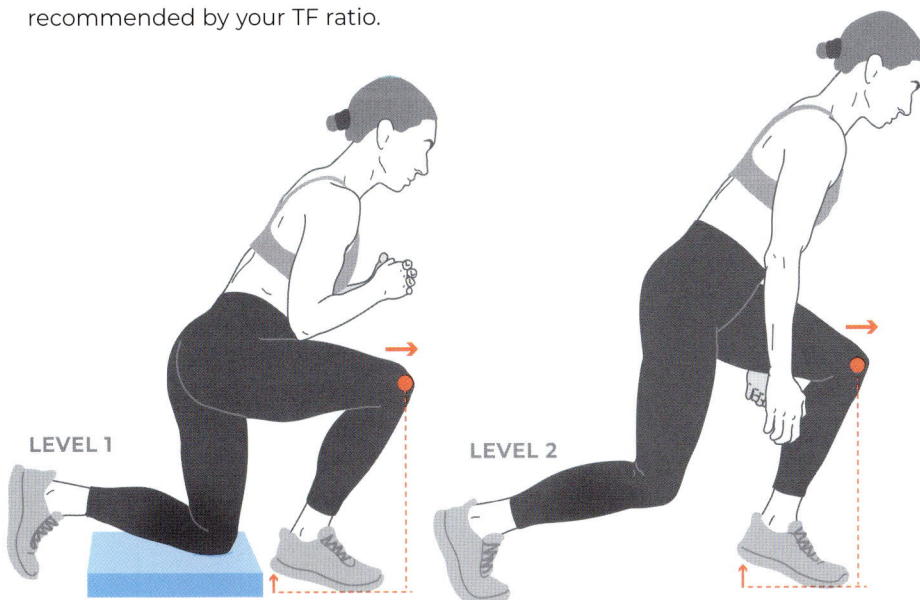

LEVEL 3

LEVEL 1

LEVEL 2

SKILL: Unilateral variations are more likely to expose imbalances or coordination deficits compared to bilateral exercises. However, the solution is gradual exposure and improved execution of these same movements. Potential indicators that lunge pattern refinement is needed include

▼ A lack of joint alignment and control or total body irradiation while performing split squats and lunges, particularly stepping variations (where transitioning from two points of contact to one and back requires dynamic control)

▼ Inconsistency in movement execution from rep to rep—such as difficulty maintaining stance, losing balance, changes in shin angle/forward knee movement, or stepping into a slightly different position each time (e.g., taking a shorter back step as fatigue sets in)

▶ Refer to the **Core Stability B (Prone) Linchpin Blueprint** (page 473) to improve pillar strength and total body stability.

▶ Use a suspension trainer or supported hand position to unload body weight as needed, allowing you to focus on full foot contact and maintaining your center of mass between both feet (rather than shifting forward over the front foot).

▶ Apply Reactive Neuromuscular Training (RNT) using a long resistance band (light):

• **Split squats & lunges:** Step your front leg into the loop so the band is around the outside of your knee to promote abduction, activate the glutes, and stabilize the pelvis. Alternatively, facing the other way so the band is around the inside of the knee promotes adduction, activating the inner thigh muscles to stabilize the pelvis in the opposite direction. If unsure which works best, video a set of reps each way and analyze which minimizes hip shift.

• **Hinge pattern development:** Stepping both feet into the loop and facing away from the anchor point to perform a hip-banded hinge is an effective way to reinforce the hinge pattern from a two-foot stance. Progressing this to a 1.5 stance hinge introduces a single-leg bias, moving toward a successful single-leg RDL.

▶ Incorporate balance exercises and unilateral supplemental movements such as glute bridges, hamstring curls, step-ups, and calf/soleus raises.

COMPENSATION: HIP SHIFT / SHOULDER TILT (UNWANTED ROTATION)

MOBILITY: Limited hip mobility can lead to a hip shift, affecting both sides or just one side when performing split squats, lunges, or single-leg RDLs. Potential mobility restrictions may present as

▼ Difficulty achieving symmetrical depth on one side compared to the other

▼ Feeling more restricted or tight on one side during stretches or warm-up movements

OPTIMIZATION STRATEGIES:

▶ Incorporate the **Hip Mobility C Linchpin Blueprint** (page 470) to address tight or short muscles around the hip joint. Customize based on specific needs, focusing on either hip flexors (front of the hip), adductors (inner thigh), or glutes.

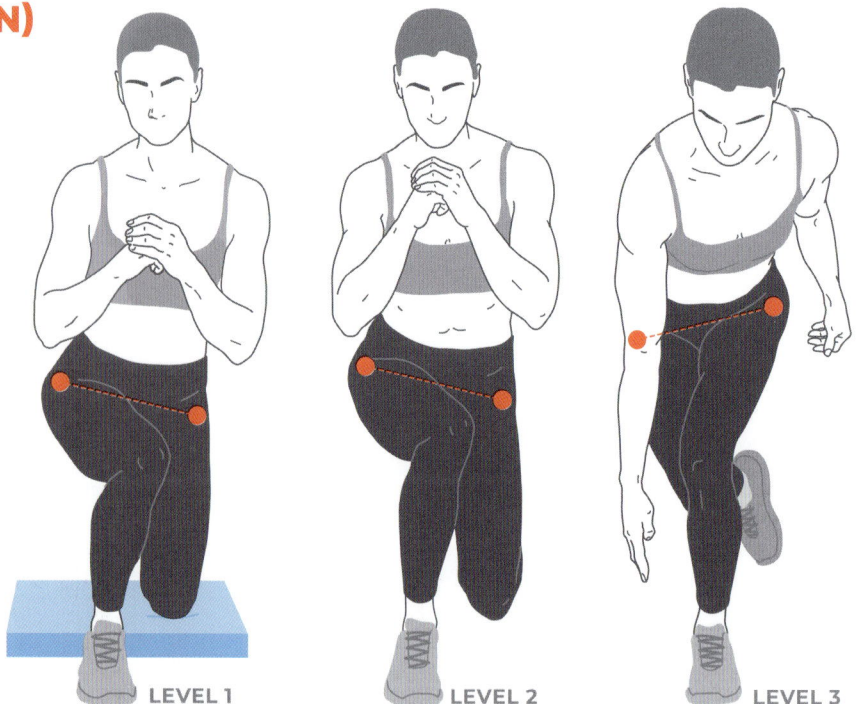

LEVEL 1   LEVEL 2   LEVEL 3

HIP SHIFT

▶ Strengthen within the authentic range you can control on each side, gradually increasing depth over time.

▶ Once competency has been established, introduce lateral split squats and lunges to address imbalances and improve mobility.

▶ Add supplemental stretches such as the half-kneeling hip flexor stretch, adductor rock-back, dynamic pigeon stretch, prone quad stretch, and supine hamstring stretch with a strap.

STABILITY: A hip shift can occur when the body compensates for poor hip centration or a lack of overall pillar stability. This may result from mismatched stances, improper setup (e.g., incorrect step or box height for step-ups or Bulgarian split squats), excessive load, or exercise variations that are not well-suited to your body. Indicators of instability include

▼ A noticeable shift, tilt, or rotation during the lowering or raising phase of the exercise

▼ Difficulty maintaining a neutral spine and stable pelvis throughout the movement

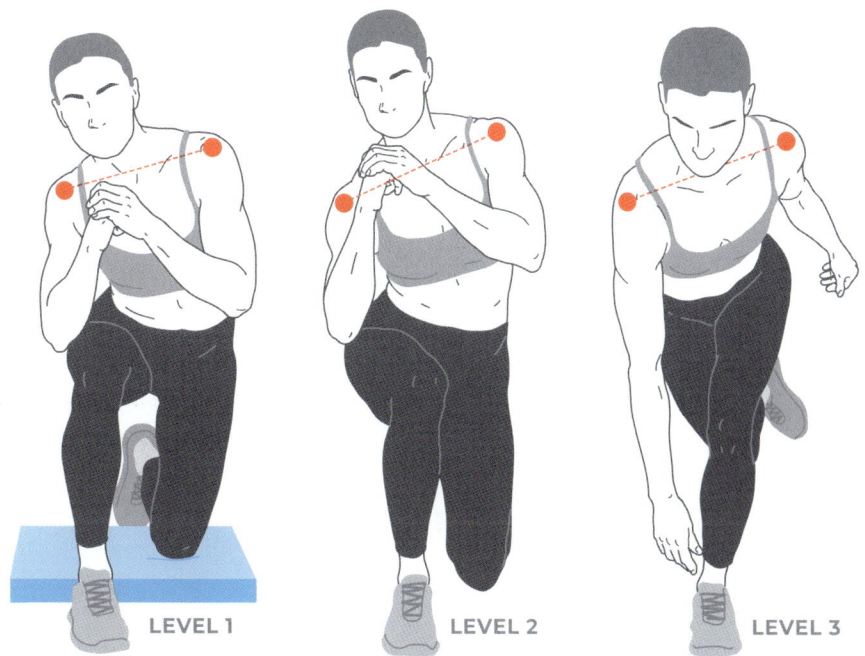

LEVEL 1   LEVEL 2   LEVEL 3

SHOULDER TILT

OPTIMIZATION STRATEGIES:

▶ Refer to the **Hip Stability B Linchpin Blueprint** (page 475) to prepare for your workout.

▶ Use the **TF Ratio Test** (page 304) to determine the appropriate amount of knee flexion and torso angle relative to your biomechanics.

▶ Apply Reactive Neuromuscular Training (RNT) using a long resistance band (light):

- **Split squats & lunges:** Step your front leg into the loop so the band is around the outside of your knee to promote abduction, activate the glutes, and stabilize the pelvis. Alternatively, if you face the other way, placing the band around the inside of your knee will promote adduction, activating the inner thigh muscles to stabilize the pelvis in the opposite direction. If unsure which works best, video a set of reps each way and analyze which minimizes the hip shift.

- **Single-leg RDL:** Since anti-rotation of the hips is a major demand in this exercise, increasing awareness of the back leg's position can be beneficial. If your right leg is the standing leg, loop a band over your right shoulder and under your left foot. In this variation, keep your back leg straight as you push your hips back into the hinge. The band provides proprioceptive feedback, helping you better control pelvic positioning.

▶ Add supplemental unilateral exercises such as side plank variations, single-leg glute bridges, hamstring curls, and slider/cable/band adduction drills or leg whips.

SKILL: Asymmetry often stems from repetitive patterns in daily life, work, or sports (e.g., always throwing, lunging, or sitting in a specific position). These habits carry over into gym movements, reinforcing imbalances. Signs of a skill gap include

▼ Struggling to control joint alignment in unilateral movement patterns

▼ Habitual compensations or biases appearing when load or speed increases, or under fatigue

OPTIMIZATION STRATEGIES:

▶ Start your session with the **Hip Stability B Linchpin Blueprint** (page 475) to address imbalances.

▶ Use the **TF Ratio Test** (page 304) to determine the appropriate amount of knee flexion and torso angle based on your structure.

▶ Regress to a single-leg variation that prioritizes movement quality and symmetry, controlling depth as needed.

▶ Focus on setup: align your stance, stabilize the pelvis by co-contracting the glutes and adductors, breathe 360 degrees, and brace to maximize intra-abdominal pressure. Maintain full-body irradiation throughout the movement to support stability and control.

LUNGE PROGRESSION PYRAMID

The lunge progression pyramid is structured to guide you through three levels of increasingly challenging variations in split-stance and single-leg movement patterns.

LEVEL 01

Level one lays the foundation with split squat variations—**bodyweight, deficit, and Bulgarian split squats**—where both feet remain in contact with the ground or a platform for added stability. This level provides the highest loading potential in the lunge progression pyramid, allowing you to develop strength, hypertrophy, and positional awareness without the complexity of stepping or shifting your base of support. By eliminating unnecessary variables, you can focus entirely on control and symmetry, establishing a rock-solid base before advancing to more dynamic variations.

LEVEL 02

Level two introduces lunges by adding movement through space, increasing the demand for dynamic stability and control. Here, you transition from two points of contact to a single-leg phase before re-establishing your base. At this level, you must demonstrate control with the **reverse lunge** through eccentric loading (deceleration) and smooth transitions before moving forward—literally. In other words, **forward lunges** and **forward walking lunges**, the next progressions up the pyramid, are more dynamic locomotion patterns that require even greater precision, force absorption, and seamless transitions. These higher-level variations are an earned progression that builds on the foundational stability established in level one.

LEVEL 03

Level three is where true single-leg training begins—only one foot remains in contact with the ground at a time, significantly increasing the challenge. This level follows a structured three-stage progression, moving from a pure hinge pattern (**single-leg RDL**) to a hybrid hinge-squat pattern (**skater squat**) before culminating in a true single-leg squat pattern (**pistol squat**). The reason for this order is simple: The more posterior chain involvement (glutes, hamstrings, and lower back), the greater the inherent stability. As you move toward a pure squat pattern, the demands on mobility, motor control, and single-leg stability increase, making the pistol squat the ultimate challenge.

Reaching level three isn't necessary for everyone. In fact, levels one and two often provide higher returns on investment in terms of strength development, progressive overload, and overall training effect. While level-three exercises offer unique benefits, they come with higher compensatory risk and lower loading potential, making them less effective as primary strength movements. This is why you rarely see single-leg RDLs, skater squats, or pistol squats programmed as key performance indicator (KPI) exercises—the heaviest, most demanding lifts performed first in a session. Instead, these variations function best as supplemental or accessory movements, supporting bilateral and split-stance KPI lifts by reinforcing movement quality, neuromuscular coordination, and functional strength at higher reps.

Rather than thinking of level three as an endpoint, view it as an advanced tool that's useful for skill development and functional hypertrophy. These movements can be particularly beneficial for individuals with low back pain or joint limitations that prevent them from loading bilateral squats or lunges effectively. In these cases, incorporating level three exercises allows you to maintain a strength stimulus while reducing spinal or joint stress.

As I've said, progressing through the pyramid isn't about leaving earlier levels behind; it's about reinforcing movement mastery at every stage. Each level serves a purpose, from developing strength to refining movement under greater dynamic demand. Whether your goal is strength, athletic performance, or injury prevention, the lunge progression pyramid provides a structured framework to advance intelligently while optimizing your mechanics along the way.

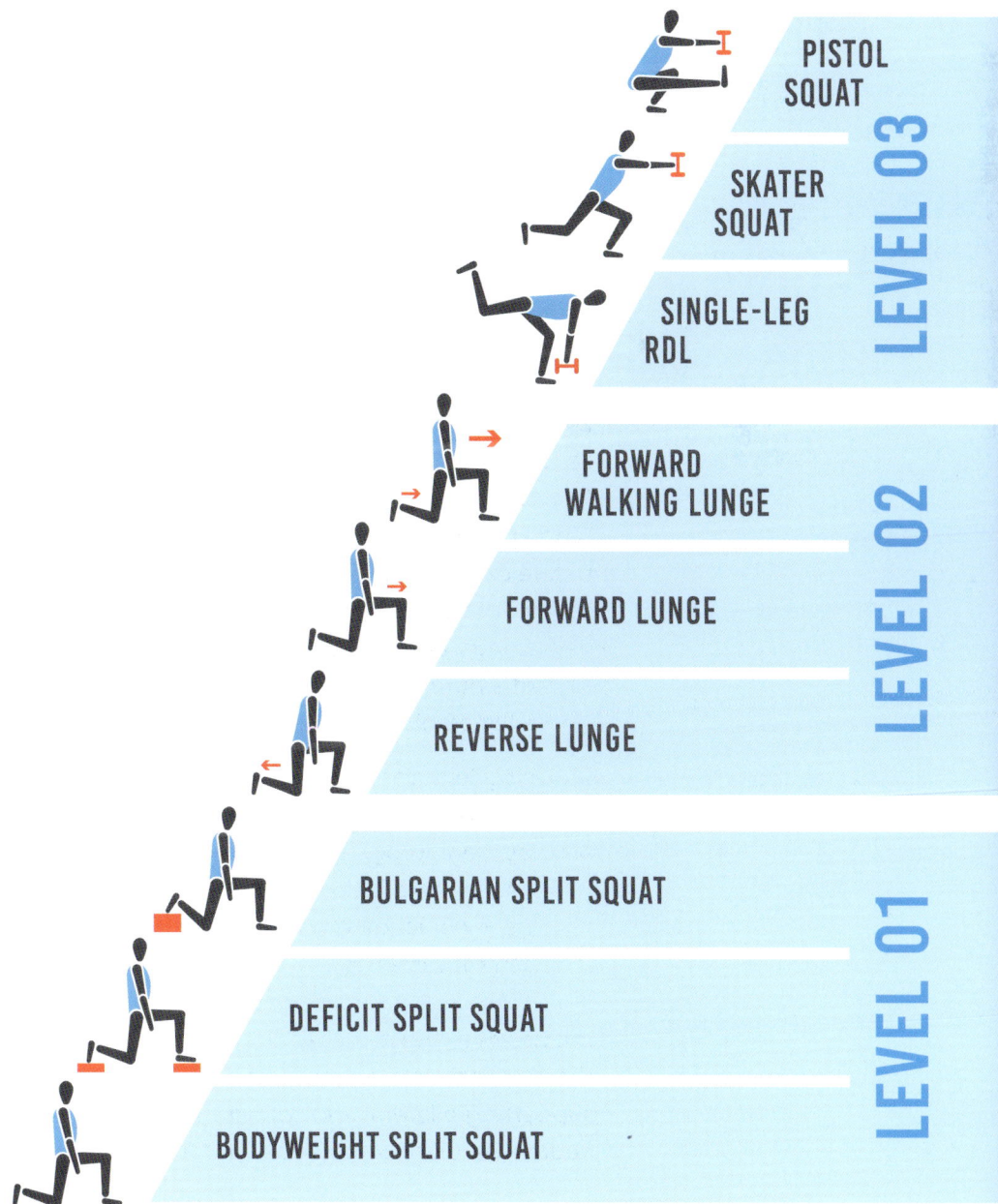

PISTOL SQUAT

SKATER SQUAT

SINGLE-LEG RDL

LEVEL 03

FORWARD WALKING LUNGE

FORWARD LUNGE

REVERSE LUNGE

LEVEL 02

BULGARIAN SPLIT SQUAT

DEFICIT SPLIT SQUAT

BODYWEIGHT SPLIT SQUAT

LEVEL 01

BODYWEIGHT SPLIT SQUAT

The bodyweight split squat is the foundation of the lunge progression pyramid, providing a stable entry point for developing balance, coordination, and control in a split stance. With both feet in contact with the ground, this movement creates the ideal environment to refine positioning, reinforce pillar stability, and ensure proper weight distribution before adding complexity or load.

While it may seem simple, the bodyweight split squat serves a crucial role: It's about mastery, not just movement. Before advancing to loaded or deficit variations, you need to establish full-body control, manage your center of mass, and eliminate unnecessary compensations. Pay attention to your balance: Can you lower and raise yourself smoothly without wobbling or shifting excessively? Are you able to maintain even weight distribution between your front and back legs? These checkpoints are key indicators that you've built the stability and motor control necessary to progress safely.

Once you meet the standards outlined in the optimization checklist, you're ready to add load to the split squat (see loading options below) and move up the pyramid.

For guidance on mastering the split squat, refer to the squat screen and optimization checklist covered earlier in the chapter.

LOADING OPTIONS FOR THE LUNGE PROGRESSION PYRAMID

When loading split-stance and single-leg movements, selecting the right strategy depends on your goals, mechanics, and experience level. The following options are listed in order of preference, starting with the most universally effective and progressing toward more targeted or situational variations.

Before adding external load, use the feel, function, perform template from the Movement Tenets chapter (pages 229–230) to determine whether you're ready to progress. If you can move through the full range of motion without compensation (Feel), maintain control and alignment under body weight (Function), and perform multiple high-quality reps with consistency (Perform), then it's time to introduce load. Prioritizing form, stability, and strength through the full range of motion before adding resistance ensures you maximize the benefits of each progression while minimizing risk.

1. Double Dumbbells at Your Sides (Farmer's Carry Position): This is the most balanced and spine-friendly way to load split-stance and single-leg exercises. With the dumbbells at your sides, the load stays close to your center of mass, reducing unnecessary strain on your lower back while maximizing stability. This setup allows for even distribution of weight and minimizes excessive forward lean, making it ideal for building strength and proficiency across all three levels.

2. Contralateral Load (Opposite Hand of the Front Leg): Holding a single dumbbell in the hand opposite the working leg creates a more targeted training effect, increasing demand on lateral stability and activating the core through the anterior oblique sling system (the central connection point between the opposite shoulder and hip that's muscularly and fascially connected through the torso). This setup improves balance and coordination while reinforcing proper hip and knee mechanics. It's particularly useful for those struggling with alignment or excessive torso lean during split squats or lunges.

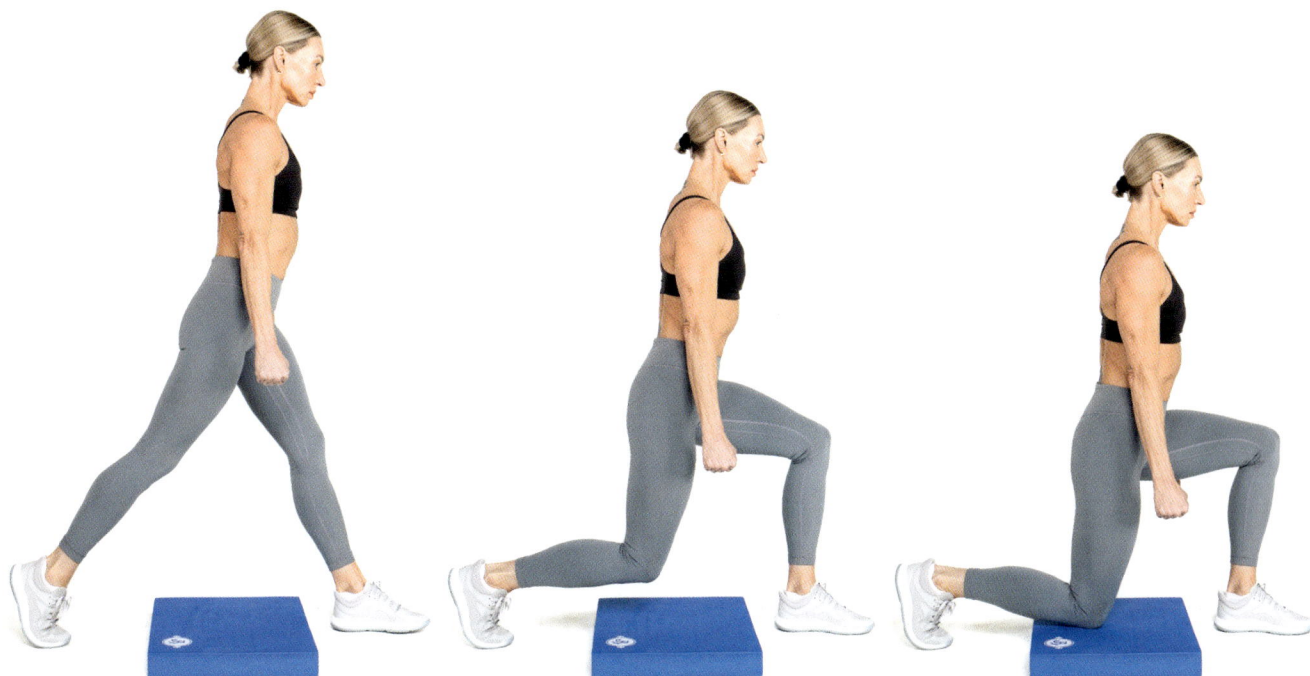

3. Goblet Position (Front Loaded): Holding a dumbbell or kettlebell in a goblet position (at chest level) shifts your center of mass forward, encouraging an upright torso and deeper range of motion. This is especially effective in early-stage progressions like deficit split squats and Bulgarian split squats, where the focus is on mastering stability and mobility. However, as load increases, the goblet position becomes less practical due to upper body fatigue and grip limitations.

4. Ipsilateral Load (Same Hand as the Working Leg): Though less common, holding a single dumbbell in the same hand as the working leg shifts the load laterally, emphasizing the anterior chain and reducing lateral stability demands. This setup is sometimes used for targeted quadriceps activation but is generally considered a novelty variation rather than a primary loading strategy.

A NOTE ON NOVELTY VARIATIONS

There are endless ways to manipulate load placement, some of which are popular on social media but lack real-world application. While variations like ipsilateral loading can serve a purpose, our focus remains on the most accessible and effective methods for building mobility, stability, and skill in split-stance and single-leg movements. Other advanced loading strategies may have value in specific programming scenarios, but they are not the foundation of this system.

By understanding how different loading positions and tools influence movement (for example, a goblet position can be performed with a dumbbell, a kettlebell, or even a landmine attachment), you can make smarter choices that align with your training goals. Master the fundamentals first, and as you progress through the lunge progression pyramid, experiment with different loading strategies to find what works best for you.

CUSTOMIZING LOAD BASED ON THE EXERCISE

Not all loading options apply equally across the pyramid. Goblet loading, for example, is only useful in levels one and two, while double dumbbells and contralateral loading provide the best carryover to heavier split-stance and single-leg work. Regardless of the variation, the key is to select a loading strategy that enhances movement quality and strength-building potential.

DEFICIT SPLIT SQUAT

The deficit split squat is the next step up in the lunge progression pyramid, increasing the challenge by expanding your range of motion. By elevating both feet on platforms, you can train the movement through a greater depth, reinforcing control, mobility, and strength in your end ranges.

There are a few variations that offer different benefits:

• **Deficit Split Squat (Double Deficit):** Elevating both feet enhances depth while maintaining a balanced weight distribution, challenging stability and strength across the full range.

• **Front-Foot-Elevated Split Squat:** Elevating only the front foot increases the range of motion while emphasizing muscular recruitment in the front leg, particularly the quads and glutes.

• **Rear-Foot-Elevated Split Squat (Bulgarian Split Squat):** Elevating only the back foot places more demand on single-leg stability, lengthens the hip flexors, and shifts the emphasis toward the front-leg musculature. *Note:* This is the next progression up the pyramid. See the following technique for a detailed breakdown.

A small elevation—typically 2 to 5 inches—is enough to provide these benefits without compromising form. Before increasing the deficit, ensure you can maintain proper knee, hip, and spine positioning without compensations, as outlined in the optimization checklist. The goal is to build strength and control through your available range, not to chase excessive depth at the expense of stability.

SETUP: Before setting up the platforms, measure your stance by lowering into a half-kneeling position. This allows you to determine the proper distance between your front and back foot to ensure optimal positioning. Your front foot should be firmly planted, and your back foot should be stable with the toes supporting your stance. Check that your hips are squared, your knee is tracking properly, and your spine remains neutral. Once you've established this position, mark where each foot lands, then position two equal-height platforms, such as weight plates or low boxes, at those points.

Step onto the front platform with both feet and go through the pillar cueing sequence to stabilize your position. Then step one foot back onto the rear

ALTERNATING VS. NON-ALTERNATING LUNGES

A key consideration in lunging is whether to alternate legs or complete all reps on one side before switching.

Non-alternating lunges, where you perform all reps on the same leg before switching, help maintain constant tension in your stabilizing muscles, particularly in the posterior and lateral chains. This sustained tension makes them ideal for building strength and hypertrophy, as the muscles remain under continuous load without interruption.

Alternating lunges, on the other hand, introduce an element of dynamic balance as you shift from one leg to the other. This movement enhances coordination and mimics real-world locomotion, making it beneficial for athletic performance, conditioning, and endurance. However, alternating lunges may reduce overall muscular tension if not performed with control, as the brief reset between steps can lessen the demand compared to non-alternating variations.

Interestingly, the non-alternating walking lunge is one of the most punishing yet underutilized variations. Because it requires rapid, repeated deceleration on the same leg before switching, it creates a training effect similar to a hard and heavy split squat set. The novelty of this stimulus alone can catch people off guard, as the relentless eccentric demand on a single leg amplifies fatigue before transitioning to the other. This makes it an excellent tool for strength and muscle development, particularly when progressive overload is the goal.

Whether you're performing non-alternating stationary lunges or walking lunges, start with your non-dominant, weaker, or lagging side first to ensure you train that leg with the highest quality while fresh. Then switch to your dominant side. But be aware that the second side will always feel harder due to the centralized training effect—heart rate (HR) and respiratory rate (RR) are already elevated, and pillar and core muscles are pre-fatigued from stabilizing during the first leg's set.

platform, stabilizing your stance before initiating the movement.

EXECUTION: Begin by lowering under control, allowing your back knee to move toward the ground or a pad. Descend smoothly and focus on even weight distribution between both legs. Avoid excessive forward knee movement or allowing your pelvis to collapse, keeping tension through your core and hips.

Descend until you reach your full range of motion while maintaining neutral alignment, then press firmly through the tripod foot of your front leg and the ball of your back foot to generate force and return to the starting position. The ascent should be smooth and controlled, with a focus on maintaining stability throughout the movement.

Between reps, maintain your positioning and reinforce your bracing sequence to ensure consistency and proper mechanics.

REAR-FOOT-ELEVATED SPLIT SQUAT (BULGARIAN SPLIT SQUAT)

The rear-foot-elevated split squat progresses the split-stance pattern by increasing the demand on the front leg. Unlike the standard split squat, where both legs contribute evenly, this variation typically shifts the workload from a 50/50 split to around 70/30, with the front leg handling the majority of the force production. Elevating the back foot extends the range of motion at the hip and knee, leading to greater muscle activation in the quads, glutes, and hamstrings. Additionally, because the load is centered over a single working limb rather than being distributed bilaterally, the exercise allows for higher load training with significantly less spinal compression, making it an ideal option for individuals with lower back limitations who still want to build strength.

This movement comes in two variations: a slight rear-foot-elevated split squat and a Bulgarian split squat. The slight elevation—typically between 2 and 12 inches—keeps the back foot actively engaged with the toes pushing into the platform, maintaining some contribution from the rear leg while reducing range of motion slightly. The Bulgarian split squat requires full rear foot elevation onto a bench (typically 15 to 18 inches high), placing an even greater emphasis on the front leg by removing active assistance from the back foot. This leads to deeper hip flexion, greater front-side loading, and a more significant stretch through the hip flexors and quads.

For those progressing up the lunge pyramid, the slight rear-foot-elevated split squat serves as a stepping stone to the Bulgarian split squat. Once you can complete controlled reps while meeting the standards covered in the optimization checklist—without relying heavily on your back leg for support—you're ready for the Bulgarian split squat.

The Bulgarian split squat is the ultimate goal of level one—and it's one of the best lower body exercises, period. It builds strength in your glutes, quads, and hamstrings while dialing in single-leg stability and mobility. The extra range of motion makes it a powerhouse movement for both athletic performance and everyday function. Plus, if back squats aren't your thing—or your lower back just isn't having it—this is one of the best ways to load up your legs without piling stress onto your spine. It's a staple for a reason.

SETUP: **Establish your ideal stance length by lowering into a half-kneeling position in front of your chosen platform.** Your front foot should be firmly planted with the knee stacked over the ankle, while your back foot rests on the platform in a stable, supportive position.

- **If using a slight elevation**, the ball of your foot remains in contact with the surface, similar to a traditional split squat.

- **If performing a Bulgarian split squat**, position the top of your foot flush with the bench (laces down).

After measuring your stance, mark your front toe position with a piece of tape or a small band to create a repeatable setup for each leg.

SLIGHT REAR-FOOT-ELEVATED SPLIT SQUAT

SETUP   EXECUTION

ECCENTRIC PHASE

CONCENTRIC PHASE

BULGARIAN SPLIT SQUAT

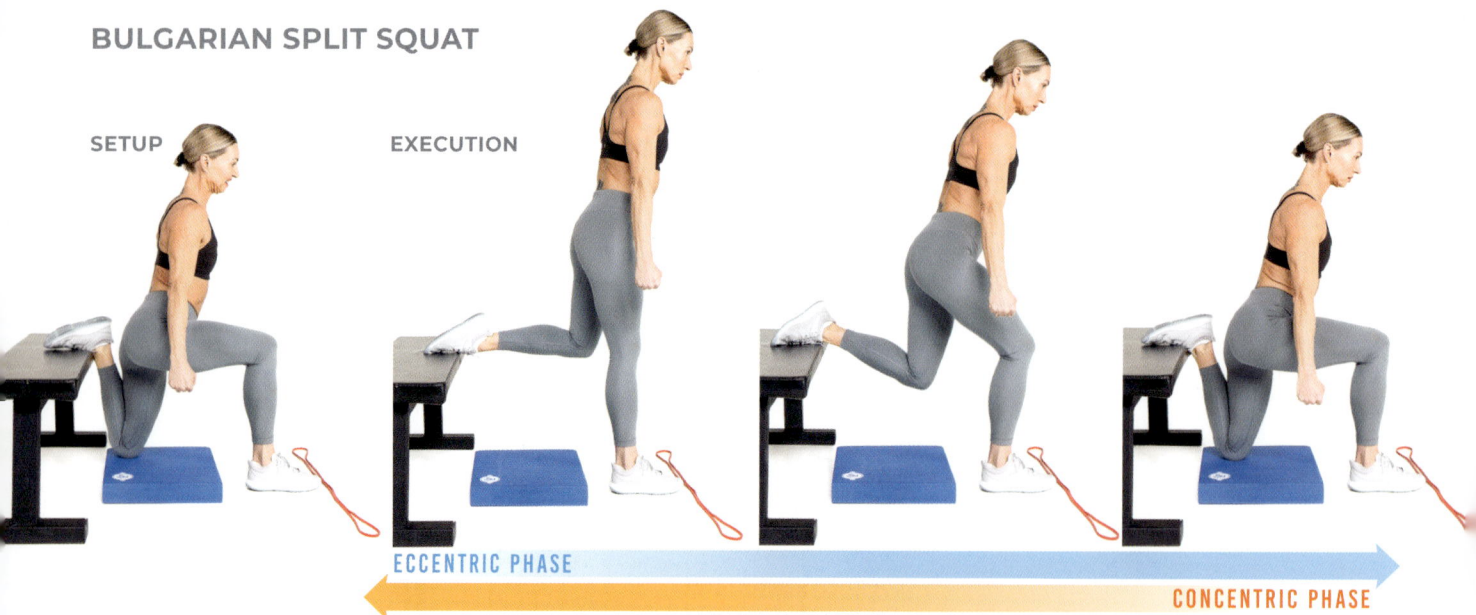

SETUP   EXECUTION

ECCENTRIC PHASE

CONCENTRIC PHASE

EXECUTION: Initiate the movement by lowering straight down, keeping your torso upright and your weight evenly distributed over the front foot. Avoid leaning excessively forward or allowing your knee to collapse inward. The goal is to move directly against gravity, descending into your full range of motion while maintaining control.

- **For a slight rear-foot-elevated split squat**, your back leg will provide some assistance, but the primary load should be on the front leg.

- **For a Bulgarian split squat**, the back leg acts as a stabilizer rather than a force producer, further isolating the working leg.

Descend until your back knee lightly taps the ground or a pad, ensuring full depth while maintaining tension. Then drive through your front foot, engaging your glutes and quads to return to the starting position. Avoid bouncing out of the bottom; each rep should be controlled, with a smooth eccentric phase and a strong, stable concentric push.

Regardless of variation, focus on a straight vertical path—no excessive swaying or shifting forward. Maintaining this A-to-B trajectory allows for maximum muscular recruitment and optimal force production, especially under heavy loads.

LEVEL
02

REVERSE LUNGE

At level two, lunges introduce movement through space, increasing the demand for dynamic stability, coordination, and strength. Unlike split squats, where both feet remain planted, lunges require a controlled transition from two points of contact to a single-leg phase before re-establishing your base. This forces you to manage deceleration during the eccentric phase and then generate enough force to powerfully accelerate back to the starting position—a critical transition that plays a key role in injury and fall prevention.

The reverse lunge serves as the foundation of level two because it allows you to build these essential skills in a stable and controlled manner. Stepping backward keeps your center of mass over your base of support longer than a forward lunge, keeping the balance demands low while reinforcing proper movement mechanics. This backward motion naturally engages the posterior chain—glutes, hamstrings, and hip stabilizers—placing less stress on the knees and making it the safest and most accessible way to introduce lunge variations.

For guidance on mastering the reverse lunge, refer to the level two screen and optimization checklist covered earlier in the chapter.

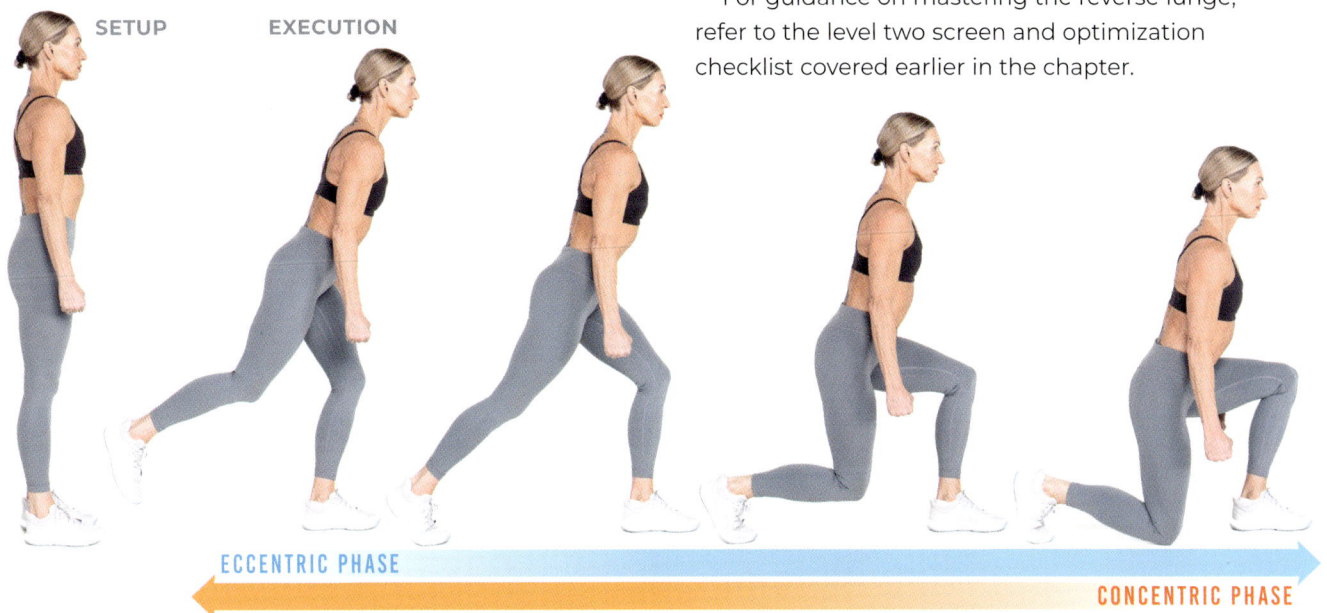

SETUP   EXECUTION

ECCENTRIC PHASE

CONCENTRIC PHASE

FORWARD LUNGE

The forward lunge isn't just a reverse lunge in the opposite direction—it's an entirely different exercise with unique demands on stability, strength, and force control. Many assume the only difference is the step, but that couldn't be further from the truth. The mechanics of the forward lunge require you to decelerate your entire body weight as you step ahead, shifting the emphasis from the posterior chain (glutes and hamstrings) to a more quadriceps-dominant movement.

This forward momentum introduces a new challenge: controlling knee flexion and maintaining alignment under load. Unlike the reverse lunge, where your back leg stabilizes the movement, stepping forward forces your lead leg to absorb the impact and control the descent. The result is more forward knee tracking, a more vertical torso position, and a significantly greater demand on the quadriceps to slow you down before you transition back to standing. This is why forward lunges tend to aggravate knee issues for some people—they place more stress directly on the knee joint, particularly if mechanics aren't dialed in.

Because of this increased demand on deceleration and control, the forward lunge is positioned after the reverse lunge in the progression pyramid. Mastering the reverse lunge first builds the necessary strength and coordination before introducing the higher-impact, forward-moving variation. The forward lunge also lays the groundwork for more advanced patterns like walking lunges and loaded dynamic variations, which further challenge stability and force production in a controlled, locomotive movement.

From a training perspective, the forward lunge has long been a staple in bodybuilding and athletic programming because of its ability to drive hypertrophy in the quadriceps. Whether you're building leg strength, improving lower body coordination, or refining your ability to decelerate and reaccelerate under control, the forward lunge is a key progression in the lunge pyramid that bridges the gap between foundational split-stance and dynamic single-leg training.

SETUP: **The setup for the forward lunge mirrors the setup for the reverse lunge.** Start by determining your optimal step length from a split squat position, ensuring that when you step forward, your knee stays aligned with your toes and your hips and spine remain neutral. **Marking your step length can help maintain precision and consistency as you string together multiple reps.**

Before moving, go through the pillar cueing sequence: Co-contract your pecs and lats, engage your glutes and adductors, take a diaphragmatic breath, and brace your core.

SETUP   EXECUTION

ECCENTRIC PHASE

CONCENTRIC PHASE

EXECUTION: Initiate the forward lunge by stepping ahead with intent, landing with control rather than allowing momentum to take over. As your foot makes contact with the ground, decelerate smoothly, allowing your front knee to track naturally over your toes. The key is to absorb force efficiently, preventing excessive knee-forward movement or instability.

Lower your back knee toward the floor in a controlled descent, aligning your torso with the angle of your front shin and resisting the urge to lean forward excessively. Your front shin should remain vertical or angled slightly forward, depending on your assessment.

To return to the starting position, drive forcefully through your front foot, using your quads and glutes to propel yourself back without relying on momentum. Ensure that the majority of the work is being done by the front leg. A common mistake is pushing off the back foot.

As you reset, re-establish your stance before initiating the next rep. Each repetition should emphasize precision in stepping, control in deceleration, and power in the return, reinforcing efficient movement and reducing unnecessary stress on the joints.

STEP DOWN BEFORE YOU STEP UP

Step-ups are often seen as a lower body staple, but they're not as easy as they look. Unlike lunges, which keep your center of mass on level ground, step-ups throw in a vertical challenge, forcing you to generate force against gravity while keeping everything locked in. That extra layer of complexity makes them a high-skill, high-stability movement with a lot of room for error. Because of this, step-ups aren't included in the lunge pyramid progression, but that doesn't mean they don't have a place in your training. When done with precision, they're a powerful tool for building single-leg strength, dialing in eccentric control, and reinforcing force production, making them a valuable accessory in a well-rounded lower body program.

But here's the thing: Most people butcher them. The biggest mistake? Skipping straight to the step-up without mastering the step-down. Think of the step-down as the foundation: If you can't control the eccentric phase on the way down, you're not going to magically clean it up on the way up. The step-down forces you to own your movement, teaching you how to absorb force, control your descent, and build the stability needed for a proper step-up.

Since step-downs and step-ups are essentially the same movement in reverse, the key is to take that slow, controlled descent from the step-down and apply it to the eccentric phase of the step-up. Rushing through reps, using momentum, or letting your knee cave in? That's how compensations creep in. Keeping it smooth and controlled is what builds strength.

Another major factor? Whether to alternate legs or stick to one side before switching. Alternating step-ups change the stability demand every rep, making it harder to refine a consistent movement pattern. Sticking to one side allows you to lock in your technique, reinforce proper mechanics, and actually get stronger where it counts.

FORWARD WALKING LUNGE

The forward walking lunge is one of the most advanced movements in the lunge progression pyramid, requiring a seamless combination of balance, coordination, and dynamic control. Unlike static lunges, this variation demands continuous motion, forcing your body to rapidly adjust and stabilize as you shift your center of mass forward with each step. Every repetition presents a new challenge—maintaining a consistent stride length, controlling deceleration, and reestablishing stability before initiating the next step.

This constant movement makes the walking lunge a true test of motor control and endurance. Unlike the forward lunge, where you step forward and then return to the starting position, the walking lunge eliminates the reset, requiring you to absorb force efficiently before propelling yourself into the next stride. This repetitive eccentric loading places a significant demand on the anterior chain— particularly the quadriceps—while also engaging the core and hip stabilizers to maintain balance throughout the sequence. Without a moment of full stabilization between reps, your ability to maintain control under fatigue is tested, reinforcing movement efficiency in real-world activities.

Beyond just lower body strength, the forward walking lunge significantly elevates heart rate and metabolic demand, making it an effective conditioning tool. The repeated shifts in weight challenge both central and peripheral fatigue,

replicating the demands of athletic movements like running, cutting, and directional changes. Even when performed with moderate loads, the combination of neuromuscular coordination and sustained time under tension makes this an incredibly taxing, yet highly rewarding, exercise.

Mastery of this movement requires progression. Beginners should start with a step-reset approach, ensuring full control before advancing to alternating steps in a continuous sequence. Whether climbing hills, hiking uneven terrain, or maneuvering through daily activities, the ability to control forward motion under load is essential. The walking lunge not only builds the foundation for higher-level single-leg training but also enhances overall movement efficiency, making it one of the most valuable exercises in your arsenal.

SETUP: Before initiating the movement, establish your optimal forward lunge stance based on your previous assessments. This ensures that when you step forward, your knee and torso stay aligned, and your movement pattern is repeatable.

Stand tall with your feet hip-width apart and go through the pillar cueing sequence. Maintain slight tension throughout your body to create stability before stepping forward. Your foot positioning should allow for smooth weight transfer as you transition from one lunge to the next.

SETUP   EXECUTION

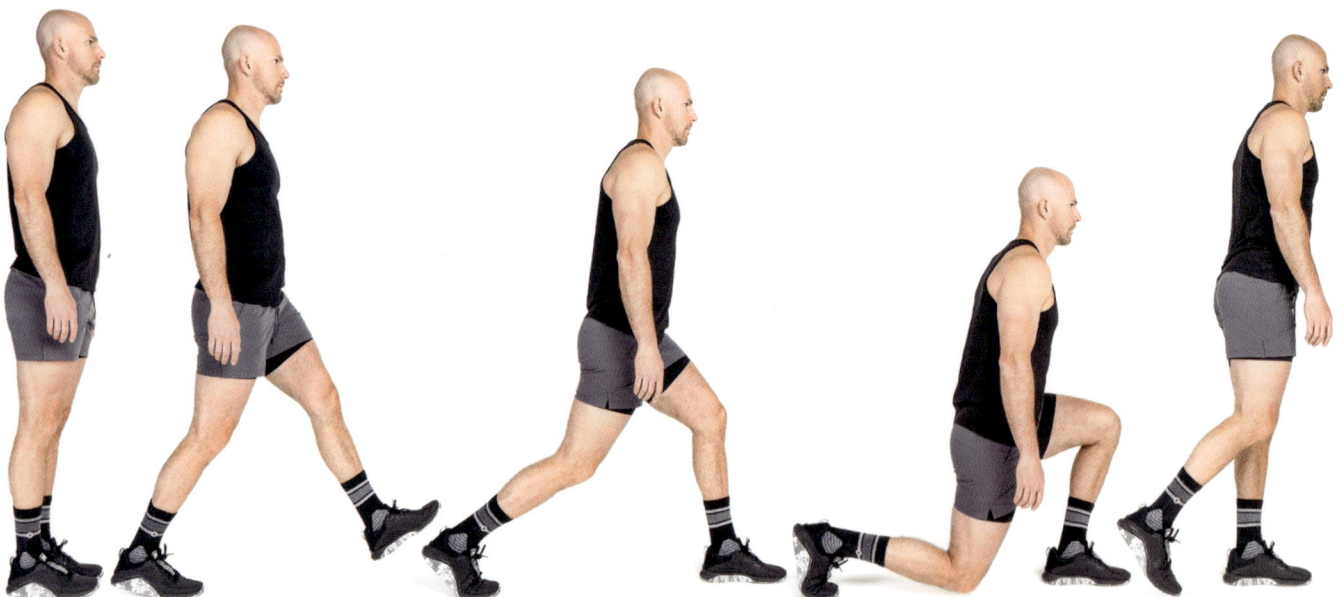

EXECUTION: Initiate the movement by stepping forward with control, planting your foot firmly on the ground. As your foot makes contact, focus on a controlled deceleration—resisting the urge to collapse into the movement. Your front knee should track in line with your toes, and your torso should stay aligned with your shin to maintain balance.

Lower into the lunge with a smooth, deliberate eccentric phase, allowing your back knee to descend toward the ground without excessive forward lean. Keep your weight evenly distributed through your front foot's tripod position while maintaining tension in your core and hips.

At the bottom of the lunge, engage your glutes and quads to push through your front foot, propelling yourself forward into the next step. The transition should be fluid, with no abrupt stopping or loss of alignment. As you step into the next lunge, maintain a steady cadence, focusing on repeatable step length, consistent posture, and smooth weight transfer.

Each rep should feel controlled and deliberate, reinforcing stability and strength as you progress through the movement.

LATERAL LUNGE

The lateral lunge isn't a pure movement pattern in the traditional sense—it's the "plus sign" in your training repertoire. While most movement occurs in the sagittal plane through asymmetrical single-leg stances (think reverse/forward lunging, walking, running, and sprinting), the lateral lunge adds a rotational, side-to-side component that challenges hip mechanics in novel ways. This movement requires extra mobility and deep end-range stability, which naturally reduces load capacity but enhances the targeted work of your adductors and lateral glutes.

Though it may not fit neatly into the category of heavy primary lifts, the lateral lunge plays a critical role in fine-tuning movement. As a high-skill, low-load exercise, it serves as a precision tool to address rotational and lateral stability, complementing the core split-stance and single-leg work that makes up the bulk of your training. Because of its lower loading potential and higher mobility demands, the lateral lunge is best performed after your primary exercises or KPIs—when strength and power work have already been prioritized. In this role, it can enhance movement efficiency, reinforce control at end ranges, and improve hip function without compromising heavier lifts.

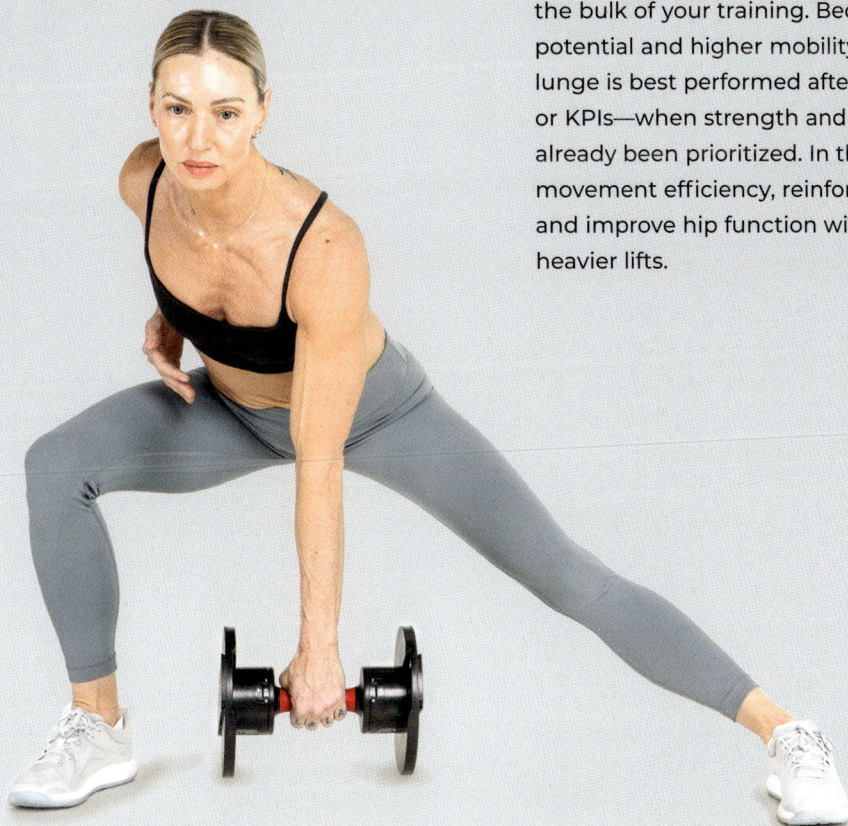

SINGLE-LEG ROMANIAN DEADLIFT (RDL)

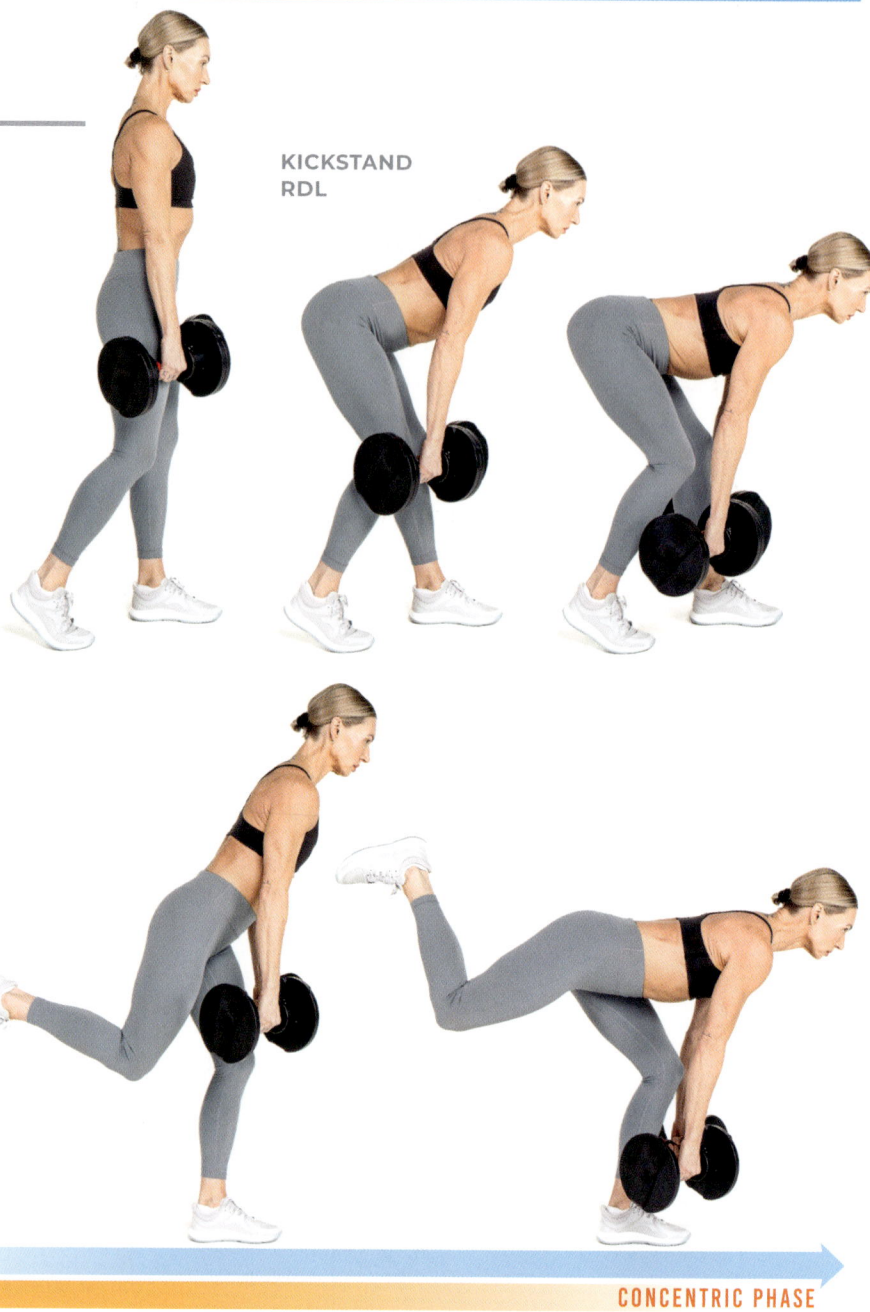

KICKSTAND RDL

SINGLE-LEG RDL

ECCENTRIC PHASE

CONCENTRIC PHASE

The single-leg Romanian deadlift (RDL) is one of the most challenging yet rewarding exercises for building unilateral strength, stability, and motor control. Unlike split-stance variations that provide extra ground contact for balance, the single-leg RDL demands total control with only one foot on the floor. That means your glutes, hamstrings, and core have to work overtime to keep your hips level, your spine neutral, and your movement smooth. Get sloppy, and you'll feel it—this movement doesn't let you fake stability.

But here's the catch: Strength isn't usually the issue when people struggle with the single-leg RDL. It's balance. Jump into it too soon, and instead of reinforcing good mechanics, you'll end up wobbling,

shifting, or compensating—none of which helps you get stronger or move better.

That's where the kickstand RDL comes in. Consider it your stepping stone from split-stance training to true single-leg work. By keeping your back foot lightly on the ground, you add just enough stability to clean up your hinge mechanics and build strength without fighting to stay upright. The goal? Gradually shift more of your weight onto your front leg while relying less and less on the back foot. Over time, you'll develop the control and coordination needed to nail a full single-leg RDL with confidence—no rotating, no compensations, just smooth, controlled movement.

SETUP: Start in a hip-width stance and go through the pillar cueing sequence.

- **If performing the kickstand RDL**, lightly position the toes of your back foot in line with the heel of your front foot—this back foot acts as a stabilizer but should not take on significant load.

- **For the single-leg RDL**, shift your weight into your front foot, lifting the back leg slightly off the ground with a small knee bend. Focus on maintaining even tension across your tripod foot to ensure stability.

EXECUTION: **Initiate the hinge by pushing your hips back while maintaining a neutral spine. Lower your torso with control.** You should feel tension in the hamstrings and glutes of your working leg.

- **In the kickstand RDL**, keep your back foot lightly grounded and your shin angled forward for balance, but ensure 90 percent of the load remains in your front leg.

- **In the single-leg RDL**, bend your knee to roughly a 90-degree angle and extend your back thigh straight behind you as a counterbalance, ensuring your hips stay level and do not rotate.

Descend until you reach your full range of motion, then drive through your front foot, engaging your glutes and hamstrings to return to a standing position. Keep each rep smooth and controlled, resisting the urge to rush or compensate with excessive knee movement.

If starting with the kickstand RDL, focus on gradually reducing weight on the back foot over time until you're ready to perform the full single-leg RDL without support.

SKATER SQUAT

ECCENTRIC PHASE

CONCENTRIC PHASE

The skater squat is a true test of single-leg control, blending elements of both a squat and a hinge into one high-skill movement. It challenges your ability to stabilize, coordinate, and generate force while managing movement in two directions—forward through the working leg and backward through the non-working leg. If your mechanics aren't dialed in, you'll feel it immediately, making it an excellent tool for refining movement quality.

But mastering this movement doesn't happen overnight. Achieving a full-range skater squat takes patience and progression. Starting with a controlled descent to a pad helps you refine your form and build confidence without collapsing at the bottom. The final stage is removing the pad entirely, demanding full eccentric control as you lower with precision and stability—a milestone that marks true mastery of this squat-hinge hybrid.

SETUP: Start in a hip-width stance, establishing a strong pillar for stability.

- If using a pad for progression, position it at a height that allows you to lightly tap your knee while maintaining full-body control.

- Holding light dumbbells at your sides can serve as a counterweight to assist with balance and control without altering the movement pattern.

EXECUTION: Initiate the movement by bending your front knee and allowing your back leg to travel backward in a smooth, controlled motion. Keep your torso at a slight forward angle while maintaining a neutral spine.

As you descend, extend your arms straight out in front of you, bringing them to shoulder height as you reach full depth. The movement of your arms should synchronize with the bending of your hips and knee.

Your back leg should travel in a coordinated arc. As you lower, let the knee track backward while keeping your foot elevated, preventing it from touching the ground. Continue lowering until your back knee either lightly taps the pad (if using one) or hovers just above the ground. Avoid collapsing or losing tension at the bottom position.

To ascend, drive forcefully through your front foot, extending your hip and knee in unison while keeping your back leg engaged and floating throughout the movement. The goal is precision, not speed. If balance remains a challenge, use a light counterweight in each hand or maintain the pad progression, gradually reducing its height over time until you can achieve a full-range skater squat with complete control.

SINGLE-LEG SQUAT (PISTOL)

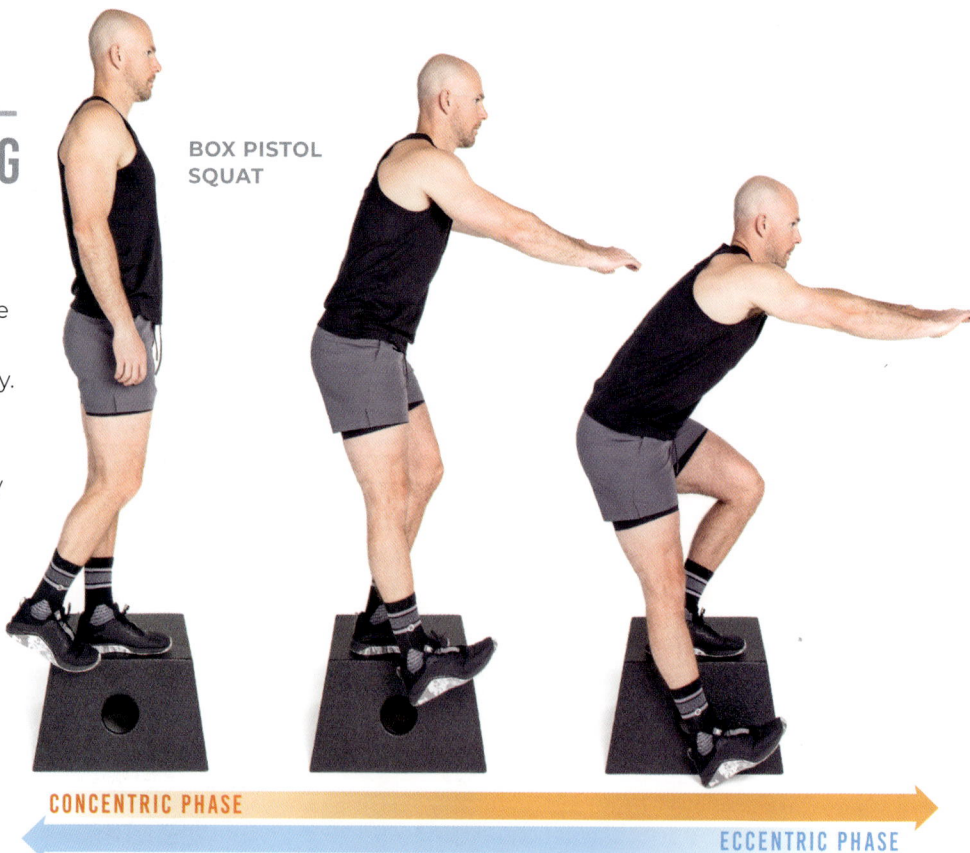

BOX PISTOL SQUAT

CONCENTRIC PHASE

ECCENTRIC PHASE

The pistol squat is the ultimate benchmark of lower body strength, balance, and mobility. No external support, no assistance—just you, gravity, and the ability to control every inch of the movement.

Unlike hinge-based variations such as the single-leg RDL and (to a lesser degree) the skater squat, the pistol squat is a pure squat pattern that shifts the focus heavily onto the anterior chain. With the quads doing the majority of the work and minimal assistance from the posterior chain, it requires exceptional relative strength to control both the descent and ascent, making it one of the hardest bodyweight movements for lower body strength and control.

That said, while the pistol squat does build strength and stability, it isn't something you'll see programmed as a key performance indicator (KPI)—the biggest, heaviest lifts that drive strength and hypertrophy. Because it demands such a high level of balance and motor control, using it as a KPI limits progressive overload, making it less effective for building strength. But when programmed as accessory work after KPI lifts, the pistol squat plays a crucial role in reinforcing single-leg stability, neuromuscular coordination, and movement integrity—without stealing energy from your bigger lifts. When used in this context, it enhances end-range mobility, balance, and control, all of which carry over to squats, lunges, and real-world movement.

Most lifters can't immediately drop into a full-depth pistol squat without compensations. Instead of forcing the movement and reinforcing bad habits, start with the box pistol squat. In this variation, you stand on a low box and gradually lower your free leg toward the ground. This allows precise control over your squat depth, helping you build strength, stability, and confidence incrementally.

Once you've developed control through that range, the next step is eliminating the box and performing the pistol squat from the ground. Since many lifters lack sufficient ankle mobility (dorsiflexion) to comfortably achieve full squat depth, you can elevate your heel using weight plates or a wedge. This slight elevation decreases the ankle mobility demands, allowing you to maintain better alignment and balance as you smoothly progress into deeper ranges of motion.

SETUP: Stand with your feet hip-width apart and then go through the pillar cueing sequence to stabilize your shoulders, hips, and core.

NOTE: *Holding light dumbbells as a counterweight can make the movement easier by shifting your center of mass forward, helping you maintain balance and control throughout the descent.*

- **For the box pistol squat**, stand on a stable, elevated surface such as a box or stacked plates with your working foot positioned near the side edge. This allows your non-working leg to extend without obstruction.

- **For the full pistol squat**, consider elevating your heel using a wedge or small weight plates. This makes it easier to maintain balance and stability while performing the full-depth pistol squat.

EXECUTION: Initiate the movement by bending at the knee and hip simultaneously, maintaining a controlled descent.

As you lower, extend your non-working leg forward with a straight knee and dorsiflexed ankle, preventing it from touching the ground. Maintain a slight forward lean to counterbalance the movement.

At the same time, extend your arms straight out in front of you, bringing them to shoulder height as you reach full depth. The movement of your arms should synchronize with the bending of your hips and knee.

Descend under control until the heel of your non-working leg touches the floor (for a box pistol) or until you reach full depth in a freestanding pistol squat. Avoid collapsing or rounding your spine excessively.

Once you reach your deepest position, drive through the mid-foot and heel of your working leg, extending your hip and knee simultaneously as you return to standing.

PISTOL SQUAT

CONCENTRIC PHASE

ECCENTRIC PHASE

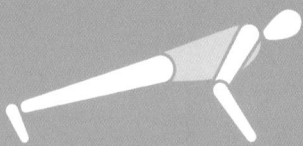

PUSH

The push is the most overtrained movement pattern—and most lifters are paying the price. Chasing heavier weights at all costs has left many with stiff shoulders and fragile foundations of strength built on poor mechanics. Combine overloaded pressing with hours spent hunched over screens, and you're primed for chronic pain and stalled progress. But pressing doesn't have to hurt. It's time to prioritize quality over quantity, build stability before strength, and master mechanics tailored to your body. This chapter guides you step-by-step to assess and refine your pressing, ensuring your shoulders stay healthy, strong, and pain-free.

Years ago, I visited an iconic flagship gym on Fifth Avenue in New York City. It was the kind of place that made you feel like you were stepping into a temple of high performance. The moment I entered, the retinal scanner at the door—yes, a retinal scanner—set the tone. Inside, marble floors gleamed under soft lighting, spiral staircases floated midair, and every detail exuded an unmatched level of fitness luxury.

As I toured the facility with the regional director, his pride was palpable. He showed me the functional training area first: sleds, turf, kettlebells—the works. Then we climbed the stairs to the main training floor, where the true extravagance came into view. Every cardio machine imaginable, dumbbell racks stretching into the horizon, and rows of machines—all pristine and state-of-the-art.

"What do you think?" he asked, gesturing toward the expansive weightlifting section. My gaze swept over the room, and I couldn't help but laugh in disbelief. "Wow," I said, shaking my head. "There are six flat bench setups and four incline bench presses. Where's the squat racks?" He pointed to the farthest corner of the floor, where a lone squat rack stood, paired with a single deadlift platform. The dim lighting gave it a neglected, almost forgotten feel.

"We gave the people what they wanted," he said with a grin, crossing his arms like he'd cracked the code of gym design.

It turned out they'd conducted a survey of their target audience—affluent, image-conscious professionals in New York City—before finalizing the layout. "What do you want to see in our flagship facility?" they'd asked. The responses were clear: benches, dumbbells, and cardio equipment dominated the wish list. Squat racks? Deadlifts? An afterthought.

"I get it," I said, trying to contain my frustration. "You're giving people what they want. But shouldn't you also give them what they need? This setup is practically an altar to the bench press."

The director shrugged. "People train what they know and what they can see in the mirror—their chest, their abs, their biceps. That's what sells memberships."

And he wasn't wrong. In fitness, we tend to gravitate toward what's familiar and visible. But as I walked through that pristine facility, it struck me that we've confused what's visible with what's vital.

The bench press, with its reputation as the king of upper body exercises, has been elevated to near-iconic status in gym culture. It dominates training programs, revered for its aesthetic and strength-building appeal. But in our obsession with this one exercise, we've neglected the foundational principles that make the push pattern effective and sustainable. This misplaced focus has led to a widespread problem: overtraining the push pattern. And the consequences go far beyond the bench press itself.

Take a moment to think about how most people spend their days—hunched over a desk, gripping a steering wheel, or staring down at a phone for hours on end. These prolonged positions train the body to accept a forward-slumped posture as its new "neutral." Your body adapts to the positions you spend the most time in, even if they're mechanically inefficient. This adaptation doesn't just affect how you sit or stand—it rewires your muscular and nervous systems, creating a baseline that favors tightness in some muscles and weakness in others. The result? Stiffness, poor mobility, and compromised neuromuscular control (the ability to coordinate muscles for smooth, efficient movement). Instead of moving in a balanced and functional way, the push pattern starts to mirror and reinforce these poor mechanics.

This imbalance creates a ripple effect. As the chest, shoulders, and neck muscles become tight and overactive, the upper back and rotator cuff muscles weaken and lose their ability to stabilize and support proper movement. Gradually, your nervous system begins to accept these poor mechanics as the default, embedding compensatory patterns that prioritize completing a movement rather than performing it correctly.

Now, add heavy bench pressing into the mix. The bench press—performed in a restricted range of motion—amplifies these existing deficits. It's an internal rotation–dominant movement, which means it reinforces tightness in the chest and lats, pulling the shoulders inward and further reducing joint mobility. Compounding the issue, the shoulder blades remain static and locked in place during the lift, unable to move freely and dynamically as they should. This lack of scapular movement places significant stress on the shoulder joint, particularly vulnerable structures like the rotator cuff, anterior deltoid, and biceps tendon. The most concerning part? These faulty mechanics and the pain they often produce eventually feel normal. Instead of building strength and resilience, the push pattern becomes a breeding ground for inefficiencies and compensations, ultimately leading to stalled progress, chronic discomfort, and, in many cases, injury.

For many lifters, this cycle feels endless. They press harder, add more weight, and train through pain, hoping sheer effort will break the plateau. But the reality is, more bench pressing isn't the solution—it's often the problem. In my years of working with clients, I've seen this scenario play out time and again: individuals dedicated to building upper body strength, yet trapped in cycles of shoulder pain, elbow flareups, and frustrating stagnation. When I suggest stepping back—reducing pressing volume, adding movement variations, and rebuilding the push pattern from the ground up—it's often met with disbelief. "But I thought more benching was the key to getting stronger," they'll say.

This reaction isn't surprising. The bench press has become symbolic of strength and upper body dominance. Stepping away from it feels counterintuitive, like abandoning progress. But here's the truth: the bench press, while valuable, captures only a narrow slice of the push pattern's potential. Its fixed hand position, static shoulder blade alignment, and restricted range of motion limit its functionality as a movement pattern. A true push pattern should allow for freedom of movement, full range of motion, and integration of multiple muscle groups working together in synergy. This integration is where exercises like the push-up excel—they operate in a closed-chain environment, demand dynamic scapular movement, and engage the entire kinetic chain.

This doesn't mean the bench press should be avoided—it means its role must be placed in context. The push pattern is far more expansive than a single exercise, and its true potential lies in addressing deficits in mobility and stability, and training it with a broader, more thoughtful approach. A well-rounded push pattern reduces pain, supports better posture, and unlocks access to ranges of motion many people have never properly trained.

So, the issue isn't with the push pattern—it's with how narrowly and incompletely it's typically trained. When you overload an imbalanced movement, neglect mobility and stability, and fail to integrate the push pattern into full-body mechanics, you rob it of its potential and inadvertently contribute to the very dysfunction you aim to avoid.

To reclaim the push pattern as a foundational movement, you must shift your perspective. It's not about chasing bigger numbers on the bench press or mindlessly repeating the same exercises—it's about refining your technique, tailoring the movement to your body, and advancing through thoughtful progressions that build strength and durability. This is the push pattern at its best: a pillar of training that merges aesthetics with sustainable pain-free function.

PUSH SCREEN

The push pattern encompasses a spectrum of motion, from horizontal pressing exercises like push-ups and bench presses to vertical movements such as overhead presses. While both planes of movement are vital for building strength and functional capacity, the horizontal plane is the best place to start—whether you're learning the push pattern for the first time or individualizing your technique.

Why focus on horizontal pressing first? Simply put, it's the most stable and accessible starting point for most people. Vertical pressing requires significant overhead mobility and shoulder stability, which can be difficult to achieve without first addressing foundational alignment and control. In contrast, horizontal pressing allows you to build these essential components in a more controlled and repeatable position. It also sets the stage for better vertical pressing mechanics down the road by modeling proper form, scapular movement, and full-body stability.

With the push-up, your hands are fixed on the ground in a closed-chain environment, which means your body must stabilize and move around those fixed points. This setup reveals how well your shoulders, core, and hips coordinate under load, exposing even minor breakdowns in form and tension.

THE LOWER PUSH SPECTRUM: WHERE DO DIPS FIT IN?

The lower portion of the push spectrum, which includes dips, is not featured in the push pattern because it places the shoulders in a deeply internally rotated, elevated, and protracted position—essentially magnifying the pain-producing compensations you're trying to avoid. While dips can be useful for those with the necessary mobility and stability, they offer no added functional benefit beyond a well-balanced horizontal and vertical push. For most lifters, dips are a high-risk, low-reward exercise that can aggravate shoulder issues, which is why they are absent from the pain-free performance program.

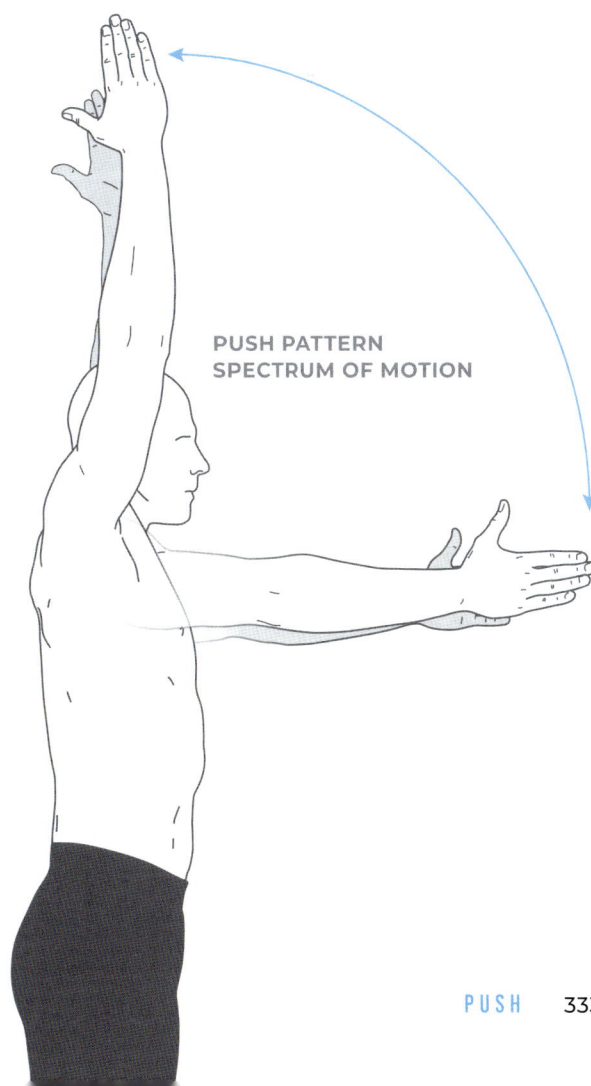

PUSH PATTERN
SPECTRUM OF MOTION

To fully understand what the push screen evaluates, let's break down the key objectives:

▼
EVALUATE JOINT ALIGNMENT AND STABILITY:

Proper push mechanics rely on optimal alignment of the pillar—shoulders, hips, and core. The push screen highlights how well these areas work together, revealing imbalances, misalignments, or compensations that could lead to inefficiencies or pain.

▼
ASSESS SCAPULAR MECHANICS:

Unlike many traditional push-up screens that focus on hand or elbow positioning, here you're placing your focus into the dynamic movement of the shoulder blades. In a closed-chain setup, the scapulae must move through protraction, retraction, elevation, depression, and rotation while stabilizing the body. Any restriction or instability often signals underlying weaknesses that can contribute to pain and poor performance.

▼
IDENTIFY FULL-BODY COORDINATION AND IRRADIATION:

The prone position demands full-body irradiation—tension radiating from the hands and feet through the core and into the hips and shoulders. This full-body engagement creates a stable platform for movement and exposes any breakdowns in coordination or tension management.

▼
HIGHLIGHT ASYMMETRIES AND WEAK LINKS:

The push screen exposes asymmetries between the left and right sides of the body, as well as weak links in the kinetic chain. These gaps often manifest as shoulder discomfort, instability, or uneven force distribution during pressing exercises.

▼
SET THE FOUNDATION FOR PROGRESSION:

Beyond identifying limitations, the push screen offers a road map for improvement. It reveals where to focus corrective efforts, how to refine technique, and how to build a strong, pain-free push pattern through intentional progressions.

SETUP: ESTABLISHING PILLAR STABILITY and PLANK POSITION

1. **Starting Position:** Begin on all fours, ensuring your wrists are directly under your elbows and your elbows are aligned beneath your shoulders. Your hands should be shoulder-width apart, with your index fingers pointing straight ahead. Spread your fingers wide to create a stable base. Position your knees hip-width apart with the bottoms of your toes pressing into the ground—avoid resting the tops of your feet on the floor.

2. **Stabilize the Pillar:** With multiple contact points on the ground (hands, knees, and toes), you can create torque at the shoulders and hips, reinforcing stability throughout the pillar. Begin at the shoulders by co-contracting your pecs and lats to stabilize the shoulder blades. Next, actively grip the floor with your hands by applying an outward spinning force into the ground— as if you're trying to "rip" it apart without letting your hands move. This generates external rotation torque that enhances irradiation, allowing the force and tension generated in your hands to transfer through your forearms and shoulders, intensifying engagement in the pecs and lats.

   With the upper body stabilized, shift your focus to the lower body. Begin by engaging your glutes to stabilize your hips. Simultaneously, activate your adductors (the muscles along your inner thighs) by slightly pressing your knees inward, creating a subtle tension that helps anchor your pelvis. Finally, engage your core as if preparing for impact—this connects your upper and lower body, creating a unified, tension-filled pillar.

3. Establish the High Plank Position: From your all-fours starting position, maintain the stability you've created through your hips, shoulders, and core. Begin by stepping one leg straight back, planting your toes firmly into the ground, followed by stepping the other leg back into a high plank position. Keep your feet hip-width apart, ensuring your toes actively grip the ground to engage the lower body and maintain balance.

As you establish the plank, focus on your body alignment. Your head, shoulders, hips, and heels should form a straight line. Avoid letting your hips sag toward the ground, which can strain your lower back, or rising above shoulder level, which disrupts the pillar's stability. Maintain a neutral spine by engaging your core, ensuring your pelvis remains level.

This position reinforces full-body stability while integrating the upper and lower body into a cohesive pillar, setting the foundation for proper push mechanics.

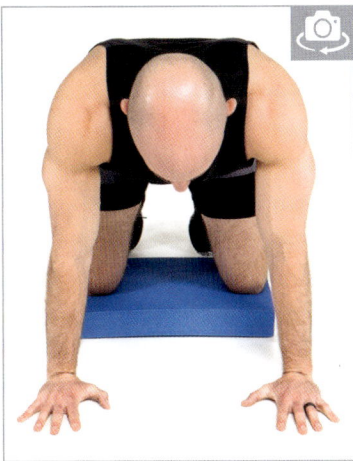

SETUP

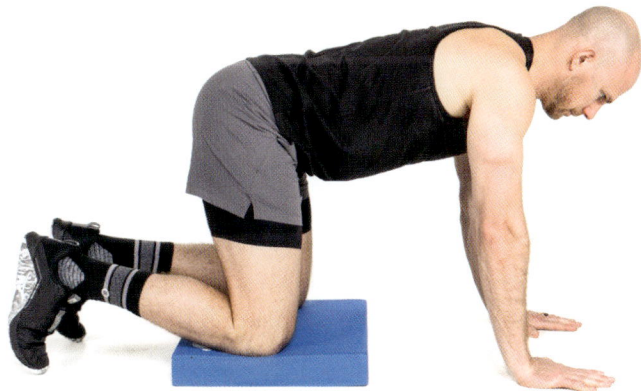

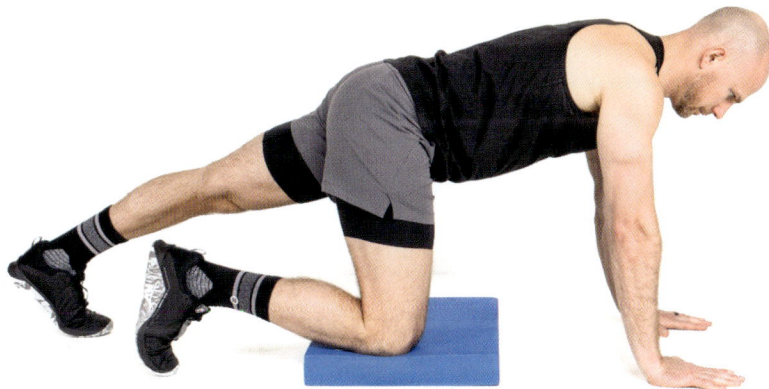

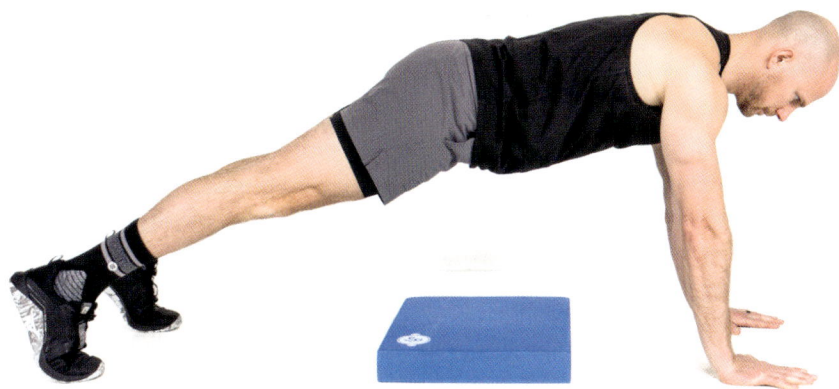

EXECUTION: PERFORMING THE PUSH-UP

Once you've established a stable plank position, the push-up begins. This phase involves controlled lowering and a powerful return, emphasizing alignment, irradiation, and full-body engagement.

Descent (Eccentric Phase): Start the descent by lowering your body as one cohesive unit, avoiding any sagging at the hips or excessive arching in your spine. Your big toes serve as a fulcrum point, anchoring your body and creating tension throughout the entire descent. This isn't just an up-and-down motion—it's a controlled arc, where your chest moves slightly forward as you lower yourself down. Keep your elbows at approximately a 45-degree angle to your torso.

As you move downward, your shoulder blades should retract, drawing together in a smooth and controlled manner. One of the most common mistakes during this phase is descending too quickly. A slow, deliberate descent isn't just about control—it's about stabilizing your upper back and shoulders, which builds strength and reinforces proper mechanics. The chest—not the stomach or hips—should lightly graze the floor to indicate your end range of motion. There's no resting at the bottom, no pause, and no loss of tension or alignment.

Ascent (Concentric Phase): From this bottom position, begin the ascent without hesitation. Maintain full-body irradiation—feel the tension radiating from your fingertips, through your shoulders, down into your core, and all the way to your toes. The big toes continue to serve as the anchor point, helping you drive upward and slightly backward as you press. Your shoulder blades should protract, moving slightly apart, as you rise. Maintain the same 45-degree elbow angle as you ascend, resisting the temptation to flare them outward or collapse inward. As your body returns to the plank position, your shoulders, core, and hips should remain stable and aligned, with no sagging, twisting, or rotation.

Throughout both phases, every adjustment in your shoulders, core, and hips directly impacts your stability and movement efficiency. Losing control in any one of these areas creates compensations that ripple through the rest of your body. Many people mistakenly focus only on the pressing phase, but the lowering phase is equally—if not more—important for building control, stability, and strength.

HAND-ELEVATED PUSH-UP

If performing a full push-up from the floor feels too challenging, elevate your hands on a sturdy surface like a bench (16 to 18 inches high) to reduce the load. Follow the same setup cues and execution mechanics covered above.

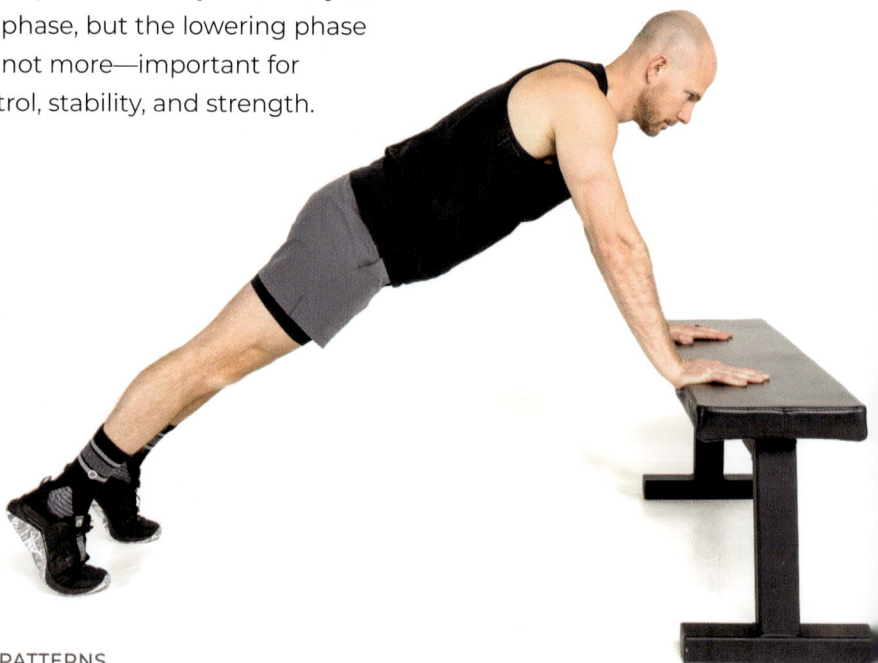

ECCENTRIC PHASE

CONCENTRIC PHASE

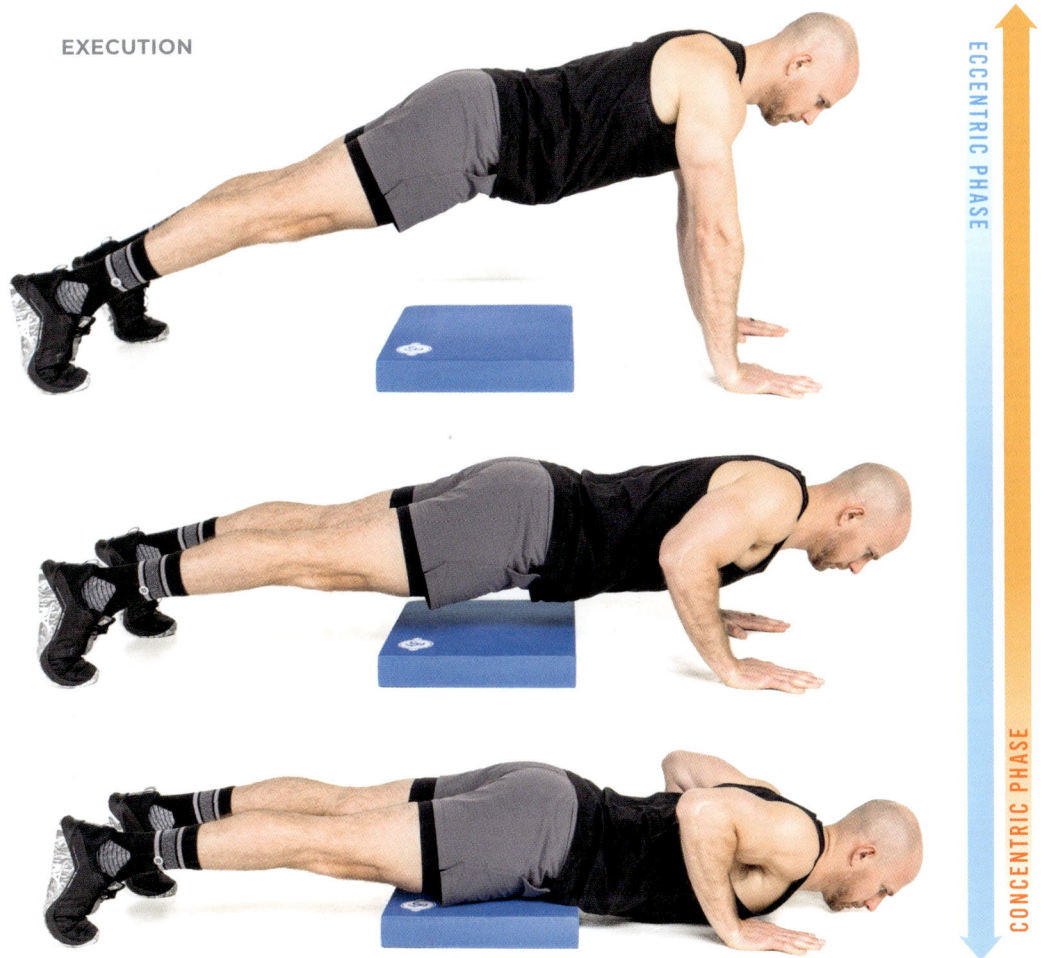

OPTIMIZATION CHECKLIST

For many, the push screen serves as a wake-up call. People who can confidently bench press impressive weight are often surprised to find themselves struggling with bodyweight push-ups when held to the standards outlined in the optimization checklist. This moment challenges common assumptions about strength, highlighting that raw power alone isn't enough to compensate for deficits in mobility, stability, and skill. Strength without control is like horsepower without steering—it can't be fully harnessed or directed where it's needed most.

At its core, the push screen isn't just about performing a push-up. It's about analyzing how your body moves, identifying where breakdowns occur, and developing a plan to address those weaknesses. Each repetition becomes an opportunity to refine your mechanics and build a stronger foundation. The better your foundation, the more effectively you'll be able to build strength—not just in the gym, but in every pressing motion you perform in daily life.

To make the most of this process, the next step is to record yourself performing the push-up from both a front and side perspective. These angles provide a clear visual reference, allowing you to compare your form against the optimization checklist standards. By analyzing your body position, scapular movement, and overall quality of motion, you'll gain valuable insights into where adjustments are needed and how to refine your push pattern for optimal performance.

✓ NEUTRAL SPINE

Maintaining a neutral spine during the push-up ensures your pillar stays stable and aligned throughout the movement. While some natural curvature in the spine is normal, the goal is to avoid excessive arching (overextension) or rounding (flexion) in the lower back, which compromises core stability and places unnecessary stress on the spine. A neutral spine allows the shoulders, core, and hips to work together effectively, creating a solid pillar for force transfer during the push.

✓ NO UNWANTED ROTATION

Avoiding rotation during the push-up means keeping your torso level and aligned from shoulders to hips. Rotation often occurs when one side of the body compensates for weakness or instability, causing the hips or shoulders to twist. Proper alignment ensures both sides of the body contribute evenly to the movement, minimizing imbalances and maximizing efficiency and control.

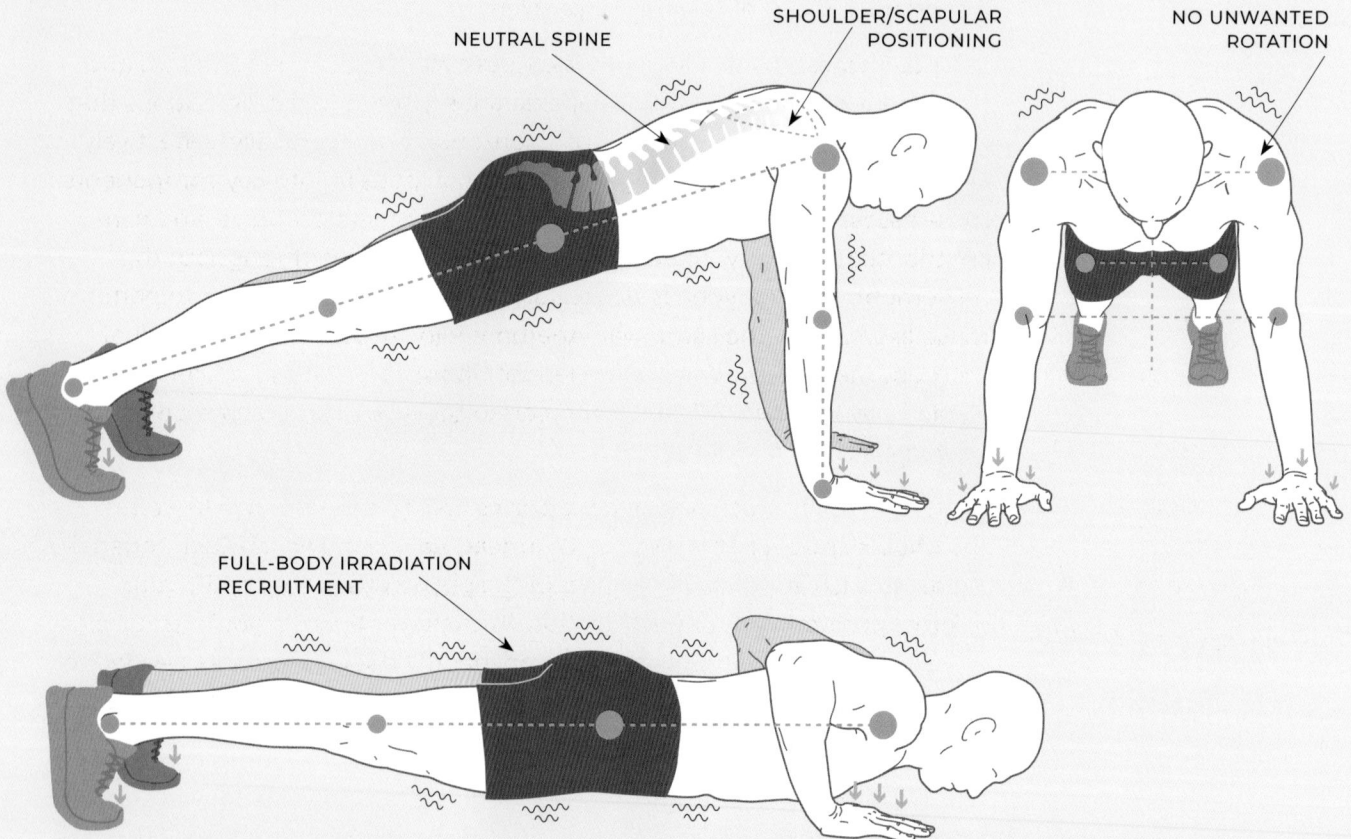

NEUTRAL SPINE

SHOULDER/SCAPULAR
POSITIONING

NO UNWANTED
ROTATION

FULL-BODY IRRADIATION
RECRUITMENT

✓ FULL-BODY IRRADIATION RECRUITMENT

Full-body irradiation refers to creating tension throughout the entire body by actively gripping the floor with your hands, pressing through your toes, and engaging your core, glutes, and shoulders. This intentional tension stabilizes your body against gravity, preventing energy leaks and enhancing strength and control throughout the push-up. It's not just about your chest or arms—it's about integrating your entire body into one cohesive unit.

✓ SHOULDER/SCAPULAR POSITIONING

Proper shoulder and scapular positioning means allowing the shoulder blades to move dynamically—protracting, retracting, elevating, and depressing—as you lower and press during the push-up. Your shoulders should not shrug up toward your ears or collapse inward. Instead, they should remain stable and coordinated, with the scapulae smoothly gliding across the rib cage to support the arms and torso. This movement pattern reduces strain on the shoulder joints and optimizes force transfer during the exercise.

NOTE: *If your hips tend to sag (lower) or pike (rise) during push-ups, it could be a sign of insufficient core stability. To correct this, focus on full-body irradiation as described above. If the issue persists, refer to the Core Stability B (Prone) Linchpin Blueprint on page 473 for a deeper dive into buttressing pillar stability.*

PUSH ASSESSMENT

Shoulder pain is one of the most common complaints among lifters, particularly during exercises like the barbell bench press. The fixed hand and shoulder blade positions required by a barbell, combined with a lack of pillar stability, often create a perfect storm for discomfort and dysfunction. But pinpointing the root cause isn't always straightforward. Is it poor execution, a lack of stability, or an underlying structural limitation? Without a clear assessment process, it's easy to fall into guesswork, repeatedly addressing symptoms instead of solving the problem.

The push assessments eliminate this guesswork by examining the unique movement qualities, structural considerations, and mobility limitations that influence your ability to press—both horizontally and vertically—effectively and without pain. By breaking down the push pattern into key components, these assessments highlight how well your shoulders, scapulae, and core contribute to stability, alignment, and force production throughout the movement. Not everyone is structurally or functionally equipped to perform these exercises in the same way. Anatomy, joint structure, and individual anthropometric differences (limb lengths, bone structure, and joint angles) all play a role in how efficiently and comfortably you can execute pressing movements.

This is where the push assessment proves essential. It uses two key tests: the **Shoulder Scour Test** and the **Overhead Range of Motion Test**. Together, these tests isolate a specific aspect of the push pattern to identify your optimal position and range of motion. With these findings, you'll gain a clear picture of your movement capacity and identify the adjustments needed to optimize your push mechanics so that you can build mobility, stability, and skill in a way that aligns with your body's unique structure.

SHOULDER SCOUR TEST— DETERMINING YOUR OPTIMAL ARM PATH

The Shoulder Scour Test is a systematic assessment designed to identify your optimal arm angle for pressing movements—whether horizontal, vertical, or anywhere in between. By isolating and testing one arm at a time at specific angles, the test reveals your *humeral carrying angle*—the natural angle between your upper arm and torso—and how it influences your pressing mechanics. This insight helps pinpoint where your shoulder feels the most stable, strong, and unrestricted while also highlighting potential imbalances or asymmetries between your left and right sides.

Each step involves a controlled movement backward through specific angles, allowing you to assess your range of motion, stability, and muscular engagement at each position. To enhance accuracy, it's helpful to film yourself from both front and side angles. This provides a clear visual reference for evaluating movement quality, spotting compensatory patterns, and making informed adjustments.

At the core of this assessment is the principle of *joint centration*—the optimal alignment of the ball-and-socket shoulder joint. Proper centration creates a stable foundation for the rotator cuff to dynamically stabilize your shoulder, allowing larger muscles like the pecs, anterior deltoids, and triceps to generate pushing forces efficiently. Without joint centration, these stabilizers struggle to do their job, leading to compensatory movement patterns, increased soft tissue stress, and, eventually, chronic pain or injury. This is why the Shoulder Scour Test focuses so heavily on controlled movement and minimizing compensations—it ensures that what you're observing is authentic movement rather than a workaround for instability.

ADDRESSING ASYMMETRIES

Asymmetries between your dominant and non-dominant shoulders are completely natural—everyone has them. But if your sport or daily activities favor one side, like throwing a baseball, swinging a tennis racket, or carrying heavy loads in one hand, those imbalances become more pronounced. These repetitive patterns can create structural differences in your shoulders over time, altering your humeral carrying angle and influencing your pressing mechanics.

The **Shoulder Scour Test** helps identify these imbalances by isolating and assessing each arm individually. If you notice a discrepancy of more than 20 percent between sides—whether in range of motion, stability, or muscle engagement—it's essential to address it intelligently rather than forcing both sides into the same setup. For most people, small asymmetries are a natural part of movement and often fall within a functional range that doesn't compromise stability, alignment, or strength. These slight differences rarely cause significant compensations or stress on the joints, allowing you to press effectively without requiring adjustments. However, moderate asymmetries may require slight changes in hand positioning, grip style, or pressing angle to ensure optimal alignment and stability for each side.

For example:

- If one arm feels more stable at a narrower angle and the other prefers a wider position, you may need to adjust your arm path in open-chain exercises (e.g., dumbbell presses and cable presses) to accommodate these differences.

- In closed-chain exercises like push-ups, you might need to stagger your hand placement slightly or focus on stabilizing one side more deliberately during setup. Another effective adjustment is choosing an exercise or setup that manages depth and range of motion by using tools like parallettes or dumbbells, which allow for greater control and joint alignment.

For individuals with extreme asymmetries—often resulting from years of high-level athletics or chronic overuse—a fixed hand position on a barbell may never be optimal. These cases benefit from tools that offer freedom of movement, such as dumbbells and cables, or even specific push-up variations that allow for slight hand-angle adjustments.

However, it's important not to overreact to minor differences. True structural outliers are rare, and most people fall within a manageable range of asymmetry that can be addressed with thoughtful adjustments to pressing mechanics. The goal is always joint centration: keeping the ball-and-socket joint aligned, stable, and supported throughout your pressing movements. By focusing on pillar alignment and stability rather than forcing symmetry where it doesn't naturally exist, you'll build a stronger, safer, and more efficient push pattern tailored to your unique structure.

The goal of the Shoulder Scour Test isn't just to determine an arbitrary angle; it's to uncover your *optimal pressing mechanics*. For some, a higher humeral carrying angle (closer to 90 degrees) suggests a wider grip and pronated hand positioning. For others, a lower carrying angle (closer to 0 degrees) points to a narrower grip and a neutral hand position. Those who fall somewhere in the mid-range (around 45 degrees) enjoy more versatility, with the freedom to switch between pronated and neutral grips effectively. This optimal angle becomes your blueprint, not just for horizontal pressing but for every pressing variation—from bench presses and push-ups to overhead pressing movements.

Understanding and applying the results of the Shoulder Scour Test bridges the gap between assessment and execution. By identifying your most stable and functional arm angle, you're no longer forcing your body into standardized positions that might not align with your unique structure. Instead, you're tailoring your pressing setup to match your natural mechanics, reducing unnecessary stress on your shoulders and elbows while enhancing performance.

Here's what you're looking for in the Shoulder Scour Test:

RANGE OF MOTION:

How far your elbow travels backward at each angle without compensating through shoulder shrugging, back arching, or torso rotation. Optimal range of motion ensures your shoulder joint can move freely and efficiently through pressing motions. Restrictions at certain angles may indicate mobility limitations or structural differences that could impact your setup and execution.

STABILITY:

Your ability to maintain joint centration (optimal ball-and-socket alignment) while moving through each angle without losing control or relying on compensatory patterns. Stability serves as the foundation for strength and efficient movement. Without it, smaller muscles may overcompensate, increasing strain on soft tissues and heightening the risk of injury.

CO-CONTRACTION OF MUSCLES:

The degree to which your pecs and lats engage to stabilize your shoulder joint throughout each angle. Balanced muscular engagement creates stability and control, preventing inefficient pressing mechanics. Insufficient co-contraction can lead to compensatory patterns and increased soft tissue strain.

ASYMMETRIES BETWEEN SIDES:

Differences in range of motion, stability, or muscular engagement between your dominant and non-dominant arms. These imbalances can create compensatory patterns during pressing exercises, placing uneven stress on the shoulders and increasing injury risk. Addressing these differences helps establish a more balanced and efficient push pattern.

OPTIMAL ARM ANGLE:

The angle (0, 45, or 90 degrees) where your arm achieves the greatest range of motion, stability, and balanced muscular engagement without compensation. While testing these three positions, most people will naturally fall between 40 and 60 degrees, which is why 45 degrees serves as the default for pressing and pulling mechanics. This position optimizes joint alignment, maximizes muscle recruitment, and minimizes unnecessary stress on the shoulders—making it the most effective reference point for upper body push/pull patterns.

SHOULDER SCOUR TEST

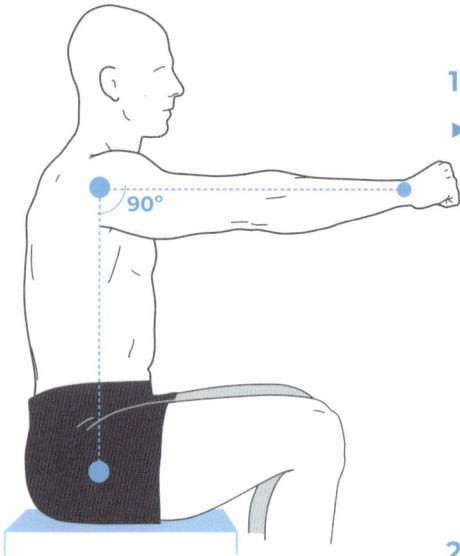

1. STARTING POSITION

▶ **Action:** Sit upright with a neutral spine. Raise one arm to shoulder height so that your humerus (upper arm) is parallel to the floor, forming a 90-degree angle with your torso. Co-contract your pecs and lats to achieve and amplify joint centration.

▶ **Goal:** Establish a stable and consistent starting position to ensure accuracy throughout the test.

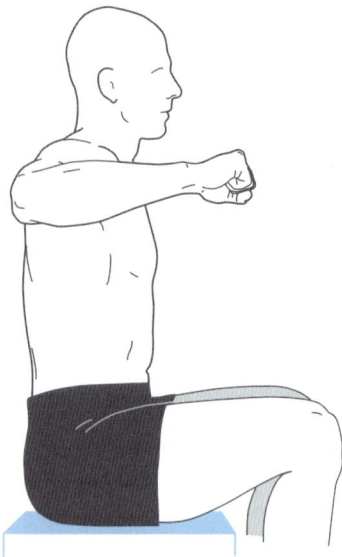

2. 90 DEGREES

▶ **Action:** With one arm raised to shoulder height, slowly pull your elbow back as far as you can while maintaining the 90-degree angle relative to your torso and co-contraction through your pecs and lats. Move with control, avoiding compensations like shrugging your shoulder, rotating your torso, or arching your lower back.

▶ **Goal:** Assess your shoulder's ability to move backward while maintaining joint centration and tension through your pecs and lats.

▶ **Observation:** Pay attention to how far back your elbow travels and whether you can maintain shoulder stability throughout the movement. Note if there is tightness, restriction, or discomfort in the shoulder joint. Observe if your range of motion feels limited or smooth and whether you lose tension through your pecs and lats.

3. 0 DEGREES

▶ **Action:** Get into the starting position. Slowly pull your elbow back while keeping your elbow close to your body, forming a 0-degree angle with your torso. As with the previous step, avoid compensations while maintaining tension in your pecs and lats to keep the shoulder joint stable.

▶ **Goal:** Assess your shoulder's ability to move through extension with your arm tight to your body. This position assesses shoulder extension mechanics in a different angle compared to the 90-degree test.

▶ **Observation:** Notice how far your elbow moves behind your torso. Does this position feel more restricted or smoother than the 90-degree test?

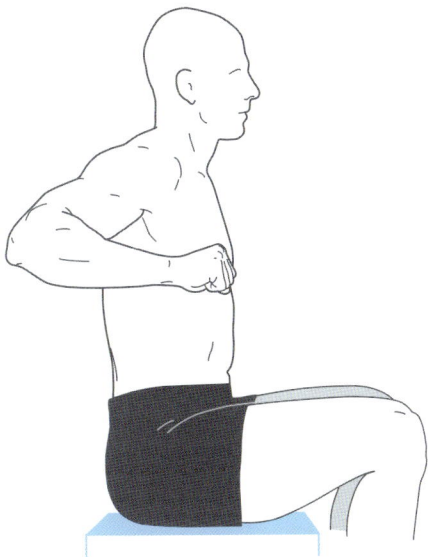

4. 45 DEGREES

▶ **Action:** Get into the starting position and then pull your arm back halfway between the 90- and 0-degree positions, forming a 45-degree angle with your torso.

▶ **Goal:** Determine your shoulder's ability to move through this middle range while maintaining joint centration and muscular co-contraction (pecs, lats, and rotator cuff working synergistically to stabilize the shoulder joint).

▶ **Observation:** Assess the smoothness of movement and overall stability in this position. Does your shoulder feel more free and stable here compared to the 0- and 90-degree positions? Do you have more range of motion?

Repeat each step with your opposite arm, noting any differences between sides.

5. ADJUST AND ASSESS

▶ **Action:** Experiment with slight adjustments above and below the 45-degree angle. Repeat the elbow extension test one arm at a time at these new positions to see how they influence your range and stability.

▶ **Goal:** Identify the angle where you achieve the greatest range of motion and shoulder stability without compensations.

▶ **Observation:** Observe how far your elbow moves back and whether the movement feels smooth or restricted. Do slight adjustments create better stability and freedom of movement? The angle where you experience the most range and control will serve as your optimal arm path for pressing and pulling.

6. TRANSFER TO THE PUSH-UP AND RETEST

▶ **Action:** Apply the findings from the Shoulder Scour Test to your push-up setup and execution.

• **Higher Carrying Angle (closer to 90°):** Wider grip, typically pronated hand positioning.

• **Lower Carrying Angle (closer to 0°):** Narrower grip, often favoring neutral hand positioning.

• **Mid-Range Angle (around 45°):** More freedom with hand positioning, allowing you to comfortably switch between neutral and pronated grips.

▶ **Goal:** Adjust your arm angle to match the optimal carrying angle identified during the assessment. Retest the push screen, adhering to the optimization checklist (neutral spine, no rotation, full-body irradiation, and proper shoulder/scapular positioning).

▶ **Observation:** Does the push-up feel smoother, more stable, and more controlled? Has anterior shoulder discomfort or instability improved? Do your shoulders, core, and hips feel more integrated and aligned? If the answer is yes, the assessment has successfully identified and corrected key limitations, setting you up for stronger, more efficient, and pain-free pressing patterns.

OVERHEAD RANGE OF MOTION TEST— DETERMINING YOUR VERTICAL PRESSING MOBILITY

The Overhead Range of Motion Test is designed to answer a critical question: Can you access the overhead position with good form? For many people, the inability to perform overhead pressing movements isn't about strength—it's about an inability to achieve proper overhead positioning in the first place. This test evaluates whether you have the mobility, stability, and motor control necessary to extend your arms fully overhead while maintaining alignment through your pillar. If you can't get into the position unweighted, it's a clear indicator that training overhead movements with weight could reinforce poor mechanics and increase your risk of pain.

This assessment is simple yet highly effective. The goal is to observe three key factors as you attempt to bring your arms overhead: range of motion, quality of movement, and pain response. Optimal range typically falls between 165 and 180 degrees, with your biceps aligned close to your ears. Beyond the range, you're looking for how smooth and symmetrical the movement appears: Do your shoulder blades glide evenly, or do they get stuck? Finally, you need to determine if achieving this position triggers pain or discomfort, which signals a deeper restriction or imbalance that needs to be addressed.

When overhead mobility is restricted, people often assume it's purely a mobility issue. They'll stretch their lats, foam-roll their upper back, and repeat this cycle without seeing any meaningful progress. While mobility limitations are common, they're only one piece of the puzzle. Stability and motor control play an equally important role. The test differentiates between a true mobility restriction, where tissues physically prevent full range of motion, and a stability or skill deficit, where the body lacks control or confidence in the overhead position.

To tease out the distinction between a mobility deficit (e.g., tight lats or thoracic immobility) and a stability or skill deficit (e.g., an inability to control or stabilize the shoulder joint through its full range of motion), the test should be performed in two positions: standing and lying down.

When standing, your body must manage gravity, pillar alignment, and core stability—all factors that challenge your ability to achieve a clean overhead position. Think of it as a functional screen. If you can get overhead with good form and no pain, then there's no need to perform the assessment lying down because you already meet the standards for training the vertical pattern.

If you can't get overhead without pain or restriction, however, you need more information to work with. More specifically, you need to determine whether it is a mobility, stability, or skill issue, which is what the supine test is for.

By transitioning to a lying position, stability is built into the system. The floor provides passive support for your spine and shoulder blades, removing the variable of motor control. If you gain range in this position compared to standing, mobility isn't the issue—it's an inability to stabilize in space. In this scenario, you will follow the Overhead Stability Linchpin Blueprint (page 474), focusing on corrective exercises (phase 3), activation drills (phase 4), and movement pattern development (phase 5) to build the necessary stability and skill before adding load or speed to the position.

Conversely, if the restriction remains the same in both positions, then mobility is likely the true limiting factor. In this case, you will implement targeted interventions to improve overhead range of motion, such as soft tissue work (phase 1) and stretching (phase 2)—both of which are covered in the Overhead Stability Linchpin Blueprint (page 474).

The tests also provide valuable insight into right-to-left discrepancies. If one arm moves freely into the overhead position while the other remains restricted, it highlights an imbalance that shouldn't be ignored. In this case, pure bilateral vertical pressing isn't ideal. Instead of forcing both arms into a compromised range, modifying the movement with angled pressing variations, such as landmine presses, allows you to train within your available range while working toward improved mobility and stability. These adjustments ensure that the body isn't compensating elsewhere—such as at the lower back or rib cage—to make up for a lack of authentic overhead motion.

It's important to remember that the goal of this assessment isn't to force a textbook-perfect 180-degree overhead position (biceps slightly behind or aligned with the ears). Most people fall somewhere between 165 and 175 degrees (biceps slightly in front of the ears), with slight variations based on individual structure and mobility. While slight limitations in overhead range aren't necessarily a problem, attempting to press with poor positioning is. External load can sometimes help "fill in" the last few degrees by providing joint compression and stabilization, but that only works when the movement pattern itself is sound. If you're forcing the position and compensating just to get overhead, adding weight is only going to make things worse.

This is where old-school thinking often leads lifters astray. Some lifters, particularly those with a strongman or powerlifting background, cling to the idea that the overhead press—particularly with a barbell—is a make-or-break lift for shoulder development. But if they can't even lift their own arms overhead without compensating, what makes them think adding load is a good idea? When they force it, they don't just struggle with the press itself—they contort their entire body to make it happen. Instead of pressing straight up, they overextend their lower back, dump their pelvis into anterior tilt, and lean into the movement. Their knees drift forward, their hips shift back, and the whole thing starts to resemble a standing bench press—except instead of using a bench for support, they're hanging off their lumbar spine.

When pressing becomes an exercise in compensating rather than reinforcing good movement patterns, the risk outweighs the reward. And while most people hyper-fixate on the shoulders in overhead work, it's the lower back that usually pays the price. Hyperextension under load can be just as detrimental as hyperflexion or excessive spinal rounding in a deadlift. Neither is ideal, especially when it breaks the foundational principles of pain-free performance.

Instead of fighting against your body, use these tests to determine where you stand—then train accordingly. Whether the focus needs to be on mobility, stability, or alternative pressing strategies, the goal is the same: pain-free, sustainable training that respects your body's natural abilities.

OVERHEAD RANGE OF MOTION TEST

STANDING

1. STARTING POSITION

▶ **Action:** Stand tall with your feet hip-width apart, maintaining a neutral spine. Let your arms hang naturally at your sides with palms facing inward and thumbs pointing forward. Go through the pillar cueing sequence to stabilize your hips, shoulders, and core.

▶ **Goal:** Establish a controlled, upright posture with a neutral and braced pillar.

2. RAISE YOUR ARMS AND ASSESS SCAPULAR ROTATION

▶ **Action:** Slowly raise both arms straight in front of your shoulders, keeping your elbows fully extended. As your arms pass 90 degrees, observe how your shoulder blades begin to rotate upward. Continue raising your arms to a full overhead position, ensuring that the scapulae move smoothly and in sync with your arms. The movement should be pure shoulder flexion, without excessive arching in the lower back or shrugging at the shoulders.

▶ **Goal:** Achieve an overhead position where your biceps align near your ears, aiming for 165 to 180 degrees of elevation. Your shoulder blades should rotate at a 2:1 ratio relative to arm elevation—meaning for every 2 degrees of arm movement past 90 degrees, the scapulae should rotate 1 degree in an upward direction. This movement should be fluid, coordinated, and symmetrical.

▶ **Observation:** Assess for any deviations, such as one arm reaching higher than the other, excessive shrugging, or an inability to reach the target range. From a side or back view, assess whether the shoulder blades rotate at the same rate and to the same extent. If one shoulder blade moves more or less than the other, or if there are abrupt shifts instead of a smooth transition, it suggests an imbalance, mobility restriction, or motor control deficiency.

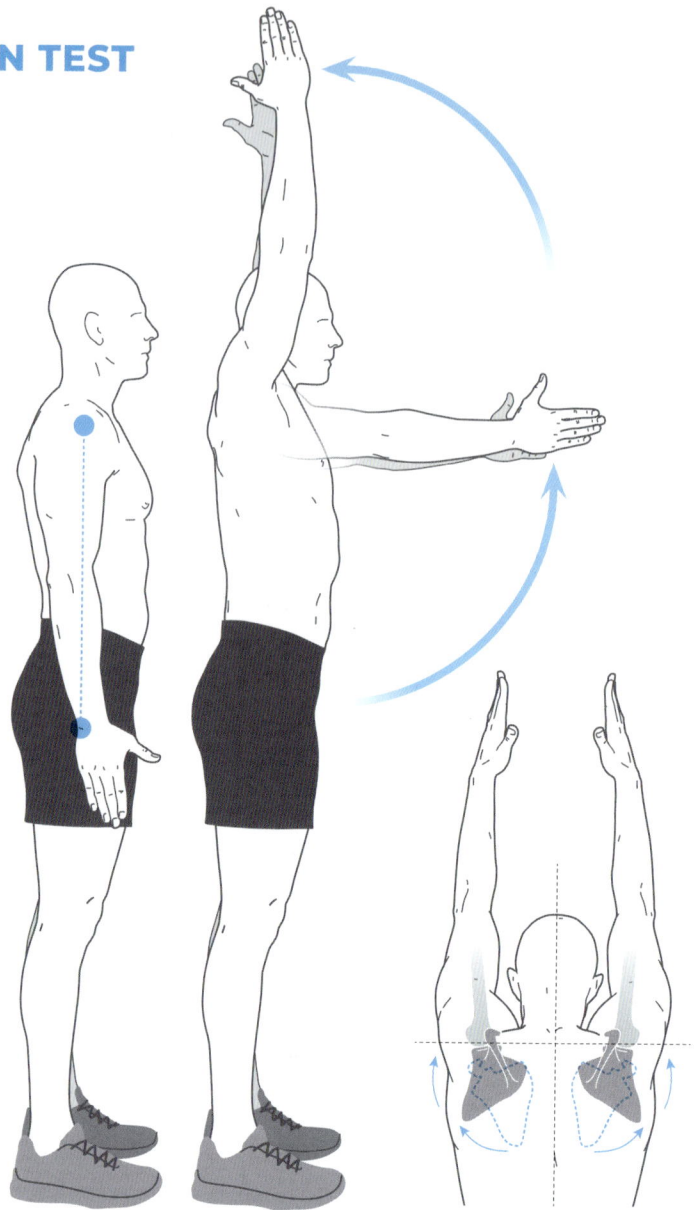

3. EVALUATE OVERHEAD POSITION

▶ **Action:** Hold the overhead position briefly to assess comfort and control.

▶ **Goal:** A high-quality overhead position should feel stable and unrestricted, with the scapulae properly rotated and no compensatory shifts in the lower back, pelvis, or neck.

▶ **Observation:** Note your position.

• **If you can achieve the overhead position without compensation,** you can train the vertical pattern and there is no need to perform the supine test.

• **If you are unable to get into the overhead position or compensation is needed to raise your arms,** perform the supine test to determine whether this issue is linked to mobility or motor control.

SUPINE

1. STARTING POSITION

▶ **Action:** Lie on your back with knees bent and feet flat on the ground. Keep your lower back in neutral contact with the floor. Position your arms at your sides with palms facing inward.

▶ **Goal:** Establish a stable, neutral position that removes the demand for postural control, allowing for a pure assessment of mobility.

▶ **Observation:** Ensure that your lower back remains neutral throughout the test. Excessive lumbar extension may falsely indicate greater shoulder mobility than is actually available.

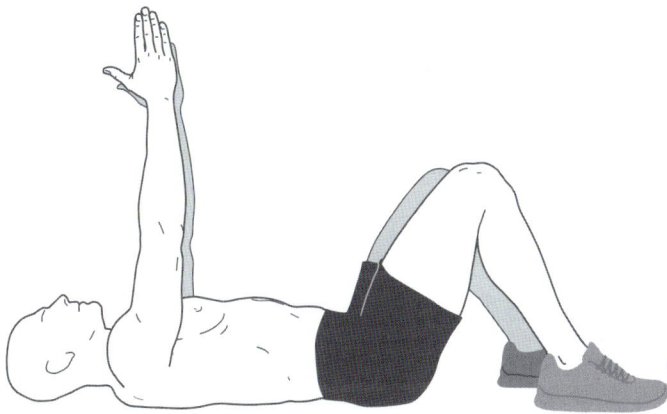

2. RAISE YOUR ARMS

▶ **Action:** Slowly raise both arms overhead while keeping your back, ribs, and shoulder blades in contact with the floor. Move with control, avoiding excessive momentum or force.

▶ **Goal:** Reach an overhead position where your arms approach 180 degrees without your rib cage lifting or the spine compensating. The movement should feel smooth and unrestricted, with no pinching or discomfort.

▶ **Observation:** Compare the supine range of motion to the standing test.

• If overhead range is significantly better in this position, the limitation is not a mobility issue but a stability or motor control deficit (see **Overhead Stability Linchpin Blueprint** on page 474).

• If the restriction remains the same in both positions, true mobility deficits (such as tight lats or thoracic stiffness) are likely the cause (see **Shoulder Mobility B (Vertical) Linchpin Blueprint** on page 472).

3. TESTING UNILATERAL OVERHEAD MOTION

▶ **Action:** If bilateral movement is limited or asymmetric, perform the test one arm at a time to assess side-to-side discrepancies. Raise one arm while keeping the other stationary.

▶ **Goal:** Identify whether one side has significantly better range of motion than the other. Single-arm testing also helps determine if asymmetries improve when movement is uncoupled from the opposite side.

▶ **Observation:** If one arm reaches full overhead while the other remains restricted, follow the vertical push progression pyramid to train within your available range while addressing asymmetrical deviations. This approach allows you to modify pressing angles, incorporate single-arm variations, and introduce exercises that help unlock overhead mobility on the restricted side without forcing compensations or reinforcing imbalances.

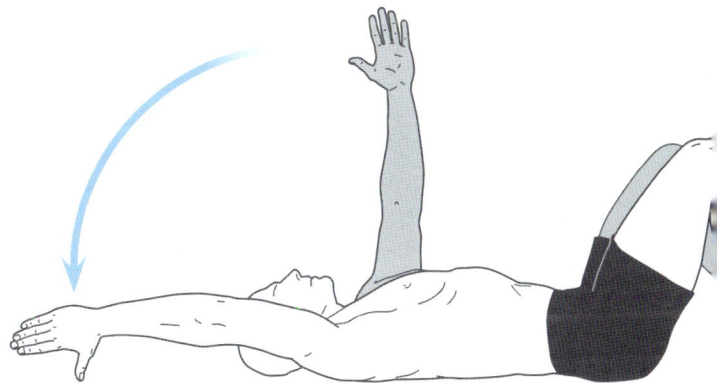

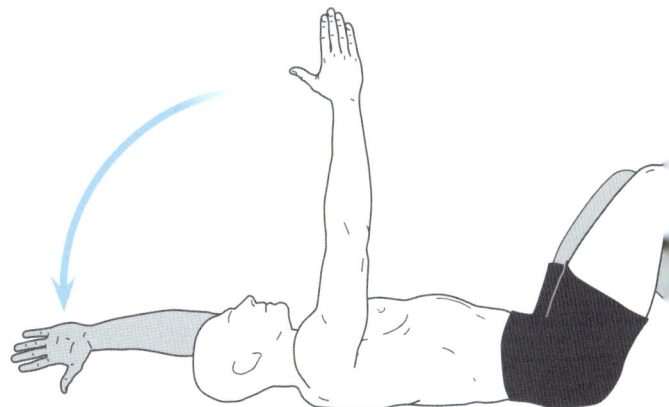

OPTIMIZATION STRATEGIES

The strategies in this section are designed to help you refine your push mechanics by directly addressing compensations found during your push screen and overhead assessment. These compensations are your body's way of working around limitations—usually related to **mobility, stability, or skill deficits**—and can eventually cause discomfort, instability, or stalled progress if ignored.

The goal here is proactive improvement. Rather than waiting until inefficiencies become painful or hinder performance, you can use targeted strategies to get ahead of these compensations, making your push movements smoother, stronger, and pain-free.

Let's break down the most common push pattern compensations and explore how targeted optimization strategies can move you closer to movement mastery.

NOTE: *Compensations observed in the push-up often appear in other pressing exercises too. Improving your push mechanics through these strategies not only addresses immediate movement faults, but also enhances your overall upper body function, creating a positive carryover into all upper body movements.*

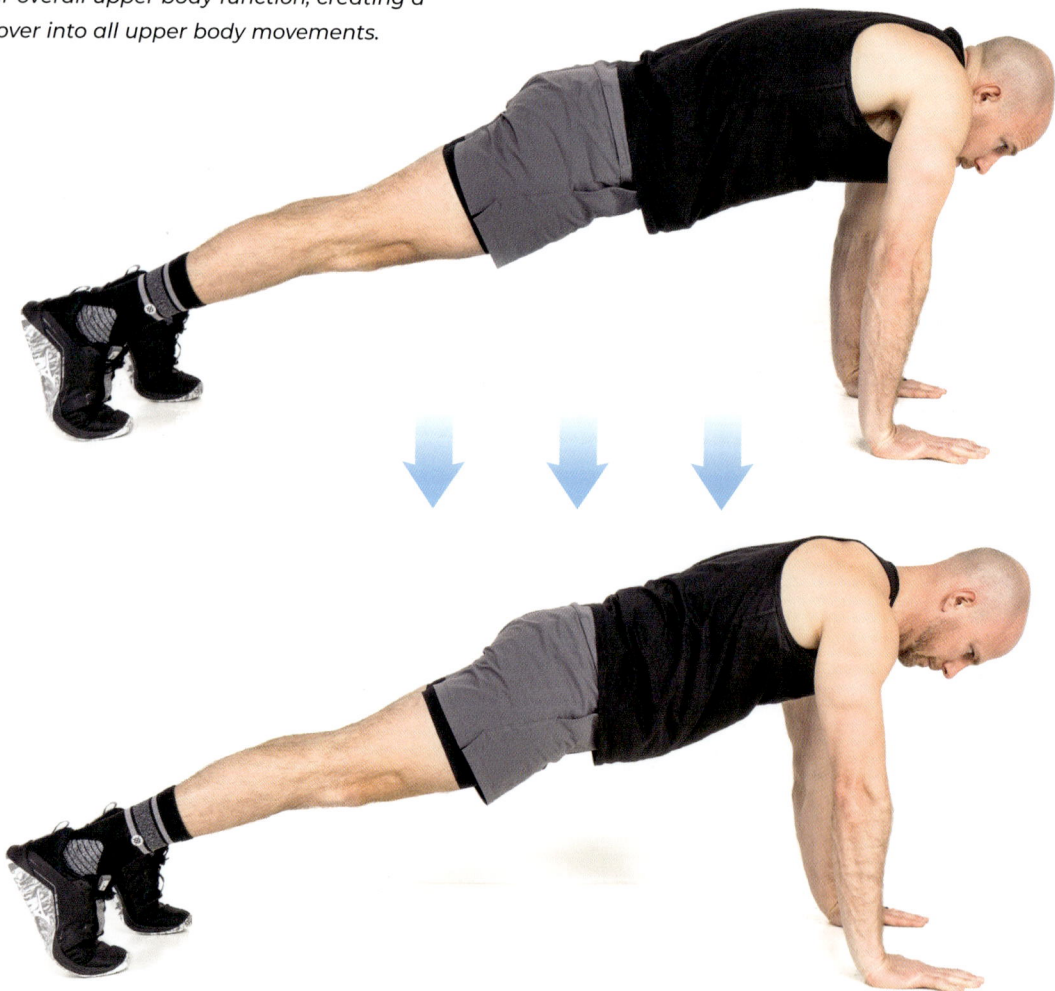

COMPENSATION: SHOULDER ELEVATION (SHOULDERS RISE OR ROUND FORWARD DURING PUSH/PRESS MOVEMENTS)

MOBILITY: Tight pecs or upper traps—often due to overtraining push movements, excessive desk work, or constantly looking down at your phone—can create muscular imbalances that inhibit proper pressing mechanics. Signs you may have a mobility restriction:

▼ Tightness across your chest or the front of your shoulders when opening your arms into a T-shape

▼ Upper trap or neck muscles feel tight or achy, and/or you constantly feel like your shoulders are creeping up toward your ears when pressing

OPTIMIZATION STRATEGIES:

▶ Perform the **Shoulder Mobility A (Horizontal) Linchpin Blueprint** (page 471), focusing on your pecs in phases 1 and 2.

▶ Choose exercises that allow you to train within a pain-free range of motion without compensation while working to improve mobility (e.g., push-ups to a pad/block or dumbbell floor presses).

▶ Audit your program to ensure a 3:1 pull-to-push ratio, incorporating pulling exercises from multiple angles with rotational movements.

▶ Incorporate post-workout stretches such as the 90/90 chest stretch and prone chest stretch, along with daily mobility drills like the quadruped thoracic spine rotation.

STABILITY: Shoulder stability involves proper rib cage positioning, scapular movement, and centration of the glenohumeral (GH) joint. Poor posture, a weak core, undertrained stabilizing muscles, or repetitive movement patterns in daily life can all contribute to an unstable shoulder joint. Challenges associated with poor stability may present as

▼ Feeling your traps in the top of the push-up (high-plank position)

▼ Anterior shoulder discomfort or difficulty achieving joint centration in pushing or pulling movements

▼ Difficulty keeping dumbbells steady during pressing exercises

OPTIMIZATION STRATEGIES:

▶ Perform the **Scapular Stability Linchpin Blueprint** (page 473).

▶ Focus on pillar setup by co-contracting the pecs and lats to stabilize the shoulders. Move slowly and with control, maintaining proper joint alignment throughout the range of motion.

▶ Use exercises that allow your hands to rotate (e.g., dumbbell presses, cable or band exercises) to encourage natural rotation and improve joint centration.

SKILL: The shoulder is the most mobile joint in the body, so there is significant range of motion available. Learning to move purposefully through different angles, with different tools, for various tasks requires smart training progression and sufficient time building competence at each stage. Without proper skill development, mobility and stability alone cannot prevent compensations. Indicators of a skill gap include

▼ Difficulty maintaining total-body irradiation, optimal shoulder and scapular positioning, or a controlled tempo (especially during the eccentric/lowering phase of a movement)

▼ Defaulting to compensatory patterns (shoulder rounding or elevation) during pressing movements

OPTIMIZATION STRATEGIES:

▶ Begin your upper body workouts with the **Scapular Stability Linchpin Blueprint** (page 473) to reinforce alignment and joint control.

▶ Use the pillar cueing sequence when setting up (see the Pillar chapter for detailed instructions for stabilizing the pillar).

▶ Regress exercise variations to control your range of motion, maintain stability, and build competency. Examples include push-ups with pads/blocks, incline push-ups, or floor presses.

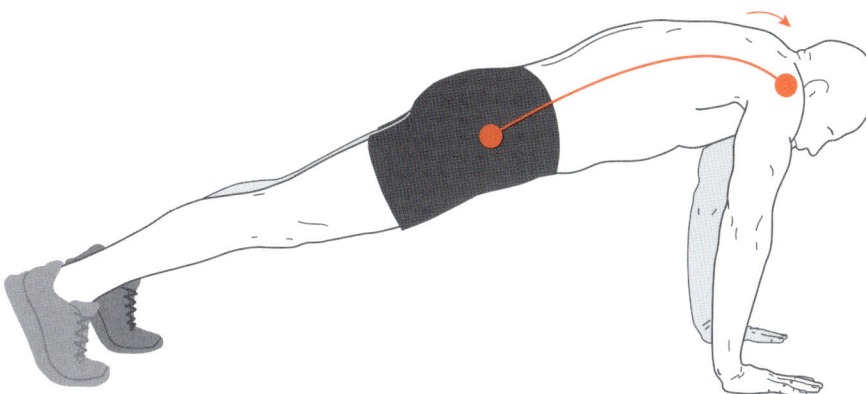

COMPENSATION: ASYMMETRY/ UNWANTED ROTATION

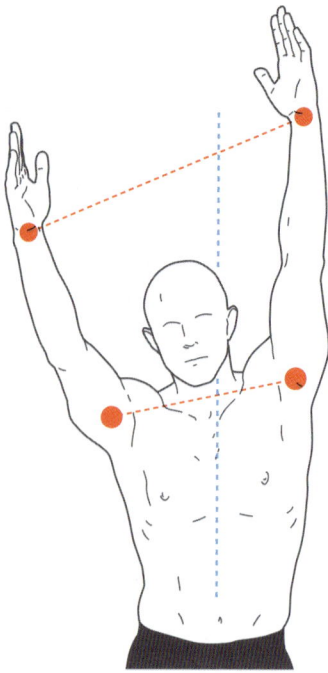

MOBILITY: Tightness or restrictions, often resulting from repetitive daily activities, desk work, or dominant-hand tasks, can lead to asymmetrical or uneven movements. You may have a mobility restriction if you

▼ Feel tightness or restriction on one side compared to the other during stretches or pressing or pulling movements

▼ One arm moves farther back than the other when performing the **Shoulder Scour Test**

OPTIMIZATION STRATEGIES:

▶ Perform the **Shoulder Mobility B (Vertical) Linchpin Blueprint** (page 472) to mobilize tight or restricted tissues.

▶ Use your authentic hand position as determined by the **Shoulder Scour Test**, allowing for slight differences in hand placement or rotation to ensure proper joint centration.

▶ Choose exercise variations that allow training within your authentic range of motion, controlling asymmetries as you improve mobility (e.g., dumbbell floor presses, push-ups to blocks/ pads to pins).

STABILITY: Since most people have a dominant side for writing and fine motor skills, it's common for one side to feel more stable than the other. This natural stability difference can be amplified by repetitive activities like racket or throwing sports, as well as previous injuries—such as a shoulder dislocation—which often reduce strength, confidence, and joint control. These experiences reinforce asymmetrical patterns, increasing the likelihood of instability or imbalance between sides. Indicators of instability include

▼ One shoulder feeling less stable or weaker during pressing or pulling movements

▼ Difficulty co-contracting pecs and lats equally, resulting in uneven muscle activation between sides

OPTIMIZATION STRATEGIES:

▶ Perform the **Overhead Stability Linchpin Blueprint** (page 474).

▶ Pay close attention to pillar setup by co-contracting your pecs and lats to stabilize your shoulders. Use a slow, controlled tempo through the full range of motion to maintain joint alignment and control.

▶ In dumbbell, kettlebell, or cable exercises, focus on squeezing your grip tighter to increase irradiation and enhance stability in the arm and shoulder.

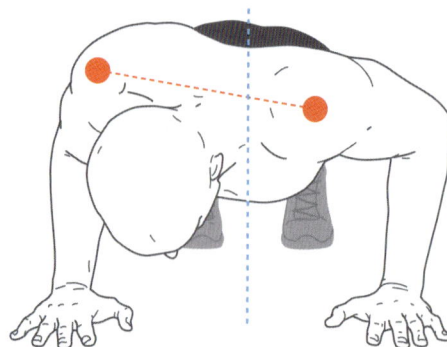

SKILL: Repetitive movement creates ingrained motor patterns— whether optimal or suboptimal— which means that your dominant side may naturally feel stronger, more stable, and more coordinated than your non-dominant side. When learning a new movement or refining technique, this imbalance can lead to one side taking over, disrupting symmetry in pressing patterns. Signs of a skill gap include

▼ Unequal stability or strength between sides when performing push or press exercises

▼ One elbow or side of your torso dropping faster or lower than the other

OPTIMIZATION STRATEGIES:

▶ Perform the **Overhead Stability Linchpin Blueprint** (page 474).

▶ Use supported exercises like the machine chest press or control the depth of movement to maintain symmetry and alignment as you refine your pressing mechanics.

▶ Pay attention to pillar setup by co-contracting your pecs and lats to stabilize your shoulders. Move slowly and deliberately, performing each repetition with full-body control and joint alignment before progressing in load or complexity.

▶ Develop proficiency with lighter loads before progressing to ensure even strength and movement quality on both sides.

▶ Incorporate unilateral (single-arm) dumbbell exercises into your routine to target and build proficiency on your weaker side.

COMPENSATION: ELBOWS FLARING OUT

MOBILITY: Tight pecs or lats can force your body to adjust its natural movement patterns, altering your humeral carrying angle to find an "easier" way to complete the exercise. Instead of maintaining optimal alignment, your body compensates by flaring your elbows outward, often leading to shoulder instability and inefficient force production. Indicators of mobility restrictions include

▼ Difficulty maintaining proper elbow position due to tightness or restriction in the chest or lats

▼ Feeling tension or tightness in the chest or front of the shoulders when lowering into a push-up position (or performing the **Shoulder Scour Test**)

OPTIMIZATION STRATEGIES:

▶ Perform the **Shoulder Mobility A (Horizontal) Linchpin Blueprint** (page 471) to address tight pecs or **Shoulder Mobility B (Vertical) Linchpin Blueprint** (page 472) to address tight lats.

▶ Perform the **Shoulder Scour Test** and set up your push-up with the ideal humeral carrying angle determined from the assessment. You can also experiment with adjusting your hand position slightly (rotating your hands inward or outward) to help alleviate restrictions.

▶ Regress the push-up by elevating your hands or manage your depth by placing a pad or plate beneath your chest, ensuring you work within the range of motion you can control.

STABILITY: The shoulder is the most mobile joint in the body, but without dynamic stability, it struggles to produce and sustain force efficiently. If your shoulder blades fail to stabilize relative to your rib cage, or if the humeral head lacks centration, your elbows will naturally flare outward as a compensation strategy. Challenges associated with poor stability may present as

▼ Difficulty activating your lats and core in the high plank and press setup positions

▼ Fingers and palms losing contact with the ground during push-ups, preventing a strong base of support

OPTIMIZATION STRATEGIES:

▶ Perform the **Overhead Stability Linchpin Blueprint** (page 474) to improve lat activation.

▶ Use the humeral carrying angle determined by the **Shoulder Scour Test** to optimize joint alignment and range of motion.

▶ Focus on pillar setup and co-contracting your pecs and lats to stabilize your shoulders. Use a slow, controlled tempo through the full range of motion, maintaining control and alignment.

▶ Regress the push-up to an elevated push-up or limit depth using a pad or plate under your chest to maintain proper mechanics while reinforcing shoulder stability.

SKILL: Maintaining proper alignment and full-body irradiation can be challenging. If your elbows flare, it may signal a lack of coordination, especially under load or stress. Signs of a skill gap include

▼ Difficulty maintaining total-body tension and stable shoulder/elbow alignment throughout the push-up, especially when descending or pushing up from the bottom position

▼ Loss of full palm-to-ground contact as you lower, especially as fatigue accumulates or when moving quickly

OPTIMIZATION STRATEGIES:

▶ Perform the **Overhead Stability Linchpin Blueprint** (page 474).

▶ Set up your pillar carefully, using the ideal humeral carrying angle from your **Shoulder Scour Test**. Focus on maintaining a strong brace and full-body irradiation during the movement.

▶ Regress the push-up to an elevated push-up or control the depth by placing a pad or plate under your chest to maintain consistent alignment and proper technique while building your skill and capacity.

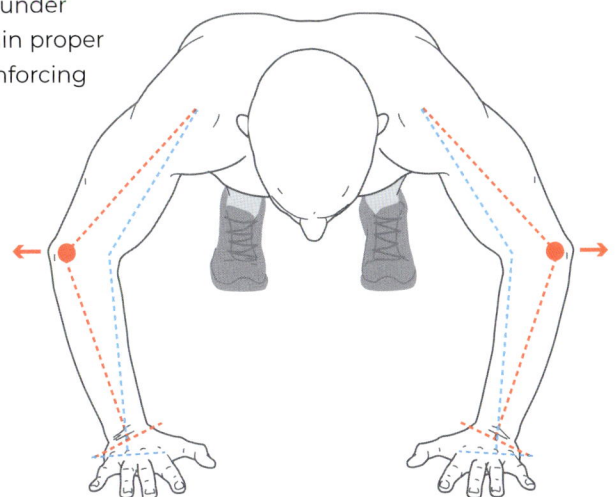

COMPENSATION: LOW BACK ARCH/RIB FLARE (VERTICAL PRESS)

MOBILITY: In the vertical pressing pattern, lat tightness is the most common mobility restriction, which you can uncover in the Overhead Range of Motion Test. The lats connect the humerus to the mid and lower back. When restricted, they limit shoulder flexion, contribute to internal rotation, and cause excessive rib flare and lumbar hyperextension during overhead movements. Signs you may have a mobility restriction include

▼ Difficulty achieving overhead positions without arching your lower back, which does not improve when lying supine during the push assessment

▼ Tightness or discomfort in your lower back during overhead pressing exercises

OPTIMIZATION STRATEGIES:

▶ Perform the **Shoulder Mobility B (Vertical) Linchpin Blueprint** (page 472), targeting the lats in phases 1 and 2.

▶ Choose pressing variations that allow you to train within a pain-free and stable range of motion. For example, you could perform landmine presses or incline presses that reduce overhead demand.

▶ Include mobility drills such as dumbbell pullovers or single-arm cable rows with rotation, staying within a pain-free range.

▶ Finish workouts with a mobility focus, such as foam rolling your lats, hinged T-spine extension and lat stretches, quadruped lat stretch, or child's pose variations.

STABILITY: Poor stability at the shoulder, rib cage, or core can lead to compensations such as lumbar hyperextension and rib flare. If your range of motion improves when performing the supine portion of the Overhead Range of Motion Test, this suggests that scapular stability is the primary limitation. Other indicators of instability include

▼ Difficulty maintaining core engagement or scapular control when pressing overhead

▼ Chronic stiffness in the traps and neck

▼ Shoulders elevating toward the ears during vertical pressing exercises

OPTIMIZATION STRATEGIES:

▶ Perform the **Overhead Stability Linchpin Blueprint** (page 474).

▶ Adjust your humeral angle to match your ideal pressing position based on the **Shoulder Scour Test**.

▶ Allow your wrists and arms to rotate naturally as you press overhead. Dumbbells provide more freedom of movement compared to barbells, which can improve joint centration and comfort.

▶ Manage your range of motion and pressing angles to match your pain-free, stable, and available positions. Unilateral exercises (one arm at a time) can help each shoulder move within its best "groove." If direct overhead pressing is problematic, consider angled alternatives like landmine presses or incline presses.

SKILL: When developing overhead pressing mechanics—whether as a beginner, after an injury, or following poor training habits—coordinating movement between the shoulder blades, thoracic spine, and glenohumeral joint can be challenging. A lack of movement awareness or control can lead to compensations like excessive rib flare or lumbar hyperextension, especially when load, speed, or fatigue increases. Without proper neuromuscular coordination, the body may default to using the lower back for stability instead of maintaining proper pillar alignment. Signs of a skill gap include

▼ Difficulty maintaining shoulder and spinal alignment during push/pull exercises

▼ Feeling weak or unstable at specific ranges of motion

OPTIMIZATION STRATEGIES:

▶ Perform the **Overhead Stability Linchpin Blueprint** (page 474) to reinforce postural awareness and strengthen underdeveloped stabilizing muscles in the posterior shoulder.

▶ Master horizontal push and pull variations at various angles before progressing to the vertical plane.

▶ Pay attention to pillar setup by co-contracting your pecs and lats to stabilize your shoulders. Use a slow, controlled tempo to maintain joint alignment and control.

▶ Use exercise variations that allow your hands to rotate, such as dumbbell presses or unilateral pressing movements, which enable better control and individualized movement quality for each shoulder. Adjust range of motion as needed to remain pain-free; gradually increase range as you gain skill and stability.

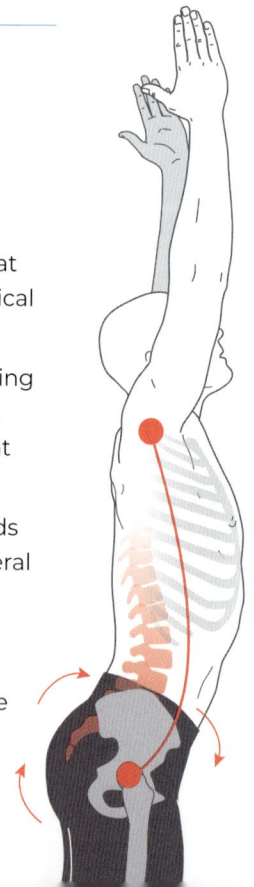

PUSH PROGRESSION PYRAMID

The push progression pyramid is about building real, lasting strength—not just loading up the bar and hoping for the best. Too many lifters chase bigger numbers without thinking about how they're moving, then wonder why their shoulders feel like junk or their progress suddenly stalls. Jumping straight into heavy barbell pressing without earning the position is like slamming the gas pedal on a car with bad alignment—eventually, something breaks down. By building mobility, stability, and skill in the right order, you're setting yourself up for pain-free, sustainable progress that actually goes somewhere.

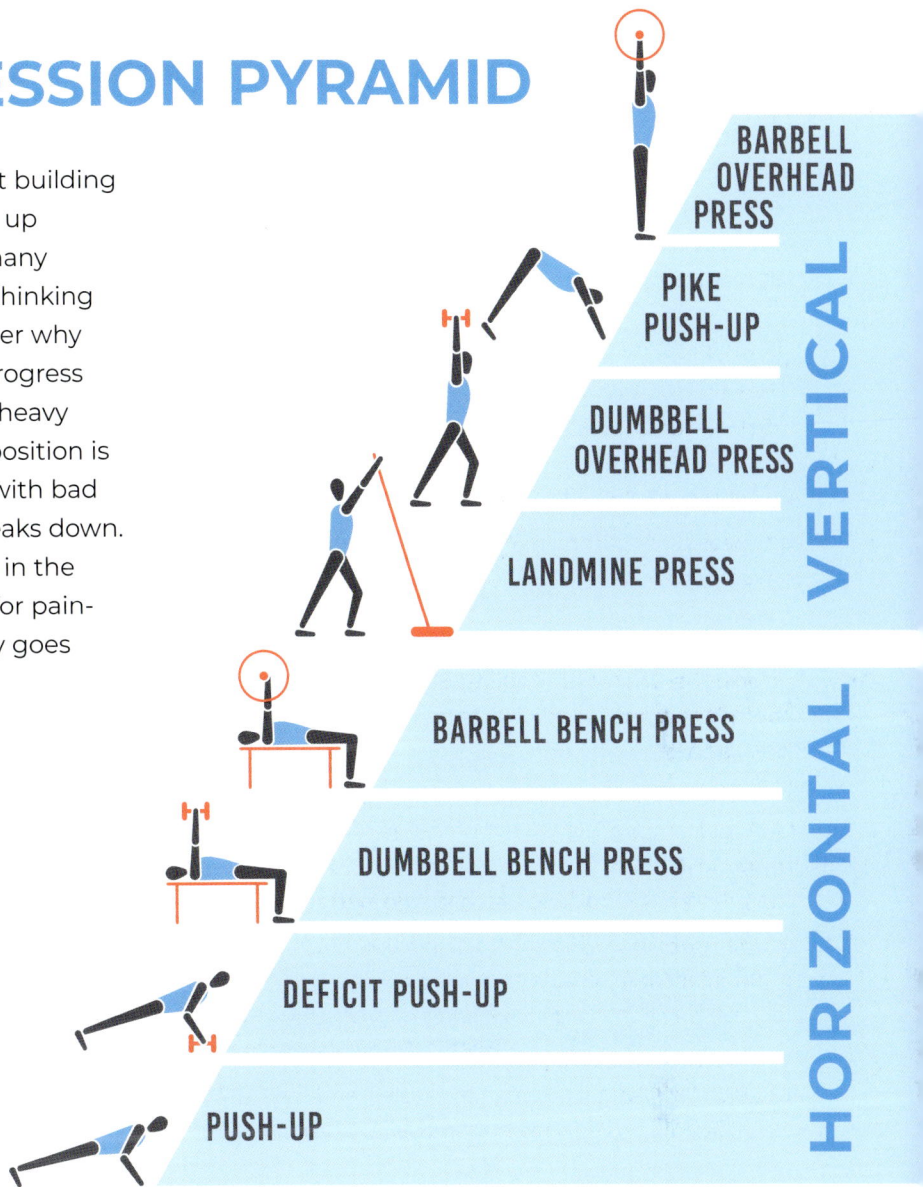

BARBELL OVERHEAD PRESS

PIKE PUSH-UP

DUMBBELL OVERHEAD PRESS

LANDMINE PRESS

VERTICAL

BARBELL BENCH PRESS

DUMBBELL BENCH PRESS

DEFICIT PUSH-UP

PUSH-UP

HORIZONTAL

The push pattern is divided into two primary categories: horizontal push and vertical push. Horizontal pressing is inherently more stable, making it easier to develop strength and control while keeping the shoulders and pillar engaged in a supported position. As movement shifts to the vertical plane, the demands on shoulder mobility, scapular control, and full-body stability increase dramatically. This is why vertical pressing tends to be more problematic—especially for those who lack the ability to achieve a clean overhead position without compensating through the lower back, rib cage, or pelvis.

The horizontal push progression starts with **push-ups**, which serve as both the movement screen and the foundation for pressing mechanics. Many lifters overlook push-ups, but they provide one of the best full-body pressing challenges by integrating scapular movement, pillar stability, and irradiation (tension throughout the entire body)—something a bench press alone cannot replicate.

Deficit push-ups are next in the progression, increasing the range of motion and reinforcing strength through a deeper stretch at the bottom position. This added depth challenges end-range strength while improving scapular mobility and reinforcing pressing mechanics before transitioning to open-chain, pillar-supported supine variations.

Once proficiency is built in the push-up and deficit variations, which can be loaded or unloaded, the progression shifts to **dumbbell bench pressing**. As an open-chain movement, the dumbbells allow for greater freedom of movement at the wrists and shoulders while maintaining external stability from a fixed surface, such as a bench. This transition reduces the full-body stabilization demands of push-ups, allowing for more targeted muscle and strength development through higher loads.

Next, **barbell bench pressing** enters the picture. This is where loading potential is highest, but it also comes with the greatest demands on joint stability. Unlike push-ups or dumbbell pressing, the barbell locks the hands into a fixed position, preventing rotation and natural scapular movement, which increases stress on the shoulders. By the time you reach this phase, you've built the mobility, stability, and skill necessary to handle these demands while maintaining clean mechanics.

Pressing strength doesn't stop at the horizontal plane. The push progression pyramid extends into vertical pressing, where the demands on mobility, scapular control, and full-body stability increase significantly. Just as horizontal pressing follows a structured path from body weight to external loading, vertical pressing progresses through a sequence designed to develop overhead strength safely and effectively.

Instead of jumping directly into an overhead barbell press, the pyramid begins with the **landmine press**—a semi-vertical pattern that provides a safe, effective transition into true overhead pressing. The landmine press offers built-in stability and compression, making it one of the most accessible vertical press variations for individuals with limited overhead mobility. From here, the progression moves into **single-arm dumbbell pressing**, performed in asymmetrical lower body stances (such as half-kneeling) to enhance stability and improve shoulder mechanics. Once single-arm control is established, split-stance and bilateral dumbbell pressing are introduced, reinforcing overhead strength while allowing slight degrees of rotation and scapular movement to minimize joint stress.

At this stage, vertical pressing takes a unique detour into **pike push-ups**—an often neglected but highly valuable closed-chain exercise where the hands are fixed to the ground, promoting scapular rotation and full-body control. The pike push-up allows for adjustments in pressing angle, enabling exercises to work within their available range before progressing to a full vertical position.

Finally, at the top of the pyramid, the **barbell overhead press** is the most advanced and demanding variation, requiring precise control of the shoulder blades and the ability to manage load in a fully extended position with no external support. If weak links exist, this movement will expose them quickly, often leading to pain and dysfunction.

The push progression pyramid is not about rushing to the heaviest lifts; it's about mastering each step and progressing intelligently. By following this structured approach, you develop the mobility, stability, and skill necessary to push without pain, allowing for long-term progress rather than short-term gains followed by breakdowns. Whether your goal is strength development, athletic performance, or injury prevention, this framework provides a clear, logical path to success, reinforcing strong mechanics at every stage.

HORIZONTAL PUSH

PUSH-UP

The push-up is the foundation of the horizontal push progression because it's a true full-body pressing movement that integrates the shoulders, core, and lower body into a single, coordinated effort. Unlike a bench press, where you're supported by a fixed surface, the push-up demands that you stabilize your entire body against gravity while maintaining control through your pillar. There's no hiding weaknesses here. If you lack core stability, shoulder control, or full-body tension, the push-up will expose it.

One of the biggest advantages of starting with push-ups is that they allow for natural scapular movement. Because your hands are fixed to the ground, your shoulder blades are free to protract (move apart) and retract (move together) with each rep, mimicking the natural mechanics of the shoulder girdle during pressing movements. This dynamic movement pattern strengthens the stabilizing muscles around the scapulae, reinforcing proper positioning and reducing the risk of shoulder impingements or compensatory movement patterns.

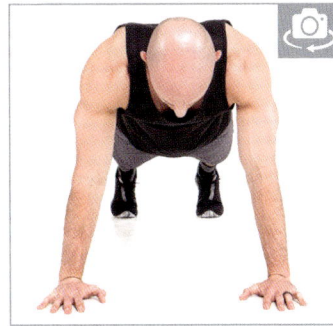

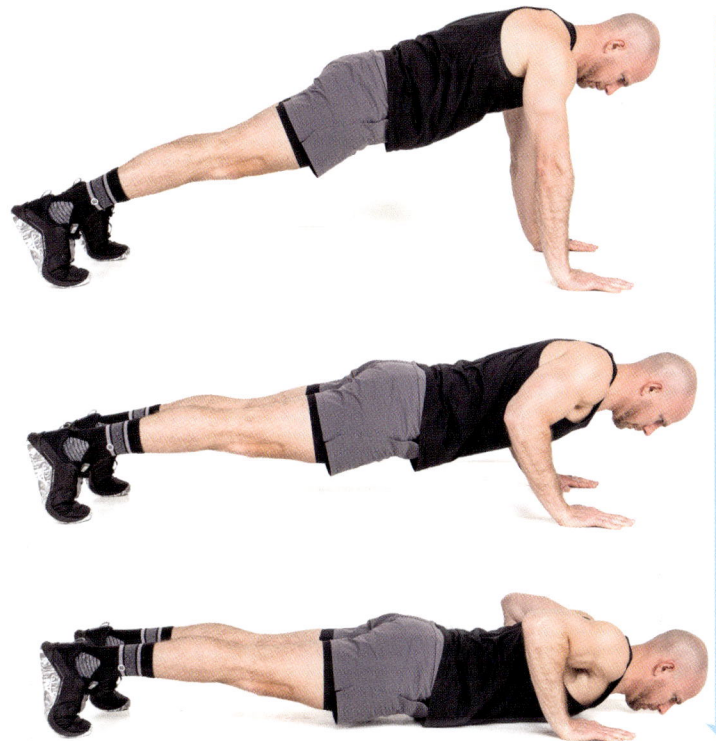

ECCENTRIC PHASE

CONCENTRIC PHASE

OPEN- VS. CLOSED-CHAIN PUSH PATTERNS: IT'S NOT THAT SIMPLE

When most people hear open vs. closed chain, they picture something straightforward—like a leg extension (open chain) vs. a squat (closed chain). In the lower body, this concept is fairly cut-and-dried. But when it comes to the upper body push pattern, it's not so simple. That's because the shoulder complex is highly dynamic, involving four different joints that must work in unison to control mobility and stability.

Instead of just thinking "hands fixed (closed chain) vs. hands moving through space (open chain)," we have to factor in scapular movement as well. This adds a third category that isn't typically part of the open vs. closed chain conversation:

- **Closed-chain pushes:** Hands are fixed on a surface (push-ups), allowing for natural scapular movement.

- **Fixed shoulder blades open-chain pushes:** Hands move freely through space while the shoulder blades remain relatively fixed (barbell bench press).

- **Dynamic shoulder blades open-chain pushes:** Hands move through space and the scapulae remain mobile (dumbbell overhead press, single-arm landmine press).

This is why upper body pushing mechanics aren't as black-and-white as they are in the lower body. The key differentiating factor is not just whether the hands are fixed or free but how the scapulae are allowed to move (or restricted). The push progression is structured to build scapular control, stability, and mobility along with pressing strength.

This matters because before you introduce heavy pressing variations—where the scapulae are more restricted due to contact with a bench—you need to earn the ability to control them through their full range of motion. Developing scapular strength and coordination in an environment where they can move freely ensures better mechanics when transitioning to more restrictive movements like barbell bench pressing. Jumping straight to heavy pressing without this foundation can lead to poor scapular control, limited mobility, and eventual breakdowns in the shoulders and upper body.

Progressing the push-up follows a simple but effective approach that leverages body angle and load manipulation. Just as the push-up screen introduces hands-elevated variations to accommodate strength deficits, the training progression uses graded elevation to fine-tune difficulty. Instead of immediately jumping to a flat-ground push-up, elevating the hands slightly—on plates, a bench, or a box—allows you to find the right level of challenge while reinforcing your ideal form. The key is to adjust elevation incrementally, reducing the angle as strength improves. A Smith machine can be particularly effective, offering precise height adjustments to make progressions controlled and repeatable.

For some, the challenge isn't just strength; it's **discomfort in the wrists**. Wrist pain can make push-ups feel awkward or even impossible, but the solution isn't to skip them altogether. Instead, modifying hand positioning can alleviate strain and make the movement more accessible. Using a neutral grip—with dumbbells or parallettes—or a slant board like a squat wedge reduces wrist extension and places the joints in a stronger, more comfortable position. This small adjustment keeps the focus where it should be—on building pressing strength and full-body control—without unnecessary joint stress.

Like all pyramid progressions, the push-up isn't just a beginner exercise; it's a fundamental skill that builds pressing strength, reinforces full-body pillar stability, and carries over into every pressing movement.

For guidance on how to perform the push-up, refer to the push screen and optimization checklist covered earlier in the chapter.

LOADING THE PUSH-UP

Push-ups are traditionally seen as a bodyweight-only exercise, but if you're treating them as nothing more than an unweighted movement, you're missing out on one of the most scalable and effective pressing variations in your program. Just like any other key performance indicator (KPI) lift, push-ups can—and should—be progressively loaded once bodyweight strength is locked in. The goal isn't just to complete more reps but to build strength in the horizontal push pattern using strategic external resistance.

The most effective way to load the push-up is to position a weight plate directly over the lower thoracic and lumbar spine. This placement ensures that load is evenly distributed through the pillar, allowing you to maintain proper mechanics without compromising scapular movement. One mistake to avoid is placing the weight too high on the upper back, directly over the shoulder blades. This inhibits natural scapular motion—one of the biggest benefits of push-ups in the first place—turning what should be a fluid, integrated movement into a restricted, compensatory pattern.

If plates aren't an option, other variations include band-resisted push-ups, where a resistance band is looped around the back and anchored under the hands for progressive tension throughout the range of motion. Sandbags or chains can also be used, as they conform to the body and allow for a more comfortable, even distribution of weight. The key is to apply load in a way that reinforces stability and alignment, allowing for strength development without compromising shoulder or core integrity.

Once bodyweight push-ups are consistent and technically sound, progressive loading is the next logical step to build strength, increase time under tension, and continue advancing through the push-up pyramid. Whether using plates, bands, or weighted implements, the principles remain the same: control the movement, maintain pillar stability, and reinforce proper mechanics under load.

DEFICIT PUSH-UP

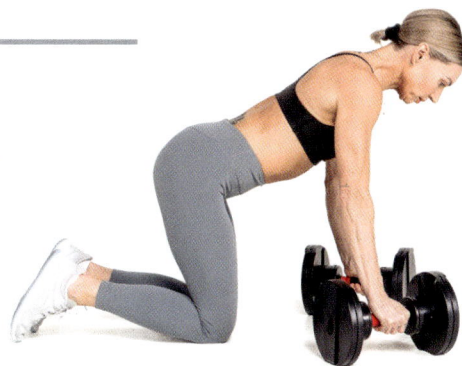

The deficit push-up is the next logical progression in the push pyramid because it extends the range of motion, allowing you to complete the horizontal push pattern through a fuller, more authentic movement. Standard push-ups, by nature, are a partial-range-of-motion exercise—the chest meets the ground before the shoulders can fully extend, limiting the amount of humeral extension and horizontal abduction at the shoulder joint. By elevating the hands on a stable surface, such as bumper plates, parallettes, or dumbbells, the deficit push-up creates the space needed to move through a greater range while maintaining full-body stability and control.

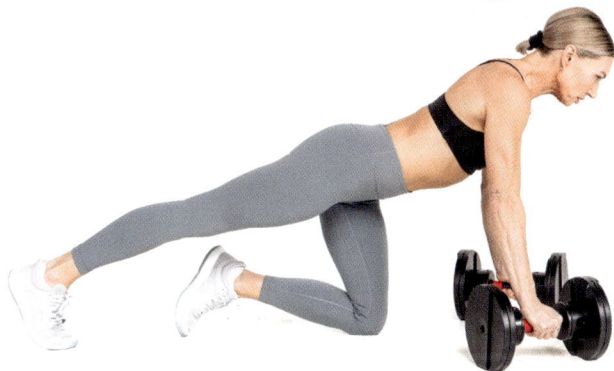

This additional range isn't about mindlessly dropping deeper into the movement—it's about accessing your true, active end range under load. Just because you can sink deeper into a stretch without weight doesn't mean you can own that position under tension. A proper deficit push-up reinforces control in the bottom position, ensuring that your shoulders remain packed, your scapulae move naturally, and no compensations (like excessive forward shoulder dumping) occur. This is where the Shoulder Scour Test proves essential. Your available range of motion in humeral extension—tested during the assessment—determines the depth of your deficit. Most people benefit from a modest increase of 2 to 5 inches, which is the size of a standard bumper plate. Beyond this, you're likely relying on passive structural support rather than actively controlling the movement through muscular engagement. Just like with loading, more isn't always better; forcing excessive range at the expense of control does more harm than good.

EXECUTION

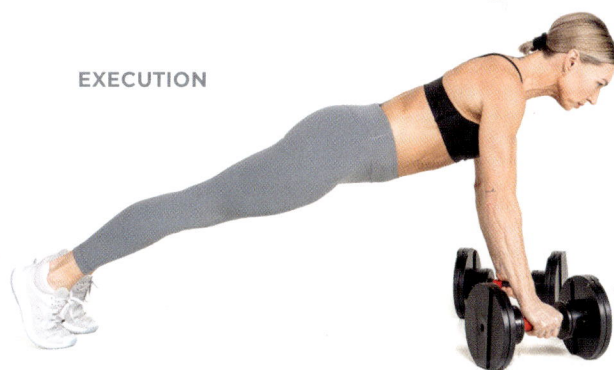

The deficit push-up follows the same setup and execution guidelines as the standard push-up, as outlined in the push screen and optimization checklist. The key distinction is to actively clench the handles or bell, engaging your hands, forearms, and shoulders to create full-body tension for improved stability and force transfer.

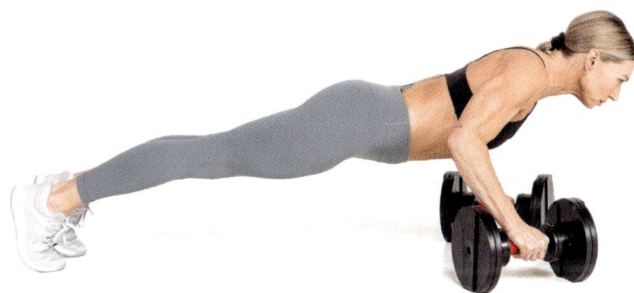

Using kettlebells can offer additional benefits, as their rounded surface allows for slight wrist extension while maintaining a natural grip position. This setup provides a stable yet responsive surface, making it easier to maintain the humeral carrying angle and control depth. Smaller or larger kettlebells can be used to adjust the deficit, tailoring the range of motion to individual mobility and strength levels.

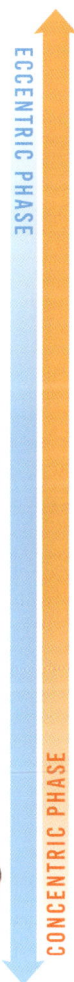

ECCENTRIC PHASE

CONCENTRIC PHASE

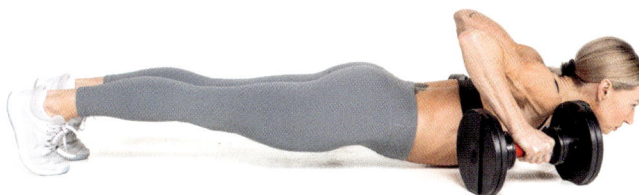

If the increased depth is too challenging, placing a pad under the dumbbells or kettlebells can reduce the range slightly while maintaining proper mechanics. This ensures that the movement remains effective while allowing for progressive adaptation.

DUMBBELL BENCH PRESS

The dumbbell bench press marks a key transition in the push progression pyramid, shifting from a closed-chain movement, like the push-up, to an open-chain press with external loading. While this move allows for greater loading potential, it also introduces new demands on shoulder stability and positioning.

In a push-up, the hands are fixed while the shoulder blades remain free to move dynamically, engaging the upper back and lats as stabilizers. This dynamic stability is essential because when you transition to an open-chain press, where your back is supported and your scapulae are fixed against a bench, you lose that freedom of movement. Without proper activation and stability in the shoulder blades, force leaks occur, leading to compensations at the glenohumeral joint that often manifest as chronic front-sided shoulder pain.

By reinforcing dynamic stability in the push-up variations, the shoulder complex becomes more resilient and prepared to handle the demands of static stability in the dumbbell bench press. This foundation allows you to maintain strong, active scapular positioning against the bench, maximizing pressing strength while reducing stress on your shoulders. The stronger and more stable you are in free-moving patterns, the more control and power you can generate in a supported, loaded press.

Beyond its role as a transitional movement, the dumbbell bench press offers significant advantages in terms of loading potential and movement variability. While the push-up can be loaded, scaling external resistance is far simpler with dumbbells, making progressive overload more accessible and measurable. The independent movement of each arm also helps address imbalances, ensuring that one side isn't compensating for the other. Additionally, dumbbells provide greater freedom at the wrists and shoulders, allowing for a more natural pressing path and reducing joint stress compared to a barbell. This adaptability makes the dumbbell bench press a highly effective tool for building upper body strength while reinforcing stability and control. By mastering this movement, you develop the foundation needed to transition into heavier barbell pressing with confidence and efficiency.

SETUP: The dumbbell bench press starts before you even get on the bench. The way you pick up and position the dumbbells matters, especially as the weights get heavier. Instead of carelessly hoisting them into position, use a split-stance lunge to lift each dumbbell from the floor or rack while maintaining a strong, neutral spine. Stand with control, then sit back onto the bench with the dumbbells resting on your knees.

ECCENTRIC PHASE

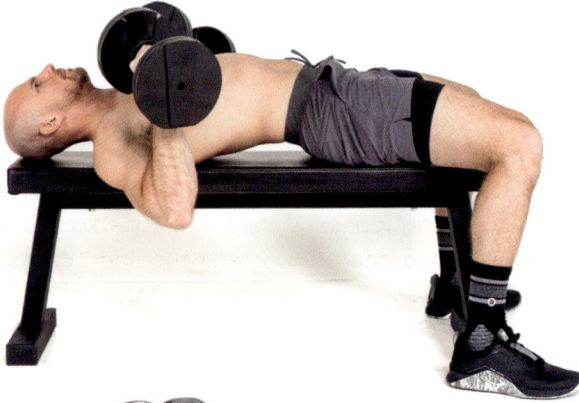

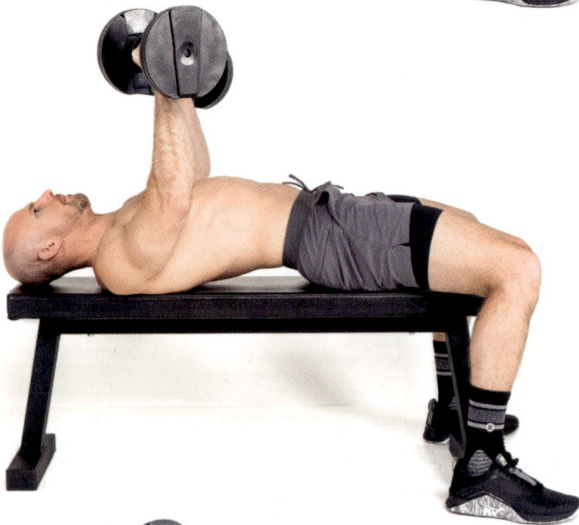

CONCENTRIC PHASE

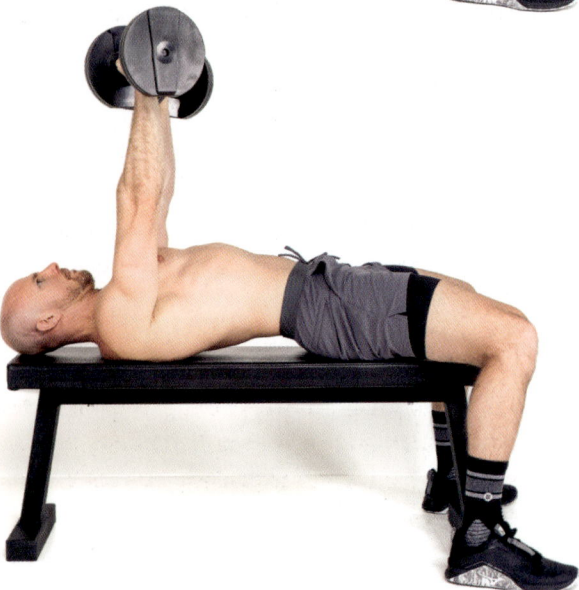

Once seated, set your pillar stability by engaging your core, locking your shoulders into position, and rooting your feet to the floor. From this position, **use an explosive knee drive to hike each dumbbell into place one side at a time, ensuring they land in your authentic humeral carrying angle**—not too flared, not too tucked.

As soon as the dumbbells are in place, lean back in a controlled manner, using your core to stabilize as you transition into the lying position. As your back meets the bench, **establish a slight natural arch by keeping your upper back and glutes in contact with the bench while allowing a small gap in the lower back.** This arch enhances force transfer and prevents excessive strain on your shoulders.

Your shoulder blades should be retracted, depressed, and locked down into the bench. Think about driving the spine of the scapula into the pad, creating a strong, supported base.

EXECUTION: Once the dumbbells are in position, the first rep starts as a press. Maintain a strong brace and drive your feet into the ground to keep full-body tension as you initiate the upward movement. As you press the dumbbells upward, focus on a fluid transition: **First, extend your arms fully in a controlled, explosive drive; then, as you begin the eccentric phase, slowly lower the weight with deliberate control**, ensuring that every inch of the descent is monitored and smooth.

Throughout the press and lowering phases, **allow for natural rotation at the wrists and shoulders, aiming for a grip that lands somewhere between neutral and pronated (45-degree angle).** The dumbbells should travel through a full range of motion, with your elbows dipping just below your torso without compromising scapular positioning or straining the shoulder joint. The emphasis is on controlled movement—don't force the depth simply for the sake of range. Precision is key.

At the bottom of the eccentric phase, **maintain lat engagement and upper back tension by actively pressing your shoulder blades into the bench.** This ensures that the movement remains a true press rather than a loose, disconnected action. Avoid letting your shoulders roll forward or losing scapular alignment. Once your shoulder blades begin to elevate and protract, any force leaks will compromise stability.

As you drive back into the press, think about pushing your back into the bench as much as you push the dumbbells upward. This dual focus reinforces stability at the shoulder joint and maximizes strength output, all while allowing for natural hand rotation and maintaining locked-down scapulae throughout the full range of motion.

WHAT ABOUT INCLINE PRESSES?

Incline presses are one of those exercises that seem to exist in a gray area—somewhere between horizontal and vertical pressing. They aren't a formal step in the push progression, but they still hold value when programmed correctly. So where do they fit in?

Mechanically, incline presses below 45 degrees fall under horizontal pressing because the scapular mechanics and joint positioning remain the same as a flat press. That's why they typically enter the progression after the flat barbell bench press. But once the incline exceeds 45 degrees, it transitions to a vertical press, meaning the shoulder mechanics shift, the muscular demands change, and the movement starts behaving more like an overhead press.

This is why most incline pressing falls within the 15-to-30-degree range—it preserves optimal scapular depression, retraction, and downward rotation while maintaining a natural humeral carrying angle. In fact, a 15-degree (slight) incline is often the sweet spot. It allows for proper positioning of the scapulae and feels more natural for most lifters compared to a traditional flat bench.

On the other hand, pressing above 45 degrees with a fixed shoulder blade position can be problematic. With the scapulae unable to move freely, it restricts the natural mechanics of the glenohumeral joint, limiting force production. That's why pressing at high inclines is not KPI progression and should be approached with caution, especially when using barbells or machines that lock the scapulae into place.

So, while high incline presses aren't a core progression in the push pattern, they have a place in programming—especially in undertrained angles that are often neglected. If there's one incline press that works well for nearly everyone, it's the slight incline (15 degrees)—low enough to preserve proper pressing mechanics but high enough to introduce a new stimulus.

BARBELL BENCH PRESS

ECCENTRIC PHASE

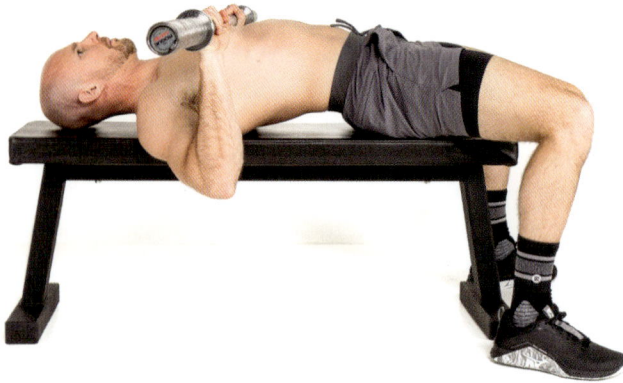

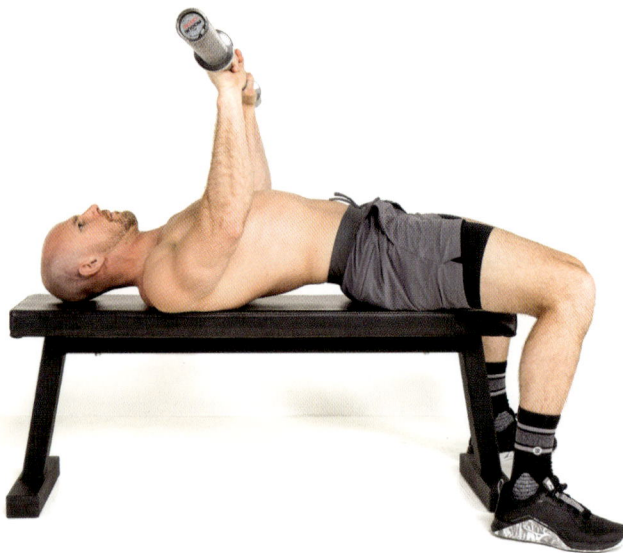

CONCENTRIC PHASE

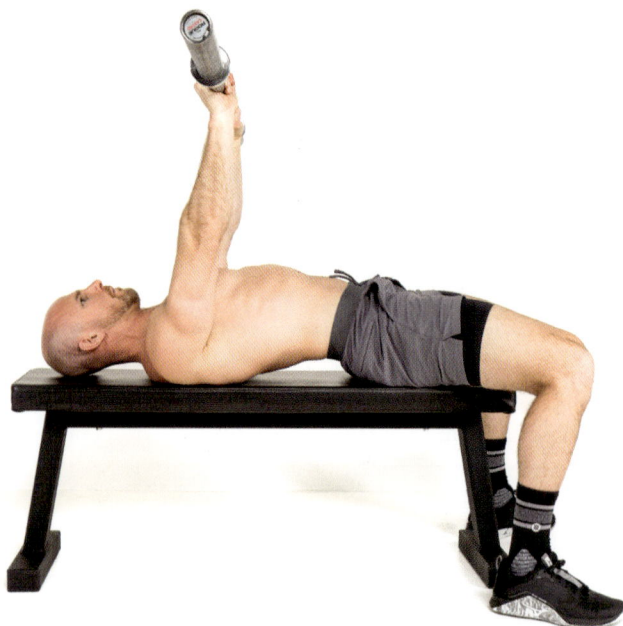

The barbell bench press sits at the peak of the horizontal push progression pyramid, not because it's the most important pressing exercise but because it offers the highest loading potential—provided the necessary strength, stability, and mechanics are in place. Unlike previous progressions, where the hands and shoulders have some degree of freedom, the barbell locks everything in a fixed position. This rigidity makes it an exceptional tool for developing maximal strength, but it also amplifies any underlying weaknesses or imbalances. Without proper preparation, it can quickly become a source of inefficiency, discomfort, or even injury.

The bench press is often viewed as the gold standard of upper body pressing, but it's also the least forgiving. While it rewards stability and control, it demands near-perfect execution to prevent compensatory patterns from creeping in. That's why it's not something you just jump into—it's a movement that has to be earned.

One of the biggest transitions from dumbbell to barbell pressing is the lack of independent arm movement. Dumbbells allow for slight variations in wrist, elbow, and shoulder positioning, naturally accommodating individual structure and movement preferences. The barbell, on the other hand, forces both arms into the same path, which means any existing asymmetries or weaknesses become much harder to mask. If you haven't built the necessary stability, control, and muscular balance through push-ups and dumbbell pressing, the barbell will expose every weak link. This is why the earlier progressions aren't just stepping stones—they're prerequisites.

While the fixed hand position may seem limiting, it provides a unique advantage: the ability to generate and maintain full-body tension before initiating the lift. Because you unrack the bar from a stable position, you can preload your pillar, engage your breath bracing sequence, and establish a rock-solid foundation before the first rep. Unlike dumbbells, which require dynamic stabilization just to get into position, the barbell allows for a controlled setup with maximal tension. This makes it the most efficient tool for developing absolute strength in the horizontal push pattern.

That said, just because the barbell bench press is at the top of the pyramid doesn't mean it's mandatory. Strength isn't defined by a single exercise, and if barbell pressing isn't the right fit—due to mobility restrictions, joint pain, or individual biomechanics—previous progressions can still build impressive upper body strength. Powerlifters and strength sport athletes may need to bench as part of competition, but for everyone else, it's a tool, not a requirement. Whether it belongs in your program depends on your goals, movement quality, and ability to execute it without compensation. If you can check those boxes, the barbell bench press offers an unparalleled opportunity to push heavy weight with precision and efficiency.

SETUP: Success with the barbell bench press starts before you even unrack the bar. First, **adjust the J-hooks to an appropriate height—typically 1 to 2 inches below your locked-out arm position** while maintaining a retracted and depressed shoulder position. This allows for a controlled unrack without forcing the bar too high (which can cause excessive protraction) or too low (which turns the unrack into a triceps extension). Since every gym's equipment is slightly different, test the setup each time you train, especially when using a new rack.

Once the rack height is set, **actively set your shoulder blades—depress and retract them into the bench, locking them in place.** You may need to slide slightly upward toward the head of the bench to achieve full scapular compression against the pad. This position should feel secure, ensuring your upper back is fully engaged before initiating the press.

Next, establish your lower body positioning. **Your feet should be set in your squat stance—typically shoulder-width apart with slight toe abduction.** This stance maximizes torque and centration at the hips, helping to stabilize the pelvis and create a strong foundation for the press. Your shins should remain roughly vertical to the ground, with the knees driving outward to create tension. This setup enables optimal leg drive, transferring force from the lower body into the upper body for a more powerful press.

With your body anchored, focus on bracing. Take a deep breath through your nose, expanding 360 degrees around your core. This intra-abdominal pressure reinforces lumbar and thoracic stability, preventing excessive spinal movement under load. Exhale slightly through your mouth to reinforce core tension while keeping your rib cage stacked over your pelvis. **All components—shoulder setup, foot positioning, and breath—must be locked in simultaneously before you unrack the bar.**

EXECUTION: With your body set, reach up and grip the bar. **The ideal hand position is roughly shoulder-width apart, with your thumbs aligned with the acromion** (the bony prominence at the top of the shoulder where the clavicle meets the scapula). Use a full grip, wrapping your fingers securely around the bar. Rather than focusing on external rotation cues like "rip the bar apart" or "rotate the hands outward," prioritize grip irradiation—squeezing the bar as hard as possible. This tension radiates from your hands into your forearms, shoulders, and upper back, reinforcing stability and maximizing strength output.

Unrack the bar with control, moving it 2 to 3 inches forward from the J-hooks into position over your chest. Avoid excessive movement—racking too far back can cause instability, while unracking too forcefully can disrupt your setup. Once the bar is positioned, **begin the eccentric phase by actively rowing the bar down to your chest.** This isn't a passive drop—your lats should be engaged, pulling the bar downward while maintaining scapular compression into the bench. The goal is to keep constant tension in the posterior chain, allowing for a controlled descent.

Lower the bar until it makes light contact with your chest. Depth should be dictated by individual mobility and humeral carrying angle, but in general, full range of motion is encouraged unless pain or structural limitations prevent it. At the bottom, your shoulder blades should remain locked down, with no elevation or protraction. The scapulae shifting forward or upward indicates a loss of stability and potential force leaks.

From the bottom position, **initiate the press by driving your back into the bench**, not just by pressing the bar upward. This reinforces scapular positioning and maximizes force transfer through your upper body. The bar should move in a straight line—this is not the old-school "nipples to eyes" trajectory. A strong setup will naturally guide the bar along an efficient path without excessive horizontal movement.

Maintain a natural arch. Your lumbar spine should maintain its natural lordotic curve, but without excessive hyperextension. **Your hips must remain in contact with the bench**—lifting the hips may increase pressure through your shoulders but compromises core engagement, reducing overall stability. While some arching is necessary for optimal shoulder mechanics, the goal is to reinforce strong, stable positioning, not artificially exaggerate spinal extension.

VERTICAL PUSH

LANDMINE PRESS

The landmine press marks the transition from horizontal to vertical pressing in the push progression pyramid. While the barbell bench press allows for maximum load potential through a fixed and stable setup, the landmine press strips away external support, forcing the body to manage stability in a dynamic environment. It's a humbling shift—many lifters who can bench press massive weight struggle with even light loads in a single-arm landmine press. The reason? It exposes weaknesses that bilateral, fixed-position pressing often masks. Without a bench or symmetrical stance to provide structure, the body must coordinate movement through multiple planes while stabilizing against gravity—just like it has to in nearly every real-world and athletic setting.

Unlike traditional overhead pressing, which demands significant shoulder mobility, the landmine press follows an arced path, placing the shoulder in a more joint-friendly position. This makes it an ideal entry point for vertical pressing, especially for those with limited overhead range of motion. It also offers a built-in regression-progression system, accommodating asymmetries between the left and right sides. Because the angle of the press can be adjusted, the landmine allows for a customized approach that meets individuals where they are rather than forcing them into a rigid overhead position that may not be accessible.

The base variation of the landmine press starts in a half-kneeling position, with the pressing arm on the same side as the down leg. This setup minimizes lower body variables, creating a stable foundation for the upper body to execute the movement with control. It also aligns the pressing path closer to a 45-degree angle—between a pure horizontal and a vertical press—offering a smooth transition from the patterns developed earlier in the pyramid. As proficiency increases, the movement progresses to a standing split stance, introducing greater stability demands and full-body integration.

While the landmine press is positioned higher up the pyramid due to its greater motor control demands, it doesn't have to come later in training. Because it represents the foundation of vertical pressing, many lifters can transition directly from push-ups to the landmine press. Its combination of an adjustable press angle, unilateral loading, and full-body integration makes it an excellent tool for improving pressing strength, enhancing scapular mechanics, and reinforcing stability in ways that traditional overhead presses often neglect. Whether as a primary movement or a strategic accessory, it remains a staple for developing strong, pain-free vertical pressing mechanics.

SETUP: The landmine press begins with a stable lower body position to establish a strong base for pressing.

- **For the half-kneeling landmine press**, position yourself with one knee down and the other foot forward in a 90/90 stance—the front knee directly over the ankle and the back knee directly under the hip, with toes dorsiflexed and pressing into the ground. The key here is active engagement: Your glutes and adductors must co-contract to stabilize your pelvis and prevent unwanted movement. A common mistake is to go passive in the lower body, which compromises force transfer and reduces pressing efficiency. Think of this position as a strong "scissor" stance, where your feet actively drive inward but your hips stay centered.

- **For the standing landmine press**, take a split stance with your back foot positioned slightly behind your body for balance. This variation introduces more full-body coordination and vertical force application compared to the half-kneeling version, which provides more inherent stability.

Once positioned, the pickup phase is crucial. The landmine should be elevated slightly (such as resting on a bumper plate) to make for a smoother clean into position. To lift the bar into place, **grip the landmine collar with both hands, using a slight rotational clean to guide it to the front rack position**. Your pressing hand should finish with the thumb facing back, ensuring the bar tracks naturally through the movement. Your non-working arm should remain active, moving into extension as you press.

EXECUTION: With the landmine securely in position at shoulder height, engage your core, lats, and opposite-side glute to create full-body tension. The landmine press follows a semicircular pressing arc, not a straight line like a traditional overhead press. This unique path makes it more joint friendly while reinforcing optimal scapular mechanics.

Begin the press by driving the bar up and slightly forward, maintaining a stable, braced torso throughout the movement. The landmine's built-in compressional force naturally encourages a strong shoulder position, allowing the scapula to upwardly rotate and stabilize dynamically.

The **non-working arm should remain engaged**, either by resisting rotation or actively moving to assist in the range of motion. In more advanced variations, rotating your torso slightly can help increase overhead range and shoulder mobility.

As the bar reaches full extension, avoid excessive leaning or arching through the lower back. Instead, maintain pillar tension and let the bar path dictate the natural lean that occurs.

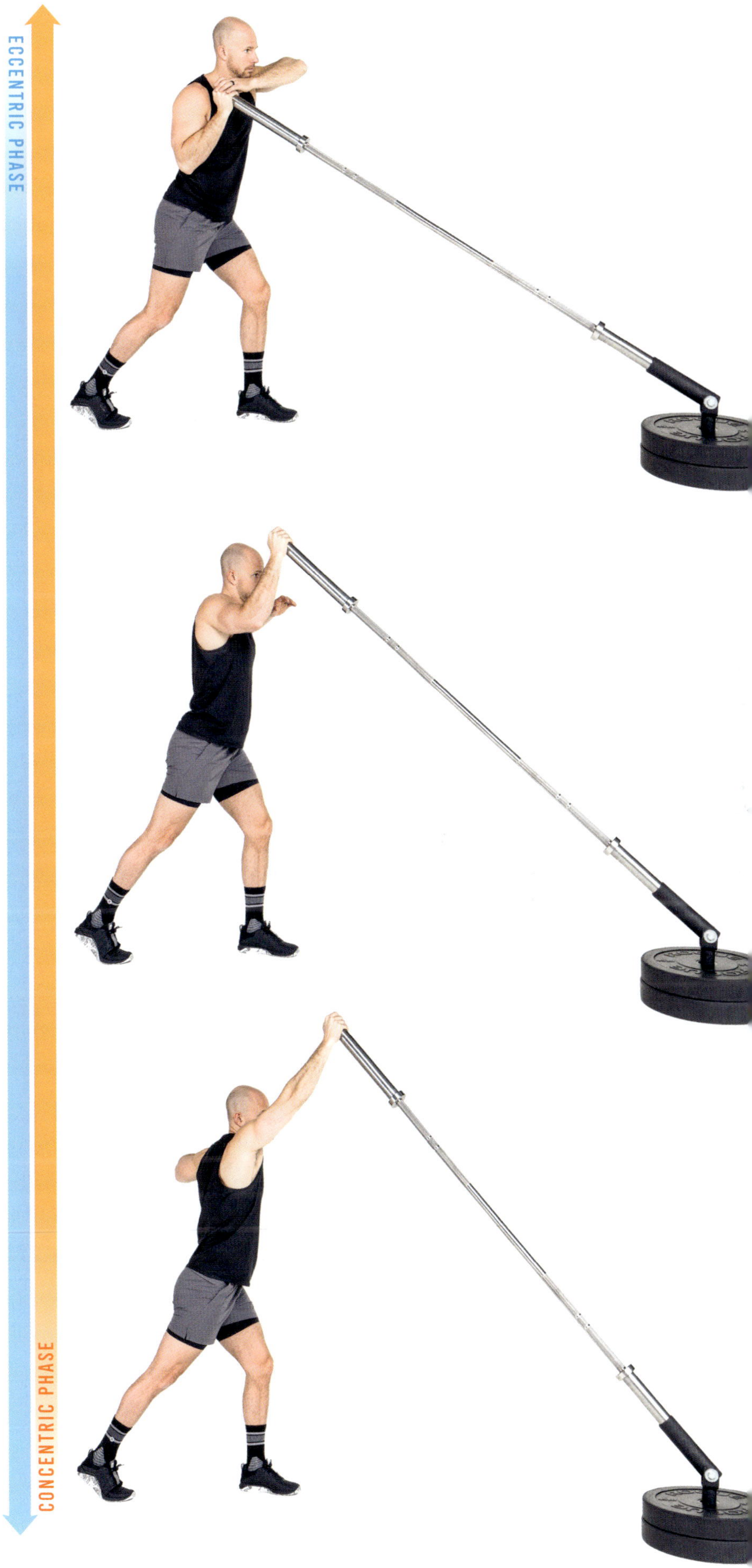

ECCENTRIC PHASE

CONCENTRIC PHASE

DUMBBELL OVERHEAD PRESS

The dumbbell overhead press is the first true vertical push in the progression pyramid. Unlike the landmine press, which follows an arced pressing path and provides built-in stability, the dumbbell overhead press requires the body to move against gravity in a fully vertical plane, increasing the demand on shoulder mobility, core stability, and full-body control. Because of these added challenges, it's not an exercise you jump into without earning the necessary movement prerequisites. The transition from the landmine to the dumbbell press is a deliberate one, designed to build pressing mechanics in a way that minimizes compensatory patterns and promotes long-term joint health.

To bridge this gap, the progression starts with a **single-arm dumbbell press in a half-kneeling position**. Training one arm at a time allows for greater range of motion by accommodating natural asymmetries, preventing the body from forcing itself into an unnatural overhead position. The half-kneeling stance further enhances control by limiting lower body variables, forcing the core and shoulders to stabilize the movement independently.

Once a strong, stable press is established unilaterally, the next step is the **bilateral dumbbell press from the same half-kneeling position**. This variation introduces greater loading potential while maintaining the core stability benefits of the kneeling stance.

From here, the progression shifts to a **standing split stance, first with a single arm, then with both arms pressing together**. The staggered stance offers a blend of stability and dynamic control, ensuring that the movement remains well integrated before advancing to a fully upright position. Finally, the peak of this phase is the **bilateral standing dumbbell press**, performed in a power stance with feet hip-width apart. This is the most demanding variation, as it requires maximum core engagement, postural stability, and shoulder control to maintain proper alignment throughout the press.

Structuring the dumbbell overhead press progression in this way—moving from unilateral to bilateral, kneeling to standing—gives the body the opportunity to develop strength and mobility in a controlled, stepwise manner that reinforces optimal mechanics while preventing common faults like excessive lumbar extension, scapular compensation, and uneven pressing patterns.

SETUP: The overhead dumbbell progression moves from half-kneeling to a split stance to a bilateral standing position.

1. For the half-kneeling dumbbell press, start with the same-side knee down as the pressing arm. Your front knee should be at 90 degrees with the ankle directly under the knee. Your back knee is also at 90 degrees, with the foot dorsiflexed and toes pressing into the ground. Brace your core, glutes, and adductors to stabilize your pelvis, ensuring that the movement stays truly overhead rather than compensating with lumbar extension. Grip the dumbbell with both hands and clean it just outside the shoulder, securing it in a neutral position. Release the support hand and either place it on your hip or extend it outward for balance. Maintain an authentic humeral carrying angle with the pressing arm, ensuring your shoulder remains in a strong, stable position.

2. Once your single-arm pressing mechanics are strong, transition to bilateral pressing in the same half-kneeling stance. Grip both dumbbells from the floor, cleaning them to the rack position just outside your shoulders. Maintain the same lower body engagement and core bracing, ensuring that both dumbbells move symmetrically overhead.

3. Move into a split stance by performing a controlled split squat to pick up the dumbbell(s) from the floor.

- **For a single-arm press**, grip the dumbbell with both hands, brace, and clean it to the rack position at shoulder height before releasing the support hand. Maintain an authentic humeral carrying angle with your pressing arm while the opposite hand rests on your hip or extends outward for balance. This unilateral press reinforces scapular control, core integrity, and dynamic stabilization.

- **For a bilateral press**, grip both dumbbells and clean them into position using a strong brace from the split squat. Secure them just outside your shoulders, maintaining a stable, neutral shoulder position. Pressing with both arms increases the coordination and postural demands, as the body must remain braced and upright while controlling the load overhead. The split stance allows for an integrated full-body press while minimizing compensation through excessive spinal extension.

4. The final variation is performed standing with feet hip-width apart, demanding maximum full-body tension to control the movement. Clean both dumbbells into position, ensuring your core is fully braced and your lats are engaged to prevent excessive spinal extension. Without the inherent stability of a kneeling or split stance, this variation requires a high level of postural control, reinforcing stability across the entire kinetic chain.

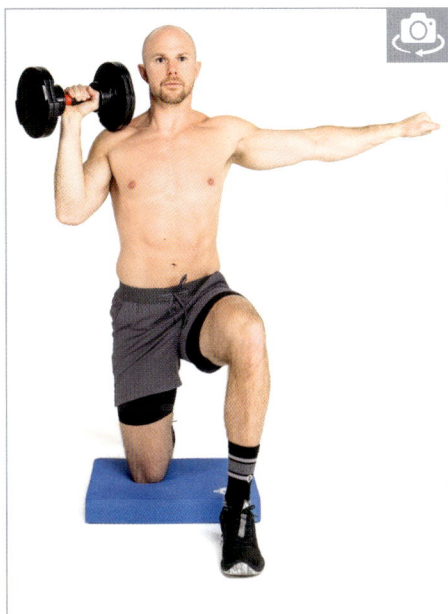

HALF KNEELING

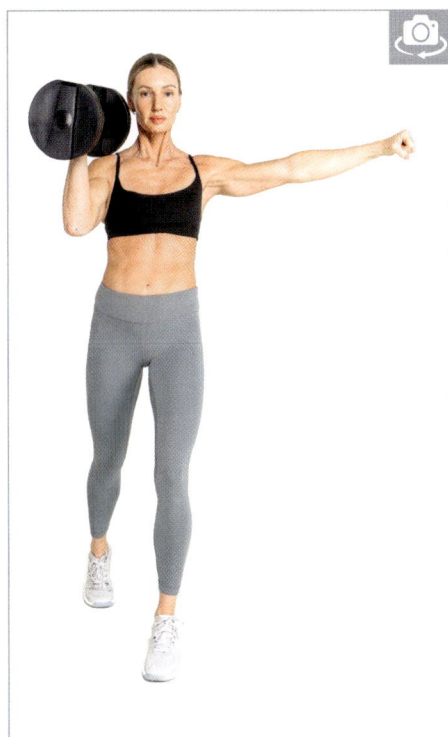

CONCENTRIC PHASE

ECCENTRIC PHASE

SPLIT STANCE

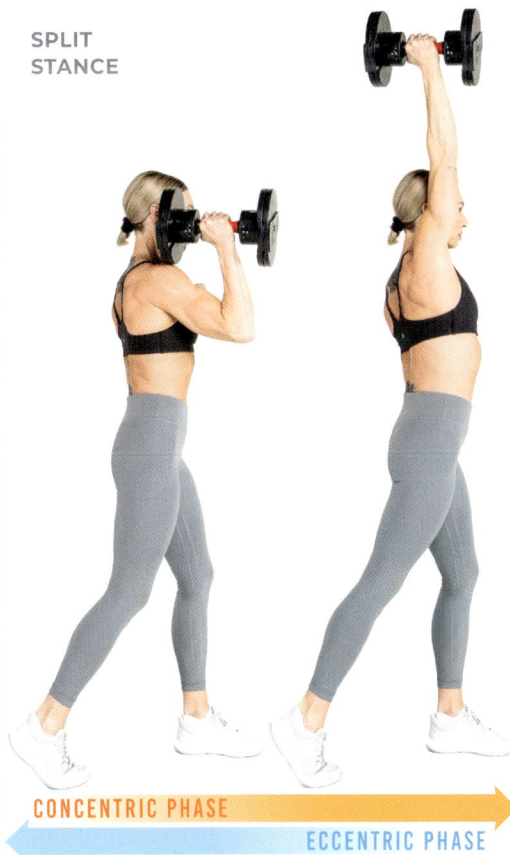

BILATERAL STANCE

CONCENTRIC PHASE

ECCENTRIC PHASE

CONCENTRIC PHASE

ECCENTRIC PHASE

EXECUTION: Press the dumbbell(s) directly overhead in a controlled vertical path, allowing for natural rotation at the wrists and shoulders. Your hands should track into a slightly neutral to pronated grip as they reach the top.

Fully extend your arms without locking out aggressively or shrugging your shoulders excessively. Keep tension in your upper back and lats to maintain scapular control.

Lower the dumbbell(s) slowly, ensuring your elbows track naturally and don't flare out excessively. The eccentric phase should reinforce control and should not be rushed.

Throughout the movement, avoid compensating with spinal extension. If you feel your lower back arching too much, reset your brace and reduce the weight if needed.

For bilateral presses, both arms should move symmetrically, maintaining even tension throughout.

PIKE PUSH-UP

ECCENTRIC PHASE

CONCENTRIC PHASE

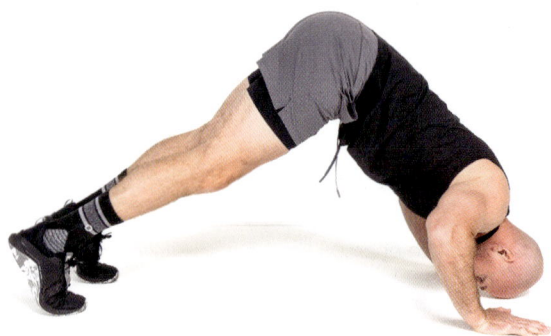

DEFICIT PIKE PUSH-UP

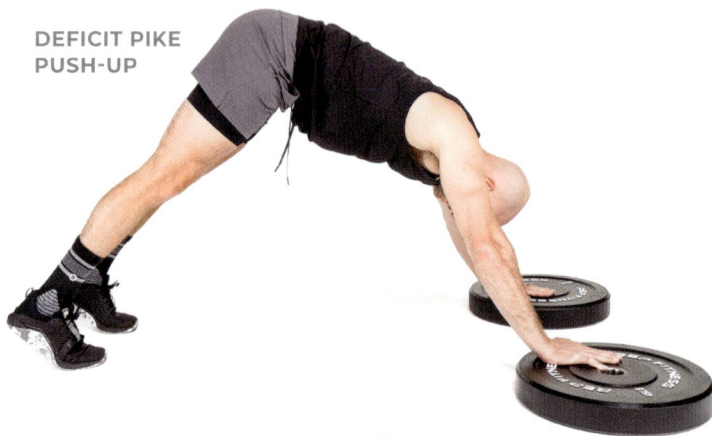

FEET-ELEVATED PIKE PUSH-UP

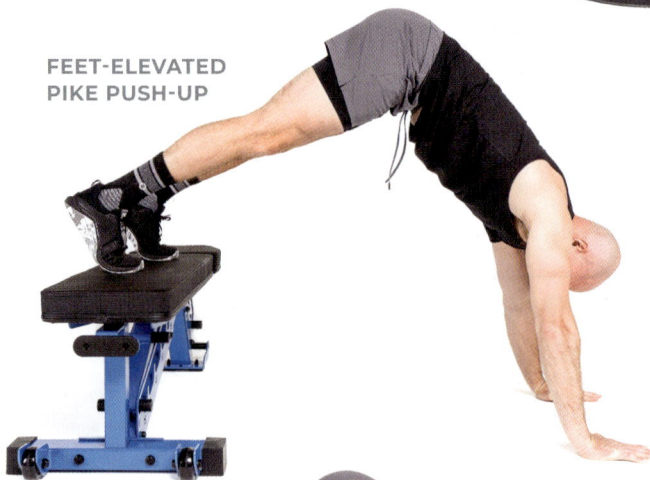

FEET-ELEVATED DEFICIT PIKE PUSH-UP

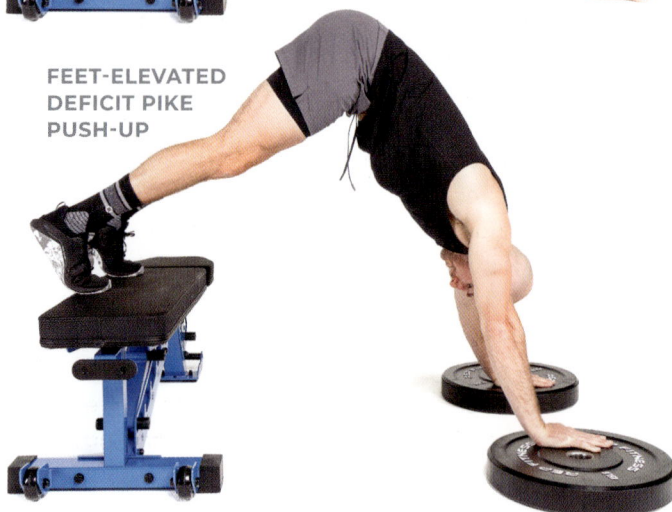

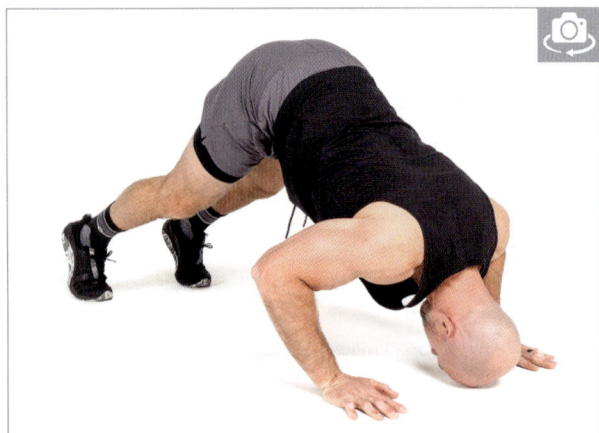

The pike push-up represents a key shift in the vertical push progression, introducing a closed-chain movement where the hands remain fixed on the ground. Unlike earlier progressions that focus on pressing external loads, this variation forces the body to stabilize itself in an inverted position, emphasizing shoulder strength, scapular control, and full-body tension in a way that traditional overhead pressing does not.

The most notable difference between the pike push-up and other overhead variations is the body positioning and angle of force application. Instead of pressing with the hips extended, the movement requires a hip-hinged posture, positioning the torso at a downward angle. This creates a unique challenge, as you must learn to control your center of mass against gravity while reinforcing proper shoulder mechanics and overhead stability.

This progression follows the dumbbell overhead press because, while both reinforce overhead pressing mechanics, the pike push-up requires greater full-body integration and positional awareness. With hands and feet fixed in place, there's no external load to stabilize, meaning the body must manage all movement demands internally.

What's more, unlike the landmine or dumbbell press, the pike push-up doesn't allow for single-arm work—making it less adaptable for individuals who lack bilateral overhead mobility. For those who struggle with full overhead positioning, unilateral variations are often a better option to maintain proper mechanics while building strength in the vertical plane.

To make the most of this movement, the pike push-up offers two key progressions that allow you to scale the challenge and maximize effectiveness. The standard variation, performed with hands on the floor, is the starting point, reinforcing scapular control, core stability, and overhead pressing strength while keeping the range of motion manageable. For those with solid mechanics, deficit pike push-ups—where the hands are elevated on boxes, parallettes, or plates—extend the range of motion, demanding greater strength and control in the bottom position. This extended range mimics the depth required in more advanced overhead pressing variations, reinforcing strength where most lifters are weakest.

The pike push-up also serves as a natural entry point for handstand push-up progressions. However, it's not an exercise that I program or recommend for most people. While the handstand push-up is often viewed as the ultimate bodyweight overhead press, its setup introduces significant instability and a steep learning curve. The risk of failing—whether due to lack of balance, improper mechanics, or insufficient strength—often outweighs the reward. The pike push-up, by contrast, delivers the same pressing benefits in a controlled environment, allowing you to develop overhead strength, shoulder stability, and movement proficiency without unnecessary risk.

By integrating both standard and deficit pike push-ups into a training program, you can progressively challenge your pressing strength and stability, ensuring a safe, structured path to vertical pressing mastery—without the need for high-risk movements.

SETUP: The pike push-up starts from the **same base push-up position** used in the horizontal push pattern screen. Begin in a strong plank position, rooting your hands into the ground and stabilizing your shoulders, hips, and core. From here, **actively press your hands into the floor and shift your hips back**, creating a posterior translation until you achieve **approximately 90 degrees of hip flexion**. Ideally, your knees should remain straight, but real-world coaching experience suggests that a slight bend (up to 20 degrees) is common to help maintain optimal spinal alignment and control. Your feet should remain active and firmly planted into the ground.

At the top position, your **biceps should be aligned next to your ears**, your neck and chest should maintain a neutral position, and your spine should be stacked properly to create a strong overhead pressing angle. This is your starting point before initiating the eccentric phase of the movement.

EXECUTION: From the pike position, eccentrically **lower your body by bending your elbows**, controlling your descent toward the floor. Your head serves as the limiting factor, approaching the ground at the bottom range. Instead of simply letting gravity pull you down, **actively drive your hands into the floor as you descend** to maintain tension throughout the movement.

Once you reach the bottom, press forcefully into the ground, driving yourself back up to the starting position while maintaining a stable and controlled movement pattern. The goal is to train as close to a pure vertical pressing motion as possible while keeping the pillar engaged.

PROGRESSIONS: For those with sufficient strength and skill, elevating the feet on a box increases the verticality of the press, making it a more demanding overhead variation. This shifts the center of mass and places greater emphasis on the shoulders and upper body, closely mimicking the mechanics of a handstand push-up.

A further progression is the feet-elevated deficit pike push-up, which allows for a greater range of motion by elevating the hands on parallettes, boxes, or weight plates. This works similarly to the deficit push-up, but because the head is the limiting factor rather than the chest, a significant elevation (up to 12 inches) may be necessary to achieve a full and complete range of motion. To maintain balance and control, the deficit pike push-up is best performed with both feet and hands elevated, ensuring a true vertical pressing angle while minimizing compensatory movements.

BARBELL OVERHEAD PRESS

The barbell overhead press sits at the peak of the vertical push progression pyramid—not because it's a mandatory exercise but because it places the highest demands on mobility, stability, and skill. In theory, it's one of the most comprehensive full-body pressing movements. The load is positioned as far from the ground as possible, requiring extensive bracing, pillar stability, and force transfer from the lower body through the core and into the shoulders. But in practice, it's one of the most challenging lifts for most people to execute safely and effectively.

The biggest issue? Few lifters have the necessary prerequisites to press a barbell overhead without compensations. This isn't just about shoulder strength— it's about thoracic mobility, scapular control, core stability, and maintaining proper alignment under load. Any deficiency in these areas leads to compensations that not only diminish performance but also significantly increase the risk of pain. Yet I see lifters attempt to go straight from minimal overhead training to heavy barbell pressing without first developing the foundational components necessary to execute it optimally.

Beyond mobility and stability constraints, the bar path itself adds another layer of complexity. Unlike dumbbells, which allow for natural wrist and shoulder rotation, the barbell locks the hands into a fixed position, making it more difficult to navigate around the head without altering mechanics.

This is why, for many lifters, reaching the top of the vertical push progression pyramid isn't necessary. While the movement represents the most advanced expression of overhead pressing, it's also the one that lifters typically struggle with the most. As the load moves farther from the ground, any weak links—mobility restrictions, strength imbalances, or poor motor control—are exposed.

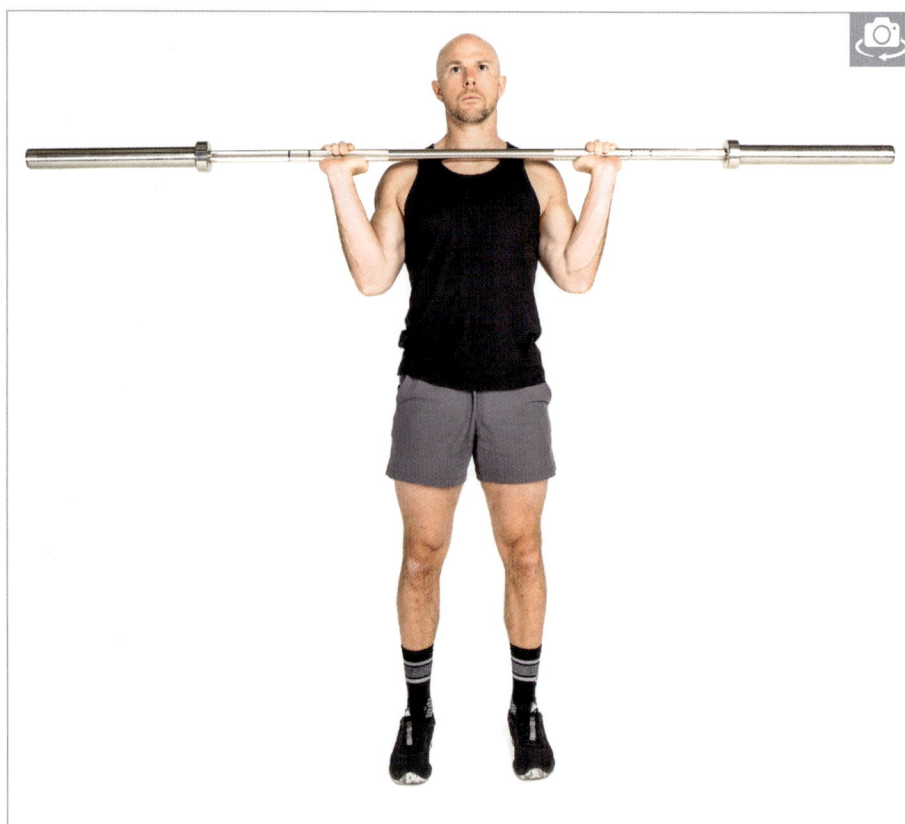

Anyone who has trained with me knows that I'm not a huge fan of barbell overhead pressing. If there was one pattern at the top of the pyramid that I almost never program, it would be this one, due to the factors I just mentioned. The goal isn't necessarily to get here—many times, you don't have to. If you're training the push and pull patterns correctly, you can build the same strength and function without forcing a movement that doesn't suit your mechanics.

The barbell overhead press sits at the top of the pyramid for a reason. Pressing overhead should reinforce movement patterns that enhance stability, muscle development, and function—not magnify weaknesses that can lead to pain. If pressing a barbell overhead forces compensations, there are plenty of alternative pressing movements that build strength with less risk. Just because a movement is possible doesn't mean it's the right choice—especially if it comes at the cost of long-term function and joint health.

BARBELL OVERHEAD PRESS

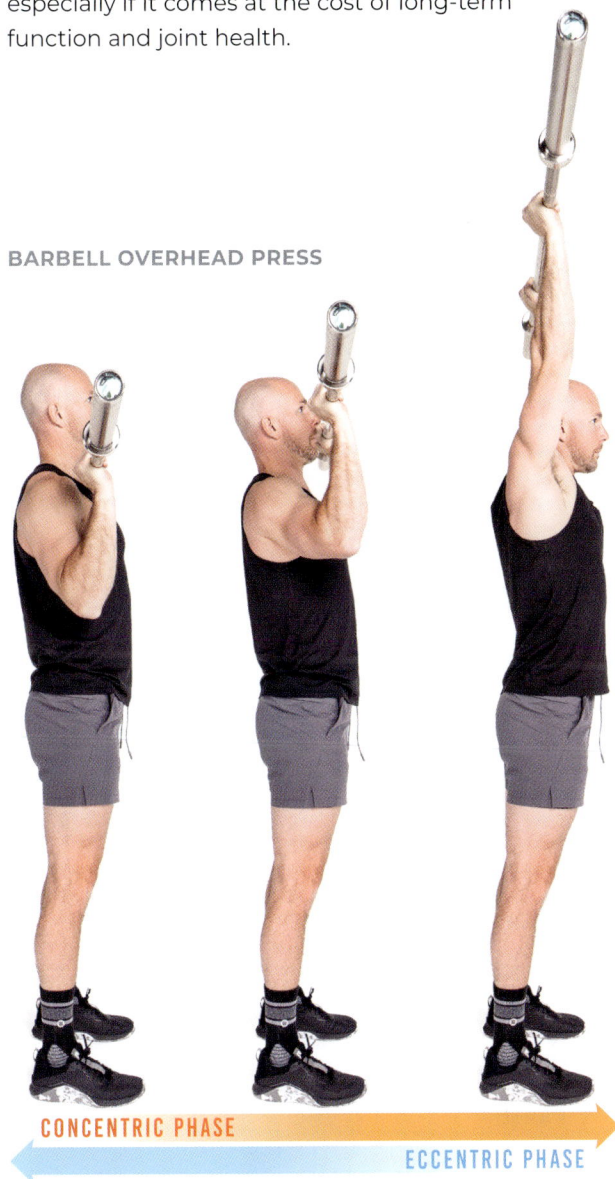

CONCENTRIC PHASE

ECCENTRIC PHASE

SETUP: To optimize the setup, **start by placing the barbell on safeties within a power rack, about 2 inches below unracking height**. This eliminates the need for an inefficient backward step and allows for a smoother, more controlled start. **Stand with your feet hip-width apart in a power stance.** Engage your glutes and adductors, ensuring a strong, stable lower body foundation. Set your pecs and shoulders, take a deep breath, brace your core, and only then grip the bar.

Hand positioning mirrors the bench press setup, with the wrists aligned just outside the acromion (the bony ridge at the top of the shoulder). This ensures an authentic humeral carrying angle while maintaining vertical alignment. Grip the bar with a full grip, wrapping your thumbs around for maximum security.

When ready, **perform a small eighth-of-a-squat to lift the bar off the safeties**, locking into position before pressing. This prevents unnecessary movement and maintains full-body tension from the start.

EXECUTION: After unracking and stabilizing the bar, initiate the press with full-body engagement, maintaining core rigidity and scapular stability. **Drive the bar overhead in a pure vertical path**, ensuring that you prioritize movement efficiency over compensation.

A key challenge with the barbell overhead press is navigating around your head while keeping the bar path straight. Instead of excessively arching your lower back or shifting your torso forward, **slightly retract your neck as you press**, allowing the bar to pass without obstruction. **As the bar clears your head, return to a neutral neck position**, keeping your gaze slightly upward to maintain alignment. This small adjustment prevents unwanted spinal extension while preserving a strong, stacked position.

At lockout, **ensure that your biceps are aligned with your ears**, with the bar positioned directly over your mid-foot for optimal balance. Avoid excessive shoulder elevation or leaning backward, as both compromise stability and force output. Control the descent, lowering the bar directly back to the starting position and maintaining core engagement to prevent any breakdown in posture.

Upon completing the set, lower the bar directly onto the safeties rather than navigating a step forward; this minimizes instability and reduces the risk of losing position.

PULL

The pull is the most misunderstood movement pattern—because most lifters never truly learn what effective pulling actually involves. It's not as simple as pulling weight up or toward you; it's a coordinated action that relies on precise shoulder rotation, smooth scapular glide, and a freely moving thoracic spine. But when these subtle mechanics are ignored, the shoulders stiffen, traps take over, and the neck and upper back pay the price—problems only worsened by hours spent slouched at a desk. This chapter clears the confusion, providing a framework to restore full shoulder function, improve movement efficiency, and unlock the true power of your pull—without compensations or pain.

When I was 15, sports were my whole world. Football, baseball, basketball—I played them all, bouncing from one season to the next, fueled by youthful energy and a competitive drive. At the time, I never thought much about why movement and athleticism felt so natural. But looking back now, it's clear that my greatest influence wasn't raw talent or determination alone—it was my dad.

He wasn't your typical sports dad shouting clichés from the sidelines. He was a local legend—the athletic director for the Williamsville Central School District, overseeing 26 schools in western New York where I grew up. For 34 years, he shaped athletic departments across the district, including three powerhouse high school programs. He was also in charge of health curriculum and, on top of all that, served as a professor at the University of Buffalo. UB and my high school were in the same district, so his influence spanned seamlessly between both institutions.

The countless hours my dad invested in coaching me gave me a distinct advantage in every sport I played. One summer, he introduced me to someone who would change my training forever: Ed Fitzsimmons, a well-respected athletic performance coach and UB's strength and conditioning coordinator.

My dad described Coach Ed as someone who "does things a little differently." At the time, I wasn't exactly sure what that meant, but I was eager to learn. While I had experience lifting weights, I was mostly just going through the motions—doing it simply because that's what athletes did and what my dad encouraged. I hadn't yet developed an understanding of proper form or the nuances of intelligent program design. Meeting Coach Ed changed all that.

Ed was responsible for Olympic sport strength and conditioning—that meant everything except football. The football strength coaches were the celebrated big shots, earning higher paychecks and training athletes in top-tier facilities. They were the "it" guys. Meanwhile, Coach Ed was quietly working in the shadows, viewed skeptically by the football coaches because he emphasized a different style of training. Rather than just bench pressing, squatting, and deadlifting, Ed prioritized functional movements, mobility, warm-ups, and prehab exercises. He championed "functional training" long before it became a buzzword.

I vividly remember one of my first encounters with Coach Ed. My dad, Ed, and I had stepped into the football team's impressive weight room at UB's stadium, waiting for the team to finish a session. I stood next to Ed, watching as the players lifted—bench pressing and jammer pressing heavy loads. Push, push, push. The weights clanged noisily, each rep driven by ego and bravado.

Ed hated everything about it—the poor form, rounded shoulders, strained necks, and flailing bodies with reduced range of motion. These athletes could barely stand straight after lifting. Their training created stiff, immobile bodies more akin to wooden 2x4s than dynamic, athletic machines. He found this personally offensive because, to him, proper technique and balanced training were everything. Watching that session, he shared his philosophy with me: "It takes more than a big bench press to be a great athlete. You need a smarter plan, one that prioritizes movement quality, balance, and long-term performance."

From day one, Coach Ed drilled a simple principle into me: For every push, there must be a pull.

Under his guidance, I strictly followed a one-to-one push-to-pull ratio—bench presses balanced by rows, overhead presses paired with pull-ups. But it wasn't just about the ratio. Coach Ed emphasized moving with good form, intention, and purpose in every rep. It seems simple—even obvious—but at the time, no one else trained this way.

While other athletes hammered their chests, neglecting their backs and sacrificing quality for ego, I felt like I'd discovered a secret weapon: a balanced, intelligent approach to pain-free, functional strength training. My performance improved rapidly, my body grew stronger, and I experienced fewer injuries.

For years, I relied on that formula. It worked brilliantly. When I transitioned from athlete to coach, I confidently passed those same principles along to my clients, sure the approach would continue to hold up. But over time, I began noticing a troubling pattern: Even athletes who diligently followed this balanced ratio with an emphasis of form were increasingly experiencing shoulder pain, neck tightness, and posture issues.

At first, I was baffled. Sports hadn't changed, and human anatomy certainly hadn't evolved overnight. Then, suddenly, it clicked: Technology had.

By 2008—the year the original iPhone was released and changed everything—screens had become ubiquitous. Smartphones and laptops dominated everyday life. People, athletes included, spent countless hours hunched forward, their shoulders rounded, necks craned, upper backs rigid and locked into place. The old one-to-one ratio simply

couldn't counteract these new sedentary demands, no matter how well the athletes moved.

I remember precisely when this realization hit home. I was treating a professional athlete during a manual therapy session, and while I was working to undo the stiffness caused by his forward-rounded posture, he sat texting on his phone. His shoulders were so protracted, his upper back so locked forward, it was as if his body had forgotten how to extend. This wasn't just bad posture—it showed just how ingrained these patterns had become, even in someone whose livelihood depended on optimal movement.

It became clear: The pull of modern life was relentless, indiscriminately affecting everyone. Even elite athletes weren't immune. Without intentional, proactive effort, these destructive patterns would persist, undermining performance and longevity.

The old one-to-one ratio clearly wasn't enough anymore. I needed a better solution. Initially, I introduced a two-to-one pull-to-push ratio, emphasizing rows, pull-ups, face pulls, and band pull-aparts. Results were immediate: Shoulder pain decreased, posture improved, and athletes moved better. But screen time continued rising, eventually surpassing 11 hours daily for many people, and even two-to-one wasn't sufficient.

Today, I advocate a three-to-one pull-to-push ratio—a shift that may seem extreme at first, but it's proven to be one of the most impactful changes I've ever made. For every push movement, perform three pulling movements, factoring in all reps equally—warm-ups, recovery, and actual training sessions alike (more on this in Part 4). It's a total volume approach—not about load, but about consistently counteracting poor posture patterns.

This adjustment directly addresses the challenges of modern life, where forward-dominant postures create imbalances that not only affect how you move and feel but also contribute to chronic neck and shoulder pain in so many people.

Here's why pulling exercises—and this ratio—are so effective:

Restore joint neutrality: Pulling movements help re-center the shoulder joint, reducing strain on the soft tissues and restoring its natural alignment. This improves overall joint health and maximizes stability and muscle engagement.

Improve thoracic mobility: Rows, face pulls, and other pulling variations promote thoracic extension, which counters the forward-rounded postures caused by hours of sitting or screen use.

Strengthen the upper back: Pulling exercises build strength in the scapular stabilizers, traps, rhomboids, and rear delts, enhancing posture and stability for nearly every movement.

Enhance range of motion: Regular training of pulling patterns re-establishes lost ranges of motion, allowing the body to access and stabilize positions it may not have used in years.

Develop "muscle armor": Consistently training pulling patterns with optimal form builds a robust, resilient upper back that supports both static and dynamic movements and protects against injury.

Prevent overtraining the push pattern: Emphasizing pulling movements helps offset and reverse the overuse of push-dominant patterns, which are common in both training and daily life.

Coach Ed's advice from years ago resonates stronger than ever: "Strength alone isn't enough. You need balance." In today's world, where screens dominate our posture and pushing exercises dominate gym culture, his wisdom holds even greater weight. It's not just about lifting heavy—it's about restoring balance to your body.

But remember—the ratio alone is not the complete solution. Performing three-to-one pulling exercises with poor technique can be just as harmful as neglecting pulling entirely.

True progress comes from a movement mastery mindset, where your goal is to rebuild your entire pattern of movement. Only by training intentionally—ensuring pulling exercises are tailored to your individual needs with thoughtful screens, assessments, and progressions—can you build lasting pain-free performance.

PULL SCREEN

The pull screen is an essential test for evaluating pulling mechanics and uncovering hidden movement inefficiencies. Built around the inverted row, it creates a controlled yet challenging environment to assess how well your shoulders, shoulder blades, thoracic cage, and arms move as one coordinated unit. Think of it as a dynamic checkup to see if your upper body is working smoothly while your lower body provides a strong, stable foundation, anchored firmly to the ground through your feet. Done right, it reveals exactly where your movement quality can improve, setting you up for greater strength, efficiency, and performance.

Similar to the push pattern, pulling movements exist on a spectrum, ranging from horizontal pulls, like inverted rows, to vertical pulls, like pull-ups. For screening purposes, the inverted row strikes a perfect balance between load and accessibility, allowing enough resistance to expose movement flaws without overwhelming the system.

The benefits of the inverted row for screening include

▼ BALANCED LOADING:
The 45-degree angle provides just enough resistance to challenge the pulling pattern while keeping movement quality intact. Unlike fully horizontal rows, which can be too demanding for some, this position ensures that strength deficits don't overshadow movement evaluation.

▼ FREEDOM OF MOTION:
The use of rings allows for natural wrist and shoulder external rotation, enhancing stability and reducing unnecessary strain on the joints and soft tissue.

▼ ACCESSIBILITY:
Most individuals, regardless of strength level, can perform a ring row at this angle, making it an effective and inclusive screening tool.

▼ FULL RANGE OF MOTION:
The inverted row allows for a complete movement arc, providing a clear view of how the shoulder joint and scapula perform throughout the pull.

▼ ADJUSTABLE DIFFICULTY:
Foot positioning and body angle can be modified to scale the difficulty—move your feet forward (more horizontal body angle) to increase the challenge or step them back (more vertical body angle) to make it easier. This ensures people of all strength levels can perform the screen effectively without masking movement faults.

Like all movement pattern screens, the inverted row is a diagnostic tool. The goal isn't to test your strength but to observe how well you move through the pattern. A clean pull involves a smooth transition between protraction (shoulder blades gliding forward around the rib cage) and retraction (shoulder blades pulling back toward the spine), with the scapulae gliding dynamically in sync with the arms and thoracic cage.

Consider a chronic bench presser attempting the pull screen. More often than not, they'll default to what they know: locking their scapulae down and back rather than allowing a natural protraction-retraction rhythm. Instead of working as an integrated system, their body essentially hits the brakes mid-movement, restricting scapular motion and limiting full extension and flexion at the glenohumeral joint. This rigidity prevents the shoulder blades from rotating freely, reducing pulling efficiency and increasing compensatory stress elsewhere in the system. The pull screen exposes these habits, making it clear where improvements are needed.

SETUP: BODY ANGLE and POSITION

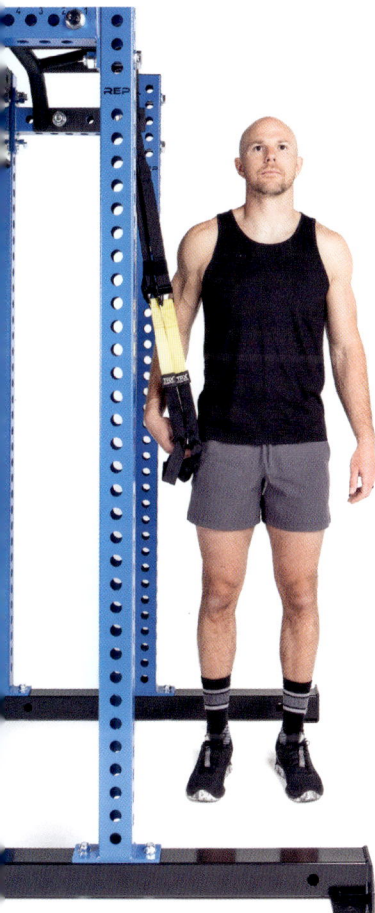

The pull screen begins with a proper setup to ensure the movement is both effective and diagnostic. The ideal setup uses a suspension trainer or gymnastic rings, which allow for natural rotation of the hands and better alignment throughout the pull. Follow these steps to set up the screen for optimal results:

1. **Height:** Position the suspension trainer or rings at hip height. This setup creates a 45-degree angle for the pull, providing just enough load to challenge the movement without overloading it or introducing compensations.

2. **Body Positioning:** There are two ways to set up for the inverted row. The first is to form your grip on the suspension trainer, sit on the ground, and then get into reverse plank position by driving your heels into the ground while extending your knees and hips. The second is to position your feet in front of the anchor point, spaced about hip-width apart, then lean back until your body forms a straight line from head to heels. Both setups create a reverse plank at approximately a 45-degree angle. Here are some key elements to focus on:

   - Maintain alignment from the shoulders, core, and hips, ensuring your spine is neutral.

   - Start with your arms fully extended with palms pronated (facing down or away from your body).

   - Adjust the difficulty by walking your feet forward, increasing the load to make it more difficult, or walking your feet back to reduce load, making the movement easier.

3. **Create Tension and Stability:** The pull screen requires proper irradiation (whole-body tension) to stabilize the movement and evaluate the mechanics accurately:

   - Co-contract the pecs and lats. Grip the handles or rings firmly. This creates tension that feeds up the chain, enhancing stability at the shoulders and core.

   - Co-contract your glutes and adductors while driving your heels into the ground.

   - Take in a big breath and lock down your core.

EXECUTION: PERFORMING THE PULL

Once the setup is established, the pull screen evaluates how efficiently your upper body coordinates scapular movement, joint centration, and muscular engagement throughout the pulling motion.

Initiating the Pull (Concentric Phase): Drive your elbows back into the same humeral carrying angle determined by the push assessment while maintaining a straight-line posture from head to heels.

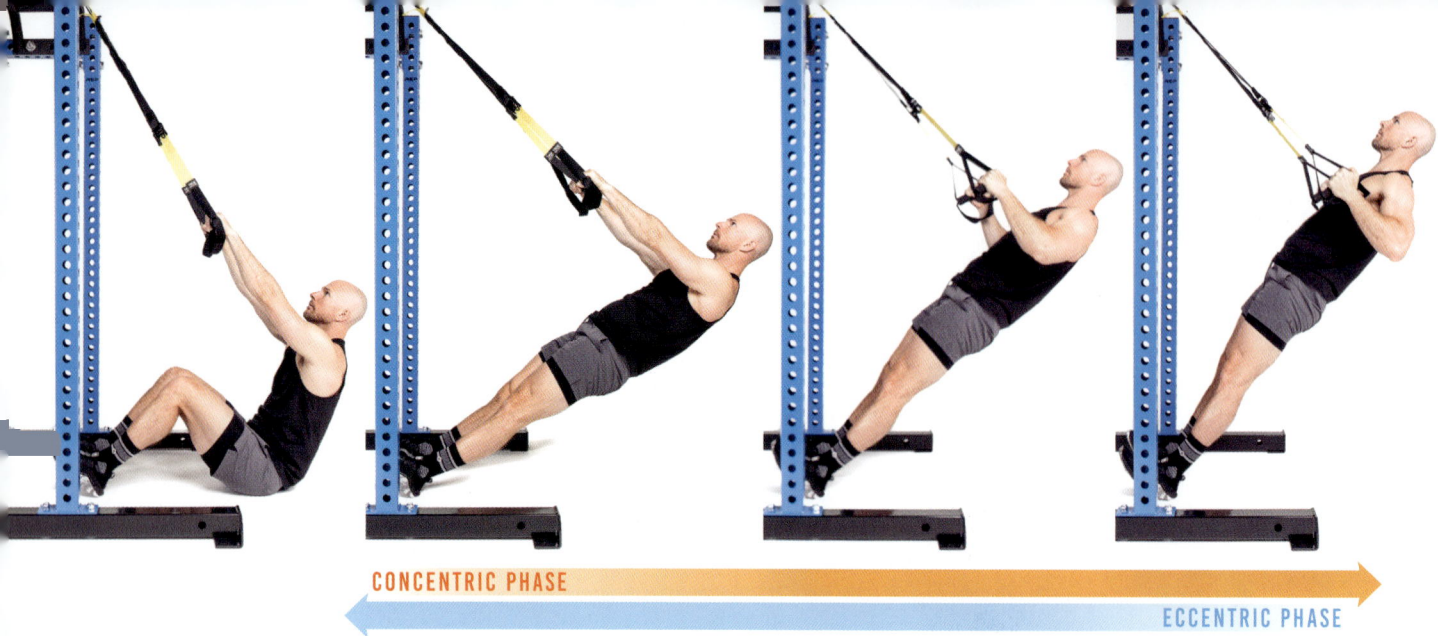

CONCENTRIC PHASE

ECCENTRIC PHASE

Allow your shoulder blades to retract smoothly, gliding along the rib cage without excessive shrugging or stiffness.

As you pull, allow your hands to rotate naturally. This rotation reflects external rotation at the shoulder joint, providing valuable insights into scapular movement and humeral carrying angles. Avoid over-cueing this aspect—it's more important to observe how your body moves naturally.

As you reach the top position, your chest should move toward the handles without your shoulders rounding forward, low back arching, or hips sagging.

Lowering with Control (Eccentric Phase): Reverse the motion by slowly extending your arms, resisting the urge to drop into the bottom position too quickly.

Let the scapulae protract naturally, ensuring smooth movement rather than rigidly holding them back.

Maintain core engagement throughout, preventing your lower back from hyperextending or your hips from dropping.

Throughout both phases, the goal is to observe whether your shoulders, scapulae, and thoracic cage work together in an integrated pattern or if compensations disrupt smooth movement.

OPTIMIZATION CHECKLIST

The pull optimization checklist fine-tunes the small but critical details that make the difference between smooth, pain-free pulling and movement patterns that create unnecessary strain or inefficiency.

By focusing on key components—keeping a neutral spinal position, controlling unwanted rotation, coordinating smooth scapular movement, aligning your shoulders properly, and maintaining full-body tension—you'll create a rock-solid foundation for stronger, safer, and more effective pulling across the entire movement spectrum. Treat this checklist as an extension of the pull screen, recording yourself from multiple angles to get a clear picture of how your body moves and what you need to improve.

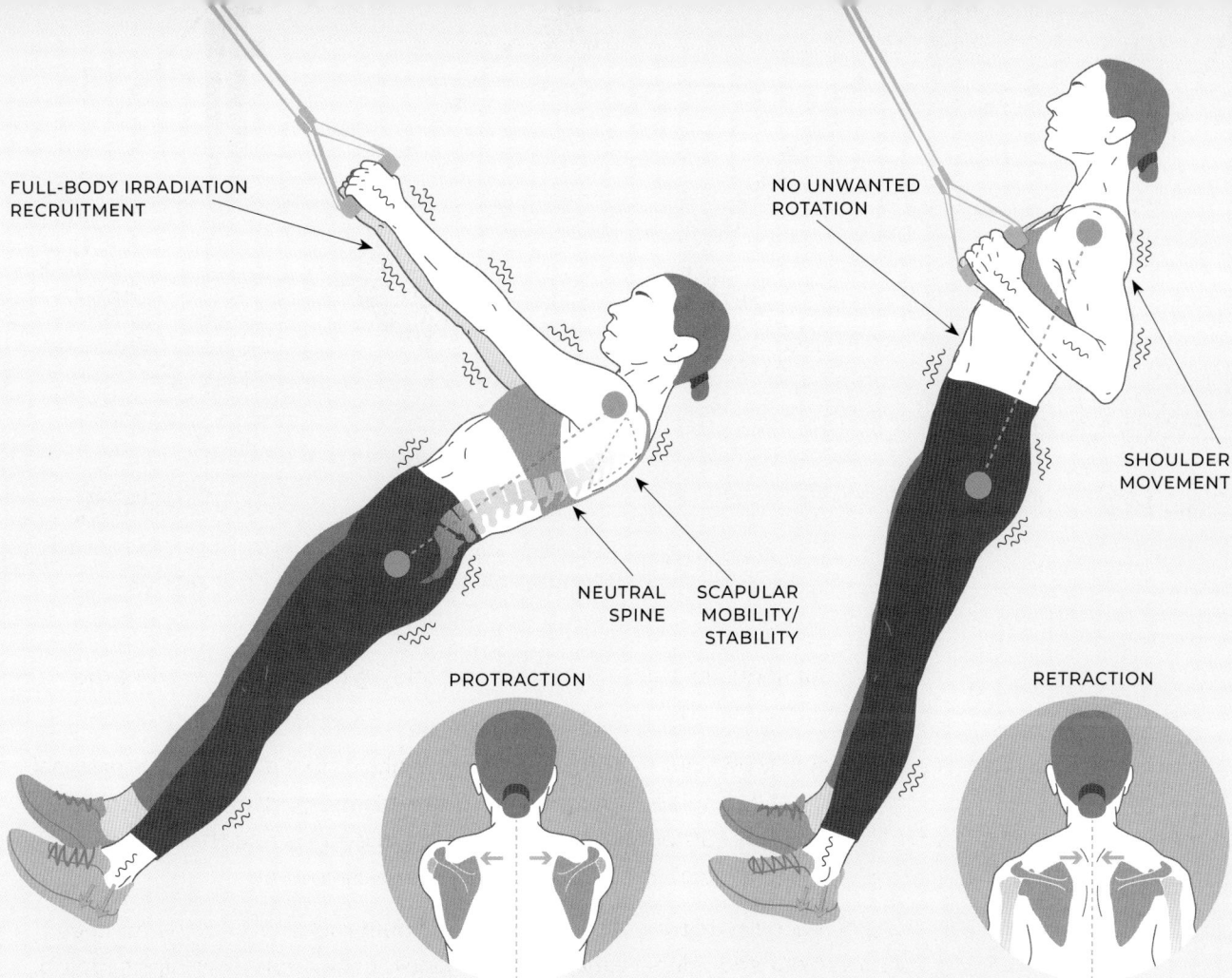

FULL-BODY IRRADIATION RECRUITMENT

NO UNWANTED ROTATION

SHOULDER MOVEMENT

NEUTRAL SPINE

SCAPULAR MOBILITY/ STABILITY

PROTRACTION

RETRACTION

✓ NEUTRAL SPINE

A neutral spine sets the foundation for an efficient pull. Excessive arching, rounding, or sagging in the lower back signals a loss of pillar control, disrupting how force transfers through the body. Stability here isn't just about posture—it determines whether the upper body can generate strength without energy leaking through unnecessary movement. When reviewing your pull screen, check for any deviations that suggest instability. The body should stay rigid from head to heels, aligned without excessive shifting or compensations.

✓ NO UNWANTED ROTATION

During the pull screen, observe whether your torso remains stable throughout the movement. Any twisting, tilting, or shifting means the body is redirecting force to make up for a lack of control elsewhere. The goal is a clean, controlled pull, where both sides of the body move in unison without unnecessary adjustments.

✓ SCAPULAR MOBILITY/ STABILITY

Scapular movement is the engine of an efficient pull. If the scapulae remain locked in place or don't move in sync with the arms, pulling strength is restricted, and unnecessary strain builds elsewhere. Smoothness and control are key. Instead of forcing the shoulder blades "down and back" at all times, let them move naturally through their full range—shifting forward into protraction as you extend your arms and pulling back into retraction as you initiate the row. This natural rhythm allows for full range of motion and optimal force production.

✓ SHOULDER MOVEMENT

Shoulder positioning dictates whether the pull is efficient or compensatory. An ideal pull keeps the shoulders centered within the joint, moving naturally with the arms without excessive shrugging. If the shoulders elevate or round forward at any point in the movement, it's a sign that the traps and anterior chain are taking over rather than the lats, traps, and rhomboids working together in balance.

✓ FULL-BODY IRRADIATION RECRUITMENT

A strong pull requires total-body engagement. The grip is the first point of engagement—a strong grip creates tension that radiates upward, stabilizing the shoulders and core. The lower body must stay engaged as well, with heels pressing into the ground and glutes maintaining tension to prevent energy leaks. Without full-body irradiation, force is lost, revealing compensations that reduce muscle engagement and amplify joint strain.

PULL ASSESSMENT

Your ability to pull with strength and control comes down to how well your body coordinates movement across multiple joints. But pulling is more than just moving weight from point A to point B—it's a dynamic, full-body process driven by scapular movement, thoracic extension, and, the most misunderstood element, rotation. The shoulder blades don't just retract and protract; they glide, tilt, and rotate in sync with the upper back, allowing for smooth, powerful movement. Yet rotation is rarely trained the way it should be, leading to stiffness, imbalances, and plateaus that lifters struggle to fix—because they don't even realize it's missing.

SCAPULAR MOVEMENT

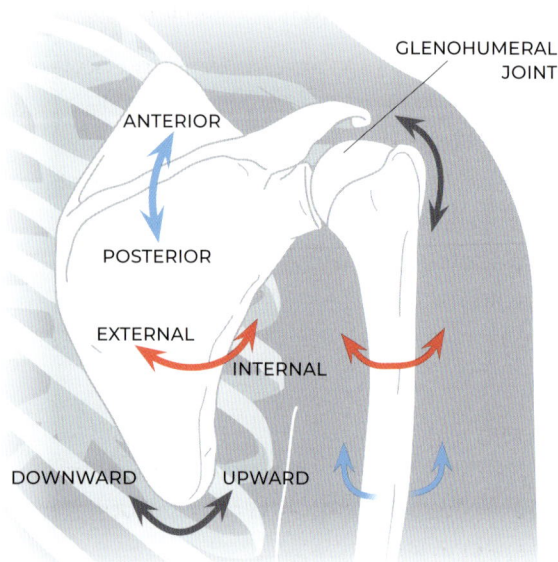

Rotation is pivotal to functional pulling movements. Without rotation, pulls become rigid and lose their unique value. But when rotation is properly integrated, pulling becomes a synergistic movement pattern essential for reversing poor posture, improving shoulder health, and enhancing overall performance. **Think of pulling exercises like daily multivitamins for your shoulders—rotation ensures you absorb all the benefits.** When rotation is restricted, the body compensates, often by hiking the shoulders up, rolling them forward, or forcing movement from the wrong areas. These inefficiencies not only weaken your pull but also increase stress on the neck, traps, and front of the shoulders, leading to imbalances and potential pain over time.

THE PUSH ASSESSMENT APPLIES TO THE PULL

In the previous chapter, you performed the push assessment to determine how your shoulders naturally align and move—specifically your humeral carrying angle and overhead mobility.

Your humeral carrying angle—the arm position identified in the push assessment—translates directly to pulling movements. The same position your arms take at the bottom of a push-up is the one they should follow at the finish of a row. Maintaining this angle keeps your shoulders in a strong, stable position, reducing unnecessary strain and allowing better control. If the assessment revealed weaknesses or restrictions, they'll show up in pulling exercises too, impacting everything from shoulder blade movement to how effectively you engage your back muscles.

Your overhead mobility findings also carry over to vertical pulling. If you struggled to reach a full overhead position without compensation, movements like pull-ups and lat pulldowns will expose the same limitations. Before progressing with overhead pulls, use your assessment results to determine whether the limitation stems from mobility, stability, or both. If mobility improves in a supported position, the focus shifts to strengthening stability and coordination (see **Shoulder Stability Linchpin Blueprint** on page 474). If your range remains restricted in both tests, mobility must be addressed by implementing the **Overhead Stability Linchpin Blueprint** (page 474).

THORACIC SPINE ROTATION

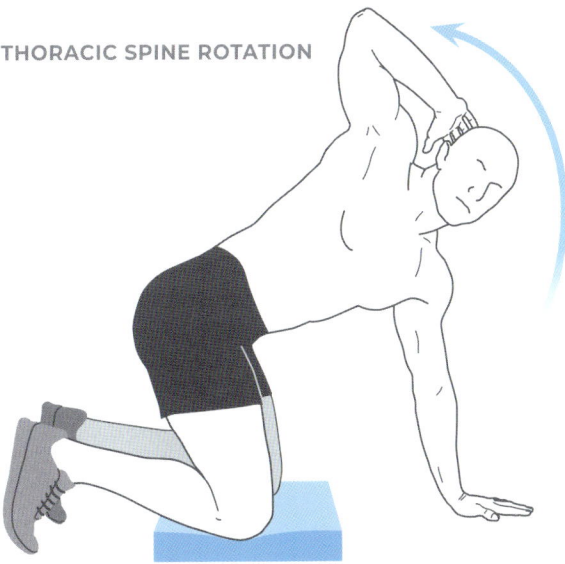

The pull assessment breaks this down clearly with two key tests: **thoracic spine rotation** and **total shoulder rotational arc**.

The first evaluates how freely your thoracic spine can rotate—a crucial function that allows your shoulder blades to move through their full range. If thoracic rotation is restricted, your shoulders are forced to overwork, leading to inefficient movement and increased joint strain. The second test assesses the total rotational arc of motion at the shoulder joint, measuring internal and external rotation. This determines how much natural rotation your shoulder can handle, directly impacting exercise selection, grip positioning, and movement quality in pulling exercises.

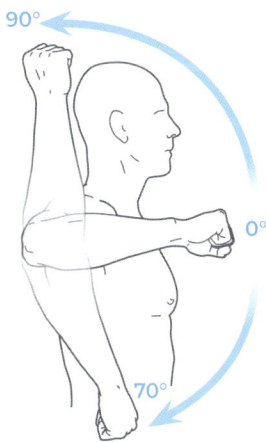

In pain-free performance, effective training revolves around restoring proper movement. That's why we prioritize pulling variations that reinforce full-range rotation rather than movements that lock the shoulder blades into fixed positions and encourage compensations. Modern life isn't doing your posture any favors—hours spent at desks and on screens stiffen your thoracic spine, making it harder for your shoulders and upper back to function properly. Training through full rotation counteracts this stiffness, improves mobility, and ensures the right muscles drive the movement rather than overloading your joints.

By performing these assessments, you'll pinpoint exactly where restrictions exist and what needs to be addressed. Whether the issue is mobility, stability, or a combination of both, the results will guide you toward the appropriate Linchpin Blueprint to improve your specific limitations.

90°

0°

70°

SHOULDER
ROTATIONAL ARC

THORACIC ROTATION TEST— UNLOCKING SHOULDER MOBILITY

The thoracic spine—the segment of your upper back between your neck and lumbar spine—is crucial for healthy, pain-free shoulder movement. Think of it as the foundation for everything your upper body does, from reaching overhead to pulling open a heavy door. How well you can extend (straighten up) and rotate this part of your spine determines how smoothly your shoulder blades glide, which in turn impacts how effectively your shoulders move.

But here's the thing: everyone's thoracic spine is different. Age, activity levels, and even daily habits shape how much mobility you have. As you get older, the spine naturally rounds forward a bit more—a posture called kyphosis—which can make extending your upper back more challenging. Combine that natural aging process with today's sedentary lifestyles—hours spent slouched over phones and computers—and it's no wonder so many people experience stiff shoulders and limited upper back movement. When your thoracic spine becomes rigid, your shoulder blades lose their freedom, making pulling exercises (like rows and pull-ups) and everyday tasks more difficult and less effective.

That's why the thoracic rotation test is such an important assessment. It measures how well you can rotate and extend your upper back, shining a light on potential restrictions that can limit shoulder function. While the initial pull screen looks at symmetrical movement—pulling with both arms simultaneously—in reality, we rarely move that way outside the gym. Most daily activities involve single-arm movements, which naturally engage rotation in your thoracic spine. That's the beauty of unilateral (one-sided) pulling exercises: they automatically unlock your body's natural rotational capabilities, tapping into your spine's true potential.

During this thoracic rotation test, you'll rotate purely from your thoracic spine and shoulders, not from twisting your hips or lower back. If your movement feels smooth, balanced, and free, that's fantastic—it means your thoracic spine is moving well enough to support your pulling exercises without limitations. But if you feel stiffness, uneven rotation, or if your body feels like it's fighting to move, that signals a potential issue. At that point, you need a deeper understanding of whether your restriction is caused by a lack of mobility (tightness or stiffness) or a lack of stability (weakness or poor control).

To pinpoint the exact problem, you'll perform a second test that immobilizes your shoulder blade and shoulder joint, isolating movement entirely to your thoracic spine. This step helps clarify whether your thoracic spine itself is restricted, or if the issue lies more in your shoulder blade coordination.

If rotation remains restricted, you'll prioritize thoracic mobility strategies—drills like thoracic extensions, rotations, and side-lying mobility exercises.

If rotation improves, your limitation is scapular control, and your strategy shifts toward activation and stability drills to improve shoulder blade smoothness and coordination.

If both tests are restricted, you'll combine both strategies to fully unlock your pulling potential.

Just like in the push assessment, the thoracic rotation test follows an "if this, then that" model. If you demonstrate adequate thoracic mobility, there's no need to move on to the second test. But if your mobility is limited, the second test is essential for identifying exactly what you need to prioritize.

T-SPINE AND SCAPULAR ROTATION

1. STARTING POSITION

▶ **Action:** Begin in a quadruped position with your knees directly beneath your hips. Position your feet so the balls of your feet and toes rest flat on the ground, with your heels pointing upward. The wrists, elbows, and shoulders should be aligned at shoulder width, with fingers pointing forward. Place one hand lightly on the back of your neck.

▶ **Goal:** Establish a neutral spine, brace your core, and prepare your body for controlled rotation without compensating through the lower back or pelvis.

▶ **Observation:** This position sets the foundation for the movement. If maintaining a neutral spine and braced core feels difficult, it may indicate a lack of baseline stability.

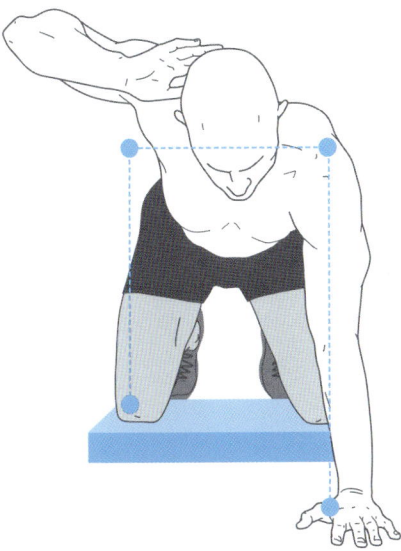

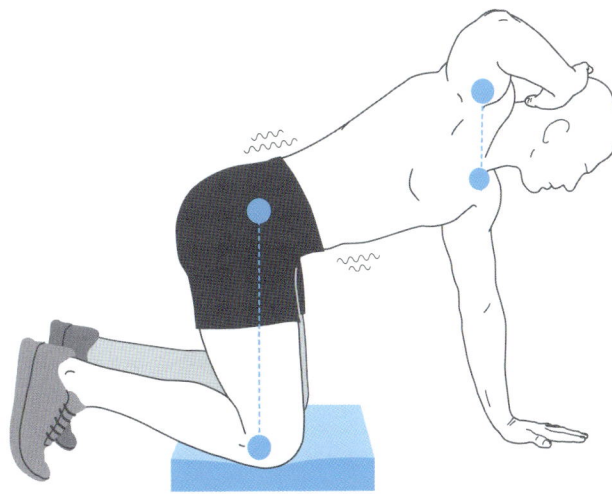

2. THORACIC FLEXION WITH ROTATION

▶ **Action:** Lower the elbow of your raised arm toward the opposite elbow while maintaining pillar stability. Avoid shifting your hips or rounding your lower back.

▶ **Goal:** Create a starting position that maximizes the range of motion from the thoracic spine while keeping the rest of the body engaged.

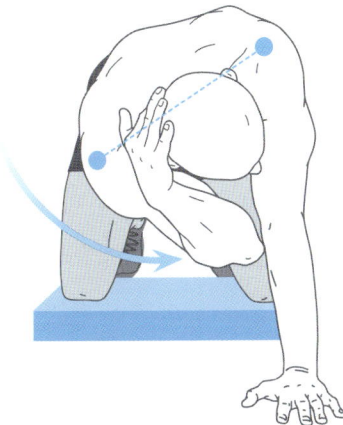

▶ **Observation:** Most individuals should reach elbow to elbow with ease. Struggling here may suggest limitations in thoracic mobility or an inability to separate upper back movement from the lumbar spine. It's important to remember that, during pulling movements—especially unilateral rows and high rows—the thoracic cage should be free to explore its complete range of motion. Although modern sedentary postures often cause the thoracic spine to become chronically rounded (flexed forward), healthy pulling mechanics require the thoracic spine to flex as well as extend.

3. THORACIC EXTENSION WITH ROTATION

▶ **Action:** Rotate your torso upward, leading with your elbow. Focus on generating movement through the thoracic spine, ensuring your hips and lumbar spine remain stable. Continue rotating until reaching end range, ideally beyond 45 degrees with your elbow approaching near your centerline.

▶ **Goal:** Assess the ability to extend and rotate the thoracic spine while maintaining pillar stability. The movement should be smooth and controlled, with the shoulder blade moving freely.

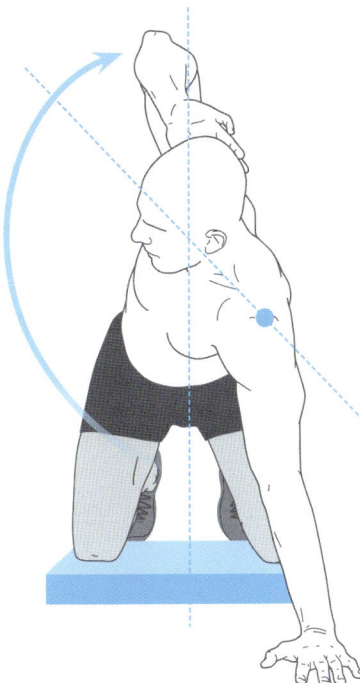

▶ **Observation:** A full range of motion not only improves rotation during single-arm rows and overhead pulling but also helps prevent compensations that come from a lack of rotational mobility. When rotation is restricted, your body will find a way to work around it—usually by shifting stress to your lower back, shrugging the shoulders, or forcing movement from the wrong areas.

• If your movement is smooth, symmetrical, and coordinated through a full range of motion, you're good to go.

• If you notice limited or uneven rotation, the next step is figuring out whether the restriction is due to limited thoracic mobility, a lack of scapular control, or both.

ISOLATED T-SPINE ROTATION

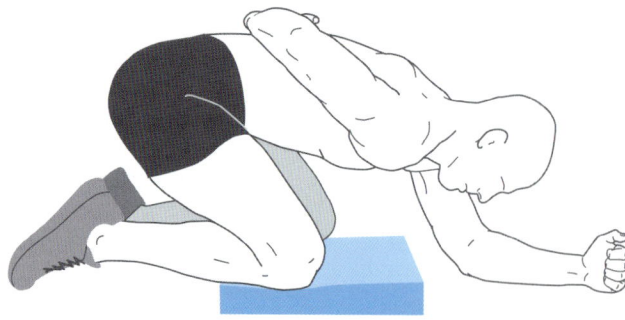

Perform each step on both sides of your body before moving on to the second test. Note any differences between your left and right sides. Then repeat the process for the second test, again testing both sides fully and comparing your results.

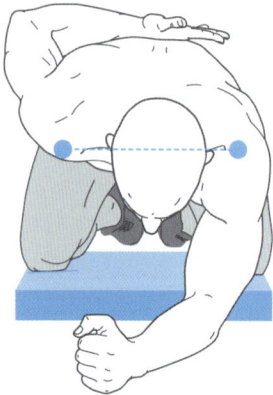

1. STARTING POSITION

▶ **Action:** Begin in a quadruped position. Point your toes down with the tops of your feet flush with the ground and shift your hips back (butt to heels) into a slight posterior pelvic tilt to lock the lumbar spine in place. Place your forearm on the ground to the inside of your knee. Position your free hand on your lower back (with the knuckles flush against your back as if being handcuffed) and move it toward your shoulder blades—this upward movement fully protracts the scapula, securing it in place and ensuring the rotation comes exclusively from your thoracic spine.

▶ **Goal:** Restrict movement at the scapula, glenohumeral joint, and lower back to isolate thoracic rotation.

▶ **Observation:** This locked setup differentiates thoracic mobility limitations from scapular control deficits, making it easier to determine whether you need the **T-Spine Mobility Linchpin Blueprint**, the **Scapular Control Linchpin Blueprint**, or a combination of both.

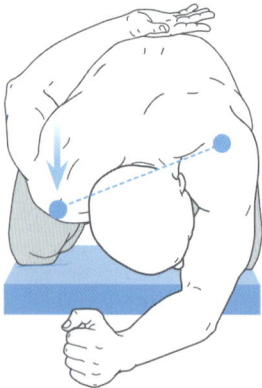

2. THORACIC FLEXION WITH ROTATION

▶ **Action:** Lower the shoulder of your "handcuffed" arm—positioned behind your back—toward your grounded elbow.

▶ **Goal:** Isolate and assess pure thoracic flexion without compensating through the shoulder blade.

▶ **Observation:** Many people aren't limited in this range due to lack of mobility; they're limited by poor control or coordination, often a result of living in chronically flexed postures. While extension often gets the spotlight in strength training, healthy pulling mechanics require both thoracic flexion and extension. Flexion allows for proper scapular glide and spinal segmentation during the eccentric and mid-range phases of a pull, while extension supports retraction and finishing the movement with control. You need both to move well and train the back effectively.

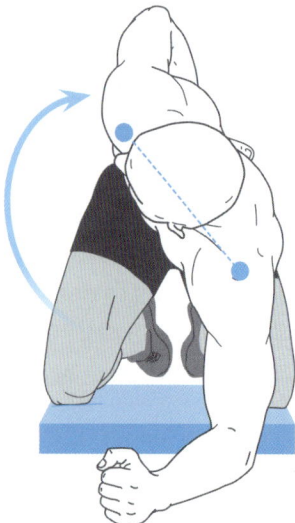

3. THORACIC EXTENSION WITH ROTATION

▶ **Action:** Rotate your torso, opening toward the ceiling. Keep your forearm planted on the ground and your opposite hand locked in position behind your back. The movement should come exclusively from the thoracic spine, with no compensation from the lower back or shoulder blade. Compare your range of motion to the previous test and note any differences.

- ▶ **Goal:** Identify whether your rotation limitation is due to restricted thoracic mobility or poor scapular control.

- ▶ **Observation:** This test provides a crucial piece of the puzzle—helping you pinpoint the root cause of movement restrictions so you can target the right solution and eliminate compensations before they lead to pain or hinder performance.

• If rotation remains significantly restricted, thoracic mobility is the primary issue, and you'll need to follow the **T-Spine Mobility Linchpin Blueprint** (page 471).

• If rotation improves noticeably in this locked position, the restriction is likely due to scapular control and stability deficits. In this case, you should follow the **Scapular Stability Linchpin Blueprint** (page 473), focusing on activation and stability drills to improve shoulder blade movement.

• If both thoracic mobility and scapular control appear limited, you'll need a combined approach, integrating both blueprints to unlock full movement potential and restore optimal pulling mechanics.

INTERNAL AND EXTERNAL ROTATION TEST —DETERMINING YOUR SHOULDERS' FUNCTIONAL ROTATIONAL ARC of MOTION

Every pulling movement naturally follows a path of shoulder rotation. As you pull, your shoulder transitions fluidly from internal rotation (where your arm rotates inward toward your body) to external rotation (where your arm rotates outward, away from your body). Your total ability to move smoothly between these two points—your shoulder's functional arc—determines how efficiently you can transfer force, maintain stability, and keep your joints healthy.

This test assesses how much total shoulder rotation you have access to, specifically at your glenohumeral joint (shoulder joint). Think of your shoulder's rotation like a dial: the wider the arc, the more versatile your pulling movements become. A wide rotational arc gives you the freedom to safely perform a variety of pulls with less restriction. On the other hand, a narrow arc limits your movement options, often leading your body to compensate with your neck, traps, or chest muscles when venturing outside your available range, creating unwanted joint stress and potential discomfort.

Previously, you assessed your thoracic spine's ability to rotate. Now you'll isolate the shoulder joint to see how much rotation your shoulder truly has. These two assessments complement each other closely—if your thoracic spine is limited, your shoulders will likely compensate, and vice versa.

By assessing both internal and external rotation, you'll get a clear picture of how well your shoulders move and where you may need adjustments. Your results will shape everything from your setup and grip positioning to the pulling variations you should prioritize, modify, or avoid—all based on your pain-free, natural range. Simply put, knowing your shoulder rotation arc helps you play to your strengths, address limitations, and fine-tune your training strategies to build stronger, healthier shoulders.

1. STARTING POSITION

▶ **Action:** Lie on your back with your upper arm resting on the ground at your humeral carrying angle (the arm angle identified during your push assessment). Your elbow should bend to roughly 90 degrees, with your forearm pointing straight toward the ceiling. Keep your shoulder blades flat on the ground. Position your feet flat with your knees bent—this wedges your torso securely into the ground and stabilizes your shoulders.

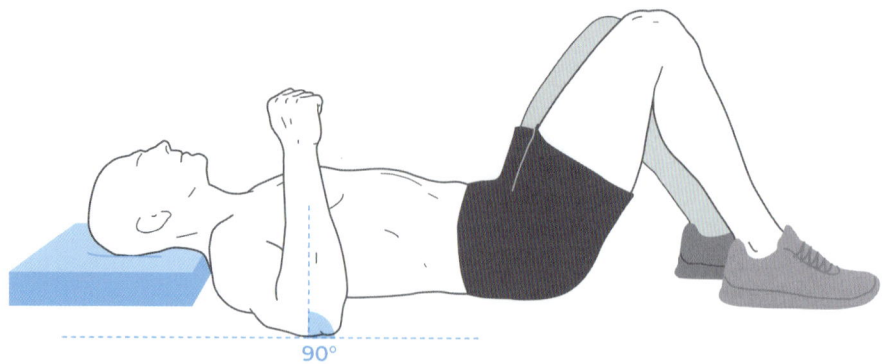

▶ **Goal:** Establish a stable, neutral shoulder position to isolate rotation at the glenohumeral joint. This setup ensures that movement occurs purely at the shoulder, without compensation from the scapula or thoracic spine.

2. EXTERNAL ROTATION

▶ **Action:** Keeping your elbow bent at 90 degrees, slowly rotate your forearm backward toward the floor. Keep your upper arm and shoulder blade stationary. Stop as soon as you feel resistance or tightness.

▶ **Goal:** Test your shoulder's ability to rotate outward (external rotation) without compensations.

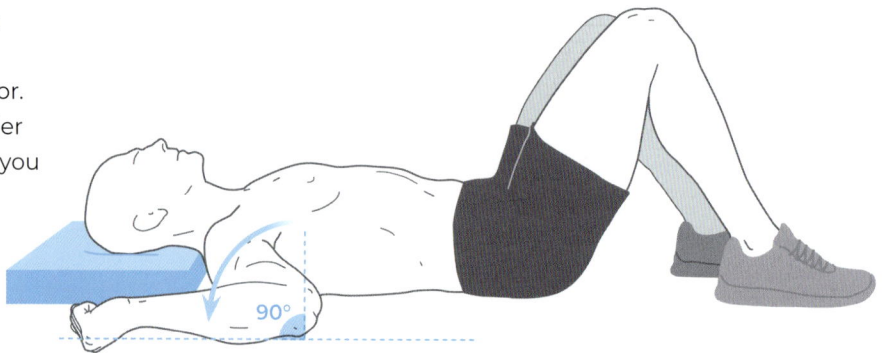

▶ **Observation:**

• **Ideal Range (around 90 degrees):** The back of your hand comfortably touches or nearly touches the floor without strain. This indicates excellent external rotation, allowing you to safely perform overhead pulls (e.g., pull-ups, overhead presses). However, having sufficient mobility alone does not guarantee that you're prepared for vertical pulling. Adequate strength, stability, and motor control are also essential. While this test confirms your theoretical rotational capacity for overhead movements, you still need to test your overhead mobility using the Overhead Range of Motion Test (page 346) and safely progress your stability and skill through the pull progression pyramid before jumping into vertical pulling exercises.

• **Acceptable Range (around 70 degrees):** Your hand is within 1 to 2 inches of the floor. You can still safely perform most pulling exercises, but you might need slight modifications to overhead or rotational patterns. The most practical adjustment involves training overhead pulling movements with a neutral grip (instead of wide pronated or supinated grips) or performing pulls at slightly angled positions—such as high angle rows—where your available range of around 70 degrees matches the positional demands of the exercise.

• **Limited Range:** Your hand remains several inches above the floor (greater than 2 inches), signaling restricted external rotation. Lack of external rotation at the shoulder makes vertical pulls and high-angle rows problematic due to mobility deficits, preventing safe access to these movements. Prioritize horizontal pull variations and emphasize your shoulder mobility linchpin blueprints to gradually restore external rotation, eventually allowing you to safely progress back into overhead and high angle pulling exercises.

3. INTERNAL ROTATION

▶ **Action:** From the same starting position, rotate your forearm forward toward the floor, again maintaining the 90-degree elbow bend. Keep your upper arm and shoulder blade locked in place.

▶ **Goal:** Test your shoulder's inward rotational capacity (internal rotation) without compensations.

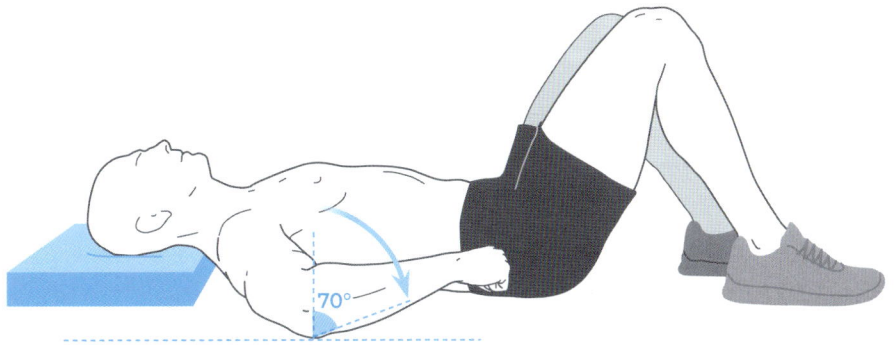

▶ **Observation:**

• **Ideal Range (over 70 degrees):** Your palm comfortably moves toward the floor, ending approximately 3 to 4 inches from the ground. This allows you to safely perform vertical pull variations (e.g., pull-ups, lat pulldowns) without excessive joint strain.

• **Acceptable Range (around 45 degrees):** Your hand reaches roughly halfway toward the floor. You can manage vertical pulls, but you may notice tension or compensations when using narrow or pronated (overhand) grips.

• **Limited Range:** Your hand moves very little, staying high above the floor. This significant restriction often results in compensations—like rounded shoulders, chest activation, or neck tightness—during overhead pulling movements. You'll need to prioritize the shoulder mobility linchpin blueprints before progressing to advanced pulling patterns.

4. INTERPRETING YOUR RESULTS

Your total rotational arc—the combined internal and external rotation—determines your overall shoulder rotation capacity:

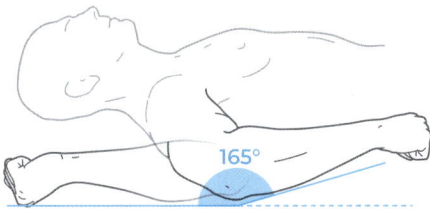

• **Wide Arc (Ideal: 165 degrees or more):** You have excellent rotation, meaning your shoulders can safely handle various pulling movements, grips, and angles with less risk of compensations. Your aim is to maintain and strengthen this capacity.

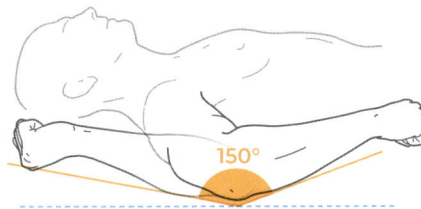

• **Moderate Arc (Acceptable: around 150 degrees):** You can still perform most pulls comfortably, but certain advanced or narrow-grip vertical pulling exercises like pull-ups and lat pulldowns might create discomfort or compensations. Prioritize targeted mobility and stability drills to expand your range safely.

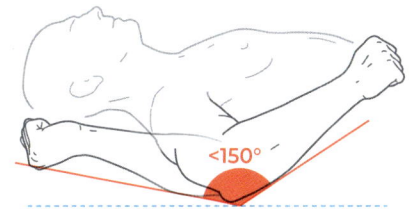

• **Narrow Arc (Limited: below 150 degrees):** You're more vulnerable to compensations—such as overusing your neck, traps, or pecs—during pulling movements, especially overhead. You'll benefit from combined interventions—thoracic mobility, shoulder mobility, and scapular stability linchpin blueprints—to progressively widen your safe pulling range.

THREE KEYS TO LONG-TERM SHOULDER HEALTH

Keeping your shoulders pain-free and strong isn't complicated—but it does require intentional training. If you want shoulders that not only move well but also last a lifetime, you need to focus on these three fundamentals:

1. ACCESS YOUR FULL RANGE OF MOTION

If you can't comfortably move into a position, your body will find a way around it—and that's where problems start. Compensation patterns kick in, shifting stress to areas that aren't meant to handle it, often leading to pain or injury.

What happens when you prioritize it?
You restore natural movement, allowing your shoulders to function efficiently, distribute stress properly, and handle a variety of movements without unnecessary strain. This means smoother, stronger reps, better posture, and reduced injury risk.

What happens when you ignore it?
Your shoulders lock down, forcing movement into the wrong places—your neck, traps, lower back, or even elbows and wrists. This often leads to chronic tightness, and nagging pain, especially with overhead or rotational movements.

Example: Think of trying to do a pull-up with limited shoulder mobility—you might make it work, but at what cost? You'll likely overuse your traps, crane your neck, arch through your lower back, and flare your elbows out. Over time, this catches up to you in the form of pain, impingements, or decreased performance.

2. TRAIN ACROSS ALL PLANES OF MOTION WITH ROTATION

Your shoulders aren't just built to move up and down or front to back—they're designed for rotation and multidirectional movement. If you only train in a single plane (e.g., pressing and pulling straight forward and back), you leave weak spots in your mobility, stability, and strength.

What happens when you prioritize it?
You develop well-rounded, resilient shoulders that can handle unexpected movements, different angles, and real-world demands. Training through multiple planes enhances coordination, reduces risk of injury, and improves athleticism.

What happens when you ignore it?
You become stiff and fragile outside your comfort zone. Your body is strong in a straight line, but the second you have to move at an angle—whether reaching for something in daily life or absorbing a force in sports—you're at a higher risk for strain or injury.

Example: If you never incorporate rotation, your ability to control your scapulae in real-world movements will suffer. Try moving your arm without rotating from your shoulder in anything outside of the usual gym patterns, and you'll find that it's impossible.

3. BUILD STRENGTH THROUGH ALL POSITIONS

Mobility is only useful if you can control it. Once you can comfortably access a position, you need to reinforce it with stability and strength—this is what keeps your shoulders from breaking down under stress.

What happens when you prioritize it?
You turn flexibility into usable strength—meaning you don't just have the ability to reach a position, but you can own it under load. This makes your shoulders more functional, adaptable, and durable.

What happens when you ignore it?
You might be mobile, but you're weak in those end ranges, making you vulnerable when stress is applied. This is why so many people feel fine until they add weight or speed and then suddenly experience pain or strain in their shoulders.

Example: Imagine being able to passively reach overhead, but the second you load a heavy overhead press, your form crumbles. Or maybe you can stretch into a deep row, but under resistance, you can't control the movement without compensating. If you don't build strength through those positions, your mobility is just a party trick, not a real advantage.

THE TAKEAWAY

Your shoulders need a balance of mobility, stability, movement variety, and strength to stay pain-free and high-performing for the long haul. If you're missing even one of these three components, your training (and your body) will eventually hit a wall. But when you combine all three, you create shoulders that are ready for anything life throws at you.

OPTIMIZATION STRATEGIES

The optimization strategies in this section will fine-tune your pull mechanics by directly addressing the mobility, stability, and skill issues you identified during your pull screen and assessment—as well as those that may surface when you perform exercises within the pull pattern pyramid. Think of compensations as your body's clever (but ultimately unsustainable) way of navigating underlying limitations. Ignore these subtle signs, and you'll likely face nagging pain in your shoulders, lower back, or neck and stalled progress down the road.

Your mission here is straightforward: Get ahead of problems before they start. By proactively targeting your weakest links, you'll establish smoother, stronger, and pain-free pulling mechanics that feel as good as they look.

Let's dive into the most common compensations seen in horizontal pulls (rows) and vertical pulls (overhead variations). We'll uncover exactly why these compensations occur and pinpoint targeted solutions you can apply immediately.

COMPENSATION: SHOULDERS ELEVATING/SHRUGGING (AND/OR INAPPROPRIATE SCAPULAR POSITION OR RHYTHM)

MOBILITY: Sitting, driving, texting, and generally living with shoulders rounded forward can result in chronically tight pecs, lats, and upper traps. These restrictions directly limit your shoulder complex's full rotational and overhead movement, negatively impacting both horizontal (rows) and vertical (pull-ups, pulldowns) pull exercises. Signs you may have a mobility restriction:

▼ Tightness or restriction in your chest or anterior shoulders when opening your arms wide to a T-shape or reaching overhead (as determined by the **Overhead Range of Motion Test** on page 346)

▼ Persistent upper trap tightness, stiffness in your neck, or trap dominance in pushing or pulling exercises

OPTIMIZATION STRATEGIES:

▶ Perform the **Shoulder Mobility A (Horizontal) Linchpin Blueprint** (page 471):

▶ Match your pulling angle and exercise selection to your current available range of motion. For example:

- **Horizontal:** Choose clearly defined range of motion endpoints that allow for optimal form and stability.

- **Vertical:** Opt for high-angle cable rows or single-arm variations that allow slight thoracic rotation instead of strict overhead patterns.

- Utilize your humeral carrying angle identified during the **Shoulder Scour Test** (page 342) to optimize range without compensation.

STABILITY: Everyday posture and training habits (overemphasizing push and neglecting pulls) often result in weak, unstable posterior shoulders and scapulae. Without sufficient posterior stability, the upper traps compensate, causing stiffness, neck pain, or poor control in your pull patterns. Challenges associated with poor stability may present as

▼ Difficulty engaging your mid-back, lats, or rear shoulders during pulls

▼ Upper traps or grip prematurely fatiguing, overshadowing your target pulling muscles

▼ Inability to consistently maintain good shoulder positioning and joint centration

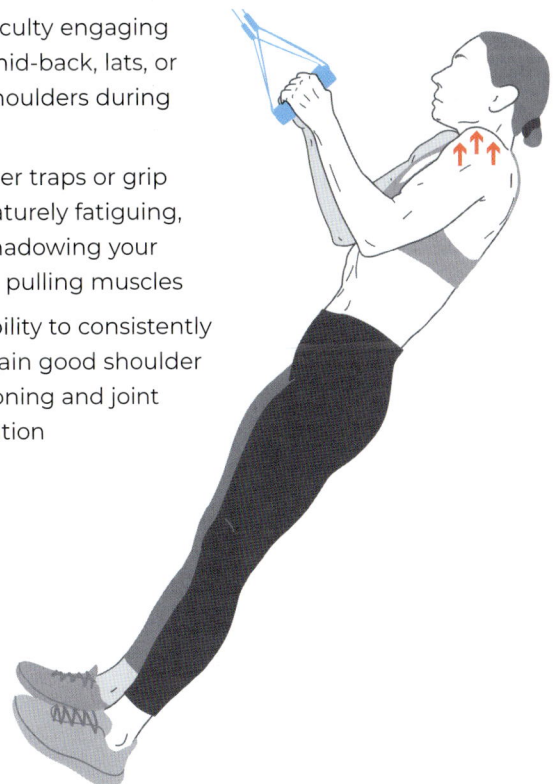

▶ Perform the **Scapular Stability Linchpin Blueprint** (page 473).

▶ Before initiating pulls, always set your pillar position by co-contracting pecs and lats, breathing and bracing effectively, and performing reps slowly and intentionally, within your controlled range of motion.

▶ Use regressed horizontal and vertical pulling variations:

- **Horizontal:** Set the suspension trainer higher, increasing the angle of your body to reduce the demand. Perform single arm row variations with light weight.

- **Vertical:** Prioritize half-kneeling single-arm pulldowns or kneeling high-angle rows.

▶ **Perform the "Scapular J" as a practice drill:** Set up like an inverted row, but keep your arms straight. Move only your shoulder blades by retracting them down and back, then gently protracting forward. Perform 8–10 reps at an angle that avoids upper trap activation. This establishes a critical mind-muscle connection, allowing you to initiate your rows properly from the scapulae.

SKILL: The shoulder joint is exceptionally dynamic and requires precise coordination for optimal function—something often compromised by rounded postures and sedentary lifestyles. Particularly for beginners or individuals working through chronic pain or discomfort, mastering consistent technique can be challenging. Indicators of a skill gap include

▼ Difficulty maintaining full-body tension (irradiation) and controlled, consistent tempo, particularly during eccentric (lowering) phases

▼ Inconsistency in pulling positions—such as variable hand placement during rows or inconsistent bar placement during pulldowns—without deliberate intent

OPTIMIZATION STRATEGIES:

▶ Alternate between the **Scapular Stability Linchpin Blueprint** (page 473) and **Core Stability A (Supine) Linchpin Blueprint** (page 472).

▶ Choose bilateral movements first to improve positional control and resist unwanted rotation. Once consistency and skill improve, progress toward unilateral exercises.

▶ Prioritize the pillar cueing sequence by co-contracting your pecs and lats to ensure shoulder joint centration. If you compensate, reduce the range of motion until you develop the motor control to maintain neutral shoulder positioning.

▶ **Perform the "Scapular J" as a practice drill** (see the description in the stability optimization strategies).

COMPENSATION: RIB FLARE/ LOW BACK ARCH

MOBILITY: Although rib flare and low-back arching typically aren't mobility issues in horizontal pulls, overhead pulling exercises reveal these limitations clearly. Excessive sitting and slouched postures can shorten and tighten your lats, limiting your ability to reach overhead without compensation. Mobility restrictions may present as

▼ Tightness in your lats when reaching overhead or pinching in the front of your shoulder

▼ Difficulty taking deep, full breaths due to restricted rib cage movement

▼ Pressure or tightness in your lower back when pressing or pulling overhead

OPTIMIZATION STRATEGIES:

▶ Perform the **Shoulder Mobility B (Vertical) Linchpin Blueprint** (page 472).

▶ Perform the **Overhead Range of Motion Test** (page 346) to determine whether the restriction stems from a true mobility deficit or is more related to a stability limitation.

▶ Swap overhead pulling movements (lat pulldowns, pull-ups) for high-angle cable or band rows to better match your current overhead mobility. Attempting to load positions you can't comfortably access increases shoulder strain, discomfort, and may further exaggerate compensation patterns.

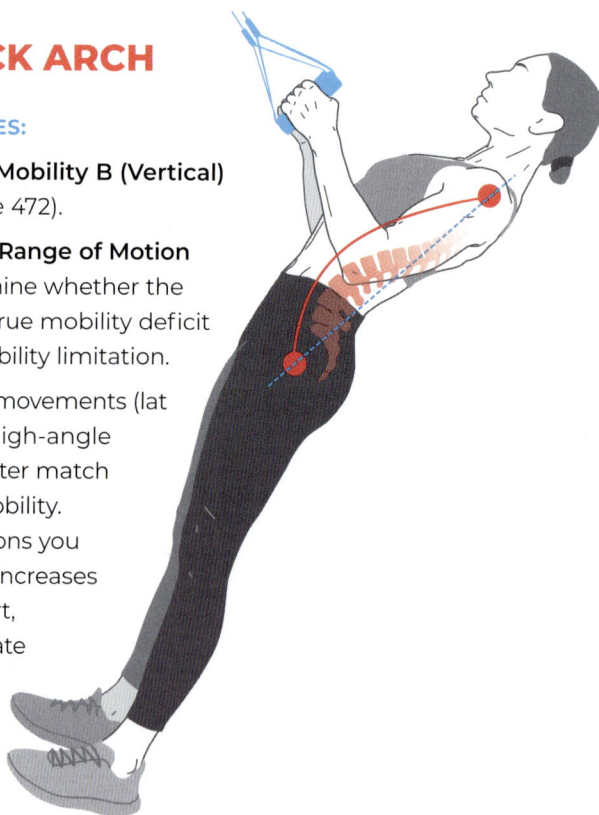

STABILITY: Poor posture, sedentary habits, or limited experience controlling your pillar can all lead to rib flare and excessive lumbar arching, affecting both horizontal and vertical pulls. Rib cage position directly impacts core stability, meaning any deficits here significantly limit your pulling mechanics and overall movement quality. You may notice:

▼ Difficulty maintaining alignment in foundational core positions like dead bugs, planks, and side planks

▼ Low-back pinching or discomfort during inverted rows or overhead pulling exercises, particularly as you approach full concentric positions

▼ Feeling the need to arch or lean back during overhead pulls (lat pulldowns, pull-ups) because it's the only position that feels stable or strong

OPTIMIZATION STRATEGIES:

▶ Regularly use the **Core Stability A (Supine) Linchpin Blueprint** (page 472) in your warm-up, emphasizing proper pillar positioning and alignment.

▶ **For horizontal pulls:**

· Use a modified setup for inverted rows. Start upright with your hands near your rib cage, your elbows pulled back, and slight tension in the straps. Set your pillar first (pelvis and rib cage stacked, pecs and lats co-contracted), then slowly walk your feet forward into your chosen angle. This allows you to find and maintain optimal posture from the start, preventing rib flare as you progressively increase the challenge over time.

▶ **For vertical pulls:**

· Prioritize high-angle cable or band rows.

· Incorporate core-strengthening exercises such as planks, side planks, Pallof presses, and hollow-body holds to reinforce strong pillar positioning, particularly as preparation for pull-ups and chin-ups.

SKILL: Both horizontal pulls (especially inverted rows) and vertical pulls (particularly chin-ups and pull-ups) place unique demands on your skill and control. Rib flare or back arching often occurs due to the unfamiliar feeling of maintaining proper alignment under these conditions. Signs of a skill gap include

▼ Difficulty controlling your body angle and resisting side-to-side sway or instability during inverted rows

▼ Unintentionally leaning backward during vertical pulling patterns, especially pull-ups

▼ Uncontrolled swinging or uneven pulling angles, indicating lack of consistency in your setup or execution

OPTIMIZATION STRATEGIES:

▶ Alternate between the **Shoulder Stability Linchpin Blueprint** (page 474) and **Core Stability A (Supine) Linchpin Blueprint** (page 472) to increase overall awareness, control, and positional stability.

▶ **For horizontal pulls:**

· Perform inverted rows at a higher body angle (more upright) or use a wider stance to increase stability and gradually build confidence and skill.

▶ **For vertical pulls:**

· Replace overhead exercises with high-angle cable or band rows until you've mastered consistent pillar positioning.

· For assisted pull-ups or chin-ups, place the assistance band under one foot (secured by crossing the opposite foot over the ankle) while maintaining a slight hollow-body position. This setup promotes a better pelvis and rib cage alignment.

· Alternatively, attach the assistance band to J-hooks rather than directly overhead, adjusting the height for optimal assistance, ensuring controlled and stable reps.

COMPENSATION: **UNWANTED ROTATION/LOSS OF SYMMETRY**

MOBILITY: Sports, hobbies, and even daily activities are frequently asymmetrical, resulting in subtle imbalances that affect your training—especially in pushing and pulling exercises. Signs you may have a mobility restriction:

▼ Tightness or restricted range of motion on one side when performing push or pull movements

▼ Increased discomfort, tightness, or a deeper stretch sensation on one side during phases 1 and 2 of your warm-up

OPTIMIZATION STRATEGIES:

▶ Perform the **Shoulder Mobility A (Horizontal) Linchpin Blueprint** (page 471).

▶ Ensure your initial setup is balanced and symmetrical by following the pillar cueing sequence (page 34). Move slowly and deliberately, staying within the range where symmetry can be maintained. Over time, you'll expand this symmetrical range through consistent mobility-focused warm-ups, workouts, and cool-down routines.

STABILITY: It's common to see differences in shoulder and scapular stability between sides, particularly if you have a clear dominant hand. Sports, repetitive tasks, or daily habits often reinforce strength and stability differences, resulting in noticeable asymmetries when performing pulls. Challenges associated with poor stability may present as

▼ Greater strength, control, or endurance on your dominant side, enabling more high-quality repetitions

▼ Earlier fatigue or difficulty controlling the eccentric (lowering) phase on your weaker side, potentially causing rotation or loss of symmetry

OPTIMIZATION STRATEGIES:

▶ Incorporate the **Scapular Stability Linchpin Blueprint** (page 473).

▶ Add core-focused exercises such as planks, side planks, and Pallof press variations, as well as rear-delt isolation drills near the end of your workouts, to further improve shoulder stability.

SKILL: Asymmetry and unwanted rotation frequently surface when you lack familiarity or confidence with certain pulling exercises, particularly when using functional training tools or when moving under heavier loads, higher speeds, or fatigue. Signs of a skill gap include

▼ Difficulty maintaining controlled, even reps

▼ Increasing rotation or loss of balance as you introduce greater intensity, load, or when approaching fatigue

UNWANTED
ROTATION/
LOSS OF
SYMMETRY

OPTIMIZATION STRATEGIES:

▶ Regularly perform the **Shoulder Stability Linchpin Blueprint** (page 474) and **Core Stability B (Prone) Linchpin Blueprint** (page 473) to enhance total-body coordination and control.

▶ Prioritize the pillar cueing sequence by co-contracting your pecs and lats to ensure shoulder joint centration. If you compensate, reduce the range of motion until you develop the motor control to maintain symmetry.

▶ Slow down your repetitions, focusing on maintaining optimal alignment and tension throughout each rep, particularly in the eccentric (lowering) phase.

▶ Perform inverted rows at a higher angle or with a wider stance, progressively increasing the difficulty only as you gain confidence and skill.

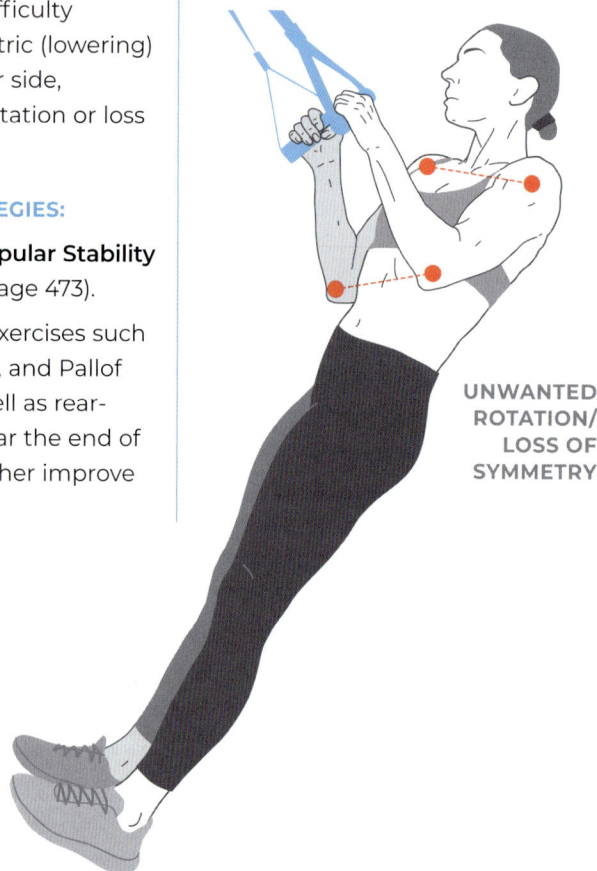

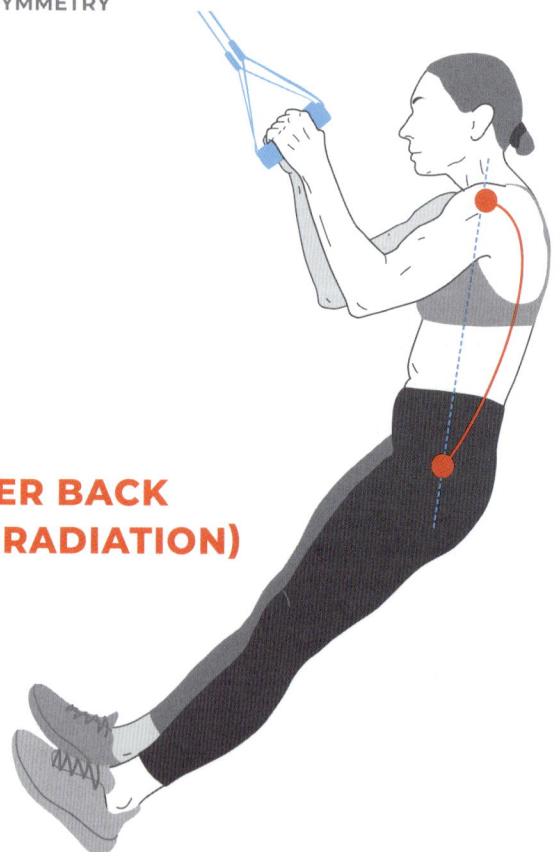

COMPENSATION: HIPS SAGGING/UPPER BACK ROUNDING (LOSS OF TOTAL-BODY IRRADIATION)

MOBILITY: Prolonged sitting can cause tight hips and limited thoracic spine extension, preventing you from fully engaging your posterior chain (glutes, hamstrings, spinal erectors, mid-back muscles). As a result, your hips may sag and your upper back might round forward as your body searches for alternative ways to gain stability or increased range of motion.

Signs you may have a mobility restriction:

▼ Tightness in your quads or pressure in your lower back when attempting to fully extend your hips

▼ Hips noticeably sagging, causing your body alignment to deviate from a straight line

▼ Abs excessively activating to "assist" the pull, indicating a compensatory flexing of your core

▼ Minimal glute and posterior chain engagement, causing difficulty maintaining the proper reverse plank position

OPTIMIZATION STRATEGIES:

▶ Perform the **Hip Mobility A Linchpin Blueprint** (page 469) if you primarily experience hip tightness and lower body restrictions.

▶ Perform the **T-Spine Mobility Linchpin Blueprint** (page 471) if upper back rounding and thoracic restrictions are more prominent.

▶ If both compensations occur, alternate between these two blueprints regularly to comprehensively address mobility restrictions.

▶ Set your feet hip-width apart, co-contract your glutes and adductors, and lengthen your spine. Squeeze your glutes actively to maintain hip extension and a neutral spine position.

▶ Focus on "getting tall" during the exercise setup, creating length from your heels through the back of your head.

▶ Allow your hands to naturally rotate during the pull, and maintain gentle chin retraction to support neutral spinal alignment throughout each repetition.

STABILITY: Sedentary habits weaken postural stabilizers and diminish scapular stability. As these crucial muscles become less effective at maintaining posture, your body may compensate by rounding your upper back or allowing your hips to sag. This instability leads to inefficient movement patterns and poor muscular engagement during pulling exercises. Challenges associated with poor stability may present as

▼ Feeling loose, disconnected, or like only your arms are working during pulling exercises

▼ Upper traps dominating during pulling movements, or frequently experiencing premature fatigue in your shoulders, biceps, or grip

▼ Struggling to feel engagement in your mid/upper back, lats, or posterior shoulders

OPTIMIZATION STRATEGIES:

▶ Perform the **Core Stability B (Prone) Linchpin Blueprint** (page 473) if hips sagging and core weakness are your main concerns.

▶ Perform the **Scapular Stability Linchpin Blueprint** (page 473) if upper back rounding, scapular instability, or trap dominance is more prominent.

▶ If both compensations occur, alternate between these two blueprints to comprehensively rebuild stability.

▶ **Perform the "Scapular J" as a practice drill:** Set up like an inverted row but keep your arms straight. Move only your shoulder blades by retracting them down and back, then gently protracting forward. Perform 8–10 reps at an angle that avoids upper trap activation. This establishes a critical mind-muscle connection, allowing you to initiate your rows properly from the scapulae.

SKILL: Suspension trainers (inverted rows) shift your body's center of mass into unfamiliar angles and positions, making it challenging for new users to maintain alignment and stability. Initially, you might experience apprehension or difficulty controlling the body's position, causing your hips to sag or your upper back to round. Indicators of a skill gap include

▼ Feeling uncomfortable or unstable leaning back into a full reverse plank on the suspension trainer

▼ Body swaying side to side, or the straps feeling uneven, making stable positioning challenging

▼ Struggling with body control throughout the exercise, especially during fatigue or increased load

OPTIMIZATION STRATEGIES:

▶ Implement either the **Scapular Stability Linchpin Blueprint** (page 473) or the **Core Stability B (Prone) Linchpin Blueprint** (page 473) to build confidence and increase stability awareness. Alternate these blueprints depending on which compensations appear most frequently.

▶ Slow down your repetitions, focusing on maintaining optimal alignment and tension throughout each rep, particularly in the eccentric (lowering) phase.

▶ Perform inverted rows at a higher angle or with a wider stance, progressively increasing the difficulty only as you gain confidence and skill.

▶ **Perform the "Scapular J" as a practice drill** (see the description in the stability optimization strategies).

PULL PROGRESSION PYRAMID

The pull progression pyramid is designed to build strong, pain-free pulling mechanics by developing mobility, stability, and skill in the right order. The pyramid starts with horizontal pulling, where the body has more stability and control, and gradually progresses toward vertical pulls, which demand higher levels of scapular coordination, thoracic mobility, and core engagement. This order isn't arbitrary—it mirrors how the body naturally develops pulling strength and motor control. By reinforcing movement quality in stable positions before layering in complexity, you create a foundation that supports sustainable progress without breakdowns.

At the base of the pyramid is the **inverted row**, the foundation of the pull pattern. Think of it as the opposite action of a push-up—the only difference is the direction of force. With both feet grounded, the inverted row offers the highest level of stability while reinforcing full-body coordination. Holding a straight-line position from heels to head builds anti-flexion core strength, while the free-moving hands allow for natural scapular motion and arm rotation. This movement sets the stage for all pulling variations by teaching you how to engage your posterior chain, control your shoulder blades, and maintain proper tension throughout the pull.

The next step introduces **single-arm row variations**, which allow for greater rotation of the thoracic spine, scapula, and shoulder. Unlike the bilateral inverted row, which stabilizes the torso in a neutral position, single-arm rows incorporate natural rotation, providing a more dynamic movement pattern. This is critical for training real-world pulling mechanics, as no pulling motion in sports or daily life happens in a perfectly rigid bilateral position. By learning to rotate efficiently, you increase range of motion and develop a more adaptable, resilient pull pattern.

Building on this, the **bent-over row progression** shifts the pull pattern into a more functional and transferable position. Unlike previous variations that provided external support (such as the ground or a bench), the bent-over row requires you to stabilize through your own structure, reinforcing strength in an isometric, hip-hinged stance. This positioning carries over directly to movements that require sustained postural control, such as maintaining stability while carrying, picking something up, or generating force from a bent-over position. Training the pull pattern in a hinge not only strengthens the upper back but also enhances full-body coordination, reinforcing the pillar control needed for more advanced pulling movements.

The next step up the pyramid is **high-angle rows**, which begin shifting the pull pattern toward the vertical plane. These variations, performed at approximately 45 degrees, introduce more vertical scapular mechanics while maintaining elements of horizontal pulling. This progression bridges the gap between rows and true vertical pulling, preparing the body for the increased demands of overhead movements. As the angle of pull changes, so do the muscle recruitment patterns—high-angle rows emphasize lat engagement and scapular depression (drawing the shoulder blades down and away from the ears), laying the groundwork for vertical pulling strength.

With a strong base of horizontal and angled pulling, the progression moves into **lat pulldowns**, marking the transition to true vertical pulling. This shift introduces new demands on scapular mechanics and pillar stability, reinforcing the movement patterns required for overhead pulling. While often overlooked as a functional exercise, the lat pulldown plays a critical role in developing the control and strength needed before advancing to the highest-level pulling exercise.

At the top of the pyramid is the **pull-up**, the ultimate test of upper body strength, stability, and coordination. Unlike all previous progressions, the pull-up removes external support, demanding complete control over the pillar. The lack of ground contact increases the challenge significantly, making it essential to have mastered the previous steps before progressing. The pull-up is one of the most butchered movements in training, often performed with excessive swinging, rib flare, and poor scapular mechanics. However, when earned through proper progression, it becomes a powerful tool for long-term strength development, athletic performance, and pain-free pulling.

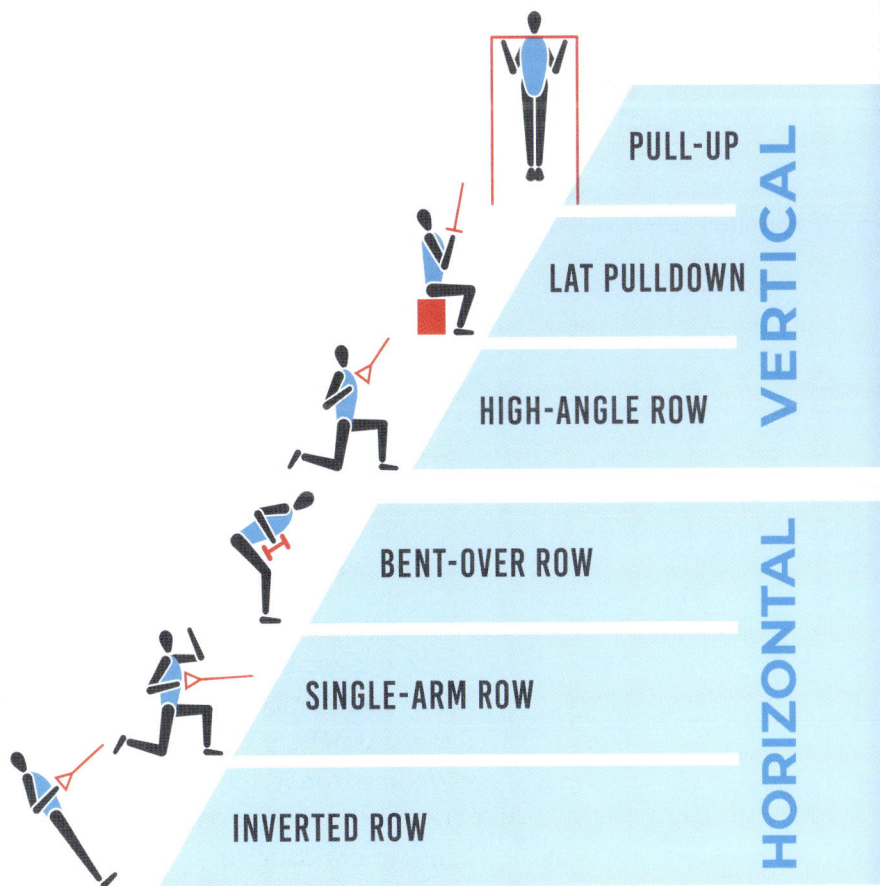

PULL-UP

LAT PULLDOWN

HIGH-ANGLE ROW

BENT-OVER ROW

SINGLE-ARM ROW

INVERTED ROW

VERTICAL

HORIZONTAL

WHAT ABOUT FACE PULLS?

If you've trained with me, you already know—you're going to be doing face pulls forever. Face pulls are a staple, and for good reason. They're one of the best movements for shoulder health, scapular control, and upper back activation. But here's the thing—face pulls are not part of the primary pulling pattern we've been building in this progression.

Unlike the key performance indicator (KPI) pulls, face pulls don't train the natural humeral carrying angle found in your push-pull assessment. Instead, they're performed in a more isolated force plane, targeting the posterior shoulder and upper back while removing the lat as a primary driver. This makes them highly effective for posterior shoulder activation improving function but not a loadable KPI movement like rows, pulldowns, and pull-ups.

So where do they belong? Face pulls should be a permanent fixture in your warm-ups for upper body training and can be used as an accessory exercise in hypertrophy-focused programming. Think of them in the same category as rear delt flies, band pull-aparts, and other direct upper back work—valuable for reinforcing movement quality, but not a replacement for heavy, compound pulling exercises.

HORIZONTAL PULL

INVERTED ROW

More than a screening tool, the inverted row is the foundation for learning and progressing the pull pattern. With your feet planted, you gain the support needed to integrate your entire body while reinforcing natural shoulder and scapular mechanics. This full-body engagement makes it one of the most effective and accessible ways to develop pulling competency and strength.

What makes the inverted row so valuable is its versatility. It can be adjusted to match any strength level and progressed in multiple ways to keep training effective and challenging. Whether you're refining hand positioning, adjusting your body angle, or adding load, the inverted row remains a core KPI exercise (key performance indicator— meaning it serves as a foundational exercise that

CONCENTRIC PHASE

ECCENTRIC PHASE

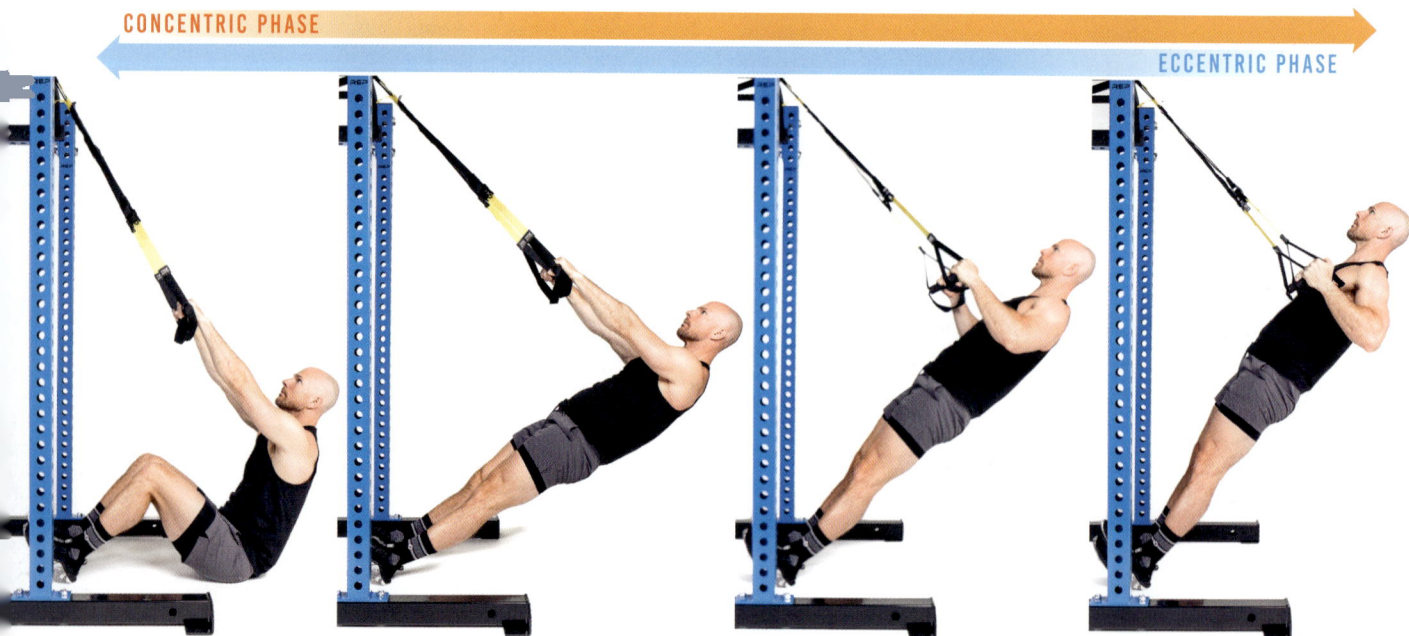

directly translates to overall pulling strength, back muscle development, and postural restoration).

Here's how to fine-tune your setup and execution for maximum benefit:

- **Equipment Selection and Hand Positioning:** The ideal implement for inverted rows is a suspension trainer such as TRX straps or rings. These tools provide the degrees of freedom needed for natural rotation through the arms and hands while allowing the shoulders and scapulae to move through a full range of motion. When necessary, a fixed bar in a rack or a Smith machine can be used, but it does not allow the same rotational mechanics. Regardless of the equipment used, maintaining full-body tension and a stable pillar position is essential for maximizing the benefits of the movement.

- **Foot Positioning and Stability:** A common mistake in the inverted row is performing the movement with bent knees and flat feet, which reduces posterior chain engagement. Instead, maintain a straight-line position from heels to head to create the necessary tension throughout your body. Ideally, your heels should press into a stable surface to provide a solid fulcrum for force transfer. Gain additional support by planting your toes against a wall or using a squat wedge to ensure a neutral ankle position. The more surface contact your feet have, the greater the stability, which enhances strength up the chain.

- **Adjusting Difficulty and Progressions:** One of the defining features of the inverted row is its scalability. Adjusting the angle of your body relative to the ground directly influences the difficulty. The more parallel your torso is to the ground, the greater the loading on your upper body. Conversely, a more upright position reduces the demand, making the movement easier. The key is to select a height that remains challenging enough to stimulate adaptation rather than simply going through the motions.

Once you've reached a position where your body is parallel to the ground and your feet are elevated—such as on a 12- to 16-inch box—you can further progress the movement by adding external load. Just like weighted push-ups, you can introduce resistance by placing a weight plate, chains, or a sandbag over your hips and lower torso.

For additional setup and execution details, refer to the pull screen and optimization checklist covered earlier in the chapter.

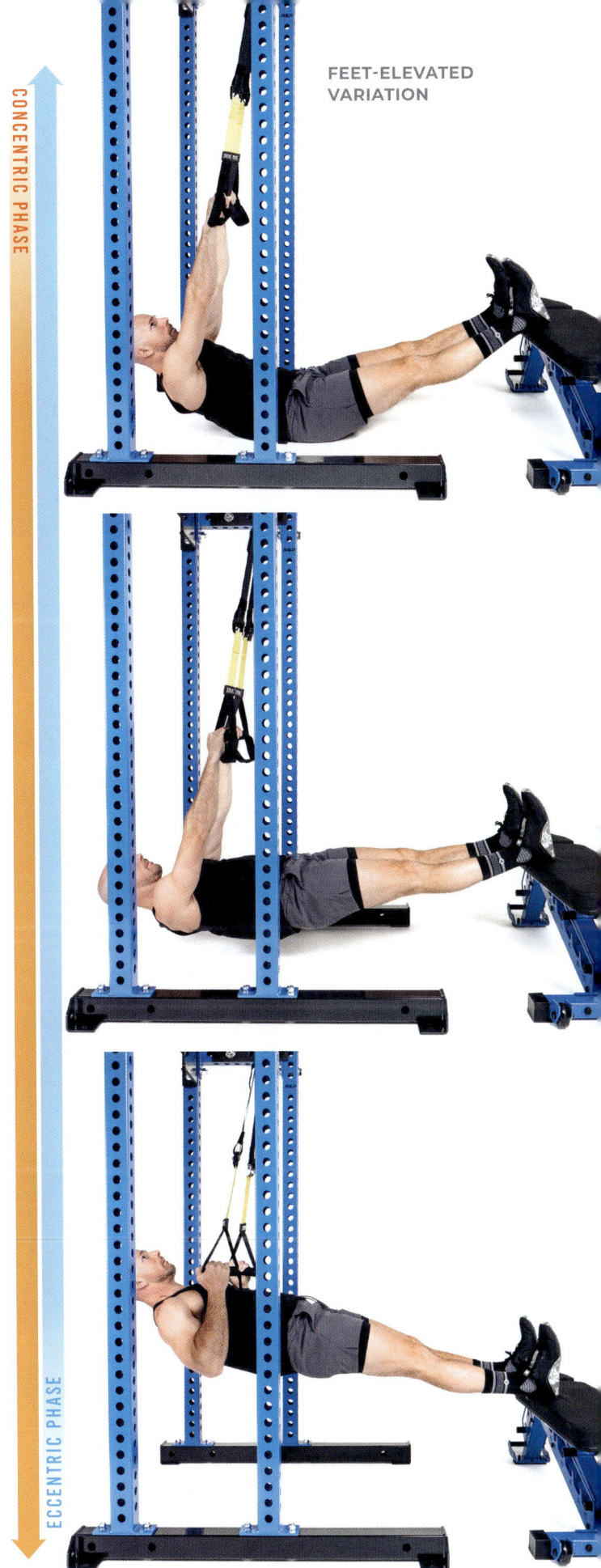

CONCENTRIC PHASE

ECCENTRIC PHASE

FEET-ELEVATED VARIATION

SINGLE-ARM ROW

The single-arm row is one of the most versatile and effective pulling exercises, making it a staple at every stage of training. Unlike bilateral rowing variations, single-arm rows allow for a more natural movement pattern, integrating thoracic spine rotation, scapular movement, and a full range of motion at the shoulder. This dynamic approach maximizes posterior shoulder and back muscle targeting, improves mobility, and reinforces postural control—all while allowing you to tailor the movement to your unique needs. By adjusting body positioning, stance, and load implement (dumbbell, kettlebell, or cable), you can emphasize different aspects of the pull, accommodate movement restrictions, and progressively challenge pillar strength and stability. Here are some considerations when progressing the single-arm row:

• **Foundational Progression:** *Three-Point Bench Row:* Provides the most stability by anchoring the body with a bench, allowing you to focus on controlled pulling mechanics, full range of motion, and scapular movement. Ideal for reinforcing proper positioning and building strength before progressing to less stable variations.

• **Intermediate Progression:** *Hinged Supported Row:* Removes one point of external stability, requiring more core and hip engagement. The kickstand stance shifts greater responsibility to the lower body while maintaining some upper body support, making it a logical next step toward more dynamic rowing.

• **Advanced Progression:** *Half-Kneeling Cable Row:* Introduces rotational freedom while maintaining a stable lower body base. This variation increases the demand for pillar stability and controlled thoracic rotation, helping to refine movement coordination in preparation for upright, unsupported pulls.

• **Highest Coordination Demand:** *Standing Cable Row:* The most dynamic variation, removing all external support and requiring full-body stability. This variation reinforces anti-rotational strength, postural control, and balance, making it an excellent choice for reinforcing dynamic control and coordination in an upright athletic stance.

SETUP: Single-arm rows can be performed with a dumbbell, kettlebell, or cable, with each implement affecting the movement slightly while maintaining the same fundamental mechanics.

• **Dumbbell/kettlebell rows** are the most common variations and provide a free-weight stimulus that demands core and shoulder stability while allowing for natural rotation.

• **Cable rows** offer a consistent resistance curve throughout the movement and allow for a more fluid pulling motion, reducing momentum and making it easier to control rotation.

THREE-POINT BENCH ROW

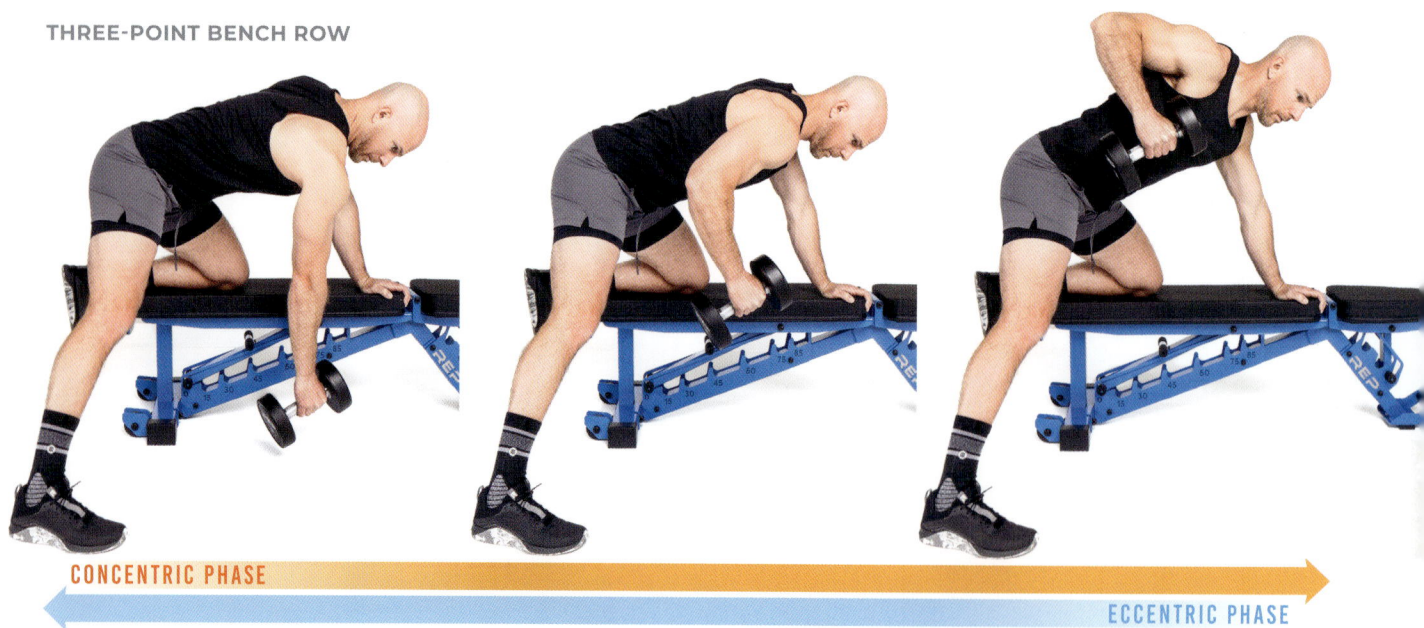

CONCENTRIC PHASE

ECCENTRIC PHASE

HINGE-SUPPORTED ROW

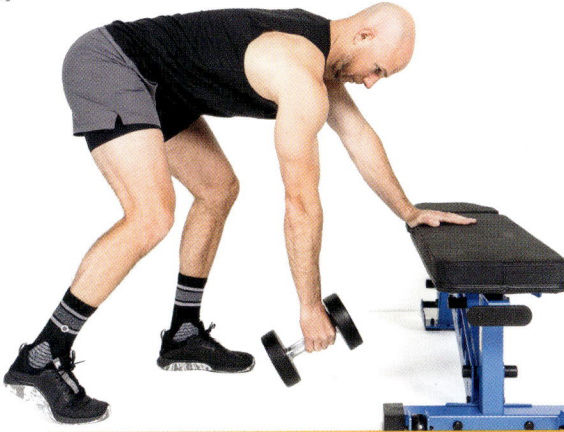

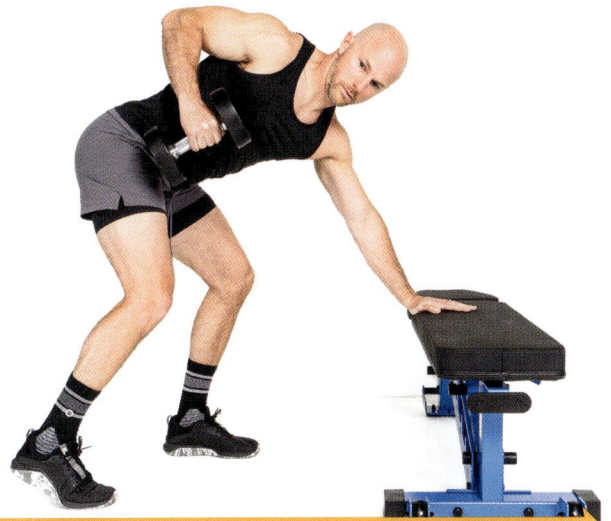

CONCENTRIC PHASE

ECCENTRIC PHASE

HALF-KNEELING CABLE ROW

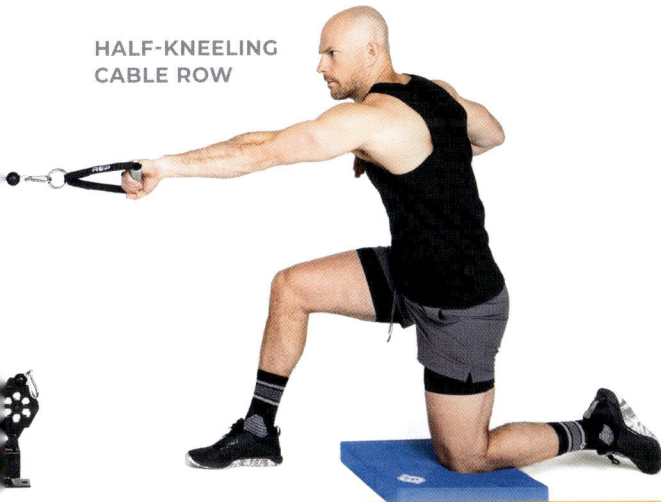

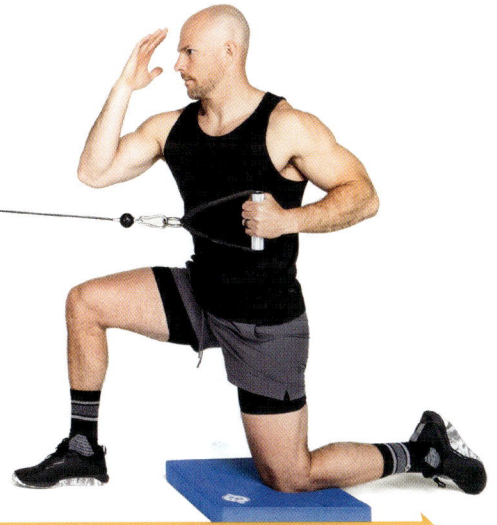

CONCENTRIC PHASE

ECCENTRIC PHASE

STANDING CABLE ROW

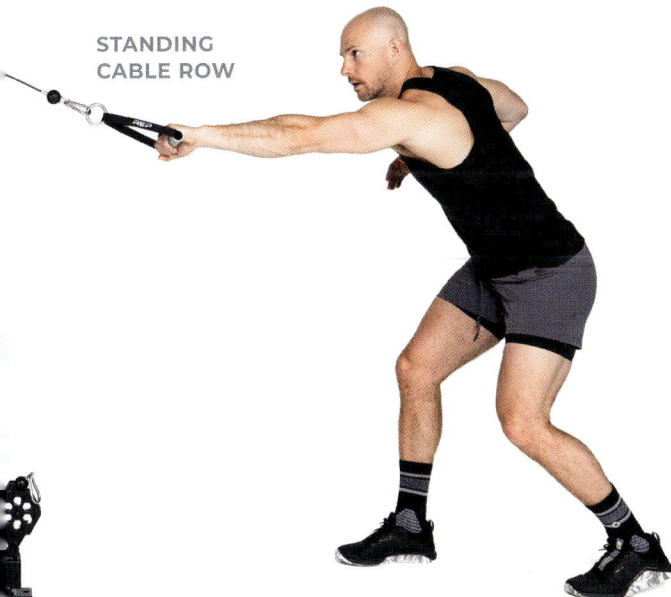

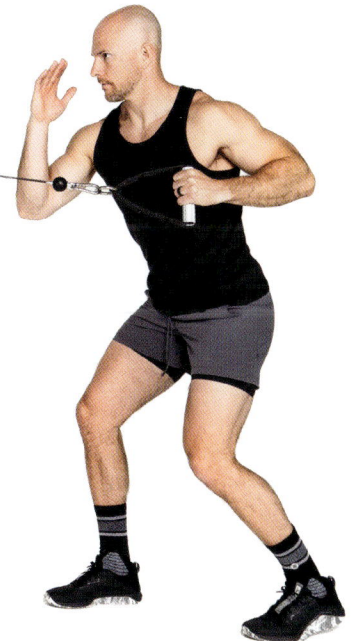

CONCENTRIC PHASE

ECCENTRIC PHASE

Each variation can be further modified based on positioning and setup:

- **For the three-point bench row with a dumbbell or kettlebell, set up with one knee and hand resting on a bench, while the opposite foot remains planted firmly on the ground.** Maintain a neutral spine and hinge at the hips to align your torso parallel to the floor. Before initiating the row, engage the pillar—think about pulling your planted foot and knee toward each other without actual movement to stabilize the hips. Simultaneously, create tension through the shoulders by co-contracting your pecs and lats, and press your planted hand into the bench without moving it. Take a deep breath and brace to lock in stability.

- **The hinged-supported row with a dumbbell or kettlebell utilizes a rack or other elevated surface for support. Position yourself in a kickstand stance, with the non-rowing foot slightly behind the supporting leg, maintaining a staggered base for balance.** Hinge at the hips, keeping your spine long and neutral, and place your non-working hand on the rack or bench. To create stability at the hips, actively press your back foot into the ground while pulling your front foot toward it without actual movement—this generates tension to anchor the lower body. For shoulder stability, co-contract your pecs and lats, and apply light pressure through your supporting hand into the rack or bench to reinforce upper body irradiation. Before initiating the row, take a deep breath and brace your core, ensuring that all movement comes from the upper body while maintaining a consistent torso angle.

- **For the half-kneeling cable row, begin in a 90/90 half-kneeling position, with the knee down on the same side as the working arm.** Your front foot should be planted firmly, with the knee stacked over the ankle to create a stable base. To stabilize your hips, co-contract your glutes and adductors. To accomplish this, lightly tuck your pelvis (this helps engage your glutes) and imagine pulling your knees together without moving them (this helps activate your adductors). For shoulder stability, co-contract your pecs and lats while pressing your non-working hand into your thigh or side. Before pulling, take a deep breath, brace your core, and ensure your ribs stay stacked over your pelvis.

- **For the standing cable row, set up in a split stance, with your front foot planted and back foot slightly behind, heel elevated.** Distribute your weight evenly between both legs, pressing the back foot into the ground while pulling the front foot back without actual movement—this activates the hips and stabilizes the lower body. To enhance shoulder stability, create tension by co-contracting the pecs and lats while keeping the shoulders square and stacked over the hips. Brace your core and take a deep breath, actively resisting excessive rotation to reinforce anti-rotational stability. This variation removes external support, requiring full-body engagement while allowing for more natural movement through the pull.

EXECUTION: Regardless of the variation, the single-arm row follows a fundamental movement sequence:

1. **Initiate the row with a dynamic, controlled pull.** Think athletic, not robotic. Avoid a slow, grinding motion; instead, generate force smoothly and explosively. As you row, maintain your authentic carrying angle (determined in the push assessment) to keep your shoulder in a natural, stable position.

2. **Integrate full-body coordination.** Your thoracic spine and shoulders should rotate in sync with the movement, based on your pull assessment findings. But just as important, the non-working arm should perform the opposite motion, mirroring a running man arm swing. This counterbalance reinforces a natural, athletic movement pattern, promoting rotation and full range of motion.

3. **Flex at the top** rather than pausing. Focus on creating a hard, active flex by squeezing your upper back and lats together. Your thoracic spine should naturally extend as you pull, reinforcing a strong, open posture without excessive shrugging or elevation at the shoulders. From this peak contraction, transition smoothly into the eccentric phase, gradually reversing the hand position into internal rotation to maximize the movement's full range.

4. **Lower the weight with control,** allowing your arm to fully extend while maintaining pillar stability. Avoid collapsing through the torso or letting your shoulder roll forward excessively.

A common mistake is keeping the movement too rigid. The single-arm row should emphasize the natural synergy between rotation and extension, fully engaging the lats and upper back.

BENT-OVER ROW

The bent-over row is a key progression in the pull pattern, advancing from supported single-arm rows to a fully self-stabilized position. Unlike previous variations, this movement requires you to maintain an isometric hip hinge while managing load through a dynamic pulling motion. This requires fatigue-resistant mechanics, meaning you need the endurance and motor control to hold a strong hinge position—without losing stability or breaking form as you pull.

When most people think of bent-over rows, they picture a loaded barbell, plates rattling, and some guy in the gym heaving the weight up like he's trying to start a lawnmower. It's a classic bodybuilding staple, often seen as a test of brute pulling strength. But here's the thing—just because it's popular doesn't mean it's the best choice for everyone.

Sure, barbell bent-over rows have their place, but they're not my go-to for building a strong, pain-free pull. Limited range of motion, a high risk of compensation (hello, low back pain), and more effective alternatives make them a tough sell as a primary movement (see the sidebar on page 402). Instead of jumping right into the most demanding and potentially injurious variation, it's best to perform bent-over row progressions that keep compensations in check while still delivering all the strength and muscle-building benefits of a loaded pull:

• **Entry Level:** *Landmine Bent-Over Row:* A stable starting point that reduces excessive movement while reinforcing proper hip hinge mechanics. With one end of the bar anchored to the ground, this setup offers built-in support, allowing for greater control and an easier introduction to the bent-over row position. This variation is ideal for developing positional awareness and hinge endurance before progressing to more dynamic, free-weight options.

However, it's important to note that the landmine row has a shorter range of motion and minimizes rotational demand. It's best used to build familiarity with the row pattern. Once you can consistently demonstrate good form—maintaining a strong hinge, neutral spine, and smooth control—it's time to progress to variations that challenge rotation and range of motion more directly.

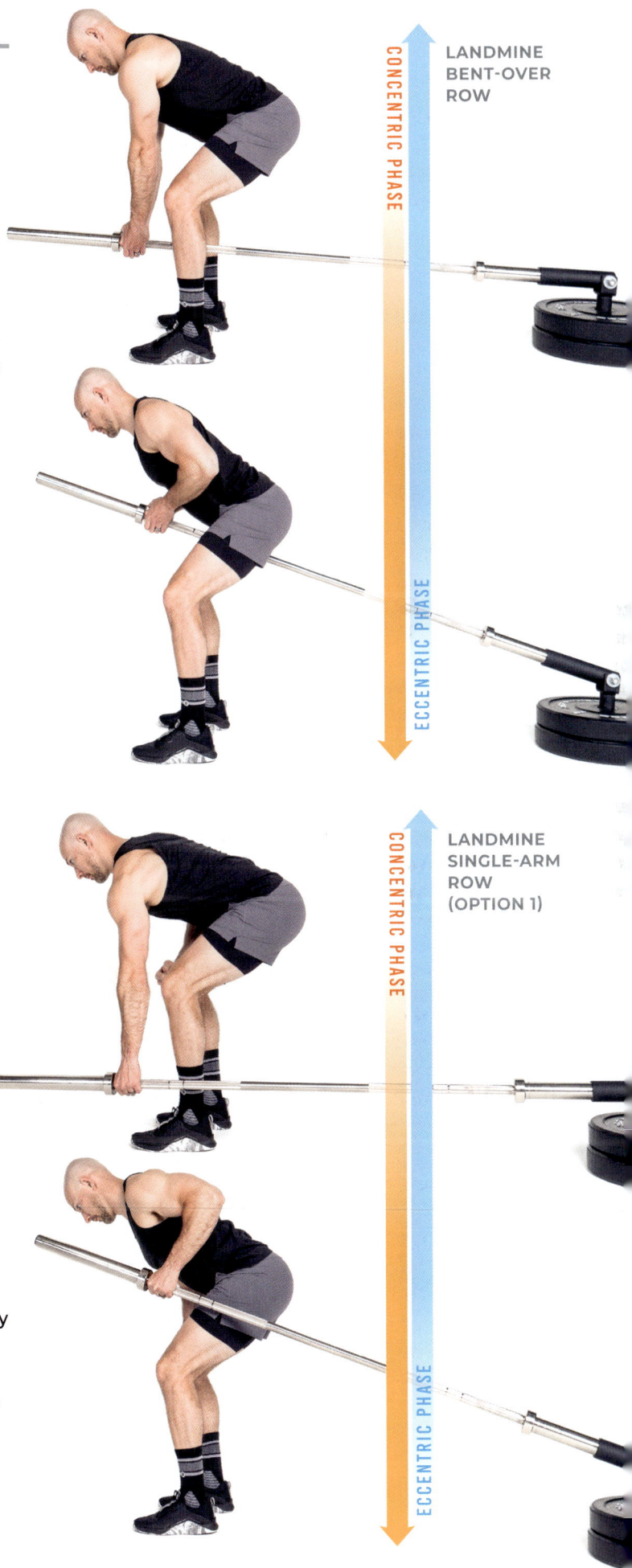

LANDMINE BENT-OVER ROW

CONCENTRIC PHASE

ECCENTRIC PHASE

LANDMINE SINGLE-ARM ROW (OPTION 1)

CONCENTRIC PHASE

ECCENTRIC PHASE

- **Asymmetrical Loading:** *Landmine Single-Arm Row:* These variations introduce asymmetrical loading, requiring the pillar to resist rotation while maintaining a strong hinge position. By rowing unilaterally, you must control rotational forces, improving pillar strength and anti-rotational stability. The single-arm landmine rows serve as an effective bridge between the supported bilateral landmine row and more advanced free-weight variations.

- **Free-Weight Progression:** *Dumbbell or Kettlebell Bent-Over Row:* Removing external stability, these variations demand full-body engagement, reinforcing hip stability and spinal endurance. It can be performed bilaterally (both arms rowing simultaneously) for higher loading potential and symmetrical strength development, or unilaterally (single-arm row) to incorporate greater rotational freedom and scapular mechanics. The unilateral variation also increases anti-rotational demands, making it a valuable tool for reinforcing asymmetrical control.

SETUP: Proper setup is the foundation of an effective bent-over row. Without a solid hip hinge and a braced pillar, tension shifts away from the upper back and into the lower spine, increasing the risk of compensation. Each variation builds on the same core principles—going through the pillar cueing sequence (see page 34) before initiating the hinge, maintaining a strong position, and controlling the pull through a full range of motion—while progressively challenging stability and motor control. Here's how to set up each variation for maximum efficiency and strength:

- **For the landmine bent-over row, set up in a hip-hinged position, with feet hip-width apart and a slight bend in the knees to maintain stability.** Hinge your hips back, allowing your torso to lower as close to parallel with the ground as your body's natural movement mechanics allow, while maintaining a neutral spine. Actively press your feet into the ground while engaging the glutes and adductors. Imagine rotating your feet outward without actual movement—this generates tension to lock in lower body stability and prevent unwanted shifting. Grip the bar with a hand-over-hand grip, stacking one hand over the other, or interlock your fingers around the barbell sleeve for a secure hold. Maintain pillar tension by co-contracting the pecs and lats, keeping the core braced to resist unnecessary movement and maximize control.

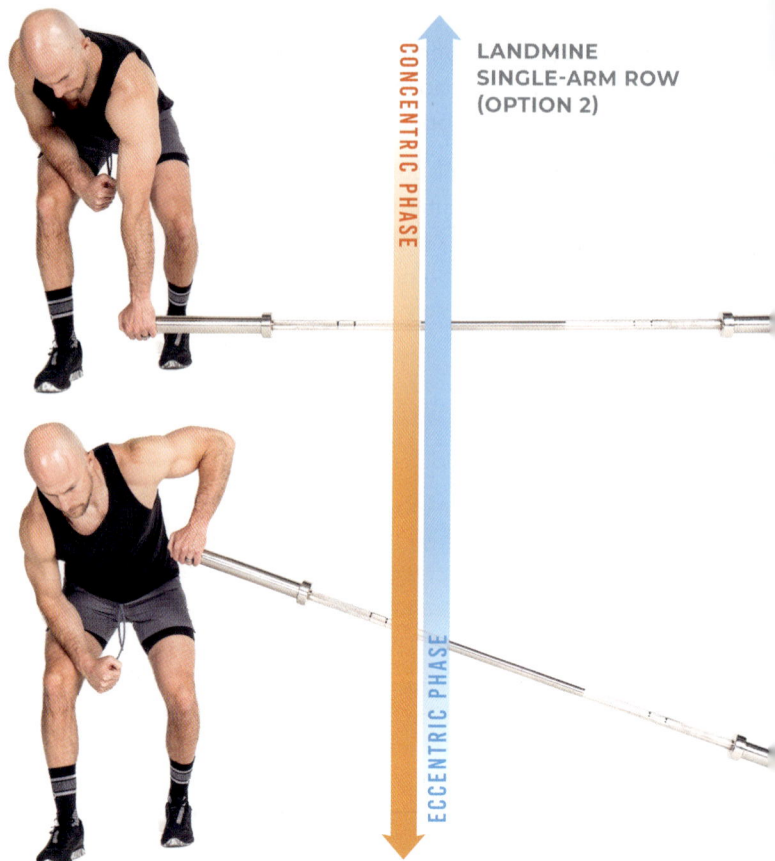

CONCENTRIC PHASE

ECCENTRIC PHASE

LANDMINE
SINGLE-ARM ROW
(OPTION 2)

- **For the landmine single-arm row, set up in the same hip-hinged position as the landmine bent-over row, maintaining a slight bend in the knees.** Unlike the previous variation, this row is performed unilaterally, requiring increased anti-rotational control through the core to prevent shifting or leaning. There are two grip options depending on bar positioning:

- If the barbell is set up parallel to your body, you'll assume a power stance—feet directly under your hips, similar to a deadlift. Grip the bar just above the sleeve with a firm, neutral grip, ensuring wrist alignment. This stance creates a more stable base and encourages a lower humeral carrying angle, which reduces the range of motion and places greater emphasis on the lats. The pull stays tight and controlled, making this variation ideal for building pure lat strength with a stable and direct pulling path.

- If the barbell is set up perpendicular to your body, you'll shift into a kickstand stance—feet hip-width apart with your back foot slightly behind you, resting on the ball of your foot in a split stance. In this setup, you'll grip the sleeve itself, allowing for a looser, more open-hand grip that encourages a natural pulling motion. This positioning promotes a higher humeral carrying angle, increasing range of motion and shifting emphasis toward the upper back. It integrates more scapular movement and thoracic extension, making it a great choice for developing postural control and total upper back strength.

- **For the free-weight bent-over row, maintain the same hip-hinged position as the previous landmine variations, ensuring a stable stance with a slight bend in the knees.** The primary difference here is that, without the anchored support of a landmine, you must rely entirely on core and posterior chain engagement to control the movement. There are two loading options depending on the training intent.

- **When performing the bilateral variation, hold a dumbbell or kettlebell in each hand with your feet directly under your hips in a power stance**—similar to your deadlift setup. This position creates a stable base for heavier loading and evenly distributes weight across both sides of the body, increasing total resistance potential. Unlike a barbell row, which can restrict range of motion and spinal movement, this setup allows for full thoracic extension and greater shoulder freedom, improving your ability to train the full range of a row pattern. It's ideal for building total back strength with a stable, symmetrical pull. However, since both sides of the body are working together, this variation offers less rotational challenge compared to unilateral rows.

- **There are two stance options for the unilateral variation. The first is performed with your feet under your hips while holding a dumbbell or kettlebell in one hand.** This increases anti-rotational demands, challenging your core and pillar stability as you resist shifting, leaning, or rotating through the pull. **If you need additional support, you can press your non-working forearm into your thigh to create a more stable base.**

- **The second option is a kickstand stance—feet hip-width apart, with the back foot slightly behind you and supported on the ball of the foot.** This offset position creates a more athletic base and shifts the challenge toward postural control and rotation management. It allows for a slightly more dynamic pull, increasing thoracic rotation, range of motion, and asymmetrical loading. It's a great progression when you want to train the upper back and core in a more sport-specific or real-world context.

FREE-WEIGHT BENT-OVER ROW (BILATERAL)

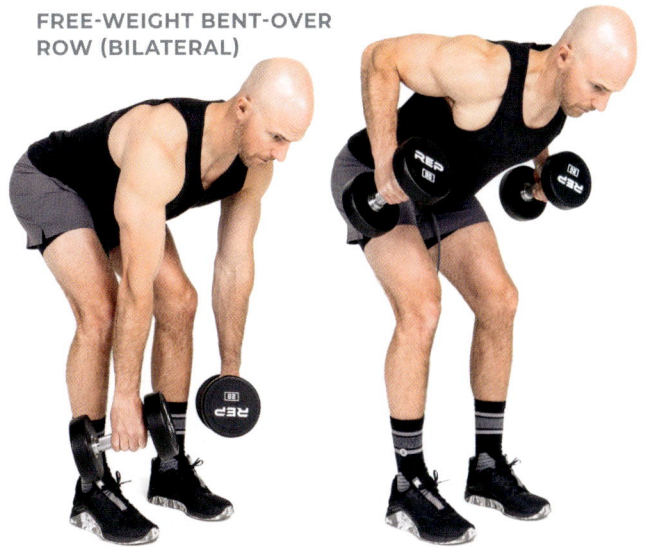

CONCENTRIC PHASE
ECCENTRIC PHASE

FREE-WEIGHT BENT-OVER ROW (UNILATERAL POWER STANCE)

CONCENTRIC PHASE
ECCENTRIC PHASE

FREE-WEIGHT BENT-OVER ROW (UNILATERAL KICKSTAND STANCE)

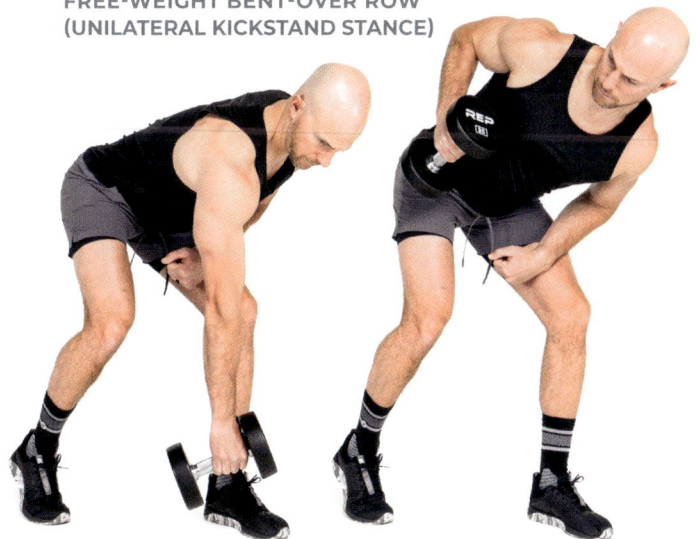

EXECUTION: No matter the variation, the execution of the bent-over row remains the same: a controlled pull, full scapular engagement, and a stable, braced position throughout. The goal is to drive movement from the upper back and lats, not the lower back or hips.

These are the key steps in executing an effective bent-over row:

1. **Initiate the row by generating force through the upper back and lats while maintaining the carrying angle determined in the push assessment.** Begin the pull with an explosive yet controlled movement, ensuring the elbows drive back along their natural path without altering the torso angle. Your spine remains fixed in the hip hinge, with no excessive movement or spinal extension, keeping all force production directed into the upper back and posterior chain.

2. **As the weight moves, allow your shoulder blades to move naturally through protraction and retraction without shrugging or elevation.**

3. **At the top, maximize the contraction by squeezing your shoulder blades together while maintaining tension through the lats and upper back.** Rather than pausing, focus on creating an active, hard flex at peak contraction while ensuring that your torso remains stable and locked in place.

4. **Lower the weight with control, maintaining eccentric tension as the arms extend fully.** Keep tension in the posterior chain, and avoid excessive torso movement, spinal rounding, or letting your shoulders collapse forward.

WHAT ABOUT BARBELL BENT-OVER ROWS, CHEST-SUPPORTED ROWS, AND SEATED ROWS?

Barbell bent-over rows are one of the most debated exercises in strength training. Bodybuilders love them, powerlifters swear by them, and plenty of people consider them a staple on back day. But I rarely include them in my programming—especially not as a KPI pull. Here's why.

The biggest issue with the barbell bent-over row is that it locks your hands and shoulder blades into a fixed position, limiting the natural rotational mechanics that make pulling patterns so effective. Unlike dumbbell, cable, or machine-based rows—where you can adjust the angle, range, and degree of rotation—the barbell variation restricts scapular movement and forces a more rigid pull pattern. This not only reduces range of motion (since the barbell hits your torso before achieving full scapular retraction), but also increases the likelihood of compensations like excessive lower back engagement or momentum-driven pulling.

Another major drawback? It's highly dependent on hinge endurance. The ability to maintain an isometric hip hinge with a heavy load while executing a dynamic pull is already challenging—add the barbell's anterior load, and the lower back becomes a common limiting factor. Even for lifters with solid hinge mechanics, fatigue sets in fast, often leading to breakdowns in form before the back muscles even reach failure.

Some argue that using a 45-degree chest support or a seal row setup solves the problem by eliminating the need for hinge endurance. But while these variations remove some of the lower back demands, they still limit range of motion—the bar stops at the bench or your torso before achieving full retraction. And if you're relying on momentum to yank the weight up, you're missing the entire point of controlled, full-range pulling.

Seated low rows, especially with a fixed close-grip attachment, fall into a similar trap. The locked hand position forces excessive internal rotation, limiting scapular movement and preventing the lats from fully engaging. That's why you rarely see this variation in my programming. Instead, I prefer setups that allow the hands to rotate freely, such as independent handle attachments, which let you adjust grip width, incorporate natural scapular mechanics, and achieve a stronger contraction.

So, what should you do instead? Simple—any row variation that allows for a full range of motion, natural scapular movement, and better load management. Dumbbell rows, landmine rows, single-arm cable rows, machine rows with independent arms—these all provide better control, greater variability, and far fewer movement restrictions.

Barbell bent-over rows, chest-supported rows, and seated rows aren't inherently bad, but they come with more drawbacks than benefits—and with better alternatives available, they don't make the cut as a KPI pull.

VERTICAL PULL

HIGH-ANGLE ROW

The high-angle row is where the pull progression starts to shift, moving beyond horizontal rows and into new movement territory. This shift is all about how the shoulders function through the pull. In previous variations like inverted rows, single-arm rows, and bent-over rows, your elbows move backward while the scapula retracts, reinforcing upper back engagement. However, once the pulling angle exceeds 45 degrees, the elbows track downward, and the lats become the dominant muscle driving the movement.

This is an important transition because the lats are the largest pulling muscle in the upper body. As the pull pattern becomes more vertical, the lats take over, making the high-angle rows a critical bridge between horizontal pulling variations and true vertical pulls like the lat pulldowns and pull-ups.

High-angle rows can be performed with cables, machines, or bands, but for key performance indicators (KPIs), cable-based variations take priority because they allow for progressive loading, consistent resistance, and a more natural pulling motion. Just like earlier pull progressions, the variations increase in difficulty based on stability and motor control demands—starting in grounded positions for more control before progressing to the more challenging standing variations:

- **Entry Level:** *Half-Kneeling High-Angle Row:* The starting variation, performed from a half-kneeling position, provides a stable base while introducing unilateral loading and controlled thoracic rotation. It's ideal for learning how to coordinate pulling mechanics with core control in a supported setup.

- **Increased Pillar Demands:** *Tall-Kneeling High-Angle Row:* Progressing from half-kneeling, the tall-kneeling position removes asymmetrical support and challenges your balance and pillar strength. Both sides of the body are now equally responsible for stability, increasing full-core activation and reducing reliance on the lower body.

UNILATERAL
HIGH-ANGLE ROW

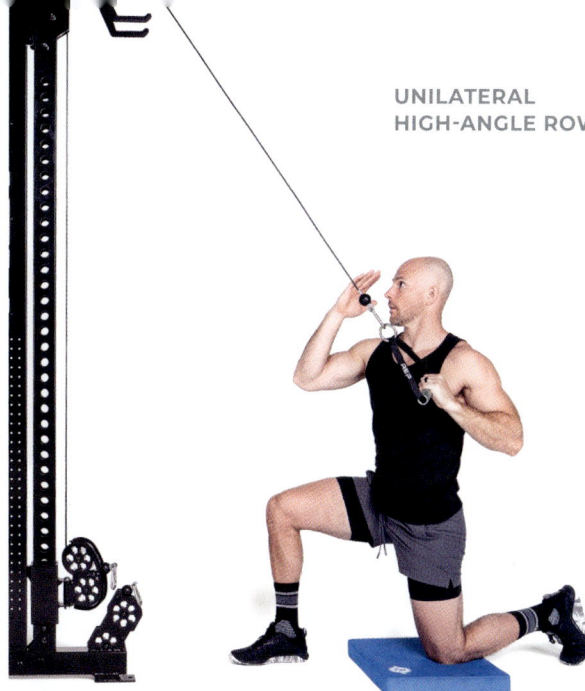

BILATERAL
HIGH-ANGLE ROW

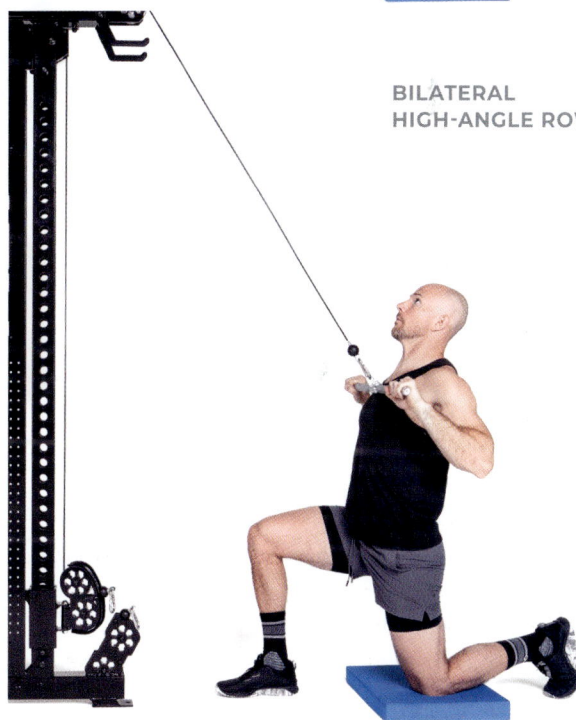

- **Full-Body Coordination:** *Standing High-Angle Row:* The most advanced variation, performed from a bilateral or kickstand stance, requires full-body stabilization. With less external support, this version introduces higher postural demands, making it an excellent transition into fully vertical pulling patterns like lat pulldowns or pull-ups.

Each of these variations can be performed bilaterally (with a straight bar or dual-handle attachment) or unilaterally (with a single handle). The bilateral variation allows for greater overall loading and symmetry across both sides of the body, similar to a traditional lat pulldown. However, it limits range of motion and removes thoracic rotation.

The unilateral variation, on the other hand, is preferred in most cases. It allows for increased rotation through the thoracic spine, more freedom of movement at the shoulder, and the opportunity to address side-to-side asymmetries. Both options are available and effective—it's up to the coach or trainee to choose the version that better aligns with the day's goals and individual movement capacity.

SETUP: All high-angle row variations are shown unilaterally (with one arm), requiring controlled rotation through the shoulder and thoracic spine while simultaneously resisting excessive movement beyond the parameters established in your assessment. Too much rotation, and you compensate. Too little, and you limit your range and muscle engagement. **Adjust the anchor point to its highest setting and position yourself so the cable forms a 45-degree angle with the ground.** To make the pull more vertical, move closer to the anchor; to create a shallower angle closer to horizontal, step farther away.

• **For the half-kneeling high-angle row, set up in a 90/90 half-kneeling position, with the knee down on the same side as the working arm.** The front foot should be planted firmly with the knee stacked over the ankle, creating a strong base. Co-contract the glutes and adductors by lightly tucking the pelvis and imagining pulling the knees together without actual movement—this enhances lower body engagement and prevents excessive spinal extension. Grip the handle with a neutral or slightly pronated grip. Maintain pillar tension by engaging the pecs and lats simultaneously, keeping the ribs stacked over the pelvis, and bracing the core before pulling.

• **When performing the tall-kneeling high-angle row, begin with both knees down, forming 90-degree angles at the knees with a neutral hip position and upright posture.** Dorsiflex your toes, pressing them into the ground. Since your base of support is now symmetrical, your core must work harder to resist excessive extension or rotation while still allowing controlled thoracic and shoulder movement during the pull.

• **For the standing high-angle row, set up in a kickstand stance by positioning the back foot slightly behind the front foot, keeping a light bend in the knees.** This staggered stance increases the challenge to pillar stability by reducing the base of support, making anti-rotational control even more critical. Ensure the ribs stay stacked over the pelvis, maintain a braced core, and engage the lats before initiating the pull.

CONCENTRIC PHASE

HALF-KNEELING HIGH-ANGLE ROW

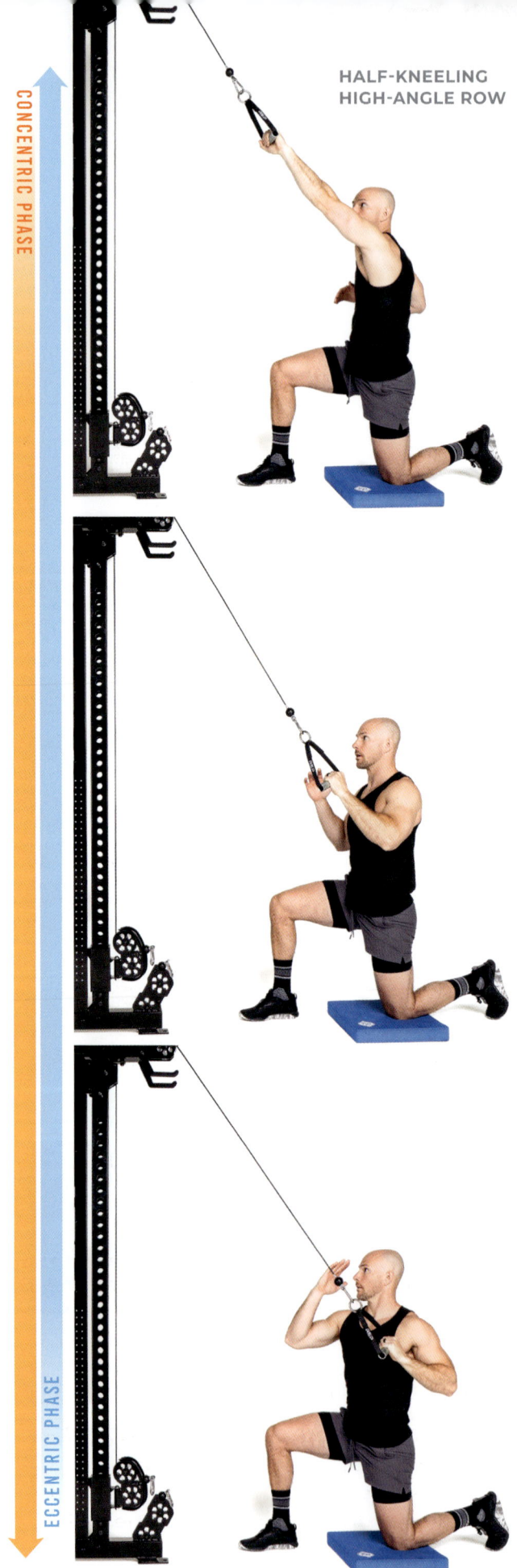

ECCENTRIC PHASE

CONCENTRIC PHASE

CONCENTRIC PHASE

ECCENTRIC PHASE

ECCENTRIC PHASE

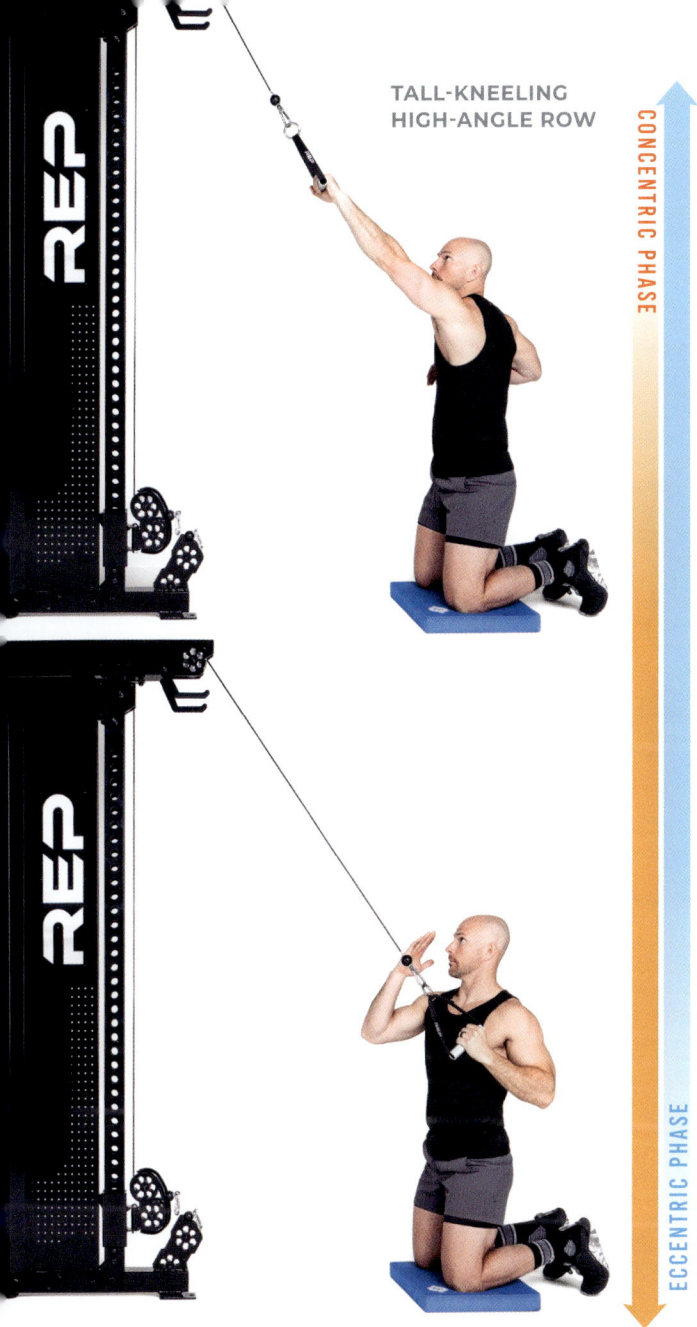

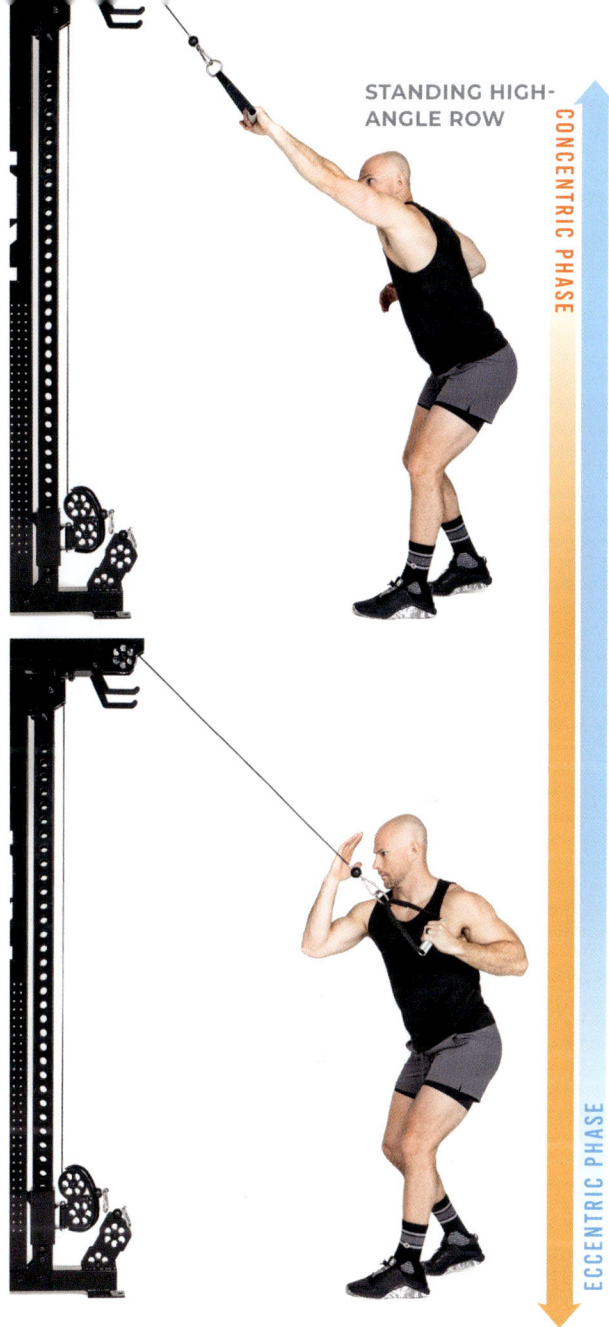

EXECUTION: Regardless of the variation, the execution of the high-angle row follows the same movement sequence:

1. Initiate the row by engaging the lats and driving the elbow back along its natural path. Since this movement shifts from internal to external rotation mechanics, the lats become the dominant movers. Keep the torso stable—avoid leaning back or compensating with momentum.

2. Control the pull by keeping the elbow aligned with your natural carrying angle (as determined in the push assessment). Allow the shoulder blade to move freely through protraction and retraction without shrugging or elevation.

3. At peak contraction, create a strong, deliberate flex by fully engaging the lats while keeping the torso locked in place. Rather than pausing, focus on maintaining full-body tension through a smooth transition into the eccentric phase.

4. Extend your arm with control through the eccentric phase. Maintain lat engagement as you fully extend your arm to ensure a stable pillar and prevent compensatory movement, such as spinal rounding, or letting your shoulder collapse forward.

LAT PULLDOWN

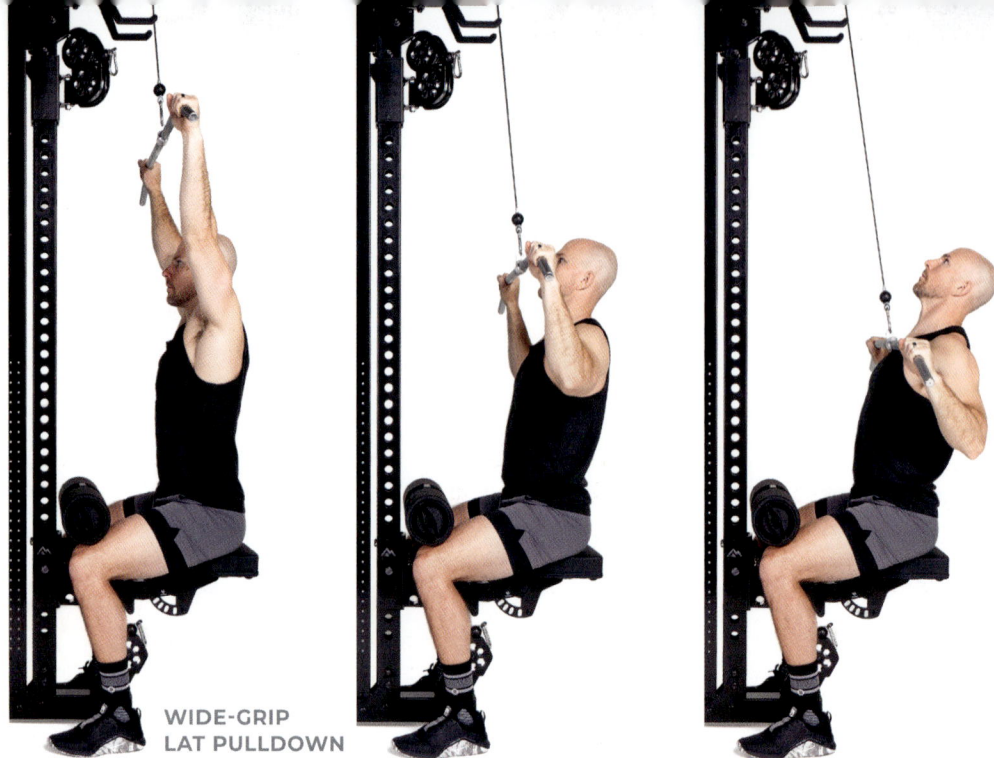

WIDE-GRIP
LAT PULLDOWN

CONCENTRIC PHASE

ECCENTRIC PHASE

The road to pull-ups starts here. The lat pulldown is the first true vertical pulling exercise in the progression, setting the foundation for the strength, control, and coordination needed to eventually move your own body weight.

While high-angle rows serve as a key bridge between horizontal and vertical pulling, they eventually hit a ceiling. As the load increases, the weight from the cable stack begins to pull you out of position, and without a stable anchor, your body weight alone isn't enough to counteract the force. At this point, the movement shifts from a test of strength to a battle for stability, limiting its effectiveness for true vertical pull development. That's where the lat pulldown comes in. It allows for progressive loading, greater lat engagement, and a direct carryover to pull-ups.

But not all lat pulldowns are created equal. Many lifters default to the classic overhand, wide-grip variation and crank out reps without much thought—but grip width, hand position, and shoulder mechanics all play a major role in how this exercise translates to functional strength. The key is to strategically progress through variations that gradually increase range of motion, control, and muscle recruitment:

- **Entry Level:** *Wide-Grip Lat Pulldown:* The starting variation that simplifies scapular mechanics by reducing rotational demands. This setup prioritizes lat engagement while limiting range of motion, making it an accessible introduction to true vertical pulling.

- **Increased Scapular Control:** *Medium-Grip Lat Pulldown:* Progressing from the wide grip, this variation allows for greater range of motion and increased scapular movement. The narrower hand position introduces more upward rotation of the shoulder blades, requiring greater control and coordination throughout the pull.

- **Peak Range and Muscle Recruitment:** *Close-Grip Supinated Lat Pulldown:* The most advanced variation, demanding the highest level of mobility. The supinated grip allows for maximum range of motion, increased lat and biceps recruitment, and full integration of thoracic extension and scapular rotation—closely mirroring the mechanics of a chin-up.

SETUP: Proper setup is critical for an effective lat pulldown. Without it, compensations—like excessive leaning, shrugging, or relying on momentum—can reduce lat activation and shift strain into the wrong areas. While each grip variation alters the movement slightly, they all follow the same fundamental principles: maintaining pillar stability, engaging the lats, and controlling the pull through a full range of motion.

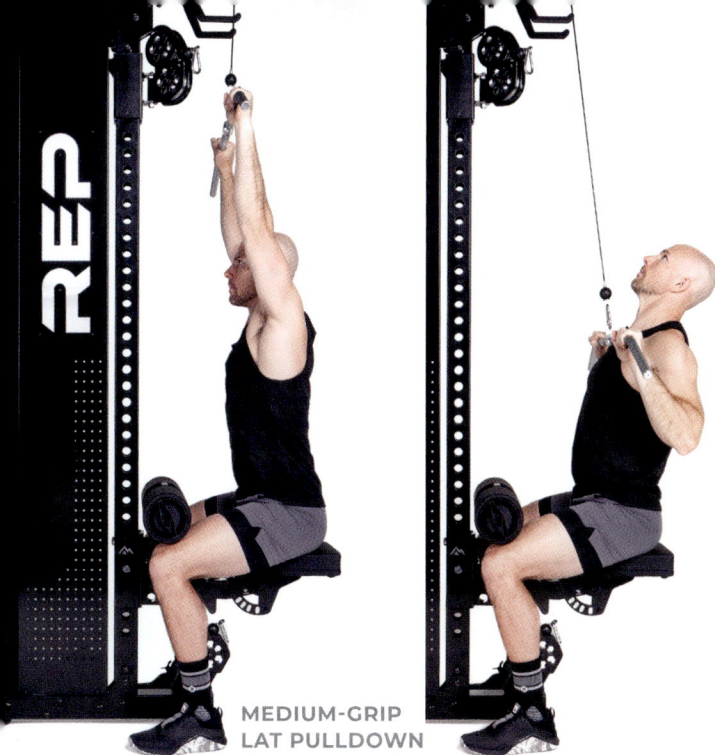

**MEDIUM-GRIP
LAT PULLDOWN**

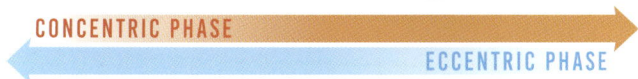

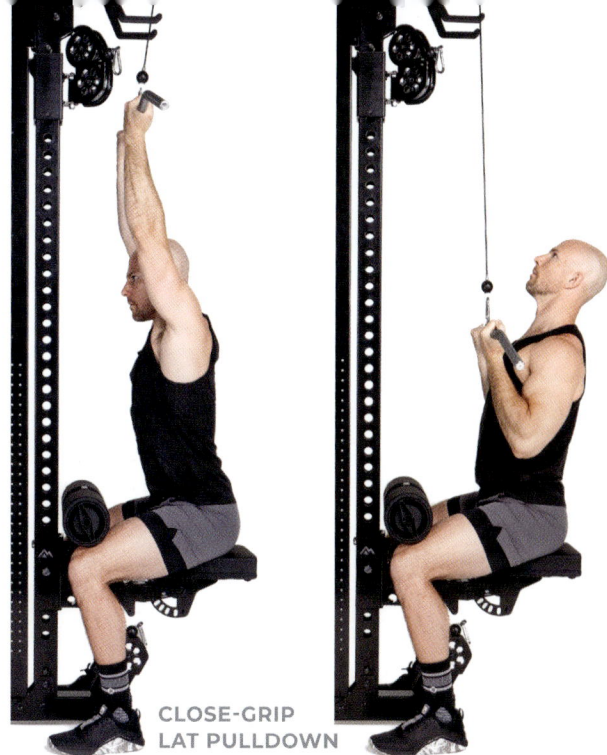

CONCENTRIC PHASE

ECCENTRIC PHASE

**CLOSE-GRIP
LAT PULLDOWN**

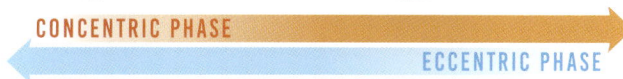

CONCENTRIC PHASE

ECCENTRIC PHASE

• **For the wide-grip lat pulldown, position yourself with the bar just within reach while seated. Grip the bar with an overhand grip, slightly wider than shoulder width.** Lean back slightly, keeping your core engaged and shoulders packed. Because this variation limits scapular movement, it simplifies the pull by keeping most of the focus on the lats.

• **For the medium-grip lat pulldown, set up in the same seated position but bring your hands in to a grip just outside shoulder width.** This variation allows for greater scapular rotation and range of motion. Keep your ribs stacked over your pelvis, maintaining a braced core while allowing your shoulder blades to move naturally as you pull.

• **For the close-grip supinated lat pulldown, use a close grip with your palms facing you.** This setup requires more mobility at the shoulders and thoracic spine while increasing the role of the biceps and upper back in the movement. Because this position demands greater mobility, focus on actively maintaining scapular control while keeping tension in the lats throughout.

Regardless of grip choice, sit tall with your feet planted and avoid excessive arching or leaning. Maintain pillar stability by engaging your core, co-contracting your pecs and lats, and positioning your shoulders in a packed but mobile position before initiating the pull.

EXECUTION: The lat pulldown should be performed with control and intent, ensuring that the lats—not momentum—drive the movement. No matter which grip variation you choose, follow these key steps:

1. Initiate the pull by engaging the lats and driving your elbows down along their natural path. Avoid using momentum or leaning excessively—this should be a controlled, lat-driven movement.

2. Control the pull by keeping your elbows tracking in line with your natural carrying angle (as determined in the push assessment). Allow your shoulder blades to move freely through protraction and retraction without excessive shrugging or elevation.

3. Actively elevate your chest toward the bar as you pull rather than just bringing the bar down to your chest. This ensures proper scapular mechanics, reinforcing downward rotation and depression.

4. At peak contraction, focus on an active flex, fully engaging your lats while keeping your torso stable. Rather than pausing, emphasize a strong squeeze at the bottom before smoothly transitioning into the eccentric phase.

5. Lower the weight with control, allowing your arms to fully extend without losing tension. Staying engaged through the full range of motion reinforces proper scapular mechanics and prevents compensatory movement.

PULL-UP

The pull-up is the peak of the pull progression—the true test of upper body pulling strength. With your feet off the ground, there's no external support to stabilize you, meaning your pillar must work as a single, braced unit to maintain control throughout the movement. This is where most people go wrong—they treat pull-ups as just another upper body exercise, letting their lower body go slack and sacrificing core engagement. But a proper pull-up is a full-body movement, and mastering it requires just as much pillar strength as it does pulling power.

Unlike lat pulldowns, where load can be adjusted incrementally, pull-ups start with a baseline resistance equal to your body weight. That means if you weigh 200 pounds, every rep is a 200-pound pull—a reality many lifters overlook. If you're not yet able to perform a strict bodyweight pull-up, that doesn't mean you're weak—it just means the movement needs to be regressed intelligently so you can build strength without compensating.

WHAT ABOUT ECCENTRIC ACCENTUATED PULL-UPS?

Pull-ups are the purest test of relative strength—the ability to produce force in proportion to your own body weight. If you can't manage your own body weight, no amount of external loading will make up for it.

What I mean is that if you lack the ability to pull your own body weight through a full range of motion, simply getting stronger in other pulling exercises—like lat pulldowns or weighted rows—won't automatically translate to a successful pull-up. You can be incredibly strong at lifting external loads, but if you don't have the relative strength to move your own body efficiently, you'll still struggle with pull-ups.

This is why prioritizing bodyweight control and proper mechanics through pull-up-specific progressions (like band-assisted pull-ups) is more effective than just getting stronger in isolated pulling movements. Strength without control won't get you over the bar—you have to train the movement as a whole, not just the muscles involved.

That's why so many "pull-up programs" fall flat, especially the ones that rely on slow eccentric lowers as a primary progression.

Here's the issue: eccentric-only work doesn't actually train the full pull-up pattern. When you jump to the bar and slowly lower yourself down, you're skipping the most critical piece—generating force from a dead hang. The hardest part of a pull-up isn't controlling the descent; it's initiating the pull while maintaining full-body tension and integrating

scapular depression, lat engagement, and core stability in one fluid motion.

Think about it—how does lengthening the muscles under load (eccentric training) directly make you stronger at the concentric action (pulling yourself up), which is where you're failing? You've broken the movement into two separate pieces and never reintegrated them. Eccentric work alone doesn't reinforce the coordination required to drive through a full pull-up, nor does it prepare you for the stability demands of completing a full rep. Without training the entire pattern, you're just delaying the inevitable frustration of getting stuck at the bottom—because you never actually built strength where you need it most.

Improving pull-ups isn't about hacking the system with one trick—it's about developing true relative strength, which comes from a combination of factors: getting stronger, refining motor control, managing body weight, and building quality movement patterns. If you're working toward your first pull-up, sticking with accommodating resistance, like band-assisted pull-ups, is a superior approach. It provides support where it's needed while still demanding full-body engagement, allowing you to train the pattern correctly while working on the foundational strength needed to progress.

There's no shortcut to mastering pull-ups. If you want to get better at them, you have to actually train the movement—not just lower yourself down and hope for the best.

Accommodating resistance, such as band-assisted pull-ups, helps smooth the transition by reducing the percentage of body weight lifted at the bottom of the movement while keeping tension in the right places. This allows you to build the necessary strength and motor control to execute full-range pull-ups with proper mechanics. Once you've developed the capacity for high-quality, controlled bodyweight reps, the next progression is weighted pull-ups—where external load is added to further drive strength adaptation and reinforce pillar stability under increased demand. Each of these variations serves as a key performance indicator (KPI), ensuring steady progress and structural integrity at every stage of the pull-up progression.

Grip selection also plays a huge role in how the movement translates to strength and muscle development. The entry point into pull-ups differs from lat pulldowns because anterior core stability becomes the biggest limiting factor. To simplify shoulder positioning and reinforce pillar stability, the pull-up progression follows a structured approach based on grip width and positioning:

- **Entry Level:** *Neutral-Grip Pull-Up:* The most accessible starting point, with a palms-facing grip that allows for optimal positioning over the center of mass. This setup minimizes excessive strain on the shoulders, making it the best introduction to vertical pulling with body weight.

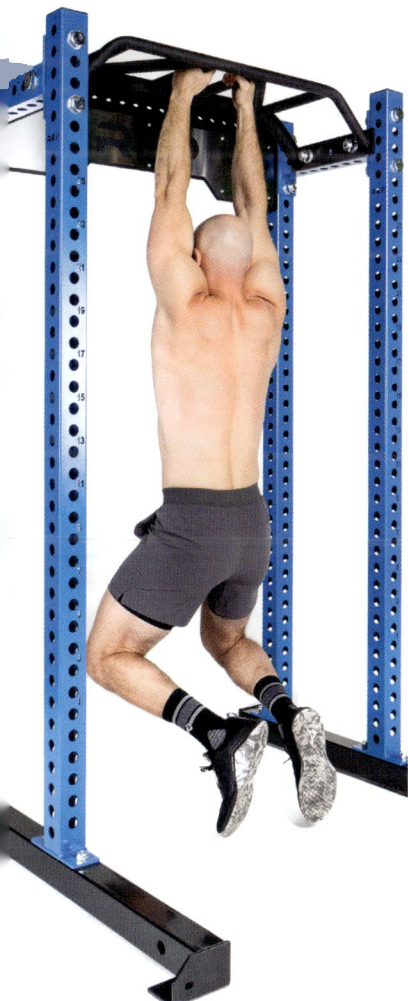

- **Increased Core and Lat Demand:** *Supinated Pull-Up (Chin-Up):* Progressing from the neutral grip, this variation shifts your center of mass slightly forward, increasing core engagement while maximizing lat and biceps activation. The supinated (palms facing your body) hand position allows for greater range of motion and increased upper back involvement.

- **Peak Motor Skill and Load Challenge:** *Wide-Grip Pull-Up:* The most challenging variation, requiring the highest level of pillar control, mobility, and strength. The wider grip moves your hands farther away from your midline, increasing torque on the shoulders and forcing the core to work overtime to prevent swinging or loss of position.

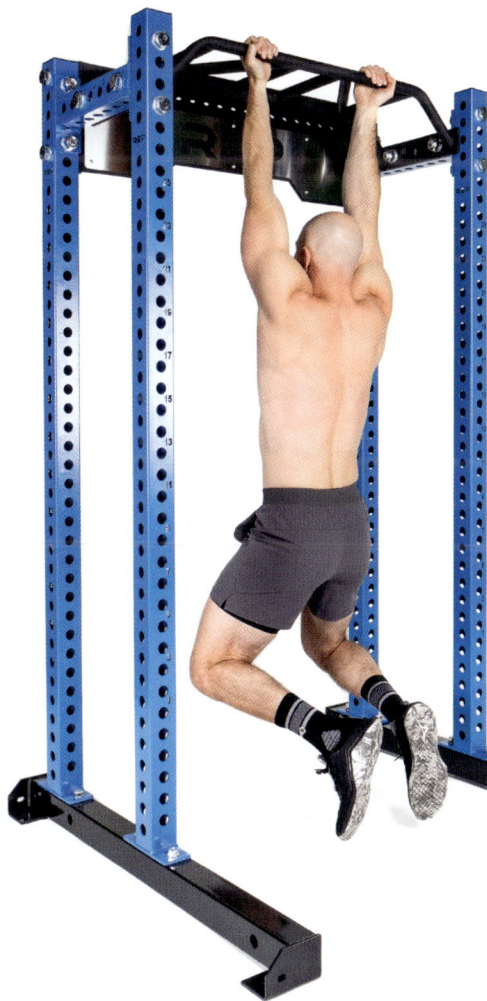

NEUTRAL-GRIP PULL-UP   SUPINATED PULL-UP (CHIN-UP)   WIDE-GRIP PULL-UP

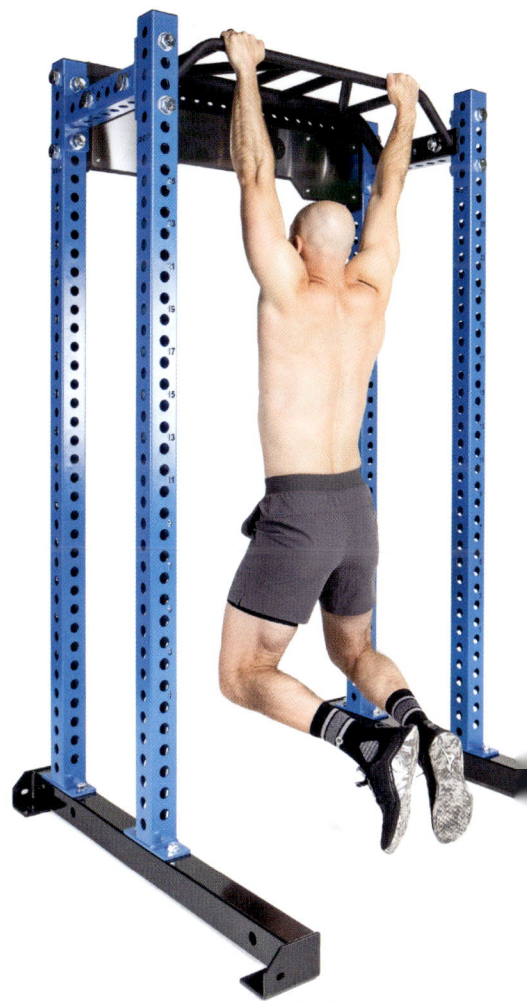

SETUP: Setting up properly for a pull-up is often overlooked, but it's one of the biggest factors in successful execution. Unlike other exercises in the pull progression, the pull-up starts with your entire body weight suspended in the air—meaning any break in positioning leads to inefficiency, poor mechanics, and joint strain. To reinforce pillar stability and optimal muscle targeting from the start, follow these key setup principles before each rep:

- **Use a bench for setup.** Avoid jumping up to the bar; instead, step up onto a box or bench to get your hands into position before lowering into a full hang. This allows you to establish pillar tension before initiating movement, just as you would with a loaded barbell squat or deadlift.

- **Establish a braced pillar before lowering into the hang.** Stand on the bench and grip the bar with your chosen hand position. Before stepping off the bench, co-contract your pecs and lats to create stable shoulders. Take a deep breath and brace before lowering yourself into a dead hang. Step off the bench one foot at a time. Co-contract your glutes and adductors with a slight posterior pelvic tilt while squeezing your legs together.

Positioning for Bodyweight vs. Weighted Variations:

- **For bodyweight pull-ups, maintain a hollow-body position—a slight 25-degree hip bend, straight knees, and toes pointed in plantarflexion.** This counterbalances the weight of your legs, preventing excessive swinging and keeping the movement controlled.

- **For weighted pull-ups, use a dip belt with either a kettlebell or weight plates. As you lower into position, bend both knees to 90 degrees, bringing your heels together behind your body.** This reduces excess movement—both from your body and the weight hanging between your legs—and ensures proper load distribution.

Regression Setup: Band-Assisted Pull-Ups

- **For looped band assistance, attach a resistance band to the pull-up bar and loop it around your foot or bent knee**, providing extra lift at the bottom while still requiring full engagement at the top.

- **For rack-assisted band setup, secure a band across the safeties of a power rack and step onto it for support.** This setup provides a more stable base, closely mimicking the body position of an unassisted pull-up. However, it requires access to a properly configured rack with adjustable safeties.

EXECUTION: A proper pull-up is not about yanking your chin over the bar—it's about moving your entire body as a single, controlled unit. Follow these steps for clean, efficient reps:

1. **Initiate the pull by driving your head toward the ceiling, not just pulling your chin over the bar.** This keeps the movement vertical and prevents compensatory swinging or neck extension. Think about pulling your sternum up rather than just bringing the bar down toward you.

2. **Maintain pillar tension throughout the ascent.** Your core, glutes, and lats should stay engaged as you drive your elbows down and back, keeping the movement fluid and controlled. Avoid excessive lean-back or overuse of momentum by swinging your legs.

3. **Adjust the range of motion based on grip selection:**
   - Neutral and supinated close grip: The bar should meet your shoulders or upper chest at peak contraction.
   - Wide-grip: The bar should align with your upper sternum, ensuring full engagement of your lats and upper back.

4. **Control the eccentric phase.** Lower yourself with control, maintaining lat tension and keeping your pillar engaged. Avoid sudden drops or relying on momentum—every phase of the rep should be deliberate and intentional.

BODYWEIGHT
PULL-UP

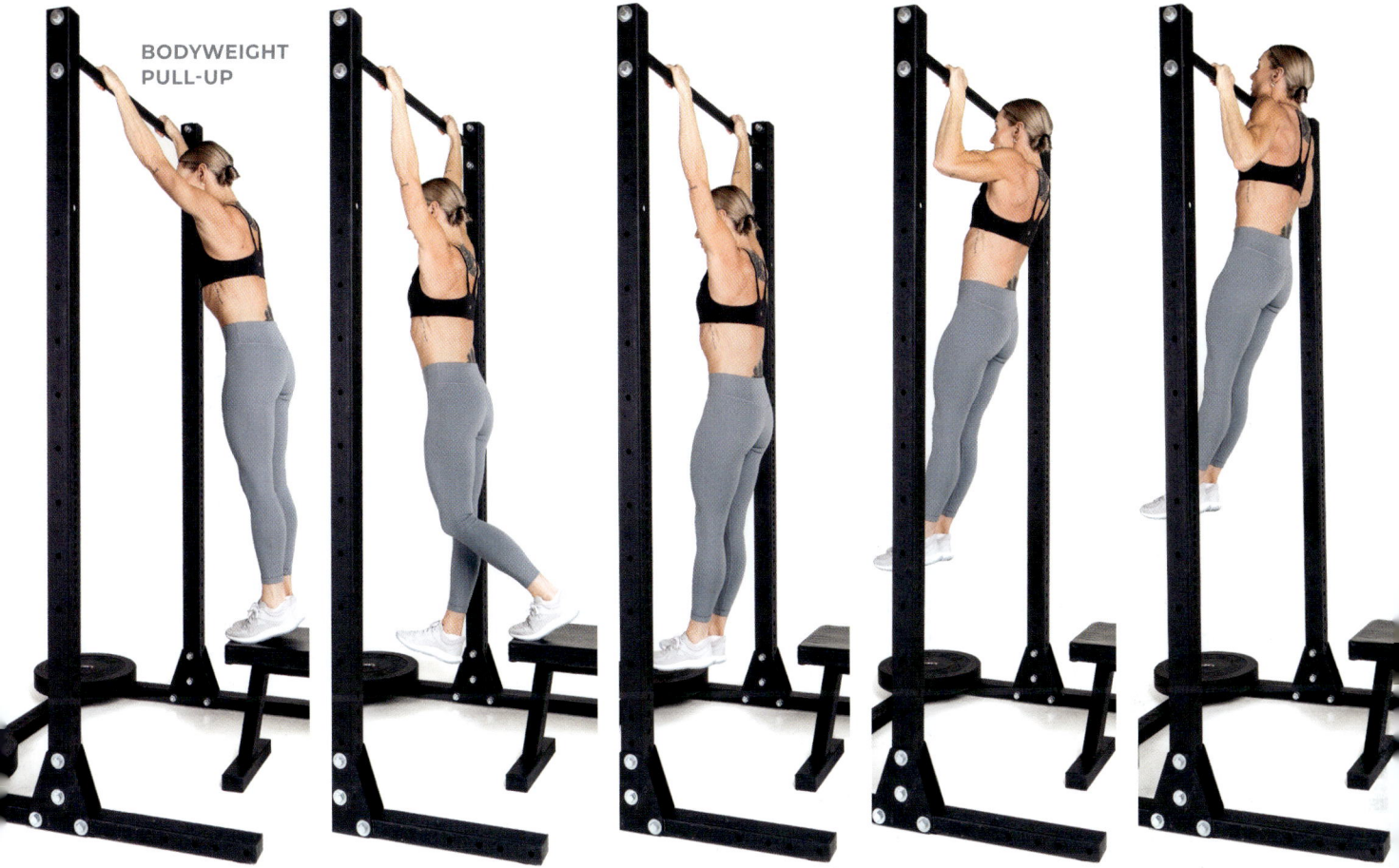

BAND-ASSISTED
PULL-UP

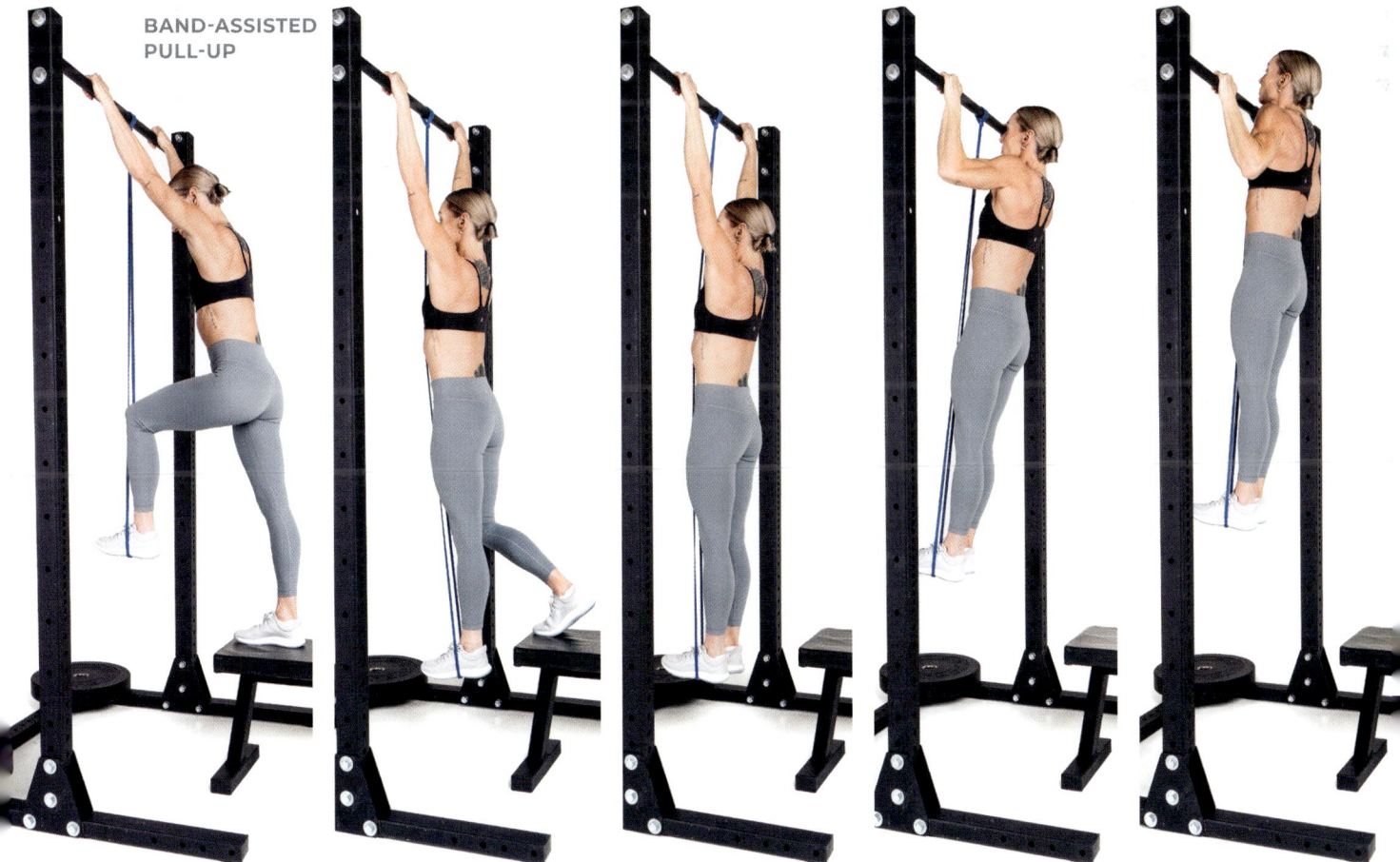

CONCENTRIC PHASE

ECCENTRIC PHASE

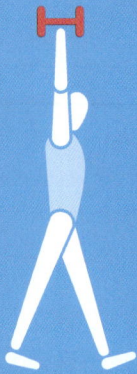

CARRY

The carry pattern is locomotion—any reciprocal action that coordinates the rhythmic swing of opposite limbs to move your body through space. While locomotion encompasses a wide variety of movements—from crawling, skipping, and walking to running and sprinting—this chapter focuses on loaded walking because it's safe, accessible, and uniquely valuable as a diagnostic tool. In the pages ahead, you'll learn how to screen and assess your carry pattern, pinpoint key compensations, and strategically target those weak links to promote movement mastery. The result? A stable, resilient pillar, stronger hips and shoulders, and a core that's ready to handle real-world demands.

Look around any park, track, or gym and you'll see it everywhere: people pounding pavement, grinding out miles on treadmills, and tallying runs on fitness trackers. We've been led to believe that running is our birthright—a natural superpower that fueled human survival. After all, we've all heard the claim that humans were "born to run." It's catchy. It feels intuitive. But it's worth asking: If running is so natural, why is it one of the most injurious activities we do? Why do even seasoned runners suffer repetitive stress injuries, nagging aches, and breakdowns that keep physical therapists busy year-round?

Here's what most people miss: Humans can run—sometimes exceptionally well—but we didn't evolve specifically for running. We were built for something else entirely. We were built to carry.

Long before ultramarathons, fitness trackers, and daily step-counting, our ancestors depended on their ability to carry moderate loads from place to place. Food, water, tools, supplies, children—carrying these essentials wasn't a luxury; it was integral to human survival. As a result, our joints, muscles, and bones evolved to support loaded locomotion, making us exceptionally efficient at transporting weight across distances.

In other words, we're not primarily runners—we're natural carriers, masterfully adapted for sustainable movement under load.

Yet despite its foundational role in our evolution, the fitness world has largely overlooked the value of intentionally training the carry pattern. Think about it: The squat, hinge, lunge, push, and pull form the backbone of nearly every effective strength program. But what about walking with weight—the very thing we evolved to do most efficiently? For most people, walking is rarely considered beyond logging daily step counts.

Don't get me wrong. Getting your daily steps in is undeniably beneficial—it's vital for general health and longevity—but mindlessly accumulating mileage won't fully tap into your body's innate capabilities or address underlying movement quality. To genuinely optimize your physical function and overall performance, you need to approach walking—especially loaded walking—as a deliberate skill worthy of purposeful training and progression.

This shift in perspective requires viewing walking not as a passive activity, but as a global movement pattern that fundamentally shapes how you interact with the world. From infancy onward, every developmental milestone—from crawling to standing upright—brings you closer to confidently balancing on two feet and skillfully carrying your body (and external loads) with fluid efficiency. Put another way, walking is more than simply putting one foot in front of the other; it seamlessly integrates all the foundational movement patterns into a single, coordinated action. With each stride, your hips and knees rhythmically flex and extend, mirroring the actions of squatting and hinging. Every step demands the single-leg stability of a lunge as your arms naturally swing in reciprocal push-and-pull harmony. At the center of this coordinated interplay is your pillar—the unified stability of your shoulders, hips, and core—synchronizing your entire body into one synergistic, functional unit.

But the effortless integration of movement you developed in childhood isn't guaranteed to last—especially in a modern world that systematically undermines it. Over time, the simple routines of daily life slowly erode your foundational patterns, layer by layer. Thoracic rotation becomes restricted, shoulders drift forward into a rounded position, and hip stability gradually deteriorates. On a leisurely stroll, these minor deviations may remain hidden, but add load, and they become impossible to ignore. Suddenly, limited upper back rotation reveals itself as hunched shoulders and compromised posture, while unstable hips result in uneven strides or difficulty maintaining proper alignment.

This is precisely why loaded carries deserve an intentional place in your training. Because the carry is a global pattern that integrates aspects of every other foundational movement, improving your carry directly translates to enhanced squats, hinges, lunges, pushes, and pulls. More importantly, intentionally loading your carry pattern is how you rebuild your natural locomotion, reversing compensations that modern life inevitably creates.

By this point, you've completed detailed screens and assessments for each foundational movement pattern, clearly identifying your linchpins—the mobility, stability, or skill deficits repeatedly limiting your performance and predisposing you to pain. Now, the carry screen and assessment serve as your final confirmation of these findings. Carrying won't just expose your weak links—it will highlight exactly which linchpins matter most, eliminating guesswork and sharpening your training focus.

Bottom line: The carry isn't something you should just casually do. It's essential training—integrating, evaluating, and optimizing every foundational pattern you work so hard to master.

THE SMARTEST WAY TO CHALLENGE AND PROGRESS THE CARRY PATTERN

The two most effective ways to challenge any movement pattern are with load or speed. When it comes to locomotion, increasing speed—such as running or sprinting—certainly has value, but it's not always safe or practical, especially if you're coming off an injury, rehabilitating pain, or addressing underlying movement deficits. That's why loaded walking serves as your safest, most effective starting point. Universally accessible and uniquely valuable, carefully loaded walking (with weights carried at your sides, as you'll do in the screen, assessment, and exercise progressions in this chapter) is appropriate for virtually anyone, regardless of fitness level, providing both a powerful assessment and a reliable performance benchmark.

As you progress toward longer durations or distances—particularly in general fitness or everyday life—you'll find shifting the load placement from your hands to your torso or pillar incredibly beneficial. Weighted vests, rucksacks, and backpacks place the load closer to your body's natural center of gravity, significantly reducing grip and arm fatigue while promoting optimal posture and pillar stability.

These alternative carries better simulate real-world demands, setting the stage for sustained cardiovascular conditioning.

From this stable foundation, you can progressively build toward more dynamic locomotion patterns. The carry pattern—defined as any reciprocal action coordinating opposite limbs to move your body from place to place—extends beyond loaded walks. Locomotion also includes running, sprinting, crawling, skipping, swimming, and lateral movements like shuffling, each demanding increased levels of stability and motor control. Incorporating these more advanced forms of locomotion training over time helps you develop greater cardiovascular capacity, muscular endurance, and high-level motor control—qualities loaded walking alone can't fully address.

Put simply, loaded carries safely establish the strength and stability you need to earn more dynamic locomotion methods. This book is dedicated to helping you build from the ground up, using loaded walking as your practical, reliable first step toward lifelong performance.

CARRY SCREEN

The carry is uniquely human—and while it's undoubtedly complex, screening your carry pattern doesn't have to be complicated. Locomotion engages every joint from your feet to your neck, but the carry screen applies the same fundamental principles you've used throughout this book. You're still evaluating your ability to effectively maintain a neutral spine, preserve symmetry between the left and right sides, and control rotation through your hips, shoulders, and torso. The key difference is that now you're actively moving from one place to another, incorporating elements of squatting, hinging, lunging, pushing, and pulling, but in smaller, subtler ranges of motion compared to the full-range movements of previous screens.

You might wonder why we begin by screening the carry pattern unloaded, especially since walking without load can mask subtle compensations. While load does amplify compensations, starting with an unloaded walk allows you to establish a baseline of your natural gait mechanics. You're first checking how you move under ideal, stress-free conditions. Once you introduce load (which you'll do in the upcoming assessment), subtle deviations become magnified and more visible, but knowing what your baseline looks like makes these deviations easier to identify and more meaningful to interpret.

To get the most from the carry screen, treat it as a step-by-step optimization checklist. Rather than getting lost in biomechanical minutiae, you'll systematically observe each region of your body as you walk naturally. Because the carry pattern integrates every other foundational movement, it's your chance to confirm previously identified linchpins, reinforce optimal mechanics, and ensure nothing critical gets overlooked.

Keep in mind that everyone's gait naturally varies—the goal isn't robotic uniformity. Instead, you're verifying that your movement aligns with the optimization principles you've already learned, setting the stage for the loaded carry assessment that follows.

SETUP AND EXECUTION

To perform the carry screen, simply walk back and forth at a distance of 20 feet for multiple reps. Record yourself from both front and back angles, as many compensations are easiest to spot from these perspectives.

Walk naturally and comfortably. The goal right now is to observe, not to correct. Don't overthink your form or try to make changes on the fly. This screen is about capturing your default movement so you can assess how you actually move, not how you think you should move. Later, you'll use the optimization checklist to evaluate what you see, breaking down joint positions from the ground up in a systematic, easy-to-follow way.

Before diving into that checklist, though, it's important to understand what optimal walking mechanics look like. That way, you'll know what to look for as you review your footage. Every step moves through two main phases: **stance** (when your foot is on the ground) and **swing** (when your foot is in the air).

HEEL STRIKE (INITIAL CONTACT)	FOOT FLAT (LOADING RESPONSE)	MID-STANCE	HEEL-OFF (TERMINAL STANCE)	TOE-OFF (PRE-SWING)	INITIAL SWING	MID-SWING	TERMINAL SWING
DOUBLE SUPPORT	SINGLE SUPPORT			DOUBLE SUPPORT	SINGLE SUPPORT		

STANCE PHASE:
The Foundation of Each Step

1. Heel Strike (Initial Contact): Land softly on your heel, keeping your knee slightly bent to absorb impact. Your opposite arm should naturally swing forward to help counterbalance the motion. Keep your spine neutral and gaze forward.

2. Foot Flat (Loading Response): Let your foot roll forward, distributing weight evenly as your whole foot makes contact with the ground. Maintain a strong, stable core to keep your pelvis level and avoid excessive side-to-side shifting.

3. Mid-Stance: Shift your weight directly over your planted foot while maintaining control. Avoid collapsing into your hip—your stance leg should feel strong and engaged. Keep your spine tall, arms swinging in rhythm, and movement smooth from one side to the other.

4. Heel-Off (Terminal Stance): Press through the ball of your foot as your heel lifts off the ground. Your back leg should stay active, preparing to push off. Stay balanced, avoiding excessive forward lean or unnecessary tension in your upper body.

5. Toe-Off (Pre-Swing): Push off the ground with intent, using your toes to propel your body forward. Let your back leg extend fully while your opposite arm swings forward. Keep the movement controlled, avoiding jerky transitions or loss of posture.

SWING PHASE:
Driving the Next Step Forward

1. Initial Swing: Lift your foot off the ground by bending your knee and driving your thigh forward. Your core should stay engaged to prevent excess twisting or swaying.

2. Mid-Swing: Let your leg move naturally forward, keeping your knee bent and hips level. Your arms should continue their natural swing, maintaining rhythm and stability.

3. Terminal Swing: Extend your leg smoothly as your foot prepares to land. Keep control as your heel lowers toward the ground, setting up for a soft, stable landing into the next step.

Walking may seem automatic, but refining these phases is key to carrying with strength and efficiency. By focusing on controlled movement, a stable pillar, and efficient weight transfer, you'll create a foundation for strong, pain-free locomotion.

Unlike previous screens that evaluate a single joint or isolated pattern, the carry screen assesses how effectively your entire body coordinates under the demands of locomotion. You'll begin by walking naturally (without load), systematically observing each region of your body to identify subtle compensations and confirm linchpins uncovered in earlier assessments.

Here's exactly what to look for at each segment, along with the linchpin blueprints you'll use to address any compensations you uncover.

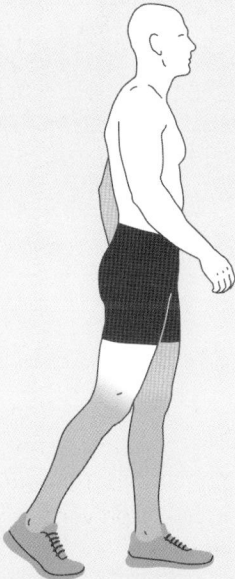

FEET AND KNEES

Watch closely as your feet strike and leave the ground. Both sides should look relatively symmetrical. Common compensations include

- Heel whip (the heel swinging excessively outward)
- Uneven push-off between right and left feet
- Knees or ankles shifting inward or outward, signaling possible hip or ankle mobility or stability issues

For most compensations, you'll choose the linchpin blueprint targeting the joint that's directly causing the unwanted movement. For example, if your heel swings outward excessively (heel whip), it typically indicates a lack of hip mobility. This happens because limited hip mobility prevents your leg from naturally moving straight forward, forcing your foot to rotate outward as compensation. In this case, you'd perform the **Hip Mobility Linchpin Blueprints** (pages 469–470).

If you notice an uneven push-off—meaning one foot appears to push off the ground differently than the other, such as leaving the ground earlier or more abruptly—begin with the **Ankle Mobility Screens** (page 246). If the test reveals limited ankle mobility, perform the **Ankle Mobility Linchpin Blueprint** (page 468). If your ankle mobility checks out, then your uneven push-off is likely due to instability in your hips, so perform the **Hip Stability Linchpin Blueprints** (page 475) instead.

Knee issues are rarely isolated; they usually originate from mobility or stability problems either above (hip) or below (ankle). If your knees or ankles consistently shift inward or outward, you'll need additional information to pinpoint the exact source. In this scenario, revisit the previous foundational screens and assessments (such as squat and lunge screens) to help clarify the root cause. Typically, you'll end up addressing these compensations with either the **Hip Stability Linchpin Blueprints** or the **Ankle Stability Linchpin Blueprint** (page 468).

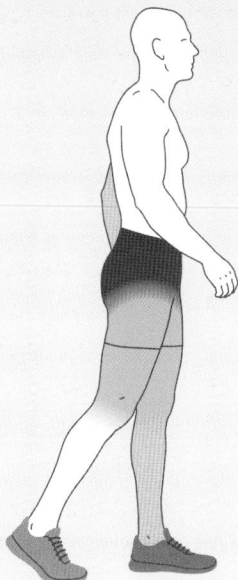

KNEES AND HIPS

The knee primarily bends and extends, but its stability depends greatly on the hip. Watch for unwanted inward collapse (valgus) or outward shifting (varus). Such deviations usually stem from hip mobility or stability deficits. Remember, your hips are the central junction of your pillar and typically have the greatest impact on gait mechanics.

If unsure whether the issue lies with your hips or ankles, prioritize your hips first, as improvements there usually translate down the chain.

Refer to the **Hip Mobility Linchpin Blueprints** if you notice restricted hip movement, specifically difficulty extending your hip behind your body (tight hip flexors) or moving your leg outward to the side (tight adductors). Choose the **Hip Stability Linchpin Blueprints** if you identify weak glutes—common signs include difficulty holding a single-leg glute bridge or maintaining proper alignment in side plank variations. You should also prioritize hip stability if your knees frequently collapse inward (without signs of ankle instability) or if you notice your pelvis shifting side-to-side excessively (without signs of core instability).

HIPS AND LUMBOPELVIC JUNCTION

Your pelvis naturally rotates slightly during walking, but excessive up-and-down movement (instead of controlled rotation) signals stability issues. Watch for uneven hip levels or excessive tilting. Common compensations include

- Excessive anterior pelvic tilt (lower back arching excessively)
- Limited hip extension, often due to insufficient stability at the lumbar-pelvic junction

Excessive lower back arching often results from limitations in either hip mobility, core stability, or both. If your pelvis frequently tilts forward excessively, creating a pronounced arch in your lower back, begin by implementing the **Core Stability Linchpin Blueprints** (pages 472–473), as core instability is a common root cause of this issue.

If you struggle specifically with fully extending your hip behind you—without significant arching of your lower back—this indicates restricted hip mobility. In this case, you should focus on the **Hip Mobility Linchpin Blueprints** (page 475).

For best results, consider alternating between both blueprints, as improvements in core stability often directly enhance your ability to achieve proper hip extension.

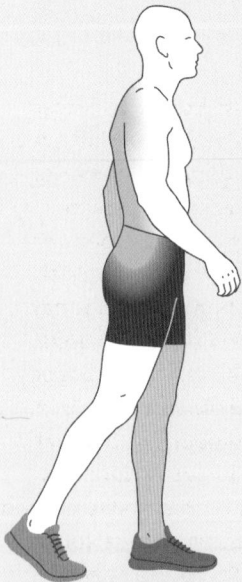

LUMBAR AND THORACIC SPINE

Ideally, your lumbar spine stays relatively stable while your thoracic spine rotates gently. Excessive lumbar rotation or noticeable stiffness in your upper back indicates limited thoracic mobility. Signs include

- Limited upper back rotation, forcing compensatory rotation at the lumbar spine
- Rounded shoulders or forward-hunched posture due to restricted thoracic extension

Limited rotation in your upper back—forcing your lower back to rotate excessively—or a forward-hunched posture with rounded shoulders typically indicates restricted thoracic mobility. If these compensations appear, immediately incorporate the **T-Spine Mobility Linchpin Blueprint** (page 471). Improving your thoracic mobility can quickly enhance your posture, reduce strain on your lower back, and significantly optimize your carry pattern.

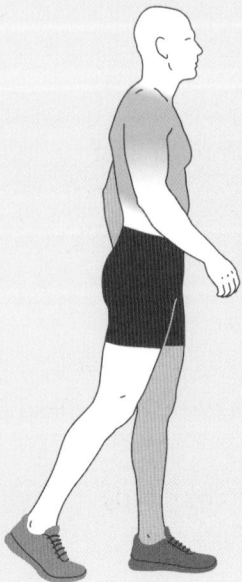

THORACIC CAGE AND SHOULDERS

Your shoulder blades should glide smoothly over your rib cage, moving symmetrically forward and backward. Restrictions often show up as uneven arm swings or excessive shoulder shrugging. Watch for

- Limited scapular protraction or retraction, causing stiffness or asymmetry in arm swing
- Excessive shoulder elevation (shrugging), indicating a lack of thoracic extension and shoulder stability

If you notice uneven arm swings or stiffness when your shoulders move, you're likely experiencing restricted thoracic mobility or limited scapular stability. Excessive shoulder shrugging, especially while carrying weight, is also a clear indicator of inadequate scapular stability and limited thoracic extension. To address these compensations, first incorporate the **T-Spine Mobility Linchpin Blueprint** (page 471) to restore proper thoracic motion and posture. Next, follow the **Scapular Stability Linchpin Blueprint** (page 473) to reinforce proper scapular positioning and strength, ensuring smooth, symmetrical shoulder movement.

ELBOWS AND WRISTS

As your arms swing naturally, your elbows should bend slightly (about 70 degrees forward, extending to about 15 degrees backward), with wrists neutral and thumbs pointing forward. Watch for stiff arms or lack of rotation in the wrists, indicating shoulder or thoracic mobility deficits. Common compensations include

- Limited arm swing range
- Excessively straight or stiff arms, showing rigidity and a lack of reciprocal motion

If your arms appear stiff, excessively straight, or have limited swing while walking, this is typically a sign of restricted thoracic mobility or poor scapular stability. A lack of smooth, reciprocal arm movement often originates from tension or stiffness in the upper back or instability in the shoulder blades. Start by performing the **T-Spine Mobility Linchpin Blueprint** (page 471) to improve upper back extension and rotation. Next, apply the **Scapular Stability Linchpin Blueprint** (page 473) to develop better control and coordination of your shoulders, helping you restore fluid, natural arm swing during walking.

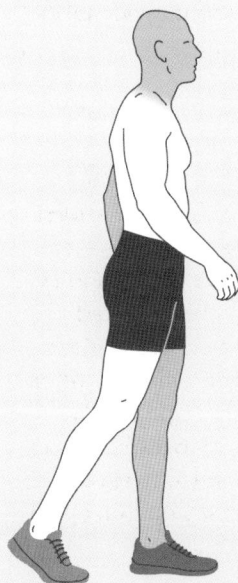

HEAD AND NECK

Your head and neck should remain stable and neutral, with eyes forward. Watch for excessive forward head posture, repetitive head bobbing, or tension in the neck. Common compensations include

- Forward chin position, indicating postural issues from lower down the chain
- Excessive head movement during gait, often a sign of poor pillar stability

If your head moves excessively or your chin juts forward as you walk, it typically indicates a postural imbalance originating lower down your body. A forward head posture often stems from stiffness in your upper back or insufficient stability around your shoulder blades and neck. Begin by addressing these issues with the **T-Spine Mobility Linchpin Blueprint** (page 471) to enhance upper back mobility, allowing your head and neck to sit naturally above your shoulders. Additionally, the **Scapular Stability Linchpin Blueprint** (page 473) will help you build stability around your shoulder blades, reducing neck tension and improving your ability to maintain a neutral head position.

PUTTING IT ALL TOGETHER

The goal of the carry screen isn't perfection; it's awareness. You may see multiple compensations, and that's normal, especially if you've identified linchpins from previous screens. Rather than becoming overwhelmed or intimidated, focus on using this information constructively.

You won't rebuild your gait by consciously "thinking" your way through it. Instead, use the carry to confirm what you've already discovered in other foundational patterns. Address the most problematic and glaring linchpins first and watch as your gait naturally improves over time.

In other words, the carry screen is designed to empower you by clearly identifying exactly where you should focus your training efforts next.

CARRY ASSESSMENT

When my clients perform a walking screen without load, they usually look fine. After all, walking involves a smaller range of motion compared to patterns like squats and lunges, so subtle compensations rarely stand out—unless they're rehabbing from a significant injury, spend most of their day hunched over screens, rarely engage in structured exercise, or have developed poor postural habits over years. But here's the catch: Simply appearing "fine" during unloaded movement isn't the goal.

The true value of the carry assessment lies in highlighting compensations that get magnified under load. Unlike the squat, hinge, lunge, push, and pull assessments—where you individualize joint angles, stance width, and setup—the carry assessment is both diagnostic and performance oriented, strategically designed to accomplish two critical objectives.

1. CONFIRM COMPENSATIONS

Because walking integrates aspects of every foundational movement pattern, previously identified linchpins from your squat, hinge, lunge, push, or pull often reemerge clearly when you perform loaded carries. For instance:

SQUAT PATTERN:
Hip mobility issues may surface as uneven side-to-side shifting.

HINGE PATTERN:
Poor lumbopelvic control may show up as excessive arching or discomfort in the low back.

LUNGE PATTERN:
Limited single-leg stability can become obvious through wobbly or asymmetrical steps.

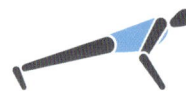

PUSH AND PULL PATTERNS:
Shoulder stability deficits often present as grip fatigue, uneven arm swing, or inability to maintain optimal posture.

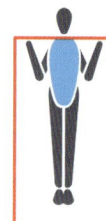

If you're concerned about walking with weight—especially if you've struggled with pain or movement limitations—you're not alone. The idea of loading a movement pattern you've never formally assessed can be daunting. But here's the good news: The carry assessment is uniquely safe, designed to highlight compensations without placing unnecessary stress on your joints or putting you at risk for injury. Here's why you should approach this assessment confidently, without concern of hurting yourself:

First, the carry assessment progresses gradually, beginning at lighter, manageable loads (50 percent of body weight) and increasing systematically only after you've confirmed proper mechanics and control. This staged approach ensures you never overload tissues or joints beyond your current capabilities.

Second, the upright posture inherent to walking places your spine, hips, and shoulders in a neutral, low-risk position. Unlike exercises such as squats and overhead presses, where joints often move through extensive ranges under load, walking naturally limits the amplitude of joint motion, placing less stress on vulnerable structures.

Third, the positioning of the load itself significantly contributes to safety. With the weights held securely at your sides, the load remains closely aligned with your body's natural center of mass and central stability line. This symmetrical placement eliminates risky leverage or torque on your joints, significantly reducing the likelihood of discomfort or injury.

Lastly—and perhaps most importantly—because walking is a self-paced, controlled movement, you have complete autonomy to adjust or stop the movement at any point. Unlike dynamic exercises that might commit you to unstable positions, you can safely drop the load if compensations begin to appear.

Together, these biomechanical advantages make the loaded carry assessment uniquely safe, precise, and effective, providing immediate clarity around your movement quality and pinpointing exactly where you should focus your attention.

In other words, walking with load brings clarity. It magnifies compensations into clear, actionable opportunities to improve your performance across all the foundational movement patterns.

2. ESTABLISH CLEAR PERFORMANCE BENCHMARKS

This assessment also offers measurable standards that give context to your pillar stability, functional strength, and overall movement quality. Whether you're coming off an injury, training for general fitness, or striving toward elite athletic performance, these benchmarks provide a meaningful way to quantify your capabilities and track your progress.

Testing yourself against clear standards isn't just insightful; it's empowering. When clients perform these tests, they're often surprised. Many discover hidden strengths, while others recognize important weaknesses they can now systematically improve. Either way, the test results create a clear, motivating path forward. You won't just know where you stand; you'll know precisely what to do next.

But the value of performance metrics extends far beyond training motivation. Research consistently links the qualities measured in loaded carries—grip strength, pillar stability, and overall functional capacity—to improved longevity and reduced injury risk. For example:

▶ Grip Strength and Longevity: Multiple studies have found grip strength to be a powerful indicator of overall health and lifespan. A comprehensive 2015 study published in *The Lancet* showed that individuals with stronger grips had lower risk of cardiovascular disease, improved functional independence, and significantly increased life expectancy compared to those with weaker grips.[1] Simply put, grip strength reflects how well you'll age and thrive.

▶ Pillar Stability and Injury Prevention: Your pillar—the integrated strength and coordination of your shoulders, hips, and core—is critical to maintaining balance, preventing falls, and avoiding chronic pain, especially later in life. A systematic review published in *Sports Health* (2013) found evidence that targeted core stability training significantly reduces injury risk, particularly in the lower extremities.[2]

▶ **Functional Strength for Lifelong Independence:** Maintaining strength in fundamental movements like loaded carries directly supports a higher quality of life as you age. Extensive longitudinal research published in the *Journals of Gerontology* (2016) found that strength—more than muscle mass alone—is strongly associated with lower mortality risk and could be beneficial for extending lifespan.[3]

Setting clear performance benchmarks isn't just about improving your fitness or strength numbers—it's about building an unbreakable body. When you enhance your grip strength, solidify your pillar stability, and elevate your overall functional capacity, you're actively setting yourself up for decades of healthy movement and physical freedom at every stage of life.

ASSESSMENT LEVELS AND WHAT THEY MEAN

Performing the carry assessment is straightforward, effective, and safe. You'll perform a bilateral farmer's carry at three progressively challenging levels—50, 100, and 200 percent of your body weight—each for a duration of 30 seconds.

You might wonder why we test loaded carries at these particular percentages. Here's the rationale:

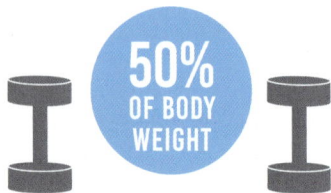

50% OF BODY WEIGHT

100% OF BODY WEIGHT

200% OF BODY WEIGHT

This initial benchmark represents the minimum effective dose needed to assess basic pillar stability and control. At half your body weight, the load is manageable enough to clearly highlight foundational movement quality without overwhelming your system—perfect for individuals returning from injury, managing chronic pain, or new to loaded carries.

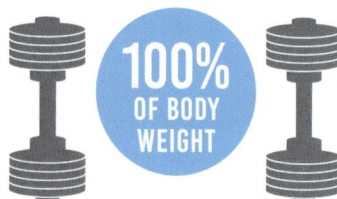

Carrying your own body weight evenly distributed at your sides is a meaningful measure of functional strength and stability. This load represents a key performance baseline that every healthy, active person should strive to achieve. Meeting this standard indicates you've established solid pillar integration, movement symmetry, and functional competency.

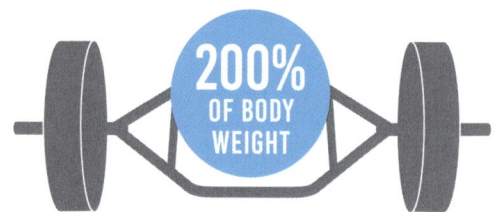

Doubling your body weight serves as an aspirational, elite-level benchmark. It's intended primarily for advanced athletes and highly trained individuals seeking maximal performance. This isn't a must-reach standard for everyone. Consider it a motivating challenge rather than a necessary indicator of good movement quality or pain-free performance.

The 30-second duration for all three levels further enhances this balance. Shorter intervals would overly emphasize maximal strength and risk compromising safety, especially at the heaviest loads. Conversely, longer durations shift toward muscular endurance rather than stability and functional strength. At 30 seconds, the test mirrors the total time under tension experienced during a typical strength training set (8 to 15 reps), ensuring relevance and accessibility for everyone.

Here's exactly what each assessment level measures, who it's designed for, and what it means for your training.

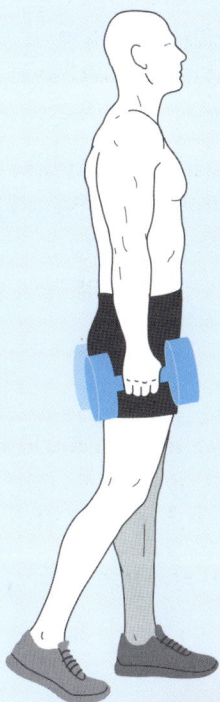

LEVEL 01 REHABILITATION STANDARD

WHO IT'S FOR: Individuals recovering from injury, rehabbing pain, or transitioning back into regular activity or training.

WHAT YOU'RE TESTING: Basic competence and foundational pillar strength at minimal loads.

WHAT IT MEANS FOR YOU:

- Successfully maintaining mechanics indicates readiness for more challenging loads and broader training.
- Visible compensations suggest revisiting your linchpins—especially core bracing, or hip and shoulder stability—prioritizing focused work until you comfortably meet this standard.

25% PER HAND

50% BODY WEIGHT TOTAL

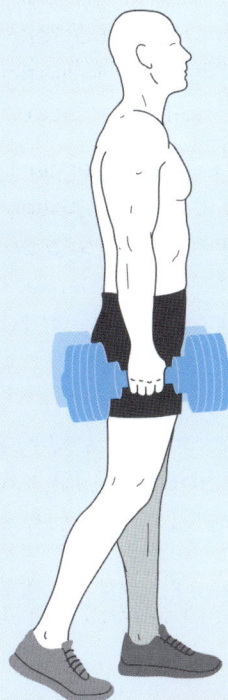

LEVEL 02 GENERAL FITNESS STANDARD

WHO IT'S FOR: Fitness enthusiasts who value health, longevity, and optimal physical function.

WHAT YOU'RE TESTING: Your ability to stabilize and control real-world loads without significant compensation. This is the baseline standard you should strive for to ensure optimal movement health.

WHAT IT MEANS FOR YOU:

- Passing this benchmark confirms your ability to safely manage everyday functional demands.
- Compensations at this stage indicate a need to revisit foundational patterns, using lighter-loaded carries and targeted pillar prep exercises until you build the requisite strength and stability.

50% PER HAND

100% BODY WEIGHT TOTAL

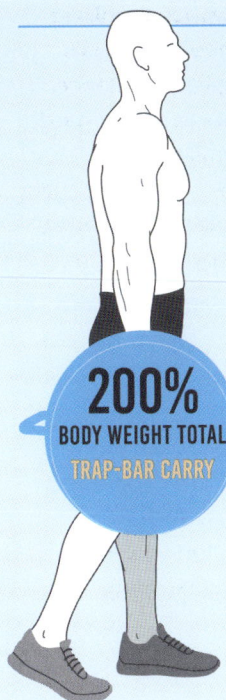

LEVEL 03 ELITE PERFORMANCE STANDARD

WHO IT'S FOR: Advanced athletes or highly trained individuals aiming for maximum strength, durability, and high-level performance.

WHAT YOU'RE TESTING: Maximum capacity to dynamically integrate pillar strength, manage significant loads, and stabilize your entire movement system under maximal challenge.

200% BODY WEIGHT TOTAL
TRAP-BAR CARRY

WHAT IT MEANS FOR YOU:

- Successfully meeting this standard indicates exceptional movement quality, impressive strength, and next-level stability—clear proof that your pillar strength and foundational patterns are exceptionally dialed in.
- For most people—even experienced lifters—this standard represents more of a stretch goal or a fun performance challenge than a requirement for pain-free, healthy movement. Not meeting this benchmark doesn't imply you're deficient in stability or mechanics; it simply reflects how demanding this elite standard truly is.
- If you fall short here, don't interpret it as a major weakness or limitation in your movement quality. Instead, treat it as motivation to continue building toward greater strength and resilience. Remember, your goal isn't necessarily to pass this test—it's to continually progress and become more capable in all your foundational patterns.

SETUP

LOADING (GETTING INTO POSITION):

LEVELS 1 AND 2:

▶ If accessible, pick weights directly from the floor using a split squat stance or a controlled hinge movement.

▶ If you have mobility restrictions or discomfort picking up weights from the floor, use two benches or boxes positioned at your sides. First, elevate each weight one at a time onto the box or bench. Next, stand between the benches, brace your pillar, and pick up the weights simultaneously to safely maintain proper alignment and avoid strain on your hips or lower back.

LEVEL 3 (Trap Bar Carry)

▶ Load a trap bar and position it on an elevated surface if needed (like bumper plates or boxes).

▶ Step inside, hinge your hips, grip firmly, brace your pillar, and stand tall with the bar, maintaining neutral alignment through your shoulders, hips, and spine.

EQUIPMENT NEEDED:
- **LEVELS 1 AND 2:** Dumbbells or kettlebells
- **LEVEL 3:** Trap bar

WHY BODY COMPOSITION MATTERS FOR RELATIVE STRENGTH

When it comes to testing relative strength—meaning strength in proportion to your body weight—it's important to acknowledge the reality of body composition. If you're carrying extra body weight, whether or not you feel comfortable with your current body composition, meeting the recommended carry benchmarks might feel challenging or even frustrating. And that's completely okay.

This assessment is designed to provide clarity and motivation, not judgment. The fact is, relative strength tests naturally favor leaner individuals, because carrying excess body weight inherently means carrying heavier weight in your hands.

But rather than viewing this as a negative, consider it as a powerful insight into where your biggest opportunities for improvement lie. Enhancing relative strength isn't just about training harder or building more muscle—it's about incrementally refining your movement skills, gradually building strength, and steadily improving your body composition over time. Small, consistent progress in any of these areas

can rapidly compound, significantly boosting your relative strength.

Think about the three assessment levels as clear checkpoints along your personal journey. If Level 2 (100 percent bodyweight carry) currently feels unattainable, don't stress—that's precisely why Level 1 exists. Begin there, using it as your achievable starting point. As your strength and skills improve, and as your body composition naturally shifts, you'll steadily move closer to that next benchmark.

If your initial results aren't where you'd like them to be, don't get discouraged. Instead, leverage these levels to set meaningful, holistic goals that align with your current abilities and goals. Your objective is to gradually progress from Level 1 toward Level 2—and perhaps eventually Level 3—by consistently getting stronger, moving better, and nudging your body composition toward a healthier, more functional place. Doing so not only improves your carry assessment results but also creates the foundation for lasting health.

1. **Shoulders:** Co-contract your pecs and lats and the handles firmly to create irradiation—this naturally centers and stabilizes your shoulders in a strong, neutral position.

2. **Hips:** Co-contract your glutes and adductors simultaneously to stabilize your pelvis. Further enhance lower body stability by gripping the ground with your feet and rotating outward without actually moving them.

3. **Breath and Brace:** Perform the Double Breath Technique (page 49), inhaling deeply into your abdomen and creating 360 degrees of tension around your core as if bracing for impact.

4. **Final Check:** Confirm your spine is tall and neutral, eyes forward, shoulders aligned directly over your hips, and weight evenly balanced through your feet before taking your first step.

EXECUTION

If compensations become obvious or posture deteriorates, immediately stop walking and carefully lower the weights by hinging your hips back and gently placing them on the ground, or safely drop them by stepping clear and guiding the weights downward without compromising your position.

1. Begin walking deliberately in a straight line at a steady, controlled pace—approximately one step per second—to maintain continuous tension and stability throughout your body. Avoid rushing; aim for smooth, purposeful strides rather than speed.

2. Maintain rhythmic breathing throughout the carry (refer to page 59) to preserve cadence, consistent intra-abdominal pressure, and optimal core stability.

3. Actively squeeze the handles and maintain tension in your shoulders, hips, and core, ensuring your spine remains neutral with every stride. Avoid swaying side to side or letting the weights pull you forward or backward.

4. When you reach the end of your space, perform a slow, controlled turn by taking small steps while maintaining alignment and tension. Avoid twisting sharply or quickly to protect your spine and joints.

5. Continue for a full 30 seconds and then lower the weights with control.

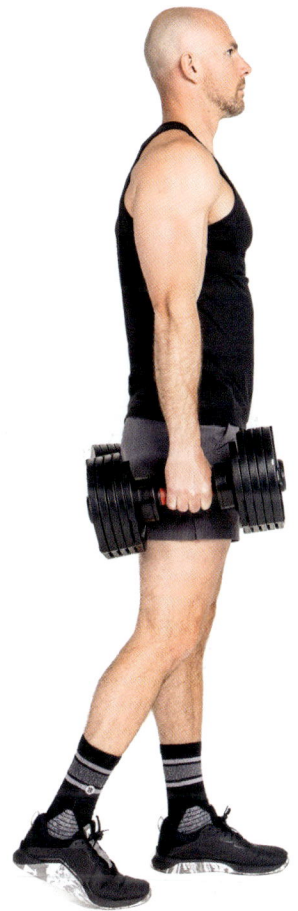

KEY TAKEAWAY

The carry assessment isn't about impressing anyone with brute strength; it's about pinpointing exactly what your body needs to move better. To reiterate, loaded carries clearly highlight your most impactful compensations, guiding your training choices and motivating steady improvement.

That said, each assessment test directly translates into powerful training strategies, meaning they can and should be used as a conditioning finisher in your workouts.

WHY GRIP MATTERS (AND WHY STRAPS MISS THE POINT)

It's rare for grip strength alone to be the true limiting factor during a loaded carry, especially at Level 1 or Level 2. More often, grip issues reflect deeper compensations—usually deficits in shoulder stability, thoracic spine mobility, or inefficient pillar mechanics. If you can't comfortably hold onto the weights, it's likely because you haven't properly activated the spiral of stability that radiates from your grip through your shoulders and core. This powerful neuromuscular connection is called the Law of Irradiation, and it ensures that when you grip something firmly, the tension spreads throughout your body, enhancing your overall stability and performance.

Using lifting straps might seem like a shortcut around weak grip, but here's why that's a mistake: straps disrupt your body's natural ability to create stability through irradiation. They bypass your grip, short-circuiting the crucial feedback loop between your hands, shoulders, and pillar. Without training your grip directly, you're leaving a significant strength and stability opportunity on the table—one that has direct, proven benefits beyond just performance in the gym.

Studies repeatedly show that stronger grip strength directly correlates with improved health span and longevity. But here's the catch: most of those studies measure grip strength with maximal-effort squeezes on a handheld dynamometer—essentially a 1-rep max test for your hands. Yet common advice for improving grip usually involves long-duration hangs from a bar, the equivalent of doing high-repetition endurance work. Trying to build maximal strength with endurance training rarely delivers results.

Loaded carries, however, bridge this gap perfectly. They train your grip under meaningful loads for moderate durations—around 15 to 30 seconds—which aligns far better with how grip strength is actually tested, measured, and used in real life. And because loaded carries naturally recruit every foundational pattern (squat, hinge, lunge, push, pull), they reinforce the full-body integration your grip was designed for in the first place.

Bottom line: Don't use straps. Let loaded carries rebuild your grip the way nature intended—by lifting, carrying, and holding onto meaningful loads.

OPTIMIZATION STRATEGIES

Unlike other patterns, there's no separate set of optimization strategies for the carry itself—because the compensations revealed here directly mirror the linchpins you've already identified in your squat, hinge, lunge, push, and pull screens. If your carry screen and assessment confirm a specific issue, such as limited hip mobility, insufficient shoulder stability, or impaired pillar control, it's your final validation to return to the optimization strategies detailed earlier in this book or address the linchpin that you identified with the targeted linchpin blueprint.

Put simply: Improving your carry means directly addressing the linchpins you've already uncovered. Train your other foundational patterns intentionally, target mobility, stability, and skill deficits as outlined in their respective chapters, and your carry performance will improve. Remember, the carry isn't isolated—it's the ultimate reflection of your overall movement quality. Optimize the individual pieces, and your global pattern follows naturally.

CARRY PROGRESSION PYRAMID

Loaded carries are one of the highest-return exercises you can do—period. But the reality is, most people have barely scratched the surface of their potential. Even if you've experimented with carrying heavy, chances are you haven't approached it systematically, let alone progressively, to build motor control, strength, and pillar stability. And that's exactly why this progression pyramid exists.

This structure not only serves as a powerful training tool but also functions as an extended assessment, allowing you to continuously uncover and refine weak links as you climb the pyramid.

Here's how it works: The carry pyramid is structured into three clear levels, each representing a progressively higher challenge in mobility, stability, and skill. The exercises within each level also move sequentially from bilateral loading (weight in both hands) to unilateral loading (weight in one hand), allowing you to steadily ramp up the challenge and pinpoint specific deficits. This structure not only serves as a powerful training tool but also functions as an extended assessment, allowing you to continuously uncover and refine weak links as you climb the pyramid.

Your starting point is the **farmer's carry**, with weights held at your sides by your hips. This places the load closest to your body's center of mass, making it the most stable variation and ideal for building initial load capacity and general strength. Bilateral loading provides symmetrical stability, while unilateral loading exposes subtle asymmetries in your lateral chain—highlighting hidden compensations in hip, core, or shoulder stability.

Once you've built a solid foundation, you'll elevate the load onto your shoulders in the **front rack carry** position. Here, the weight moves farther away from your lower body's stable base, intensifying the demands on pillar stability and thoracic extension. Your body now must manage subtle rotational and lateral forces with every step, requiring greater control. As before, you'll start with bilateral loading to build strength and confidence, then progress to unilateral loading to significantly challenge lateral stability and core control.

Finally, you'll move into the **overhead carry**, positioning the load at its most challenging point: directly overhead with arms fully extended, biceps close to your ears. Now the load is as far from your center of mass as possible, maximizing mobility, stability, and skill throughout your entire kinetic chain. Every step demands precise control, constant microadjustments through your shoulders, spine, hips, and feet, and total coordination across your body. Again, bilateral loading precedes unilateral loading, helping you identify and correct subtle asymmetries or stability deficits in your overhead motor control.

When you start with bilateral loading, the goal is straightforward: Build maximal strength, stability, and symmetry. Although bilateral carries distribute the load evenly, the reciprocal nature of walking inherently challenges your ability to manage rotation, side-to-side sway, and subtle compensations. But once you transition to unilateral loading, the challenges multiply. With a load in only one hand, your body must actively resist side bending and rotation, intensifying demands on the opposite lateral chain. For instance, a weight in your right hand significantly challenges your left-side hip, core, and shoulder stability. This makes unilateral carries a potent diagnostic tool for uncovering and addressing side-specific linchpins, pinpointing where to focus your corrective work.

Progressing through the carry pyramid isn't just about chasing heavier weights—it's about strategically matching the exercises to your unique needs and identified linchpins. Start by mastering bilateral carries at each level before moving on to unilateral variations. If your goal is general strength and performance, you'll typically use the heaviest possible loads you can control with optimal form, using timed sets (30 to 60 seconds) rather than focusing solely on distance. Timed carries help ensure consistent quality of movement rather than rushing to finish, which often triggers compensations. If you don't have the space to perform walking carries, marching in place or performing slow, controlled turns every few steps provides similar benefits.

If a particular linchpin—such as hip instability or thoracic mobility—keeps resurfacing, unilateral carries at any level can be your targeted strategy. Even with lighter loads, unilateral variations place intense demands on specific regions of your body, offering repeated exposures to challenge and correct those weak links directly.

Once you've unlocked unilateral loading at any level, you gain the option to incorporate **cross-body carry variations**, mixing load positions between left and right sides across different pyramid levels. For example, once you master unilateral front rack carries, you might carry a weight in the front rack on your right side and farmer's carry on your left. Or, having mastered unilateral overhead carries, you could carry overhead with your left hand and front rack with your right. Cross-body carries uniquely target your body's functional oblique slings and add valuable training variety beyond simply adding weight, keeping your training fresh, exciting, and challenging.

Ultimately, the carry progression pyramid is your road map for both assessing and advancing your performance. By progressing methodically from farmer's carries to front rack and finally overhead carries—and from bilateral to unilateral loading at each stage—you'll systematically build the mobility, stability, and skill you need to become strong, resilient, and truly pain-free in the way your body was meant to move.

EVERY CARRY PROGRESSION IS AN ASSESSMENT

Every carry progression—from the farmer's carry to front rack and overhead carry—are real-time assessments, instantly highlighting your most critical compensations. Watch closely for signs like uneven strides, subtle hip shifts, rib flares, excessive arching of the lower back, struggles with shoulder centration, or difficulty maintaining upright posture. Each of these compensations reveals underlying deficits that correspond directly to specific linchpin blueprints:

- **Uneven strides or lateral hip shifts:** Prioritize the **Hip Stability Linchpin Blueprints** (page 475).
- **Rib flare, excessive low back arch, or loss of pillar alignment:** Integrate the **Core Stability Linchpin Blueprints** (pages 472–473).

- **Shoulder elevation, or forward head posture (particularly in overhead carries):** Focus on the **Shoulder Stability Linchpin Blueprint** (page 474).
- **Difficulty maintaining upright posture or limited rotation through your upper back:** Use the **T-Spine Mobility Linchpin Blueprint** (page 471).

Using the carry progressions to regularly assess yourself helps ensure each exercise is purposeful—not only building strength but actively identifying and addressing the mobility, stability, or skill deficits limiting your overall performance.

FARMER'S CARRY

The farmer's carry is the foundational exercise in the carry progression pyramid, representing the simplest and safest entry point for loading the carry pattern. Because the weight is positioned directly alongside your hips—close to your body's natural center of mass—the stability demands are lower, making this variation accessible to virtually everyone. It's the ideal starting place, ensuring success while establishing a baseline of pillar strength, grip endurance, and motor control.

The bilateral farmer's carry loads both sides of the body evenly, emphasizing symmetry and building general load capacity. The unilateral variation shifts the weight to one side, significantly increasing the demands on your lateral core, hip, and shoulder stabilizers. This strategic asymmetrical loading quickly exposes subtle compensations, giving you a targeted way to address weak links and reinforce optimal mechanics.

SETUP: Select either dumbbells or kettlebells; both allow your arms to move independently, enhancing functional carry mechanics. For heavier loads or when equipment is limited, you can use a trap bar as an effective alternative.

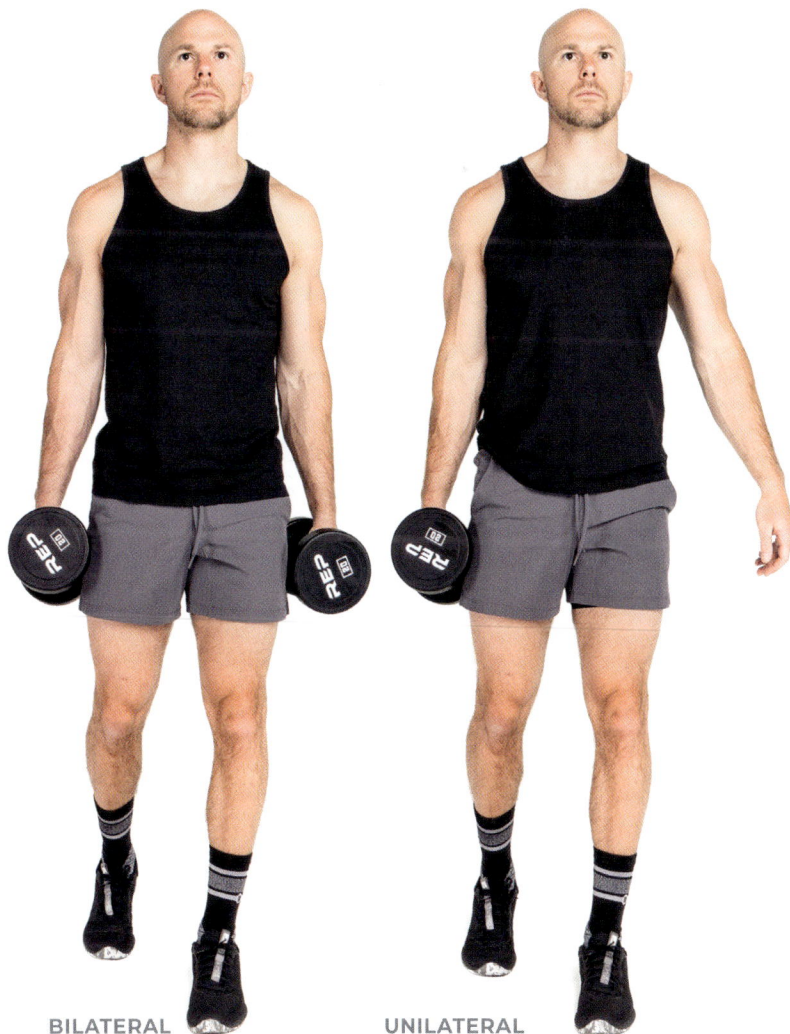

BILATERAL   UNILATERAL

For the bilateral farmer's carry, position two dumbbells or kettlebells, one on each side of you. To safely lift them, use one of two methods:

- **If you have accessible hinge or lunge mechanics, start from a half-kneeling or split stance position.** Lift both implements simultaneously from the ground, maintaining a neutral spine, braced core, and packed shoulders as you stand upright.

- **If mobility limitations prevent you from safely picking up weights from the floor, elevate the dumbbells on benches or boxes** so you can unrack them from a more comfortable height. Simply stand between two benches, grip the weights, brace, and stand up straight.

For the unilateral farmer's carry, follow the same setup protocol, but lift only a single dumbbell or kettlebell in one hand. Your unloaded arm should actively engage, either by extending slightly away from your side, contracting through your pecs and lats, or raising your arm out to a T-position for added stability. Avoid passively hanging your arm; instead, create tension through a "ghost grip," irradiating strength as if holding an actual load.

Once in position, firmly brace your pillar—actively contracting shoulders, hips, and core simultaneously—to establish maximal stability before initiating movement.

EXECUTION: With the load secured at your sides and your pillar braced, initiate a slow, controlled walk forward, maintaining an even, rhythmic gait. Your goal is to manage subtle shifts in weight distribution without sacrificing alignment or pillar integrity. Each step should feel stable and intentional, with minimal sway or rotation.

To perform the bilateral farmer's carry, walk smoothly at a steady tempo, maintaining even spacing between each step. Keep your shoulders stable, your spine neutral, and your gaze fixed straight ahead. Resist the natural tendency to rush, focusing instead on maintaining tension and control throughout your entire kinetic chain for the prescribed duration (usually 30 to 60 seconds).

With the unilateral farmer's carry, mechanics remain largely the same as the bilateral variation; unilateral loading significantly increases demands on your opposite-side stabilizers. Focus on keeping your shoulders level, resisting side-bending, and avoiding rotation toward the loaded side. The unloaded arm should actively contribute to balance by maintaining a strong, irradiated position. Expect slightly shorter carry durations and lighter loads, as unilateral carries intensify motor control demands, targeting asymmetrical compensations more directly.

In both variations, prioritize quality and control over load. This ensures maximum carryover to your foundational movement patterns and creates the ideal foundation for progressing further up the carry pyramid.

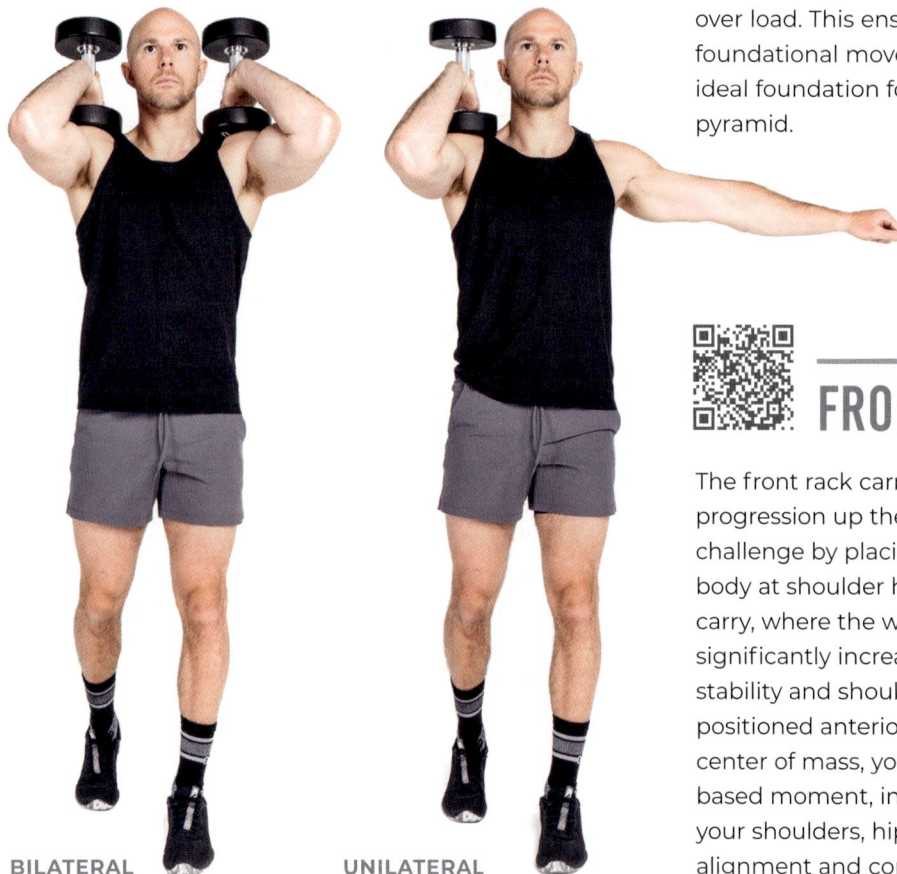

BILATERAL   UNILATERAL

FRONT RACK CARRY

The front rack carry marks the next logical progression up the carry pyramid, elevating the challenge by placing the load directly in front of your body at shoulder height. This shift from the farmer's carry, where the weight rests naturally at your sides, significantly increases the demands on your pillar stability and shoulder complex. Because the load is positioned anteriorly and slightly higher above your center of mass, your body is forced into an extension-based moment, intensifying recruitment from your shoulders, hips, and core to maintain neutral alignment and control.

The bilateral front rack carry provides balanced loading across both shoulders, emphasizing symmetrical stability and reinforcing optimal posture. Conversely, the unilateral front rack carry dramatically increases anti-rotation and lateral stability demands, challenging your pillar to resist asymmetrical loading. Both variations are strategic tools for uncovering subtle deficits in shoulder mobility, thoracic extension, and overall pillar integration, making them highly effective as both diagnostic and performance-enhancing exercises.

SETUP: Start by choosing dumbbells or kettlebells; both implements facilitate a comfortable, stable front rack position. Before initiating movement, ensure proper loading and positioning of the weights at shoulder height.

For the bilateral front rack carry, place two kettlebells or dumbbells directly in front of you on the floor. To safely bring them into the front rack position, which should mirror the humeral carrying angle determined in the push assessment (**Shoulder Scour Test** on page 342) use one of these methods:

- **Kettlebells:** Perform a kettlebell clean by initiating a powerful hip hinge, driving through your hips, and rotating the kettlebells vertically into the front rack position, allowing the kettlebell bell to rest against your anterior deltoids.

- **Dumbbells:** Use a similar hinge-plus-neutral-grip (hammer curl) movement, explosively pulling the dumbbells up and rotating them into position. The dumbbells should rest at roughly a 45-degree angle, with one end firmly against your shoulders and elbows tucked into your sides.

- **Limited mobility option:** If picking up weights from the floor is challenging, place them on an elevated surface, such as a box or bench. Use a controlled quarter-to-half-squat to unrack the weights directly into the front rack position.

For the unilateral front rack carry, follow the same loading and positioning cues as the bilateral variation, but lift only one kettlebell or dumbbell to the shoulder. Once in position, your unloaded side must actively contribute to stability. Extend your free arm slightly out to your side or maintain a strong ghost-grip to irradiate tension through your shoulder, core, and lateral hip on the unloaded side.

With the weight(s) securely in the front rack position, firmly brace your core and maximize shoulder tension by co-contracting your pecs and lats while squeezing your grips. Allowing the implement to make firm contact with your shoulders is essential—this creates a stable platform from which you can maintain optimal positioning and pillar integrity.

EXECUTION: **Once stable and braced, initiate controlled forward movement with deliberate, rhythmic steps.** Maintain constant pillar engagement, fighting to keep your spine neutral, your rib cage stacked directly over your pelvis, and your shoulders packed and down away from your ears. Actively drive your elbows down and slightly inward, reinforcing tension through your pecs and lats, ensuring your humeral carrying angle remains neutral throughout the duration of the carry.

With the bilateral front rack carry, because the load is evenly distributed, focus on symmetry and maintaining an upright torso. Resist the natural tendency to lean backward excessively; instead, actively brace through your core to manage the forward weight placement. **Your gait tempo should remain smooth, controlled, and purposeful, ensuring minimal sway, rotation, or loss of shoulder position throughout the entire carry.**

The unilateral variation significantly increases anti-rotation and lateral stability demands. Your priority is resisting rotation or lateral flexion toward the loaded side. **Maintain strong, active engagement on your unloaded side, using your arm and lateral chain muscles as stabilizers.** Your cadence might naturally slow down, as motor control demands dramatically increase. Embrace this added challenge—it highlights exactly where subtle compensations reside, allowing you to address them strategically.

Both bilateral and unilateral front rack carries provide critical feedback about your shoulder and pillar function, serving as an excellent bridge to more demanding overhead variations. Prioritize controlled movement, relentless pillar engagement, and quality positioning throughout each step, reinforcing strength and stability that translates directly into enhanced performance across all foundational patterns.

OVERHEAD CARRY

The overhead carry represents the highest point on the carry progression pyramid, elevating both load and motor control demands to their most challenging levels. Unlike the farmer's or front rack carry, the overhead carry positions the load as far away from your center of mass and base of support as possible, demanding peak levels of mobility, stability, and skill. If you're ever looking for a quick humbling experience—no matter how strong, mobile, or athletic you think you are—just walk with a moderately heavy load overhead. Within seconds, your body's weakest links become glaringly obvious, and you'll understand exactly why this progression holds the top spot on the pyramid.

Placing the load directly overhead exponentially increases the demands on your shoulder girdle, pillar stability, and thoracic spine mobility. The bilateral overhead carry requires near-perfect symmetry of movement and optimal overhead positioning, exposing any subtle restrictions in your shoulder, spine, or hips. Conversely, the unilateral overhead carry significantly challenges your pillar's anti-rotation and lateral stability capabilities, forcing you to resist compensations that may have gone unnoticed in less demanding variations. In short, if you're compensating anywhere, the overhead carry will reveal it immediately.

NOTE: *Only perform this progression if you have the mobility and stability requisites to press overhead as determined by the* **Overhead Range of Motion Test** *in the push assessment (page 346).*

SETUP: Begin by selecting dumbbells or kettlebells. Dumbbells are typically preferred due to their natural grip and balance overhead, but kettlebells can also be effective. The most critical aspect of this carry is safely and efficiently positioning the weight overhead.

For the bilateral overhead carry, place two kettlebells or dumbbells directly in front of you on the ground. To safely elevate them overhead:

- Start by performing a controlled kettlebell or dumbbell clean into the front rack position, as previously described.

- From the front rack position, perform a quick double-knee bend and drive upward with your legs—think "push press" rather than a strict shoulder press—to get the weights overhead.

- Avoid turning this into a strict press; you should always be able to overhead-carry more load than you can strict press. Use your lower body explosively to generate the momentum required to get the weights overhead safely and efficiently.

For the unilateral overhead carry, follow the loading sequence described above, but press only one dumbbell overhead.

- **For the unloaded arm, actively engage your shoulder by extending it out slightly to the side or front.** Use a strong ghost grip and irradiate tension through your pecs, lats, and core on the unloaded side. This active tension creates a stable pillar foundation that's critical for resisting rotation and lateral bending.

- Once the weight is securely overhead, establish a stable position by firmly engaging your pillar. Lock your elbows fully and align your biceps close to your ears. Your thoracic spine should remain in neutral extension, supporting a strong overhead posture.

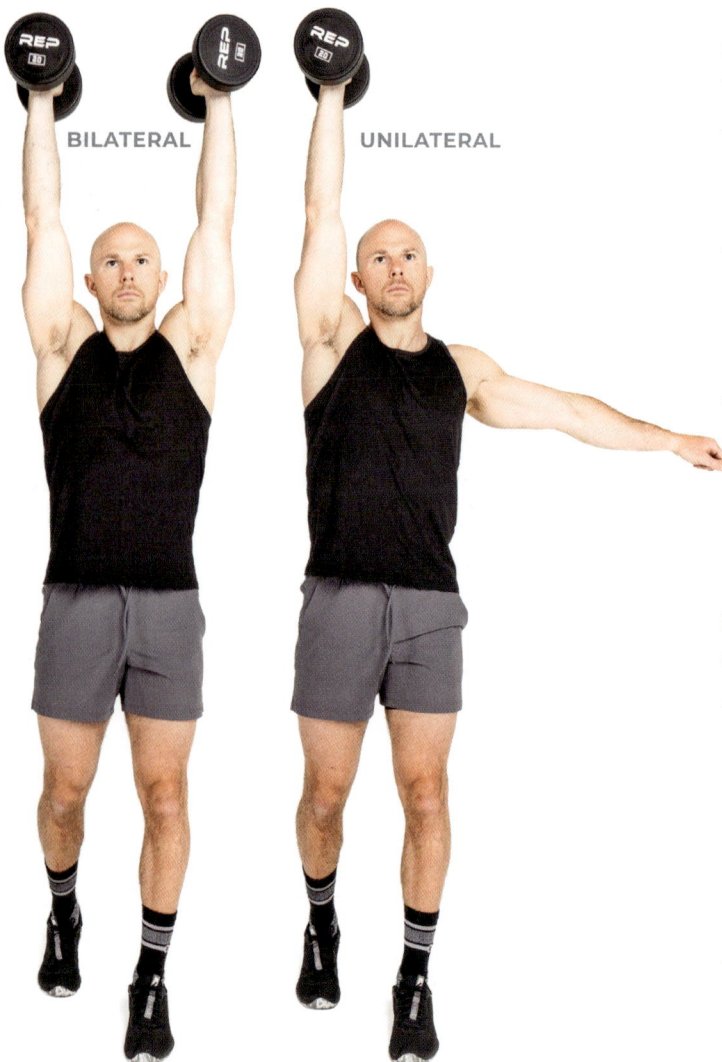

BILATERAL

UNILATERAL

EXECUTION: Begin walking forward in a controlled, deliberate manner, maintaining constant tension and stability through your entire pillar complex. **Your stride tempo should remain measured, smooth, and rhythmic.** Because the load is so far from your body's center, even small movements amplify the difficulty—expect to constantly micro-adjust to keep the load centered directly overhead.

With the bilateral overhead carry, prioritize symmetry. Resist excessive spinal extension (arching your lower back), lateral shifting, or forward leaning. Your core, hips, and shoulders should remain tightly integrated, with minimal sway or side-to-side movement. **Keep your eyes fixed straight ahead and maintain steady breathing with an emphasis on controlled exhales to reinforce your brace.** Aim to minimize compensation by consistently recalibrating pillar tension with every step.

The unilateral overhead carry is uniquely challenging, particularly in its demand for anti-rotation and lateral stability. Your primary objective here is to resist any tendency to rotate or lean away from the loaded side. You'll naturally slow down to maintain control—embrace it. Constantly re-engage tension on your unloaded side, using the active ghost-grip arm and lateral musculature to stabilize your body's alignment. **Pay close attention to maintaining vertical alignment, and consistently check yourself for subtle compensations in your hips, torso, and shoulder position.**

Both variations of the overhead carry provide invaluable feedback on your overall movement competency and help highlight mobility and stability deficits that carry over into nearly every other foundational movement pattern. Incorporating overhead carries into your training not only builds extraordinary pillar strength and stability but also offers clear diagnostic feedback, allowing you to directly target and improve your body's weakest links.

READY TO LEVEL UP? EXPLORE CROSS-BODY CARRIES

Once you've worked your way up the pyramid and demonstrated solid control with unilateral carries, you unlock the next level of challenge: cross-body variations. These involve combining different load positions— like a front rack carry on one side with a farmer's carry or overhead carry on the other.

Cross-body carries introduce asymmetrical demands that train your body's functional slings, especially the anterior and posterior oblique systems, forcing you to stabilize and coordinate across multiple planes. They're a smart way to add intensity, variety, and complexity without simply increasing load.

You can mix and match any combination of carry progressions— overhead, front rack, and farmer's— across both sides. Start with what feels stable, and progress from there.

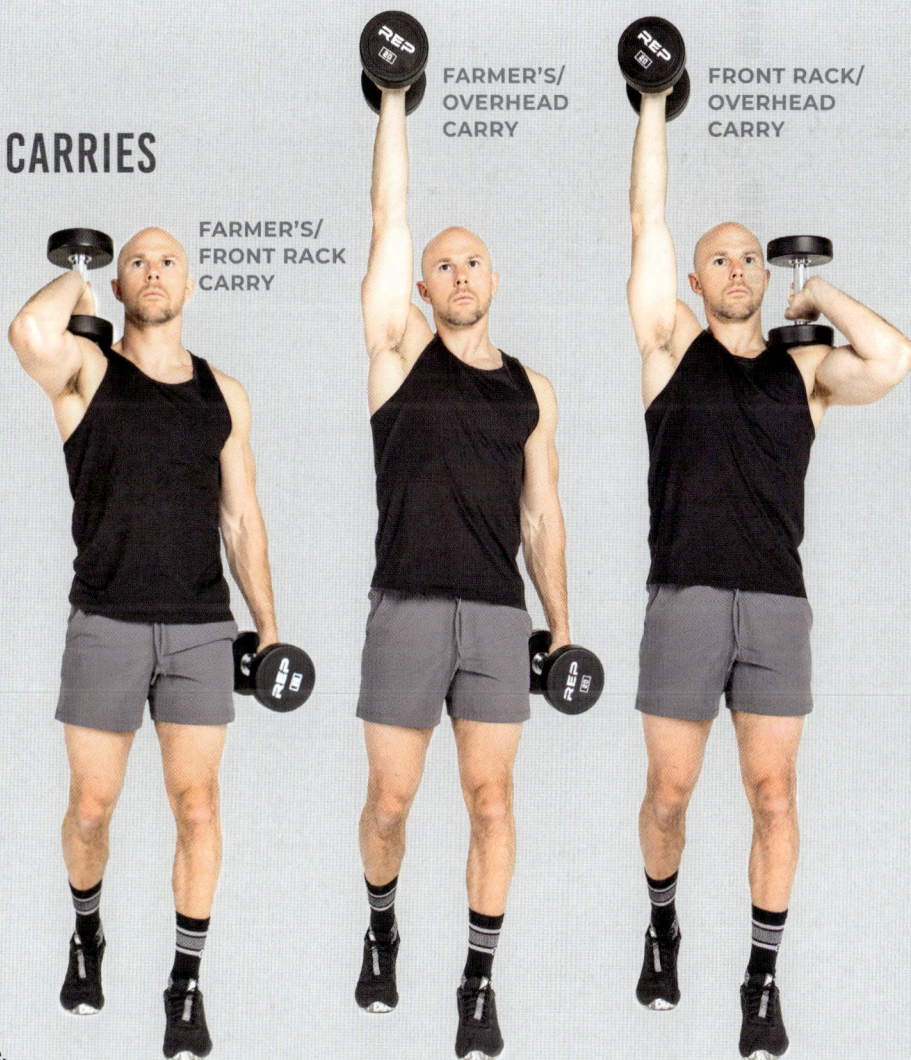

FARMER'S/ FRONT RACK CARRY

FARMER'S/ OVERHEAD CARRY

FRONT RACK/ OVERHEAD CARRY

04

PROGRAMS AND TEMPLATES

PROGRAMS AND TEMPLATES

Pain-free performance is your plan— programming is your prescription.

You can move well and still get hurt. You can have great form and still burn out. You can master the patterns and still hit a wall—if you're not programming intelligently.

Throughout this book, you've rebuilt your movement from the ground up. You've learned how to identify weak links, correct compensations, and restore the qualities that make pain-free performance possible. But even exceptional movement isn't a foolproof safeguard against pain, breakdown, or stalled progress. Lifelong performance—sustained health and pain-free function for a lifetime—requires more. It demands consistent, intentional training across all the physical characteristics that support health and longevity:

STRENGTH:
Your ability to manage and move load with control across a variety of movements, ranges, and positions. Strength gives you capacity—and capacity gives you options.

POWER:
Your ability to move fast, react efficiently, and express speed when it matters most. Power is protective. It keeps you sharp, responsive, and ready for real life.

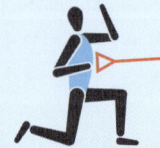

HYPERTROPHY:
Muscle is more than aesthetics. It's structural, metabolic, and functional tissue that supports everything you do. Looking good is just the bonus.

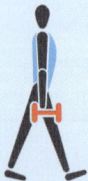

CONDITIONING:
The ability of your heart and lungs to fuel the work you do—and recover from it. A strong aerobic base is the platform your other qualities are built on.

ATHLETICISM:
Movement fluency across multiple planes, positions, and patterns. Rotation, coordination, balance, and reactivity—all combined to help you move with confidence in any direction.

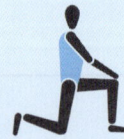

MOBILITY:
The usable range of motion you can control and apply under load. Mobility is what gives your joints freedom and your body options— without pain.

Training each of these physical characteristics is important. But the real challenge—the part most people struggle with—is knowing how to put them together in a way that promotes synergy and progress. That's what pain-free performance programming solves. It doesn't just check boxes for strength or mobility; it gives you a structure to develop all the qualities that matter, in the right amounts, at the right times—with your movement health in mind.

In this section, you'll find a practical framework for integrating each of these physical characteristics into your training. You'll get warm-up templates designed to prepare your body and mind for the demands of training, ensuring each session starts with intention instead of autopilot. You'll also get linchpin blueprints—targeted strategies you can use on recovery days to address nagging pain, improve mobility, and correct the compensation patterns that derail progress. And because everyone's schedule looks different, you'll get training programs built for various frequencies so you can stay consistent whether you train three, four, or more days per week.

All these elements are organized within a structured, progressive format that evolves with you. They're designed to help you build movement mastery, layering in challenge with precision.

And while pain-free performance is the overarching plan, your program is the prescription—your individualized strategy to train smarter, stay consistent, and address the exact needs of your body.

NOTE: *Programming is an extensive subject worthy of an entire book. Realistically, I can't cover every nuance here. Instead, my goal is to provide you with a clear, actionable starting point—the essentials that will get you moving in the right direction. With structure to follow and room to adapt, you'll be able to turn restored movement into real results, laying the foundation for lifelong performance.*

RECLAIM. REBUILD. REGAIN.

TRAINING TENETS

This chapter is where movement becomes momentum—
and where smart, sustainable training begins. The tenets in
this chapter give you a clear, no-fluff framework for building
programs that weave in all the foundational movement
patterns and physical characteristics of health and longevity.
You'll learn how to structure your workouts—taking everything
that works and showing you how to apply it, step by step. By
the end, you'll not only understand the system; you'll know how
to run it.

Before there was a system or a certification called pain-free performance, there was just the training. I was writing programs that worked—programs that produced results and kept people coming back for more. Back then, I didn't have a formalized approach or a branded method. What I had was a stack of client case studies built from real-world experiences, along with the instinct to program based on what helped people move, feel, and perform better.

I didn't realize that my approach was unconventional. I didn't know it wasn't what most coaches were doing. All I knew was that my clients were getting out of pain and hitting new personal bests—and that wasn't what I was seeing around me. It wasn't what was being taught in textbooks or shared in forums. But it was working.

At the time, it never felt revolutionary. I wasn't trying to disrupt anything. I was just doing the only thing I knew how to do: draw from everything I'd been taught and experienced— and from everyone who had mentored me—to find a better way forward. That's what led to writing hundreds of published articles, coaching Olympians and professional athletes, and certifying tens of thousands of coaches in pain-free performance—a training system that could be taught and scaled effectively.

But the programming came first. That was the original spark.

Most people think you need to master a system before you can build great programs. For me, it was the opposite. I was programming before I had all the answers—and the success of that programming is what led me to ask better questions. Why was it working so well? What were the underlying principles? How did all the components—movement quality, warm-ups,

foundational patterns—fit together to create such consistent outcomes?

This chapter is the answer to those questions. It's the bridge between the system you've just learned and the action you're about to take.

Because the truth is, programming is where it all comes together. You can master movement, dial in your form, and train pain-free—but if you're not programming with intent, you'll still hit walls. Burnout, pain, and performance plateaus aren't always caused by how you move. Often, they come down to how you train. That's where the tenets come in.

They're the principles that underpin every program I write. They reflect years of trial and error, field-testing with clients at every level— from professional athletes to everyday people just trying to feel like themselves again. And while no single program works for everyone, the framework you're about to read is designed to support anyone—at any age, any experience level, and at any stage of training.

TRAIN ALL SIX PHYSICAL CHARACTERISTICS OF HEALTH AND LONGEVITY—
HOW TO DESIGN AND STRUCTURE YOUR WORKOUTS

The goal of this system is simple: train for health, performance, and longevity without triggering pain or setting yourself back in the process.

But what that actually looks like will vary from person to person. Your needs, your movement profile, and your training history all shape how the system should be applied. That's why your program is a prescription. It's a tailored approach that delivers the right type and amount of stimulus, based on how you move and what you need most.

And that prescription only works when it targets the six physical characteristics: strength, hypertrophy, power, conditioning, athleticism, and mobility. These are the foundational qualities that help your body function better and adapt to the demands of training and life over time.

You've spent the first three parts of this book rebuilding your movement, restoring function, and laying a foundation for pain-free performance. But now comes the hard part: putting it all together.

Most people know what they should be training. But when it's time to design a complete workout that trains all six physical characteristics, many default

WAVE LOADING: THE NATURAL FLOW OF LOAD AND RECOVERY THAT SHAPES EVERY PHASE OF YOUR WORKOUT

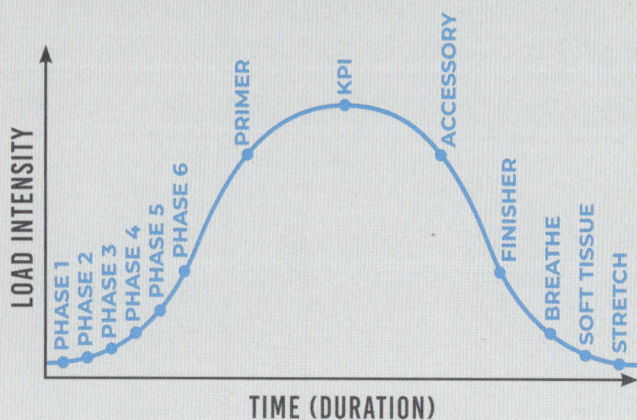

The structure of a pain-free performance session is built on a principle called wave loading. It's the process of riding a gradual curve—from low to high loading, and then back down again—matching your body's natural stress-recovery cycle.

You start in a low parasympathetic state with soft tissue work and mobility. You build into activation, dynamic movement, and finally peak in your KPI lift, where strength and load are highest. Once you've reached that peak, you don't stay there. You come down the other side of the wave, decreasing load through hypertrophy-focused accessory work, conditioning finishers, and finally recovery-focused cool-downs.

Wave loading is like surfing the rhythm of your body—gradually building load, peaking at your highest level of effort, then intentionally tapering back down. By matching each phase of your workout session to this natural ebb and flow, you strategically manage your training effort, so you finish feeling energized, recovered, and prepared for your next session.

to programs that specialize in just one. They follow powerlifting templates to build strength. Bodybuilding splits to gain muscle. Yoga classes to improve mobility. Others dive into HIIT circuits, rely on athletic drills, or get stuck in corrective routines. Each of these methods has its place, but most fail to connect the dots. When key components are neglected, the result is almost always the same: overuse, imbalance, and pain.

That's why this tenet comes first. Because the art of intelligent programming is in creating synergy—putting the pieces together in a way that builds momentum, minimizes risk, and meets you where you are.

This is where the pain-free performance system stands apart.

While most programs focus on individual characteristics, this system looks at how each component of a training session interacts with the next—and how every session connects to the bigger picture of your training plan. Nothing is random. Everything has a role.

What follows is the structure of a complete pain-free performance training session. Each phase targets one or more of the six physical characteristics while reinforcing movement quality and supporting durability over time. This means you'll be able to train like a bodybuilder without breaking down. Build strength like a powerlifter while still moving like an athlete. Condition like a CrossFitter without burning out. It works for elite performers. It works for people in pain. And it works for anyone who wants to stay capable and train for life.

This is the exact structure I use in my own training and with every program I write—because when the goal is performance that lasts, every phase matters.

1.
PRE-TRAINING PREPARATION

6-PHASE WARM-UP

SETS/REPS: Varies by phase (see "6-Phase Dynamic Warm-ups" on page 463)

REST: Minimal, if any, between exercises and phases

PURPOSE: *Prepare your body and nervous system for the demands of training by improving mobility, activating key stabilizers, and addressing weak links.*

TOTAL TIME: 10–12 minutes *Each phase should take roughly 2 minutes to complete.*

Prepare. Prevent. Perform.

Your training day starts with the 6-phase dynamic warm-up, covered in Part 2. The goal here is twofold: to unlock movement and to reinforce it. You're prepping tissues, priming the nervous system, and activating postural stabilizers while simultaneously addressing weak links and painful patterns. This is where mobility shines brightest, helping you access and control range of motion with purpose and stability. But this phase isn't just about injury prevention; it's also about readiness, designed to get your body firing on all cylinders and your mind locked in. Done right, this phase should feel like the best physical therapy session you've ever had—combined with the professional warm-up you'd expect from a high-level athlete.

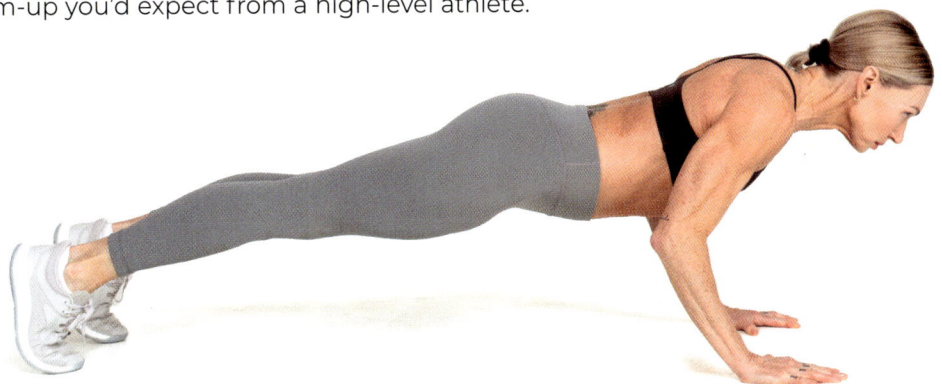

2. PRIMING AND POTENTIATION

After completing the warm-up, you don't jump straight to your heaviest lift. This next phase serves as a bridge extending the benefits of the warm-up while preparing your body and mind for higher levels of intensity and performance.

Two types of priming strategies are used in this phase: **mechanical priming** and **neurological priming**.

Mechanical priming is the more accessible of the two. It involves moderate-load, high-rep accessory exercises designed to target specific areas like the posterior shoulder, glutes, and hamstrings. The goal is to increase local blood flow, reinforce stability in vulnerable joints, and prime weak links using hypertrophy-style programming—slow eccentrics, constant tension, and a strong mind-muscle connection. This work is typically performed for 3 to 5 sets of 15 to 25 or more reps, with 30 to 45 seconds of rest between sets to maintain tissue temperature and engagement.

For example:

▶ Face pulls before bench pressing

▶ Hamstring curls before squats or lunges

▶ Hip thrusts before deadlifts

Neurological priming, on the other hand, is a more advanced strategy. It borrows from phase 6 of the warm-up and includes explosive high-speed movements like jumps, throws, and plyometric variations. These drills are ideal for developing power, speed, and reactivity—but they require a more complete movement foundation.

You'll get the most out of neurological priming when all six foundational patterns are present and pain-free and when you've developed a strong baseline of coordination, control, and motor skill. Exercises in this category are typically performed for 3 to 5 sets of 1 to 5 high-effort reps, with 30 to 45 seconds of rest between sets to maintain peak intensity and quality of movement.

Once both strategies are in your toolkit, you can combine them for even greater effect. A well-structured superset—two exercises performed back-to-back with minimal rest—is one of the best ways to fire up both your tissues and your nervous system, especially before a heavy or high-performance session.

In practice, you'll perform your neurological primer first, rest briefly (10 to 15 seconds), and then go straight into the mechanical primer. After completing both, take 30 to 45 seconds of rest before starting the next round. Repeat for the prescribed number of sets based on your readiness and training goals.

MECHANICAL PRIMING

SETS/REPS: 3–5 sets of 15–25+ constant-tension, mind-muscle connection reps

REST: 30–45 seconds between sets

PURPOSE: *Increase blood flow, reinforce stability, and activate weak links in target muscle groups—especially for those in pain or needing a more robust warm-up.*

TOTAL TIME: 5–7 minutes

NEUROLOGICAL PRIMING

SETS/REPS: 3–5 sets of 1–5 high-effort, high-speed explosive reps

REST: 30–45 seconds between sets

PURPOSE: *Fire up the nervous system, sharpen motor output, and prime the body for power and performance. Best suited for pain-free lifters with developed movement skills.*

TOTAL TIME: 5–6 minutes

NEUROLOGICAL + MECHANICAL SUPERSET

SETS/REPS: 3–5 rounds of neurological (1–5 reps) followed by mechanical (15–25+ reps)

REST: 10–15 seconds between movements, 30–45 seconds between rounds

PURPOSE: *Combine tissue prep and nervous system activation in a single sequence—bridging the gap between warm-up and performance with both control and explosiveness.*

TOTAL TIME: 6–8 minutes

3. KEY PERFORMANCE INDICATOR (KPI)

This is the centerpiece of your session—the main lift or movement pattern that drives your performance forward. It's where strength is built and tested. Where movement meets effort. But it's not just about lifting heavy loads—it's about how you strain.

Strain refers to the effort required to grind through your final concentric rep with excellent form. It's the technical challenge that occurs when a rep slows down—not because you're out of position but because you're working at your edge. This high-effort finish unlocks neurological skill development, where your brain and body learn to coordinate more efficiently, and it maximizes mechanical tension, which is critical for building true strength.

Key performance indicators (KPIs) are selected using a blend of strategy, movement quality, and self-assessment. A goblet squat might be the right fit for one person, while a barbell back squat might be right for another. One isn't better than the other—they're just different tools for different needs. The point is to choose the right tool for you, using the movement pattern pyramids to guide the overall selection process by identifying which variation is appropriate for your current ability—meaning the one you can perform *well* without pain or compensation.

On training day, that choice is refined through phase 5 of the warm-up, where you screen and rehearse the movement pattern. Think of it as a readiness check. You screen the pattern to gauge how your body feels in that moment and adjust the progression, load, or intensity accordingly. It's a dynamic decision-making process that ensures your KPI isn't just theoretically appropriate—it's functionally appropriate, today.

WHAT ABOUT A ONE-REP MAX (1RM)?

A one-rep max is often viewed as the gold standard for measuring strength. It's the ultimate test of how much force your body can produce in a single, maximal-effort rep. But in the context of pain-free performance, it's a test—not a tool we use for long-term health-focused training.

While sets of 1 to 3 reps still fall within the strength category, true **max-effort singles are rarely programmed** because most people simply don't have the movement skill, joint control, or postural stability to express maximal strength safely. They may have the potential, but without the ability to access it through clean, confident movement, a 1RM often becomes a test of compensation, not capability.

It's also worth noting that as loading gets heavier, risk increases. While strength training is remarkably safe—especially when it's programmed intelligently and performed with solid technique—true max-effort lifts carry a greater chance of injury. That's why max

testing is considered an advanced method best reserved for those with experience, clean patterns, and clear intent.

In pain-free performance, we stay within a 3-to-8-rep range for most strength work. It still produces strain, drives adaptation, and gives you measurable progress—without pushing your body past its capacity. Loads typically fall between 80 and 90 percent of your estimated 1RM, which is heavy enough to stimulate both neurological and muscular development, but light enough to maintain technical quality.

That said, there's still a time and place for a true 1RM. If you're competing in powerlifting, weightlifting, or chasing a personal benchmark, building toward it can make sense. But if your goal is to regain movement capacity, stay out of pain, and train for a lifetime of strength, chasing a one-rep max isn't necessary. And for most people, it's not even helpful.

In other words, choosing your KPI should be a deliberate pairing of pattern, progression, and purpose that reflects both your long-term training goals and your day-to-day readiness.

Once you've locked in your KPI, you'll begin with **ramp-up sets** to groove the pattern and gradually increase load. These sets are not fatiguing; they're controlled, low-rep efforts used to dial in your positioning and prepare your nervous system for the heavier work to come. The simplest way to structure

MAKING THE MOST OF YOUR REST PERIODS (FILLER SETS)

During KPI training, rest periods are longer—typically 90 seconds to 2 minutes. While that recovery time is essential, it doesn't have to mean sitting around or scrolling on your phone—especially if you're working within a tight session window.

Instead, make that rest productive. Use it to improve the very things that support your strength: mobility, joint positioning, and postural control. We call these **filler sets**—low-intensity mobility drills or positional stretches performed between KPI sets. They're specifically chosen to reinforce movement quality without adding fatigue or interfering with output.

To be clear, these aren't demanding, long-duration stretches. They are short, strategic holds—30 to 60 seconds max—focused on breathing and position. In fact, one of the golden rules of filler sets is not moving. Static positions help downshift your heart rate, lower your respiratory drive, and regulate blood flow, keeping you in a better place to lift heavy again.

And no, stretching between sets won't blunt your strength. The research is clear: Short-duration static stretching (under 1 minute) does not impair strength or power output. In some cases, it can even enhance it. You're simply getting more out of your rest window—two birds, one stone.

For example, after a heavy set of trap bar deadlifts, you might drop into a frog stretch or adductor rock-back. After pull-ups, you could hold a lat stretch that keeps you grounded and improves range. These strategies not only reinforce movement, they also help ingrain strength through length—and for more advanced lifters, they can even feel like loaded stretching, extending time under tension and reinforcing end-range control.

You don't have to do this—but if you're serious about making every minute count, it's one of the most effective ways to add value to your rest. They offer a chance to address linchpins and improve mobility, all while your nervous system resets for the next set.

This is how you build better movement without extending your session—and how you squeeze more out of the time you're already investing.

FILLER SET OPTIONS

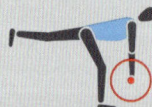

KPI LIFT	SQUAT	HINGE	LUNGE	PUSH	PULL
MOBILITY / CORRECTIVE OPTION	Half-kneeling hip flexor stretch, rear-foot-elevated hip flexor stretch, 45-degree half-kneeling hip flexor stretch, ankle dorsiflexion mobilizations, standing straight-leg calf stretch, standing bent-leg soleus stretch	Frog stretch, adductor rock-back stretch, child's pose, supine supported adductor stretch	Adductor rock-back stretch, world's greatest stretch, dynamic pigeon stretch, 90/90 shin box stretch, FABER stretch	90/90 chest stretch, single-arm pec stretch, supine T creep stretch, T-spine prayer stretch, hinged-over pec stretch	Hinged-over lat stretch, single-arm upper back stretch, child's pose, vertical hang (wrists supported)
PURPOSE	Hip, knee, and ankle mobility; decompressing lumbar spine	Hip mobility, decompressing lumbar spine, pelvic control	Thoracic spine, scapular, thoracic cage, and shoulder mobility	Improving scapular mechanics and thoracic mobility	Thoracic spine, scapular, thoracic cage, shoulder, and overhead mobility

them is to match the rep count of your working sets. For example, if your KPI calls for 3 sets of 8, your ramp-up sets should also use 8 reps as you increase the load. This consistency keeps the pattern sharp and helps you settle into the right rhythm without wasting energy.

Then you arrive at your top-end working sets—the most neurologically demanding part of your training day. These are performed for 1 to 2 sets of 3 to 8 reps, taken to or near your technical limit, which means pushing close to failure while maintaining crisp, controlled form. You should finish with 1 to 2 reps in reserve—enough to avoid compensation but still heavy enough to achieve what matters most in this phase: strain. That effort—the grind through your final clean rep—is what drives the strength adaptation you're after. Rest periods are longer here—90 seconds to 2 minutes—to allow for full recovery and ensure each set is executed with maximum intent and precision.

Most of the time, a session includes one KPI. In training programs with higher frequency (four or more days per week), this single-lift focus is ideal. It allows you to channel full effort into one main lift without accumulating unnecessary fatigue, giving your nervous system the recovery it needs between sessions.

However, in lower-frequency programs—typically two or three days per week—you often see two KPIs per session: one upper body lift and one lower body lift. In these full-body formats, KPIs can be performed separately or paired in superset fashion. For example, you might pair a dumbbell bench press (upper body push) with a trap bar deadlift (lower body hinge). When programmed this way, each lift is performed back-to-back, but you'll still rest fully between rounds to preserve output, especially when both movements are strength focused and neurologically demanding.

This strategy allows you to train both movement categories efficiently, ensuring you maintain balance across the foundational patterns, even when training volume is condensed.

4. PUMP ACCESSORIES AND PREHAB

The hardest lift is over, but the work isn't done. Now it's time to train the muscles and patterns that didn't get the spotlight during your KPI. This phase is where balance is built—through accessory work and prehab.

Pump accessories are hypertrophy-based movements. These compound or single-joint exercises are programmed with moderate loads and moderate-to-high rep ranges. The goal is to strengthen weak links, reinforce control, and drive local blood flow into key tissues. For example, if your KPI was a squat, your accessories might include a hinge and a lunge to fill in the patterns that were missed. This helps ensure all six foundational movement patterns are addressed over the course of a session or training week without creating overload in a single direction.

Prehab work, while programmed in the same block, serves a more targeted purpose. These movements tend to be lighter and more isolated, are focused on specific joints, and often zero in on commonly problematic areas—like the posterior shoulder, hips, and spine—with an emphasis on mobility, motor control, and end-range positional strength.

In practice, you often see these movements paired together. While all prehab can be considered accessory work, not all accessories qualify as prehab. The difference is load and specificity. Accessories are typically heavier and more global; prehab is lighter and more precise. When paired, prehab is often performed after the pump movement in a mini block or superset-style format.

The training frequency and split will also dictate how this phase is structured. In full-body or lower-frequency programs (two or three days per week), prehab is minimal—time and volume are prioritized for compound patterns and hypertrophy work. In higher-frequency programs (four or five days per week), you'll see more dedicated prehab integrated, especially toward the end of the session when load demands are lower and you have time to fine-tune joint position and target linchpins.

Exercise selection should follow a simple rule: Match the region and balance the pattern. On lower body days, you'll train lower body pump and prehab patterns. On upper body days, the emphasis shifts to upper body–specific work. In full-body sessions, expect to hit both. This is what makes the accessories and prehab phase so important. It's not just about the pump; it's about creating durability—building muscle, control, and strengthening the patterns that hold everything together.

QUICK TIPS FOR PROGRAMMING ACCESSORIES AND PREHAB

Accessory exercises should balance the KPI by targeting the patterns or regions *not emphasized* in your main lift.

Prehab drills support your linchpins, targeting areas like the hips, shoulders, and thoracic spine.

PAIRING EXAMPLE: *After a heavy deadlift KPI, follow with goblet squat (accessory) and physio ball hamstring curl (prehab).*

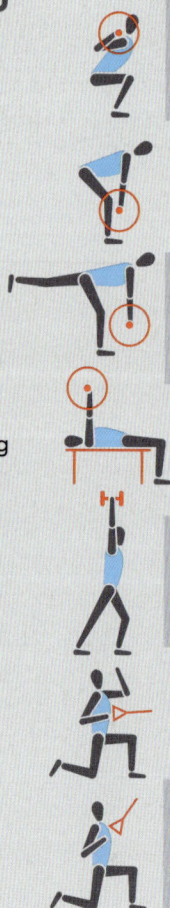

KPI LIFT	PUMP ACCESSORY (HYPERTROPHY FOCUS)	PREHAB (LINCHPIN + POSITIONAL FOCUS)
SQUAT	· Hinge (RDL variation) · Lunge (hip-dominant variation)	· Direct glute work · Direct hamstring work · Direct quad work · Direct calf work
HINGE	· Squat (front load variation) · Lunge (knee-dominant variation)	· Direct glute work · Direct hamstring work · Direct quad work · Direct erector work
LUNGE	· Squat (knee-dominant variation) · Hinge (hip-dominant variation)	· Direct glute work · Direct hamstring work · Direct quad work · Direct adductor work
PUSH (HORIZONTAL)	· Vertical push (overhead emphasis) · Vertical pull (pull-up variation) · Horizontal pull (row variation)	· Direct shoulder work · Direct upper back work · Direct arm work (triceps)
PUSH (VERTICAL)	· Horizontal push (push-up variation) · Vertical pull (pull-up variation) · Horizontal pull (row variation)	· Direct shoulder work · Direct upper back work · Direct arm work (triceps)
PULL (HORIZONTAL)	· Vertical pull (pull-up variation) · Vertical push (overhead emphasis) · Horizontal push (push-up variation)	· Direct shoulder work · Direct upper back work · Direct arm work (biceps)
PULL (VERTICAL)	· Horizontal pull (row variation) · Vertical push (overhead emphasis) · Horizontal push (press variation)	· Direct shoulder work · Direct upper back work · Direct arm work (biceps)

5.
CONDITIONING FINISHER

Every great training session ends with a final effort—and in this system, that effort targets your engine. Conditioning finishers are short, simple, and intense. They're built to elevate your heart rate and deliver a powerful cardiorespiratory training effect in just a few minutes.

But they do more than train your heart and lungs—they also leave you with an emotional payoff. They give you that satisfying sense of having worked hard and emptied the tank, which is one of the most powerful motivational tools you can tap into.

These finishers focus on safe, repeatable movement patterns and are typically structured as circuits, intervals, or time-based work sets. The goal is to finish strong, feel accomplished, and train your cardiovascular system without sacrificing the quality of your movement.

CONDITIONING FINISHER

DURATION: **20 seconds to 10 minutes of sustained effort** (varies based on circuit or interval structure)

REST: Variable—may include full recovery (1:1) or accumulated fatigue formats (2:1 or 3:1 work-to-rest ratios) depending on goal and intensity.

PURPOSE: *Elevate heart rate and improve cardiovascular efficiency while reinforcing clean, repeatable movement under fatigue. The goal is to finish strong without compromising mechanics.*

TOTAL TIME: 2–10 minutes

WHAT'S THE DIFFERENCE BETWEEN CARDIO AND CONDITIONING?

While the terms are often used interchangeably, **cardio** and **conditioning** serve distinct purposes in your training program. Understanding the difference will help you integrate both effectively to support your health, performance, and recovery.

Both cardio and conditioning have a place in your program. Cardio is your base. Conditioning is your peak. Together, they round out your health-first approach to programming.

	CARDIO	CONDITIONING
	Cardio is best used to build base endurance, support recovery between training sessions, and improve your ability to handle more volume over time. It's ideally done daily, but realistically, 3 to 4 sessions per week—often on non-lifting days—is enough to get the benefits.	*Conditioning is typically used as a finisher at the end of a workout. It's short and intense, designed to elevate heart rate, increase work capacity, and leave you with a powerful "I did something" feeling.*
DURATION	10+ minutes	20 seconds to 10 minutes
INTENSITY	Low to moderate (heart rate zones 2–3)	High (heart rate zones 4–5)
FREQUENCY	1–7 days/week (realistically 3–4)	1–3 days/week
TOTAL VOLUME	Relatively high	Relatively low
REST PERIODS	Minimal to none	Variable—depends on the goal (e.g., cumulative fatigue for longer circuits or full recovery for performance work)
TRAINING EFFECT	Enhances aerobic efficiency and recovery	Improves anaerobic capacity and work output
TRADITIONALLY	Low-intensity steady state (LISS) cardio	High-intensity interval training (HIIT)

HEART RATE TRAINING ZONES

TRAINING ZONE	% OF MAX HEART RATE	TRAINING EFFORT	TRAINING EFFECT
ZONE 5	90–100%	Maximal	Trains speed and power
ZONE 4	80–90%	Hard	Develops anaerobic capacity
ZONE 3	70–80%	Moderate	Develops aerobic capacity
ZONE 2	60–70%	Light	Builds base endurance
ZONE 1	50–60%	Very light	Enhances recovery

6. POST-TRAINING COOL-DOWN

PARASYMPATHETIC BREATHING

DURATION: 1–2 minutes

PURPOSE: *Shift your nervous system into a recovery state using deep, controlled breathing in a supported position (e.g., 90/90). Focus on full exhalation and diaphragmatic control.*

FOAM ROLLING

DURATION: 1–2 minutes per major muscle group

PURPOSE: *Use slow, controlled passes over the entire length of the tissue to reduce residual tension, promote circulation, and reinforce the parasympathetic shift initiated by breathing.*

STRETCHING

DURATION: 1–2 minutes per position

PURPOSE: *Reach an authentic end range, then maintain or gently deepen the stretch. Focus on areas that were heavily trained or that consistently show up as linchpins. Emphasize breathing, positional awareness, and relaxation.*

*REST: Minimal—only as needed to transition between phases or sides.

*TOTAL TIME: 3–8 minutes

Most people skip cool-downs. That's a mistake.

The final phase of the workout is where recovery begins. The three-phase cool-down is designed to lower your heart rate, calm your nervous system, and set the stage for physical restoration so you leave the gym in a parasympathetic state, not stuck in fight-or-flight mode.

It starts with deep, diaphragmatic breathing for 1 to 2 minutes (or until your heart and respiratory rate return to normal) using the 90/90 Parasympathetic Positional Breathing technique (see page 54) to bring your nervous system back into recovery mode.

Once your breath has begun to slow and your system has shifted gears, you move into global foam rolling, targeting the muscles that were hit hardest during the workout. Unlike the warm-up, where you oscillate on specific segments of a muscle, global foam rolling involves slow, controlled passes along the full length of the muscle for 1 to 2 minutes on each side. This not only reduces residual tension and enhances tissue recovery but also helps reinforce the parasympathetic state initiated by your breathing, making it easier to stay relaxed, grounded, and primed for recovery as you move into the final phase: stretching.

While the biphasic approach introduced in the warm-up can be used here, it may be too demanding after a high-intensity session. In those cases, default to traditional static stretching, where the goal is relaxation, not stimulation.

At this stage, your focus shifts to recovery. Choose stretches that target the areas trained most intensely or that consistently show up as linchpins in your movement. The intent is to reach an authentic end range, hold that position, and—if possible—creep deeper into the stretch by relaxing into it. Concentrate on your breathing, your position, and your ability to mentally and physically let go.

Hold each stretch for 30 seconds to 1 minute or longer, depending on how your body feels. This is your chance to lock in usable range of motion while your tissues are still warm, pliable, and receptive to change.

These three simple steps—performed with intent—can significantly reduce soreness, improve recovery, and set you up for success not only in your next session but also as you go about your day. Whether you're heading to work or just trying to stay present and pain-free, how you finish your training matters just as much as how you start.

PUTTING IT ALL TOGETHER: SETS, REPS, AND REST TIMES

When you step back and look at the full structure, you'll see that it's more than a workout; it's a system—one that's built to train every physical characteristic of health and longevity.

▼ **STRENGTH** is developed through the KPI—the heaviest, most technically demanding lift of the day.
FEELS LIKE: *Straining against load with full-body tension and control.*

▼ **HYPERTROPHY** shows up in mechanical priming, KPI work, and accessory phases to support muscle growth, joint integrity, and long-term durability.
FEELS LIKE: *A deep muscular pump and strong mind-muscle connection.*

▼ **POWER** is trained through explosive drills like jumps and throws, primarily in neurological priming and phase 6 of the warm-up.
FEELS LIKE: *Moving fast and producing force with intent and precision.*

▼ **ATHLETICISM** is expressed in dynamic movements requiring coordination, reactivity, and control—layered into the warm-up and neurological primers.
FEELS LIKE: *Full-body skill— jumping, cutting, rotating, and moving with agility.*

▼ **MOBILITY** is addressed in both the warm-up and cool-down to access, reinforce, and restore usable range of motion.
FEELS LIKE: *Stretching, breathing, and controlling end-range positions.*

▼ **CONDITIONING** is trained in the finisher, designed to challenge the cardiovascular system and enhance work capacity.
FEELS LIKE: *Elevated heart rate, physical effort, and mental grit.*

PHYSICAL CHARACTERISTIC	WHERE IT SHOWS UP	EXECUTION STYLE	HOW IT FEELS
STRENGTH	KPI (key performance indicator)	Lift heavy, move weights, strain against load	Strained and challenging
HYPERTROPHY	Mechanical priming, KPI, pump accessories	Build muscle, get a pump, reps to failure	Pumped and focused
POWER	Neurological priming (phase 2), phase 6 of warm-up	Move fast, create force, explosive movements	Fast and reactive
ATHLETICISM	Neurological priming (phase 2), phase 6 of warm-up	Jump, cut, rotate, express full-body control	Coordinated and skilled
CONDITIONING	Conditioning finisher (end of session)	Elevate the heart rate, create endurance	Breathless and energized
MOBILITY	Warm-up and cool-down	Establish full range of motion, stretch, roll	Open and mobile

PHASE	STRENGTH	POWER	HYPERTROPHY	CONDITIONING	ATHLETICISM	MOBILITY
1. PRE-TRAINING PREPARATION		■*			■*	■
2. PRIMING & POTENTIATION		■*	■*			
3. KPI (MAIN LIFT)	■		■			
4. ACCESSORIES & PREHAB			■			
5. CONDITIONING FINISHER				■		
6. POST-TRAINING COOL DOWN						■

Each phase builds on the last. Every quality complements the others. The result is a fully integrated training experience that improves how you move, feel, and perform—inside and outside of the gym.

This is how you train all six physical characteristics of health and longevity—strategically, sustainably, and without compromise.

This is your prescription for pain-free performance.

NOTE: *Asterisked phases (■*) indicate indirect or preparatory emphasis, where the characteristic is primed or reinforced, but not the central focus.*

*** POWER:** *Targeted in phase 6 of the warm-up and in phase 2 when using neurological priming methods.*

*** HYPERTROPHY:** *Emphasized in phase 2 when using mechanical priming, and consistently in phases 3 and 4.*

*** ATHLETICISM:** *Trained through dynamic, coordinated movements in phase 6 of the warm-up.*

PHASE	SETS	REPS	REST	TOTAL TIME
PRE-TRAINING PREPARATION	Varies by phase	Varies by phase	Minimal, if any, between drills	~10–12 min
PRIMING – MECHANICAL	3–5	15–25+ (constant tension)	30–45 sec between sets	~5–7 min
PRIMING – NEUROLOGICAL	3–5	1–5 (explosive)	30–45 sec between sets	~5–6 min
KPI – RAMP-UP SETS	2–4	3–5 (controlled)	30–60 sec between sets	~5–8 min
KPI – WORKING SETS	1–2	3–8 (challenging)	90 sec to 2 min between sets	~5–8 min
PUMP ACCESSORIES	2–3	15–25 (mind-muscle connection)	30 sec to 1 min between sets	~3–5 min
PREHAB	1–2	10–15 reps or time-based holds (30–60 sec)	30 sec to 1 min between sets	~3–5 min
CONDITIONING FINISHER	1	Time-based: 20 sec to 10 min	Variable (task dependent)	~2–10 min
POST-TRAINING COOL-DOWN	3 phases: breathing, foam rolling, stretching	Time-based: 1–2 min per drill	Minimal	~3–8 min

MUSCLES TRAINED IN THE FOUNDATIONAL MOVEMENT PATTERNS

Training the six foundational movement patterns ensures you're working all the major muscle groups in the body—through different ranges, angles, and functional demands.

Each pattern not only emphasizes a primary group of muscles but also activates a broader network of stabilizers and supporting tissues.

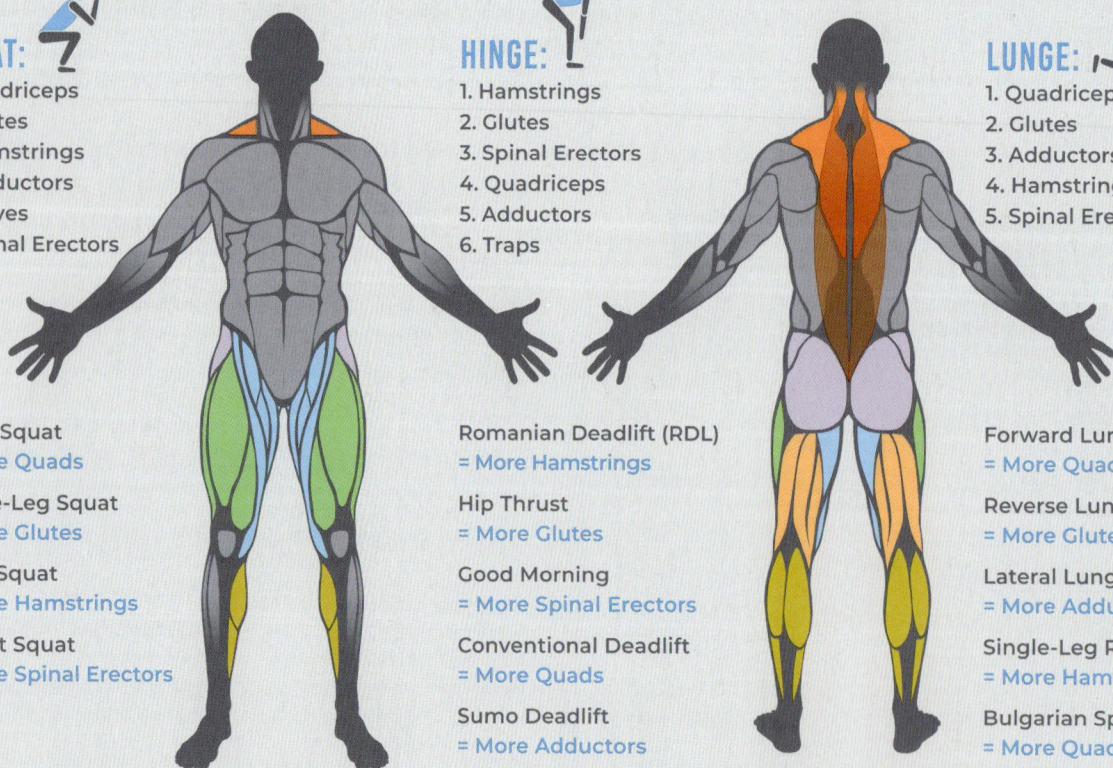

SQUAT:
1. Quadriceps
2. Glutes
3. Hamstrings
4. Adductors
5. Calves
6. Spinal Erectors

HINGE:
1. Hamstrings
2. Glutes
3. Spinal Erectors
4. Quadriceps
5. Adductors
6. Traps

LUNGE:
1. Quadriceps
2. Glutes
3. Adductors
4. Hamstrings
5. Spinal Erectors

Front Squat
= More Quads

Single-Leg Squat
= More Glutes

Back Squat
= More Hamstrings

Goblet Squat
= More Spinal Erectors

Romanian Deadlift (RDL)
= More Hamstrings

Hip Thrust
= More Glutes

Good Morning
= More Spinal Erectors

Conventional Deadlift
= More Quads

Sumo Deadlift
= More Adductors

Forward Lunge
= More Quads

Reverse Lunge
= More Glutes

Lateral Lunges
= More Adductors

Single-Leg RDL
= More Hamstrings

Bulgarian Split Squat
= More Quads

TRAIN ALL SIX FOUNDATIONAL MOVEMENT PATTERNS TWICE PER WEEK—
OPTIMIZING EXERCISE SELECTION AND RATIOS

Movement quality is the baseline, but consistent exposure is where lasting progress is made.

It's one thing to learn how to squat, hinge, lunge, push, pull, and carry with good form. It's another to train those patterns consistently, across variations, and in a way that supports your health, performance, and longevity. That's what this tenet is all about.

At the core of pain-free performance programming is a simple but powerful principle: Train every foundational movement pattern at least twice per week.

This multi-dimensional activation builds functional strength that compounds over time—especially when each pattern is trained at least twice per week. And with the right exercise variations, you can emphasize specific muscles even more, allowing you to target the areas that support your goals, movement quality, and muscular development.

Accessory and prehab work bridges the gap between function and focus. It helps fortify overlooked areas and allows you to develop muscle where it's both needed and desired, supporting pain-free performance and aesthetic goals.

PUSH:
1. Pecs
2. Anterior Delts
3. Triceps
4. Serratus Anterior
5. Traps

PULL:
1. Lats
2. Upper Back
3. Biceps
4. Rear Delts
5. Traps

UPPER BODY:
- ANTERIOR DELTOIDS
- REAR DELTOIDS
- BICEPS
- LATS
- PECTORALIS
- SPINAL ERECTORS
- SERRATUS ANTERIOR
- TRAPS
- TRICEPS
- UPPER BACK

Dumbbell Bench Press
= More Pecs

Barbell Bench Press
= More Delts

Close Grip
= More Triceps

Push-Ups
= More Serratus

Overhead
= More Traps

Pull-Ups
= More Lats

Rows
= More Upper Back

Chin-Ups
= More Biceps

Reverse Flys
= More Rear Delts

Shrugs
= More Traps

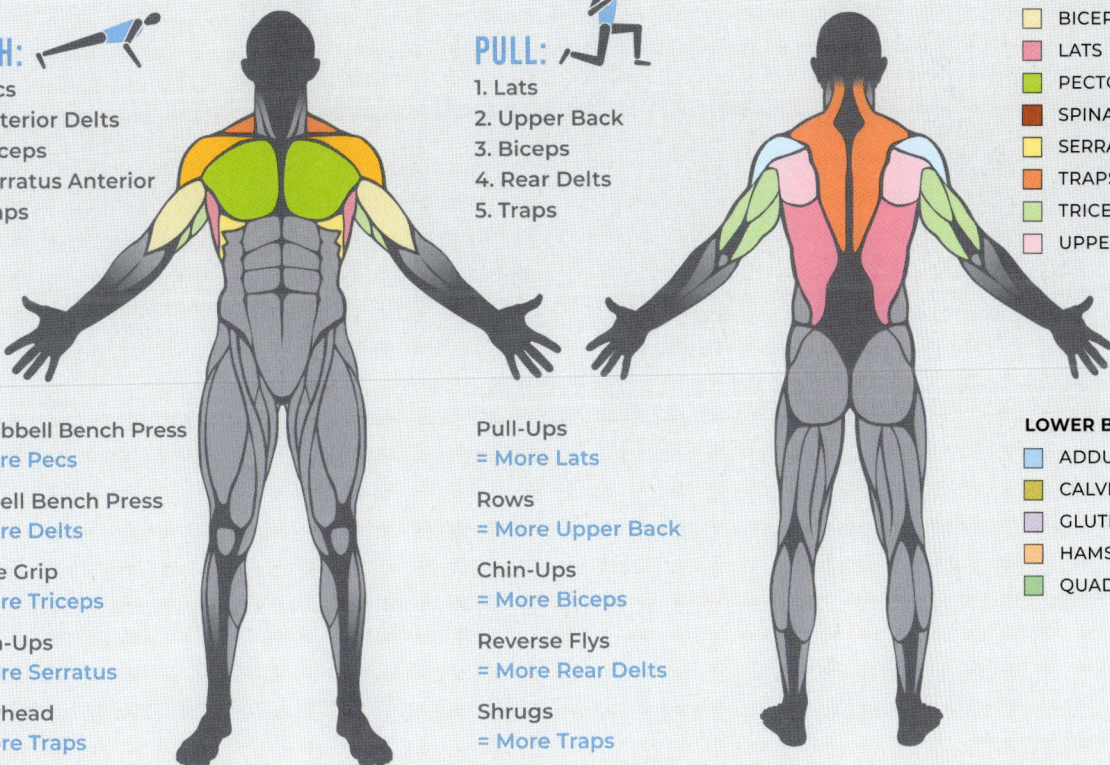

LOWER BODY:
- ADDUCTORS
- CALVES
- GLUTES
- HAMSTRINGS
- QUADRICEPS

This twice-per-week rule applies to each of the six movement patterns—squat, hinge, lunge, push, pull, and carry. These are the foundational shapes your body is designed to move through. They're not just tools for getting stronger or building muscle. They're the building blocks of function, physical autonomy, and injury-free living. And when trained regularly, they unlock both movement capacity and long-term adaptation.

But here's the challenge: just as it's difficult to program all six physical characteristics effectively, it's equally challenging to organize and train all six foundational movement patterns within a single training week. Most programs tend to overemphasize a few and neglect the rest, simply because it's easier to stick to familiar templates or repeat what's already known.

The real art—and the hard part—is combining these patterns in a way that reinforces balance, supports recovery, and avoids redundancy or overtraining. That's why we program the way we do. We've spent years refining these systems, testing them in the real world, and building templates that ensure you're not just doing the right exercises but doing them in the right combinations with the right frequency.

UNDERSTANDING THE REP RATIOS

Rep ratios refer to the intentional volume balance programmed between movement patterns to support posture, improve joint health, and reduce the likelihood of overuse or compensation. These aren't arbitrary numbers. They're built into the structure of pain-free performance to help correct common imbalances and restore movement quality—without your having to obsessively count every rep.

The following are the key rep ratios used in this system—and why they matter.

3:1 PULL-TO-PUSH RATIO (UPPER BODY)

This is one of the foundational principles of pain-free training. In a world dominated by forward posture and internal rotation, most people spend too much time pushing and not enough time pulling.

To restore balance, we recommend a 3:1 ratio of pulling to pushing. That might sound extreme, but it's automatically achieved through the warm-up, priming, KPI, and accessory work when the system is followed as designed.

More pulling improves scapular control and posture. It builds the shoulder stability that keeps you training pain-free and helps reverse the forward-dominant patterns of daily life.

2:1 HORIZONTAL-TO-VERTICAL PULLING

Within that pull-to-push ratio, we also program a 2:1 ratio of horizontal pulling to vertical pulling. Why?

Horizontal pulls—like rows—give you the ability to move with shoulder neutrality and create external rotation through scapular control. This is essential for restoring shoulder health, especially in individuals stuck in chronic internal rotation.

Vertical pulls, while excellent for strength development, rely heavily on the lats. And the lats, by nature, drive internal rotation at the shoulder—particularly during the concentric phase of the pull. When overemphasized, they can reinforce postural dysfunction instead of correcting it.

The 2:1 ratio builds a surplus of external rotation under load. That's what restores posture. And that's why we include horizontal rowing into nearly every phase of training.

To be clear, twice per week doesn't mean doing the same movement the same way twice. It means training two distinct variations within the same movement pattern across different days in your training week. For example, if you squat twice a week, you might do a goblet squat on one day and a back squat on the other day. Both are squat pattern variations, but each creates a different motor learning opportunity and training stimulus. This diversity promotes better mobility, stability, and skill acquisition without overloading a single joint or pattern.

That exposure—twice weekly—is the sweet spot for strength, hypertrophy, and motor learning. Once per week simply isn't enough. You won't get strong enough, fast enough. You won't remember what you did last week. And you certainly won't build a pattern well enough to own it. Two exposures minimum creates reinforcement without overload. Exposure means loaded training. It means KPIs, mechanical primers, and accessory work that challenges the pattern. It doesn't mean you stretched into it during a warm-up or mobilized it at the end of your session. Loaded movement is what makes the difference—and that's the standard we use when we talk about pattern exposure.

3:1 HINGE-TO-SQUAT RATIO

On the lower body side, we use a 3:1 ratio of hinging to squatting movements for total weekly volume.

This isn't because squats are bad—they're not. But your posterior chain is your powerhouse. It includes the largest and most force-producing muscles in the body—especially the glutes and hamstrings—which have the greatest potential for strength development, stability, and injury resistance.

Most people are also quad dominant, meaning they over-rely on the muscles in the front of the legs (the quadriceps) for both movement and stability. This is largely due to modern posture—hours spent sitting at desks, driving, or in semi-squat positions with hips flexed, knees bent, and the spine rounded forward. Over time, this posture creates imbalances that favor the anterior chain while leaving the posterior chain underdeveloped.

By prioritizing hinging movements, you reverse that bias. You restore balance between the front and back of the body, reinforce upright posture, and build the strength and motor control that supports performance, protects the spine, and unlocks long-term durability.

2:1 GLUTE/HAMSTRING ISOLATION TO COMPOUND HINGE

Because compound hinging (RDL or deadlifts) is so neurologically and structurally demanding, we balance that out with a 2:1 ratio of isolated glute and hamstring work to heavy hip hinge lifts.

Movements like hip thrusts, glute bridges, and hamstring curls allow us to build capacity in the posterior chain without adding stress to the spine. These are where we chase the pump—not the PR.

The logic is simple: isolate the key tissues (glutes and hamstrings) behind a strong hinge, increase training volume where it matters, and manage fatigue in the joints and nervous system.

NO CALCULATOR REQUIRED
You don't have to track these numbers manually—we've already done that for you in every program. These ratios are baked into the system, from your warm-ups to your primers and accessories.

Each program in this book is designed with that in mind.

Whether you're following a three-day full-body program or a more advanced five-day pattern-focused template, you'll hit all six patterns at least twice per week. For example:

▶ **3-day full body** trains four to six patterns per session. You'll cycle through all six patterns across each training day, giving you diversity and consistency throughout the week.

▶ A **4-day upper/lower split** allows for focused work on three patterns per day—like squatting, hinging, and lunging on a lower body day and pushing, pulling, and carrying on an upper body day—again, twice per week.

▶ A **5-day movement pattern split** prioritizes one key pattern per session as your KPI while strategically incorporating other patterns as accessory movements. This ensures each pattern is trained at least twice throughout the week.

The carry deserves special attention here. Unlike the other five movement patterns, the carry is never trained as a KPI. Instead, it plays a highly versatile and supportive role throughout the week. Carry exercises are most often integrated on upper body days—paired with pulling or pressing patterns due to their grip-intensive, shoulder-stabilizing nature. But because of their global, full-body impact, they also show up on lower body days, in finishers, or on off days when the focus shifts to cardio.

You can program the carry pattern in three primary ways:

1. **As a finisher** in high-output sessions (three- to five-day splits), where it spikes heart rate, challenges postural control, and trains full-body tension

2. **On low-intensity or off days**, often as part of walking-based or interval-style conditioning to reinforce locomotion and movement efficiency

3. **Within accessory blocks**, especially on upper body days, where it complements pulling patterns and improves grip, posture, and pillar stability

Because the carry is so adaptable, it doesn't require a standalone training day. Instead, it's woven into multiple areas of the week, allowing it to be trained at least twice, and often more. This flexible integration ensures it still meets the same frequency threshold as the other foundational patterns while complementing overall performance.

Training all six movement patterns twice per week isn't just a checklist item; it's your foundation. It's what makes the system work. It ensures that you're addressing the full spectrum of movement your body needs without overloading any one area or undertraining another.

Strength, mobility, hypertrophy, power, athleticism, and conditioning are all enhanced when you move through foundational patterns regularly.

This tenet ensures you do just that.

Train every pattern twice a week. That's your baseline.

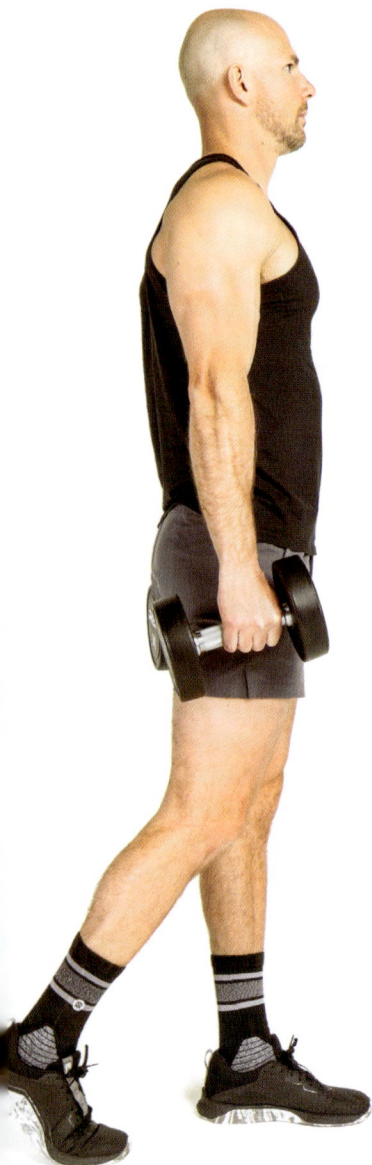

CHOOSE THE RIGHT TRAINING FREQUENCY—
BASED ON YOUR SCHEDULE, PREFERENCES, AND GOALS

The best training program is the one you can actually stick to.

When it comes to designing a program that delivers results, most people obsess over exercises and complicated periodization schemes. But one of the most important decisions you'll make—the one that determines whether your program fits your life or becomes another thing you abandon—is training frequency.

How many days per week should you train?

The answer isn't about what's ideal on paper. It's about what you can commit to consistently, week after week, without fail. That's your starting point. It's not what sounds good, what looks good, or what the textbooks or social media influencers say you should do. It's what you'll actually do.

Here's the question I ask every client: What's the number of days you can train with 100 percent consistency—even when life gets messy? If that number is three, then you train three days a week. Not because it's the most effective but because your schedule is the number one determining factor in choosing your training frequency. Not your goals. Not your preferences. Your real-life availability—and your ability to follow through.

That said, goals and preferences still matter. But they have to align with your schedule, not override it. If you prefer an upper-lower split but only have three days per week to train, that split might not be the best. If your goal is to gain muscle but you can only commit to two sessions per week, you'll need to work smart and squeeze every ounce of value out of those sessions. But let's be clear—when you're in pain, you're deconditioned, or your movement quality needs rebuilding, the only goal that matters is getting healthy. You can't build muscle, lose fat, or get stronger if you're constantly hurt or unable to move well.

That's why we don't begin with goals. We begin with reality—and work from there.

Once you've established your weekly commitment, that frequency informs the structure of your program. Each training (lifting) day has its own benefits, limitations, and design strategies. Here's how to think about them inside the pain-free performance system:

1X/WEEK

This is better than nothing, but it's not enough to create meaningful change. At most, it's an entry point—a foot in the door to consistent training. You can't build strength, muscle, power, or movement skill on one exposure per week. What you can do is create an opportunity to build buy-in and lay the groundwork for adding a second day.

2X/WEEK

This is the bare minimum to create just enough volume, movement diversity, and loading to begin stimulating progress. But you'll be walking a tightrope. It's not ideal, but it's doable—especially for beginners or those returning from injury.

3X/WEEK

This is where the magic happens. Three full-body sessions per week allow you to hit all six foundational movement patterns at least twice and start layering in meaningful work across all six physical characteristics. If you want to feel better, move better, and start building pain-free performance, this is your entry point.

4X/WEEK

At four days per week, we move into an upper/lower split. This unlocks a little more concentrated volume per session, improves recoverability, and allows for more focused work on each region and pattern. It's often the sweet spot for intermediate to advanced lifters. It also gives you room to walk, recover, and plug in mobility work on non-lifting days. If you have the time and capacity, this is one of the most sustainable and effective schedules for lifelong performance.

5X/WEEK

At five days per week, your training becomes even more specialized. You'll follow a movement pattern split—squat day, hinge day, lunge day, push day, and pull day—with each day emphasizing a distinct pattern. This increases your total volume and can allow for more hypertrophy-focused or strength-driven training. However, it does require greater attention to recovery. If your movement isn't dialed in or your life outside the gym is chaotic, this frequency can become counterproductive. But when done well, it's incredibly effective.

6–7X/WEEK

Yes, training six or seven days per week is possible, but it demands a smarter strategy, not just more work. If you're lifting five days per week, the sixth or seventh day isn't about squeezing in more volume—it's about creating balance. This is where recovery, conditioning, and movement restoration should take the lead. You can still "train" on those days, but the goal shifts. Use them for walking, low-intensity aerobic work (light carry or locomotion circuits), or following a linchpin blueprint. Refer to the **Performance Recovery System** protocol in Part 2 (page 81) to learn more about how to structure an off-day recovery workout without frying your nervous system.

In other words, the more days you're in the gym, the more intentional you need to be with programming and the types of stress you're applying. Back-to-back-to-back lifting days with no regard for movement quality, intensity, or variation will eventually catch up with you. Smart six- or seven-day training blends performance with recovery. The goal is to check every box—without checking out your nervous system.

Again, the best frequency is the one you can repeat week after week. Whether that's three, four, or five days, you need to build your program around your life—not the other way around.

Of course, even after saying that, people still ask me: "Okay, but what's the best number of days to train?"

The answer still depends.

If your schedule is wide open and your recovery is solid, **four days per week** tends to hit the sweet spot. It offers enough volume and frequency to make meaningful progress without tipping into burnout or compromising recovery. It's also the frequency I personally follow and recommend most often because it balances training with everything else that life demands—mobility work, walking, family, stress management, and all the things that make consistency possible.

And remember: More isn't always better.

Training more often does let you spread out volume and target specific patterns with more precision. But it also requires more discipline with recovery and more awareness of how you're layering stress. A three-day full-body program hits your system hard each session. A five-day pattern split spreads the load but demands more time and consistency to stay effective.

The structure of the programs in this book reflects all of that. Whether you're training three, four, or five days per week, the plans are optimized for your commitment level, movement quality, and capacity to recover. Each template aligns with the system's core tenets—training all six foundational patterns and all six physical characteristics—and does so in a way that supports your schedule.

Only after you've committed to your schedule should you consider your preferences and goals. Prefer full-body training? Start with three days. Want more focus per movement or muscle group? Go with four or five. Want to build muscle, increase strength, or improve conditioning? You'll find options for all of those in this section. You don't need to specialize to make progress. You just need to train with intent and let the structure do the work. When that happens, everything else becomes easier.

Commit to what you can do consistently. Then train smart with the time you've got.

PROGRESS LOAD, EFFORT, AND VOLUME INTELLIGENTLY—
HOW TO MAKE CONTINUAL GAINS WITHOUT THE PAIN

Consistency gets you in the door. Intelligent progression keeps you in the game.

It's easy to chase novelty in your training—new exercises, new routines, new shiny things that promise better results. But there's a problem: The more often you change your training, the harder it becomes to actually get better at anything. Progress doesn't come from doing more. It comes from doing the right things consistently, with just enough challenge to keep moving forward.

That's why every program in the pain-free performance system is built on a block-periodized model. This approach keeps things simple, strategic, and sustainable. You're not reinventing your workouts every week—you're following a four-week progression that allows your body to learn, adapt, and grow stronger with every session.

Each block is made up of four training weeks:

- ► **Week 1 is about exposure.** You're getting a feel for the exercises, the flow of the session, and the loading scheme. The goal isn't to crush yourself. It's to learn and dial in your technique: get your timing down, adjust to new movement patterns, and start exploring what you are capable of. This week functions as a built-in deload, meaning the intensity and overall training stress are intentionally lower to give your body a chance to adapt. In a new cycle, that means easing into unfamiliar movement patterns. In a repeated cycle, it gives you a chance to recover from the peak effort of Week 4 before ramping back up.

- ► **Weeks 2 and 3 are where you build.** These are your progression plays. You start adding load and pushing effort. The exercises are familiar now, which means you can focus less on figuring them out and more on executing them well.

- ► **Week 4 is your performance peak.** It's your chance to push the envelope. You go into each session knowing it's the final week of the block. This is where you go for pain-free PRs (personal records). You lift heavier and chase top-end effort—with excellent form, of course. You've earned the right to push because you've built up to it over the last three weeks.

Then the cycle resets—either by repeating or by starting a new training block with new variations and focus.

This wavelike structure is how you build progressive overload without trashing your joints or redlining your nervous system. It respects the body's need for rhythm. It acknowledges that you won't feel your best every day. And it gives you a framework to progress without relying on ego or intensity alone.

And here's the thing most people miss: Progression isn't just about adding load. It's about improving how you move. It's about how you recover. It's about showing up consistently over time.

No matter the rep range, the goal is the same: Train hard enough to stimulate change but not so hard that you can't come back and train again. We call this training to a technical limit—choosing loads that challenge you but still allow for great form and high-quality reps. Think: the hardest thing you can do well.

That's your sweet spot.

From a volume standpoint, all the programs in this book fall within moderate volume. That's on purpose. You don't need to train like a professional athlete or bodybuilder to see results. You just need the minimum effective dose to ensure consistent, compounding progress.

8-12 TOTAL WORKING SETS PER SESSION
is on the lower end (great for beginners or time-crunched lifters)

12-18 TOTAL WORKING SETS PER SESSION
is the moderate range (ideal for most people)

18-22 TOTAL WORKING SETS PER SESSION
is high volume (used occasionally, with caution and experience)

We don't need to reinvent the science here. The research has been clear for decades: These set and volume ranges work. That's why the programs in this book include predetermined sets and reps—but that's just the starting point. You still need to listen to your body. What felt great this week might feel heavy next week. If you're moving well, feeling good, and performing at a high level, you're on the right track. If not, it's time to adjust.

Progression is a long game. The biggest breakthroughs don't happen in four weeks. They happen over months and years of smart, consistent work. And that only happens when you stop chasing random intensity and start training with a purpose.

So yes, you'll repeat workouts. You'll lift similar weights. You'll do the same warm-up for weeks at a time. That's not lazy. That's strategic exposure. It's how you build the neurological skill of strength, the tissue quality of hypertrophy, the movement competency of athleticism, and the joint control of mobility—all without blowing yourself up in the process.

Progressing load, effort, and volume is what turns a workout plan into a long-term training prescription.

That's how you make gains without the pain.

TRAIN WITH PURPOSE, PRECISION, AND PERSONALIZATION—
THE MOVEMENT MASTERY MINDSET IN ACTION

PURPOSE means every set, rep, and exercise you perform has a reason.

PRECISION means doing things right.

PERSONALIZATION means acknowledging your individuality and owning your experience.

Programming is only as effective as the quality of its execution.

You can have the perfect split, the ideal rep scheme, and a textbook progression plan, but if the movements don't fit your body, your skill level, and your current capacity, it won't work. Not for long, anyway.

That's why this system isn't about blindly following a plan. It's about following a framework with the freedom to make it your own. The pain-free performance approach is rooted in movement mastery—an ongoing process of learning how to move well. And that only works when you train with purpose, precision, and personalization.

Purpose means every set, rep, and exercise you perform has a reason. You're not just doing it because it's on the page—you're doing it because it serves a function. You're working on something that moves the needle, whether it's building capacity in a key pattern, reinforcing a position that breaks down under fatigue, or strengthening a weak link that's held you back for years.

Precision means doing things right. Not perfectly, but intentionally. It's not about lifting the most weight possible. It's about lifting the most weight you can with control, consistently. It's about knowing the difference between effort and recklessness, and choosing the former every time. This mindset is what keeps your progress sustainable. It's what allows you to build intensity without sacrificing movement quality—and it's what keeps you in the game for the long haul.

Personalization means acknowledging your individuality and owning your experience. Your body is unique. Your injury history, movement limitations, and training background all shape how you respond to a program. And that's exactly why this system is built to adapt around you—not the other way around.

It's why we use movement pyramids to help you select the right variation for each pattern. It's why KPIs are relative to your skill and strength, not someone else's. It's why we offer mechanical and neurological primers based on how your body feels, and why linchpin mobility drills show up in your warm-ups and recovery work. Every piece of this program is built to support movement mastery.

And while this mindset has been woven through every tenet so far, this is where it becomes explicit: Programming is about awareness. It's about showing up, paying attention, and making decisions that reflect how your body feels today, not just what a spreadsheet says.

That's the difference between doing a workout and training.

Training with purpose is knowing why you're doing what you're doing. Training with precision is knowing how to do it well. And training with personalization ensures it's all built around you—your pain points, your linchpins, your schedule, your preferences, and your goals.

That's what the movement mastery mindset looks like in action. It's a commitment. And when you pair it with everything else—structured programming, progressive overload, smart frequency, and full-pattern training—it unlocks the results you've been chasing all along.

This is what it means to train smart. And more importantly, this is what it means to train for life.

COACHES' CORNER

COACHING THE PAIN-FREE PERFORMANCE SYSTEM

If you're a coach, trainer, or rehab professional, this isn't just a system you follow—it's a system you deliver.

The movement mastery mindset doesn't end with you. It's something you model, teach, and reinforce with every client interaction. Because your clients don't just need workouts—they need structure, clarity, and a sustainable strategy that feels safe, effective, and personalized. They need a plan that builds trust in their body again. And you're the one who can make that happen.

Pain-free performance programming gives you the framework to do exactly that, whether you're coaching in person, remotely, or in a group setting. Every element of the system is designed to be coachable, scalable, and adaptable to real-life clients with real-life challenges.

If you're working with clients remotely, this framework helps you create structure without the guesswork. KPI-based programming provides a clear foundation for tracking progress across blocks. Warm-up templates, linchpin blueprints, and recovery strategies give your clients repeatable tools that they can confidently apply on their own. And the programming tenets create consistency across distance, helping your clients build competency even when you're not in the room with them.

If you coach in a group setting, the system still works—because the principles stay the same even when the delivery changes. You can use movement pyramids to scale exercises in real time. You can assign KPI variations based on each client's ability. And you can run warm-ups, priming, and cool-downs in a way that ensures every person is getting what they need, even if the format is shared. Group doesn't mean generic. This system keeps it personalized, even in a group environment.

Whether you work with special populations, athletes, or everyday clients, this framework meets them where they are. The programming scales up or down depending on age, ability, injury history, and training goals. Whether someone is rehabbing a shoulder, rebuilding from back pain, or chasing performance goals in their sport, the structure doesn't change—the execution does. You're not reinventing your programming every time a new client walks in. You're adapting a proven system to fit their needs.

PREPARATION AND RECOVERY PROGRAMS

Pain-free training doesn't start with your first lift—and it doesn't end with your last rep. The way you prepare and recover shapes everything that happens in between.

This section includes a complete library of 6-phase dynamic warm-ups, linchpin blueprints, and cool-downs. Use them to get ready before a session. To reset your system after training. To reduce pain and improve how your body moves and functions day to day.

Aim to complete at least one of these sequences—whether it's a warm-up, linchpin blueprint, or cool-down—each day as part of your commitment to movement mastery. Think of it as a non-negotiable practice that maintains how you move, how you feel, and how well you train.

6-PHASE DYNAMIC WARM-UPS

The warm-ups in this section are structured as templates, designed to get you moving quickly and effectively. Each follows the six-phase structure and is aligned with one of the foundational movement patterns: squat, hinge, lunge, push, or pull.

These templates are meant to be used in conjunction with your training program. On any given training day, you'll select the warm-up that matches your key performance indicator (KPI)—your hardest, heaviest lift in the session. For example, if you're squatting, use a squat warm-up. If your KPI is a horizontal push like a bench press, choose the corresponding push template.

If you'd like to customize your warm-up by adding more than one exercise per phase, or if you want a deeper understanding of how to tailor it to your body, refer to Part 2. That's where you'll find detailed explanations of each warm-up phase, complete with exercise breakdowns, setup cues, and progression strategies.

Scan the QR codes throughout this section to access follow-along video playlists with demos of each exercise.

HOW TO READ SUPERSETS AND EXERCISE GROUPINGS IN THE WARM-UP CHARTS

You'll notice that some warm-up phases include more than one exercise. Here's how to follow them correctly:

- **If there are two movements labeled A and B, this is a superset.** Perform Exercise A, immediately perform Exercise B, and then repeat. Continue alternating until you've completed all sets and reps for both exercises.

- **If multiple exercises are listed without A/B labels, they are not meant to be supersetted.** Perform each drill individually in any order, following the time or set and rep guidelines provided.

This structure allows for more complete preparation—especially in full-body warm-ups and linchpin blueprints—without extending the session unnecessarily.

IMPORTANT: Complete each phase once. You do not need to repeat the entire warm-up multiple times. One pass through all six phases—completing each exercise or superset in each phase—is all it takes to prime your mind and body for better movement or recovery.

SQUAT

EQUIPMENT: Foam roller, light or medium long resistance band, light dumbbell or kettlebell

PHASE	EXERCISE	SETS/REPS/DURATION
1: SOFT TISSUE TECHNIQUES	Quadriceps (foam roller)	1m each side (30s oscillation / 30s neurological trigger point)
2: BIPHASIC POSITIONAL STRETCHING	Half-Kneeling Hip Flexor Stretch	1m each side (30s oscillation / 30s end-range hold)
3: CORRECTIVE EXERCISE	Bird Dog	30s alternating between sides
4: ACTIVATION DRILLS	Banded Glute Bridge (light or medium long resistance band)	2–3 sets of 8–10 reps
5: MOVEMENT PATTERN DEVELOPMENT	Goblet Squat (light dumbbell or kettlebell)	3 sets of 5 reps
6: CNS STIMULATION	A: Vertical Jacks B: Vertical Jump	A: 3 sets of 5 reps B: 3 sets of 1 rep Superset: Alternating between A & B

HINGE

EQUIPMENT: Foam roller, light dumbbell or kettlebell (optional)

PHASE	EXERCISE	SETS/REPS/DURATION
1: SOFT TISSUE TECHNIQUES	Adductors (foam roller)	1m each side (30s oscillation/ 30s neurological trigger point)
2: BIPHASIC POSITIONAL STRETCHING	Adductor Rock-Back	1m each side (30s oscillation / 30s end-range hold)
3: CORRECTIVE EXERCISE	Plank	1m hold
4: ACTIVATION DRILLS	Side Plank Hip Thrust (select progression from page 166)	2–3 sets of 8–10 reps
5: MOVEMENT PATTERN DEVELOPMENT	Single-Leg Romanian Deadlift (RDL) (dumbbell or kettlebell)	3 sets of 5 reps
6: CNS STIMULATION	A: Seal Jacks B: Broad Jump	A: 3 sets of 5 reps B: 3 sets of 1 rep Superset: Alternating between A & B

LUNGE

EQUIPMENT: Foam roller, med ball

PHASE	EXERCISE	SETS/REPS/DURATION
1: SOFT TISSUE TECHNIQUES	Lateral Hip/Tensor Fasciae Latae (TFL) (foam roller)	1m each side (30s oscillation / 30s neurological trigger point)
2: BIPHASIC POSITIONAL STRETCHING	Dynamic Pigeon Stretch	1m each side (30s oscillation / 30s end-range hold)
3: CORRECTIVE EXERCISE	Dead Bug (select progression from pages 143–145)	1m
4: ACTIVATION DRILLS	Single-Leg Glute Bridge	2–3 sets of 8–10 reps
5: MOVEMENT PATTERN DEVELOPMENT	Reverse Lunge	3 sets of 5 reps
6: CNS STIMULATION	A: Med Ball Slam B: Skip	A: 3 sets of 3 reps B: 3 sets of 10 reps Superset: Alternating between A & B

PUSH/PULL (HORIZONTAL)

EQUIPMENT: Foam roller, long resistance band, suspension trainer, med ball

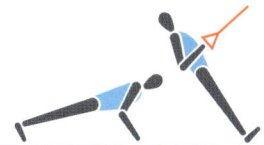

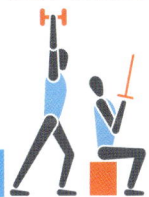

PHASE	EXERCISE	SETS/REPS/DURATION
1: SOFT TISSUE TECHNIQUES	Pectoralis Group (foam roller)	1m each side (30s oscillation / 30s neurological trigger point)
2: BIPHASIC POSITIONAL STRETCHING	90/90 Chest Stretch	1m each side (30s oscillation / 30s end-range hold)
3: CORRECTIVE EXERCISE	Quadruped T-Spine Rotation	30s each side
4: ACTIVATION DRILLS	Rusin Banded Shoulder Warm-Up (long resistance band)	2–3 sets of 10 reps for each exercise
5: MOVEMENT PATTERN DEVELOPMENT	Push-Up (push) / Inverted Row (pull) (suspension trainer)	3 sets of 5 reps
6: CNS STIMULATION	A: Seal Jacks B: Bent-Over Med Ball Press	A: 3 sets of 5 reps B: 3 sets of 3 reps Superset: Alternating between A & B

PUSH/PULL (VERTICAL)

EQUIPMENT: Foam roller, long resistance band, suspension trainer, med ball

PHASE	EXERCISE	SETS/REPS/DURATION
1: SOFT TISSUE TECHNIQUES	Thoracic Spine (foam roller)	1m (30s oscillation / 30s neurological trigger point)
2: BIPHASIC POSITIONAL STRETCHING	Hinged T-Spine Extension / Bilateral Lat Stretch (suspension trainer)	1m (30s oscillation / 30s end-range hold)
3: CORRECTIVE EXERCISE	Bird Dog	30s alternating between sides
4: ACTIVATION DRILLS	Banded Lat Pulldown (long resistance band)	2–3 sets of 8–10 reps
5: MOVEMENT PATTERN DEVELOPMENT	Single-Arm Band Press (push) / Half-Kneeling Single-Arm Band Lat Pulldown (pull) (long resistance band)	3 sets of 5 reps each side
6: CNS STIMULATION	A: Vertical Jacks B: Med Ball Slam	A: 3 sets of 5 reps B: 3 sets of 3 reps Superset: Alternating between A & B

FULL BODY A (SQUAT & PULL)

EQUIPMENT: Foam roller, long resistance band, suspension trainer, light dumbbell or kettlebell, med ball

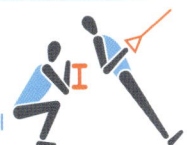

PHASE	EXERCISE	SETS/REPS/DURATION
1: SOFT TISSUE TECHNIQUES	Quadriceps & Thoracic Spine (foam roller)	1m each exercise/side (30s oscillation / 30s neurological trigger point)
2: BIPHASIC POSITIONAL STRETCHING	Half-Kneeling Hip Flexor & Hinged T-Spine / Bilateral Lat Stretch (suspension trainer)	1m each exercise/side (30s oscillation / 30s end-range hold)
3: CORRECTIVE EXERCISE	Bird Dog	30s alternating between sides
4: ACTIVATION DRILLS	A: Banded Glute Bridge B: Band Pull-Apart (long resistance band)	A: 2–3 sets of 8–10 reps B: 2–3 sets of 8–10 reps Superset: Alternating between A & B
5: MOVEMENT PATTERN DEVELOPMENT	A: Goblet Squat (dumbbell) B: Inverted Row (suspension trainer)	A: 3 sets of 5 reps B: 3 sets of 5 reps Superset: Alternating between A & B
6: CNS STIMULATION	A: Med Ball Slam B: Vertical Jump	A: 3 sets of 3 reps B: 3 sets of 1 rep Superset: Alternating between A & B

FULL BODY B (HINGE & PUSH)

EQUIPMENT: Foam roller, long resistance band, light dumbbell or kettlebell, med ball

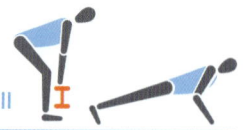

PHASE	EXERCISE	SETS/REPS/DURATION
1: SOFT TISSUE TECHNIQUES	Adductors & Thoracic Spine (foam roller)	1m each exercise/side (30s oscillation / 30s neurological trigger point)
2: BIPHASIC POSITIONAL STRETCHING	Adductor Rock-Back & 90/90 Chest Stretch	1m each exercise/side (30s oscillation / 30s end-range hold)
3: CORRECTIVE EXERCISE	Quadruped Adductor T-Spine Rotation	30s each side
4: ACTIVATION DRILLS	A: Banded Glute Bridge B: Banded Lat Pulldown (long resistance band)	A: 2–3 sets of 8–10 reps B: 2–3 sets of 8–10 reps Superset: Alternating between A & B
5: MOVEMENT PATTERN DEVELOPMENT	A: Romanian Deadlift (RDL) (dumbbell or kettlebell) B: Push-Up	A: 3 sets of 5 reps B: 3 sets of 5 reps Superset: Alternating between A & B
6: CNS STIMULATION	A: Seal Jacks B: Med Ball Rotational Chest Pass	A: 3 sets of 5 reps B: 3 sets of 3 reps Superset: Alternating between A & B

FULL BODY C (LUNGE & PULL)

EQUIPMENT: Foam roller, long resistance band, med ball

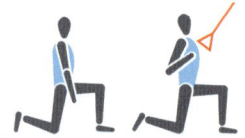

PHASE	EXERCISE	SETS/REPS/DURATION
1: SOFT TISSUE TECHNIQUES	Lateral Hip/TFL & Lats (foam roller)	1m each exercise/side (30s oscillation / 30s neurological trigger point)
2: BIPHASIC POSITIONAL STRETCHING	Dynamic Pigeon Stretch & Posterior Shoulder Stretch	1m each exercise/side (30s oscillation / 30s end-range hold)
3: CORRECTIVE EXERCISE	Plank	1m hold
4: ACTIVATION DRILLS	A: Side Plank Hip Thrust B: Band Face Pull (long resistance band)	A: 2–3 sets of 8–10 reps B: 2–3 sets of 8–10 reps Superset: Alternating between A & B
5: MOVEMENT PATTERN DEVELOPMENT	A: Reverse Lunge B: Half-Kneeling Band High-Angle Pull (long resistance band)	A: 3 sets of 5 reps B: 3 sets of 5 reps Superset: Alternating between A & B
6: CNS STIMULATION	A: Med Ball Slam B: Skip	A: 3 sets of 3 reps B: 3 sets 10 reps Superset: Alternating between A & B

LINCHPIN BLUEPRINTS

The linchpin blueprints are not your standard warm-up. They're part of the **Performance Recovery System** (page 81), which shares the same six-phase structure as the dynamic warm-ups, but with a different goal.

While the general warm-ups are best used before training to prepare your body for performance, these blueprints are geared toward movement restoration and recovery. The structure stays the same—six deliberate phases—but the emphasis shifts. You'll spend more time in soft tissue and stretching work, address multiple regions in the early phases, and use the later phases for controlled deceleration, rotation, and movement exploration. This isn't about pushing load or intensity; it's about giving your nervous system the input it needs to move and feel better.

Use these blueprints on your off days alongside cardio activities like walking or cycling, or as a secondary recovery session in the evening after a high-output morning session. They're ideal when your body feels tight, stuck, or slightly flared up and you need a systematized way to **address common pain points and mobility limitations**. They're also a valuable tool when your movement simply feels "off." You're not injured, but you're not moving well either. That's when a linchpin blueprint can act as a low-stress reset.

Unlike the training-day warm-ups, these are not built around the KPI. They're built around you. They target the compensations (weak links) that you discovered through the movement screens. Think of them as ongoing body maintenance. Not corrective in the clinical sense, but proactive. These are the patterns that break down first—and if you don't address them, they're often the ones that keep coming back.

While these blueprints can be extremely effective for navigating low-level pain or movement issues, they are not intended to replace medical advice. If you're dealing with acute pain, sudden swelling, sharp discomfort, or anything that signals a true injury, it's time to consult a licensed healthcare provider. The blueprints are meant to support long-term restoration and mobility restrictions—not provide emergency pain relief.

That said, most people are dealing not with an acute injury but rather minor pain flare-ups. It's disuse. It's decades of poor posture and skipped warm-ups culminating in a body that feels stiff, fragile, or one wrong move away from another setback. These blueprints help you fill in the gaps—with movement that re-engages the areas you've neglected and retrains your system to function the way it was built to function.

Use them regularly. Cycle them based on what your body needs. If you're feeling especially cooked and need a more relaxed, mobility-driven recovery session, you can either replace phases 5 and 6 with mobility-focused stretches and flows or skip the linchpin blueprint altogether and implement one of the cool-down templates (covered in the next section) in its place.

ANKLE MOBILITY

EQUIPMENT: Foam roller, wedge

GOOD FOR:
- Improving ankle mobility (range of motion)
- Increasing squat depth
- Alleviating knee or hip discomfort, especially if you have asymmetrical ankle mobility (one side is more restricted than the other)

PHASE	EXERCISE	SETS/REPS/DURATION
1: SOFT TISSUE TECHNIQUES	Calves, Soleus, Tibialis (foam roller)	1m each exercise/side
2: BIPHASIC POSITIONAL STRETCHING	Calf Stretch (wedge) & Half-Kneeling Soleus Stretch	1m each exercise/side
3: CORRECTIVE EXERCISE	Full Range of Motion Calf Raise (wedge)	1–2 sets of 10–15 reps
4: ACTIVATION DRILLS	Standing Tib Raise (wedge)	1–2 sets of 10–15 reps
5: MOVEMENT PATTERN DEVELOPMENT	A: Reverse Lunge (front foot on wedge) B: Heels-Elevated Bodyweight Squat	A: 3 sets of 5 reps per side B: 3 sets of 5 reps Superset: Alternating between A & B
6: CNS STIMULATION	Pogo Hops (optional: on wedge)	3 sets of 10 hops

ANKLE STABILITY

EQUIPMENT: Foam roller, massage ball, wedge

GOOD FOR:
- Ankle inversion sprain
- Unstable ankle or knee position
- Ankle or knee collapses inward or outward

PHASE	EXERCISE	SETS/REPS/DURATION
1: SOFT TISSUE TECHNIQUES	Calves (foam roller), Feet (massage ball)	1m each exercise/side
2: BIPHASIC POSITIONAL STRETCHING	Calf Stretch (wedge) & Three-Way Knee-Over-Toes Mobility	1m each exercise/side
3: CORRECTIVE EXERCISE	3D Balance Reach	1–2 sets of 10–15 reps
4: ACTIVATION DRILLS	Standing Tib Raise & Calf Raise (with ball between heels)	1–2 sets of 10–15 reps
5: MOVEMENT PATTERN DEVELOPMENT	A: Reverse Lunge (front foot on wedge) B: Heels-Elevated Bodyweight Squat	A: 3 sets of 5 reps per side B: 3 sets of 5 reps Superset: Alternating between A & B
6: CNS STIMULATION	Pogo Hops (optional: on wedge)	3 sets of 10 hops

HIP MOBILITY A

EQUIPMENT: Foam roller, long resistance band, short resistance band, light dumbbell

GOOD FOR:
- Unlocking tight hip flexors
- Improving hip extension range
- Reducing low back discomfort
- Enhancing glute activation in lower body training

PHASE	EXERCISE	SETS/REPS/DURATION
1: SOFT TISSUE TECHNIQUES	Hip Flexor, Quadriceps, TFL (foam roller)	1m each exercise/side
2: BIPHASIC POSITIONAL STRETCHING	Half-Kneeling Hip Flexor Stretch with Overhead Reach & Supine 90/90 Shin Box Positional Hold	1m each exercise/side
3: CORRECTIVE EXERCISE	Dead Bug Leg Extension & Quadruped Leg Extension	1m each exercise / alternating between sides
4: ACTIVATION DRILLS	A: Banded Glute Bridge (long resistance band) B: Side-Lying Banded Clam (short resistance band)	A: 1–2 sets of 10–15 reps B: 1–2 sets of 10–15 reps each side Superset: Alternating between A & B
5: MOVEMENT PATTERN DEVELOPMENT	A: Reverse Lunge with Reach B: Hip Banded Hinge (long resistance band)	A: 3 sets of 5 reps each side B: 3 sets of 5 reps Superset: Alternating between A & B
6: CNS STIMULATION	A: Triple Extension to Snap-Down B: Goblet March	A: 3 sets of 1 rep B: 3 sets 10–15s march Superset: Alternating between A & B

HIP MOBILITY B

EQUIPMENT: Foam roller, long resistance band, short resistance band

GOOD FOR:
- Releasing tight adductors
- Improving lateral hip mobility, especially for deep sumo or hybrid stances
- Gaining smoother, more controlled range in lateral lunges
- Managing lingering groin discomfort or returning to movement after a past groin strain

PHASE	EXERCISE	SETS/REPS/DURATION
1: SOFT TISSUE TECHNIQUES	Adductor, Hamstrings, Glutes (foam roller)	1m each exercise/side
2: BIPHASIC POSITIONAL STRETCHING	Adductor Rock-Back & Dynamic Pigeon Stretch	1m each exercise/side
3: CORRECTIVE EXERCISE	Copenhagen Side Plank Hip Drop & Dead Bug Leg Extension	30s each side & 1m alternating
4: ACTIVATION DRILLS	A: Banded Glute Bridge (long resistance band) B: Quadruped Banded Fire Hydrant (short resistance band)	A: 2–3 sets of 8–10 reps B: 2–3 sets of 8–10 reps each side Superset: Alternating between A & B
5: MOVEMENT PATTERN DEVELOPMENT	A: Alternating Lateral Lunge with Rotation Reach B: Wide-Stance (Zercher) Banded Good Morning (long resistance band)	A: 3 sets of 5 reps each side B: 3 sets of 5 reps Superset: Alternating between A & B
6: CNS STIMULATION	A: Banded Lateral Monster Walk (short resistance band) B: ¼ Speed Skaters	A: 3 sets of 15 steps each direction B: 3 sets of 10–20 alternating skaters Superset: Alternating between A & B

HIP MOBILITY C

EQUIPMENT: Foam roller, short resistance band, suspension trainer

GOOD FOR:
- Releasing tight hip rotators
- Improving knee tracking during squats, lunges, running, or stair climbing
- Reducing lateral knee discomfort
- Boosting glute engagement

PHASE	EXERCISE	SETS/REPS/DURATION
1: SOFT TISSUE TECHNIQUES	Quadriceps, TFL, Glutes (foam roller)	1m each exercise/side
2: BIPHASIC POSITIONAL STRETCHING	Half-Kneeling Hip Flexor Stretch with Overhead Reach & Supine 90/90 Shin Box Positional Hold	1m each exercise/side
3: CORRECTIVE EXERCISE	Side Plank Hold with Banded Clam & 90/90 Shin Box with Rotation Reach	30s each side & 1m alternating between sides
4: ACTIVATION DRILLS	A: Single-Leg Glute Bridge B: Quadruped Banded Fire Hydrant (short resistance band)	A: 2–3 sets of 8–10 reps each side B: 2–3 sets of 8–10 reps each side Superset: Alternating between A & B
5: MOVEMENT PATTERN DEVELOPMENT	A: Bodyweight Squat B: Suspension Trainer Reverse Lunge	A: 3 sets of 5 reps B: 3 sets of 5 reps each side Superset: Alternating between A & B
6: CNS STIMULATION	A: Snap-Down B: Low Amplitude Curtsy Hops	A: 3 sets of 3 reps B: 3 sets of 10–20 alternating hops Superset: Alternating between A & B

POSTERIOR CHAIN (HINGE) MOBILITY

EQUIPMENT: Foam roller, massage ball, wedge

GOOD FOR:
- Limited hamstring mobility
- Stiffness or tension in the lower back
- Difficulty performing hinges without rounding the spine

PHASE	EXERCISE	SETS/REPS/DURATION
1: SOFT TISSUE TECHNIQUES	Feet (massage ball), Calves, Hamstrings (foam roller)	1m each exercise/side
2: BIPHASIC POSITIONAL STRETCHING	Wedge Calf Stretch, Half-Kneeling Soleus Stretch, Hamstring Stretch	1m each exercise/side
3: CORRECTIVE EXERCISE	Active Straight-Leg Raise & Bird Dog	1m each (alternating between sides/exercises)
4: ACTIVATION DRILLS	A: Heels-Elevated Straight-Leg Hamstring Bridge B: Single-Leg 90/90 Glute Bridge	A: 2–3 sets of 8–10 reps each side B: 2–3 sets of 8–10 reps each side Superset: Alternating between A & B
5: MOVEMENT PATTERN DEVELOPMENT	Eccentric-Focused Romanian Deadlift (RDL)	3 sets of 8–10 reps
6: CNS STIMULATION	A: High Bear Crawl B: Supported Leg Swings	A: 3 sets of ~15s crawl B: 3 sets of 10 swings each leg Superset: Alternating between A & B

T-SPINE MOBILITY

EQUIPMENT: Foam roller, long resistance band, suspension trainer

GOOD FOR:
- Rounded upper back and shoulders
- Stiffness from long hours sitting
- Chronic tightness or restriction in the upper back or neck
- Rib flare (excessive arching) or compensations (like bent elbows) when reaching overhead

PHASE	EXERCISE	SETS/REPS/DURATION
1: SOFT TISSUE TECHNIQUES	Thoracic Spine & Lats (foam roller)	1m each exercise/side
2: BIPHASIC POSITIONAL STRETCHING	Hinged T-Spine Extension / Bilateral Lat Stretch (suspension trainer)	1m each exercise/side
3: CORRECTIVE EXERCISE	Bow and Arrow & Quadruped T-Spine Rotation	1m each exercise/side
4: ACTIVATION DRILLS	Rusin Tri-Set (long resistance band)	2–3 sets of 10 reps each exercise
5: MOVEMENT PATTERN DEVELOPMENT	A: Elevated Push-Up B: Bridged Banded Pullover	A: 3 sets of 5 reps B: 3 sets of 5 reps Superset: Alternating between A & B
6: CNS STIMULATION	A: Alternating Rotational Band Pull B: High Anchor Banded Kneeling Ab Crunch	A: 3 sets of 5 reps each side B: 3 sets of 20–30s Superset: Alternating between A & B

SHOULDER MOBILITY A (HORIZONTAL)

EQUIPMENT: Foam roller, long resistance band, suspension trainer

GOOD FOR:
- Forward-rounded shoulders or poor scapular positioning
- Alleviating anterior shoulder pain
- Difficulty reaching behind your body, like grabbing a wallet from your back pocket

PHASE	EXERCISE	SETS/REPS/DURATION
1: SOFT TISSUE TECHNIQUES	Pectoralis Group, Lats & T-Spine (foam roller)	1m each exercise/side
2: BIPHASIC POSITIONAL STRETCHING	90/90 Chest Stretch, Hinged T-Spine Extension & Posterior Shoulder Stretch (suspension trainer)	1m each exercise/side
3: CORRECTIVE EXERCISE	Side-Lying T-Spine Arm Sweep & Quadruped T-Spine Rotation	10 each exercise/side
4: ACTIVATION DRILLS	A: Band Internal Rotation B: Band External Rotation	A: 2–3 sets of 8–10 reps B: 2–3 sets of 8–10 reps Superset: Alternating between A & B
5: MOVEMENT PATTERN DEVELOPMENT	A: Push-Up or Elevated Push-Up B: Inverted Row (suspension trainer)	A: 3 sets of 5 reps B: 3 sets of 5 reps Superset: Alternating between A & B
6: CNS STIMULATION	A: Single-Arm Band Press with Rotation (Punch) B: Single-Arm Band Pull with Rotation (Split Stance)	A: 3 sets of 5 reps each side B: 3 sets of 5 reps each side Superset: Alternating between A & B

SHOULDER MOBILITY B (VERTICAL)

EQUIPMENT: Foam roller, long resistance band, suspension trainer

GOOD FOR:
- Limited overhead range of motion
- Tight lats restricting vertical reach
- Rib flare or shoulder elevation when attempting to reach overhead

PHASE	EXERCISE	SETS/REPS/DURATION
1: SOFT TISSUE TECHNIQUES	T-Spine, Lats, Posterior Shoulder (foam roller)	1m each exercise/side
2: BIPHASIC POSITIONAL STRETCHING	Hinged T-Spine Extension & Posterior Shoulder Stretch (suspension trainer)	1m each exercise/side
3: CORRECTIVE EXERCISE	Bird Dog & Dead Bug with Band Pullover	30s alternating between sides & 1m alternating between sides
4: ACTIVATION DRILLS	A: Banded Lat Pulldown (long resistance band) B: Kick-Throughs	A: 2–3 sets of 8–10 reps B: 2–3 sets of 8–10 reps each side Superset: Alternating between A & B
5: MOVEMENT PATTERN DEVELOPMENT	A: Single-Arm Band Press (vertical) B: High Kneeling Banded Pulldown (long resistance band)	A: 3 sets of 5 reps each side B: 3 sets of 5 reps each side Superset: Alternating between A & B
6: CNS STIMULATION	Plank to Pike Flow	3 sets of 15–30s

CORE STABILITY A (SUPINE)

EQUIPMENT: Foam roller, long resistance band, suspension trainer, light dumbbell (for Pallof Press)

GOOD FOR:
- Trouble establishing or maintaining a stable pillar position
- Ongoing or recurring low back discomfort
- Returning to movement following a previous low back injury or pregnancy
- Anterior pelvic tilt or excessive low back arching during screens or training
- Difficulty coordinating breath and movement in dead bug variations
- Poor integration between the core, pelvis, and spinal position

PHASE	EXERCISE	SETS/REPS/DURATION
1: SOFT TISSUE TECHNIQUES	Hip Flexors & Quadriceps (foam roller)	1m each exercise/side
2: BIPHASIC POSITIONAL STRETCHING	Half-Kneeling Hip Flexor Stretch, Prone Quad Stretch, Child's Pose (10 & 2)	1m each exercise/side
3: CORRECTIVE EXERCISE	Dead Bug (Opposite Arm & Leg) & Half-Kneeling Pallof Press	1m alternating between sides & 30s each side
4: ACTIVATION DRILLS	Banded Glute Bridge (long resistance band)	2–3 sets of 8–10 reps
5: MOVEMENT PATTERN DEVELOPMENT	A: Goblet Squat (light dumbbell) B: Inverted Row (suspension trainer)	A: 3 sets of 5 reps B: 3 sets of 5 reps Superset: Alternating between A & B
6: CNS STIMULATION	A: Lateral Bear Crawl B: Run in Place	A: 3 sets of 15s both directions B: 3 sets of 15s Superset: Alternating between A & B

CORE STABILITY B (PRONE)

EQUIPMENT: Foam roller, long resistance band, short resistance band, elevated surface (bench)

GOOD FOR:
- Inability to maintain a strong, stable pillar position
- Persistent low back discomfort or history of low back injury
- Returning to movement after pregnancy
- Visible anterior pelvic tilt or lumbar arching during screens
- Difficulty holding a front plank without sagging, pain, or breath control
- Poor integration between shoulders, core, and hips

PHASE	EXERCISE	SETS/REPS/DURATION
1: SOFT TISSUE TECHNIQUES	Hip Flexors, Lateral Hip (TFL), Glutes (foam roller)	1m each exercise/side
2: BIPHASIC POSITIONAL STRETCHING	Half-Kneeling Hip Flexor Stretch with Lateral Reach & Dynamic Pigeon Stretch	1m each exercise/side
3: CORRECTIVE EXERCISE	Plank (incline if needed) & Side Plank	30s each side & 1m alternating between sides
4: ACTIVATION DRILLS	A: Banded Glute Bridge (long resistance band) B: Quadruped Banded Fire Hydrant (short resistance band)	A: 2–3 sets of 8–10 reps B: 2–3 sets of 8–10 reps each side Superset: Alternating between A & B
5: MOVEMENT PATTERN DEVELOPMENT	A: Banded Hinge B: Push-Up or Elevated Push-Up	A: 3 sets of 5 reps B: 3 sets of 5 reps Superset: Alternating between A & B
6: CNS STIMULATION	A: Forward & Backward Crawl B: ¼ Speed Skaters	A: 3 sets of 15s both directions B: 3 sets of 15s alternating between sides Superset: Alternating between A & B

SCAPULAR STABILITY

EQUIPMENT: Foam roller, long resistance band, suspension trainer

GOOD FOR:
- Shoulder elevation during push or pull screens
- Overactive or tight traps during upper body exercises
- Trouble activating or feeling the mid-back and lats during pushing and pulling movements
- Scapular winging or poor control of the shoulder blades during screens or training

PHASE	EXERCISE	SETS/REPS/DURATION
1: SOFT TISSUE TECHNIQUES	Thoracic Spine, Pectoralis Group, Posterior Shoulder (foam roller)	1m each exercise/side
2: BIPHASIC POSITIONAL STRETCHING	90/90 Chest Stretch	1m each side
3: CORRECTIVE EXERCISE	Quadruped Hover & Side Plank	Accumulate 1m hold each
4: ACTIVATION DRILLS	A: Supine Band Face Pull B: Band Pull-Apart (long resistance band)	A: 2–3 sets of 8–10 reps B: 2–3 sets of 8–10 reps Superset: Alternating between A & B
5: MOVEMENT PATTERN DEVELOPMENT	A: Push-Up or Elevated Push-Up B: Inverted Row (suspension trainer)	A: 3 sets of 5 reps B: 3 sets of 5 reps Superset: Alternating between A & B
6: CNS STIMULATION	A: Plank Shoulder Taps B: Single-Arm Band Press (Punch)	A: 3 sets of 15–30s alternating sides B: 3 sets of 5 reps each side Superset: Alternating between A & B

SHOULDER STABILITY

EQUIPMENT: Foam roller, long resistance band, suspension trainer

GOOD FOR:
- Forward head-of-shoulder position
- Discomfort or pain at the front of the shoulder during pressing movements
- Difficulty stabilizing dumbbells during overhead or horizontal pressing
- Significant strength discrepancy between sides when pushing or pressing

PHASE	EXERCISE	SETS/REPS/DURATION
1: SOFT TISSUE TECHNIQUES	Thoracic Spine, Pectoralis Group, Posterior Shoulder (foam roller)	1m each exercise/side
2: BIPHASIC POSITIONAL STRETCHING	90/90 Chest Stretch	1m each side
3: CORRECTIVE EXERCISE	Dead Bug (Arm Extensions) & Bird Dog	1m alternating between sides & 30s alternating between sides
4: ACTIVATION DRILLS	A: Supine Band Face Pull and Band Pull-Apart B: Single-Arm Band External Rotation (long resistance band)	A: 2–3 sets of 8–10 reps B: 2–3 sets of 8–10 reps each side Superset: Alternating between A & B
5: MOVEMENT PATTERN DEVELOPMENT	A: Push-Up or Elevated Push-Up B: Inverted Row (suspension trainer)	A: 3 sets of 5 reps B: 3 sets of 5 reps Superset: Alternating between A & B
6: CNS STIMULATION	A: Single-Arm Banded Low to High Pull B: Plank to Pike Flow	A: 3 sets of 5 each side B: 3 sets of 15–30s Superset: Alternating between A & B

OVERHEAD STABILITY

EQUIPMENT: Foam roller, long resistance band, dumbbells or kettlebells (optional)

GOOD FOR:
- Limited overhead range of motion
- Discomfort or pain in the shoulders during vertical pressing or pulling movements

PHASE	EXERCISE	SETS/REPS/DURATION
1: SOFT TISSUE TECHNIQUES	Thoracic Spine, Lats, Posterior Shoulder (foam roller)	1m each exercise/side
2: BIPHASIC POSITIONAL STRETCHING	Kneeling Bench Overhead Prayer Stretch	1m
3: CORRECTIVE EXERCISE	Dead Bug (Arm Extensions) & Prone T & Y Fly	1m alternating between sides & 1m
4: ACTIVATION DRILLS	A: Supine Bridge Iso Band Pullover B: Diagonal Band Pull-Apart (long resistance band)	A: 2–3 sets of 8–10 reps B: 2–3 sets of 8–10 reps Superset: Alternating between A & B
5: MOVEMENT PATTERN DEVELOPMENT	A: Single-Arm Band Press B: Half-Kneeling Single-Arm High-Angle Row (long resistance band)	A: 3 sets of 5 reps each side B: 3 sets of 5 reps each side Superset: Alternating between A & B
6: CNS STIMULATION	A: Band Low Anchor Overhead March B: Plank to Pike Flow	A: 3 sets of 15–30s B: 3 sets of 15–30s Superset: Alternating between A & B

HIP STABILITY A

EQUIPMENT: Foam roller, long resistance band, short resistance band

GOOD FOR:
- Pelvic shifting or rotation during squats or lunges
- Discomfort around the lateral hip or knee
- Difficulty activating or feeling the glutes in bridges or lower body exercises

PHASE	EXERCISE	SETS/REPS/DURATION
1: SOFT TISSUE TECHNIQUES	Hip Flexor, Quadriceps, Lateral Hip (TFL) (foam roller)	1m each exercise/side
2: BIPHASIC POSITIONAL STRETCHING	Half-Kneeling Hip Flexor Stretch with Lateral Reach & 90/90 Glute Stretch	1m each exercise/side
3: CORRECTIVE EXERCISE	Plank & Bird Dog	Accumulate 1m & 30s alternating between sides
4: ACTIVATION DRILLS	A: Banded Glute Bridge (long resistance band) B: Quadruped Banded Fire Hydrant (short resistance band)	A: 2–3 sets of 8–10 reps B: 2–3 sets of 8–10 reps Superset: Alternating between A & B
5: MOVEMENT PATTERN DEVELOPMENT	A: Bodyweight Squat B: Banded Hinge	A: 3 sets of 5 reps B: 3 sets of 5 reps Superset: Alternating between A & B
6: CNS STIMULATION	A: Forward & Backward Crawl B: Narrow to Wide Hops	A: 3 sets of 15–30s both directions B: 3 sets of 15–30s Superset: Alternating between A & B

HIP STABILITY B

EQUIPMENT: Foam roller, long resistance band, short resistance band, light dumbbell or kettlebell

GOOD FOR:
- Difficulty maintaining balance in split squats, lunges, or step-ups
- One-sided discomfort in the hip or lower back
- Knee, hip, or back pain during running or other dynamic movements

PHASE	EXERCISE	SETS/REPS/DURATION
1: SOFT TISSUE TECHNIQUES	Hip Flexor, Lateral Hip (TFL), Adductor (foam roller)	1m each exercise/side
2: BIPHASIC POSITIONAL STRETCHING	Adductor Rock-Back & Dynamic Pigeon Stretch	1m each exercise/side
3: CORRECTIVE EXERCISE	Copenhagen Side Plank (short lever from knee)	Accumulate 1m each side
4: ACTIVATION DRILLS	A: Single-Leg Glute Bridge (long resistance band) B: Side-Lying Banded Clam (short resistance band)	A: 2–3 sets of 8–10 reps B: 2–3 sets of 8–10 reps Superset: Alternating between A & B
5: MOVEMENT PATTERN DEVELOPMENT	A: Lateral Lunge B: Supported Single-Leg RDL (optional: light dumbbell or kettlebell)	A: 3 sets of 5 reps each side B: 3 sets of 5 reps each side Superset: Alternating between A & B
6: CNS STIMULATION	A: Lateral Crawl B: Goblet March (light dumbbell or kettlebell)	A: 3 sets of 15–30s both directions B: 3 sets of 15–30s Superset: Alternating between A & B

COOL-DOWNS

Cool-downs don't need to be long to be effective, but they do need to be intentional. This section includes two types of cool-down templates: **post-workout cool-downs** and **mobility-focused cool-downs**.

The post-workout sequences are short on purpose. They're designed to be practical and pattern specific, giving you just enough time to restore the areas taxed most during your training session. These are ideal when you're wrapping up a workout and getting on with your day.

The mobility-focused templates go a layer deeper. They're longer and more exploratory, and they closely resemble the structure of a linchpin blueprint. You can use them at the end of a stressful day, on a rest day, or anytime you want to restore your body and improve your mobility. Think of them as a reset button for how you move and feel.

Both templates share a few core principles:

You'll start with global foam rolling—slow, deliberate passes along the full length of the muscle rather than the oscillatory work you used in your warm-up. Then you'll move into stretching, not to force range but to settle into good positions and let your tissues open up with time and breath. No biphasic methods here—just calm, stable holds.

Each template is fully customizable. You can follow it exactly as written or treat it as a starting point and adjust as needed. Swap in a drill that works better for your body. Hold a stretch longer if it feels good. Scale back if necessary. Just like your warm-ups and linchpins, these cool-downs should reflect how you feel and what you need that day.

For more detail on how the cool-down fits into the overall system, see page 83.

NOTE: *All cool-downs require a foam roller and, in some cases, a stretch strap or band (for quad and hamstring stretches) or suspension trainer (for T-spine, lat, and shoulder stretches). It's a good idea to have a foam roller on hand both in the gym and in your living room. If you don't have a stretch strap, band, or suspension trainer handy, you can modify the stretch. For example, you can use your hand to grip your foot for quad and hamstring stretches or utilize child's pose variations for T-spine, lat, and shoulder stretches.*

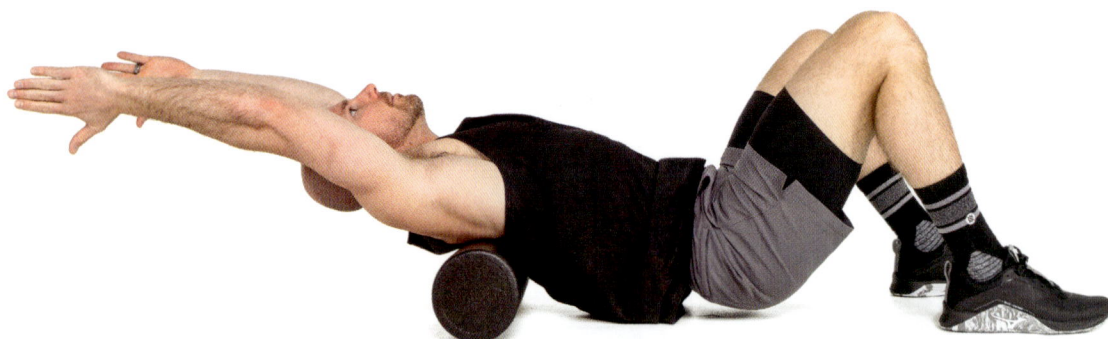

PHASE	DRILL	DURATION
SQUAT COOL-DOWN		
PARASYMPATHETIC POSITIONAL BREATHING	90/90 Supine	1–2 min
FOAM ROLL	Quadriceps	1–2 min each side
STRETCH	Prone Quad Stretch	1–2 min each side
HINGE COOL-DOWN		
PARASYMPATHETIC POSITIONAL BREATHING	90/90 Supine	1–2 min
FOAM ROLL	Hamstrings	1–2 min each side
STRETCH	Supine Hamstring Stretch with Strap	1–2 min each side
LUNGE COOL-DOWN		
PARASYMPATHETIC POSITIONAL BREATHING	90/90 Supine	1–2 min
FOAM ROLL	Adductors	1–2 min each side
STRETCH	Frog Stretch	1–2 min each side
PUSH/PULL HORIZONTAL COOL-DOWN		
PARASYMPATHETIC POSITIONAL BREATHING	90/90 Supine	1–2 min
FOAM ROLL	Pectoralis Group / Anterior Shoulder	1–2 min each side
STRETCH	Prone Chest Stretch	1–2 min each side
PUSH/PULL VERTICAL COOL-DOWN		
PARASYMPATHETIC POSITIONAL BREATHING	90/90 Supine	1–2 min
FOAM ROLL	Lats	1–2 min each side
STRETCH	Quadruped Single-Arm Lat Stretch (Child's Pose Variation)	1–2 min each side
HIP MOBILITY COOL-DOWN		
PARASYMPATHETIC POSITIONAL BREATHING	90/90 Supine	1–2 min
FOAM ROLL	Quadriceps, Hamstrings, Glutes, Adductors	1–2 min each side/region
STRETCH	Prone Quad Stretch, Hamstring Stretch with Strap, Quadruped Adductor Stretch, Dynamic Pigeon Stretch	1–2 min each side/stretch
T-SPINE MOBILITY COOL-DOWN		
PARASYMPATHETIC POSITIONAL BREATHING	90/90 Supine	1–2 min
FOAM ROLL	Thoracic Spine, Chest, Lats	1–2 min each side/region
STRETCH	Prone Chest Stretch, Hinged T-Spine Extension / Bilateral Lat Stretch, Posterior Shoulder (Alt: Child's Pose & Quadruped Single-Arm Lat Stretch)	1–2 min each side/stretch
SHOULDER MOBILITY COOL-DOWN		
PARASYMPATHETIC POSITIONAL BREATHING	90/90 Supine	1–2 min
FOAM ROLL	Thoracic Spine, Chest, Lats	1–2 min each side/region
STRETCH	Kneeling Bench Overhead Prayer Stretch, 90/90 Chest Stretch, Quadruped Single-Arm Lat Stretch	1–2 min each side/stretch

Scan the QR code to access demos of each exercise.

COOL-DOWNS

TRAINING PROGRAMS

This is where everything comes together—and your training begins.

The programs in this section are rooted in the principles you've already learned: training all six foundational movement patterns and integrating all six physical characteristics. But here, the focus shifts from principles to execution.

When it comes to choosing the right program, the first decision you'll make is frequency—that is, the number of days you will train throughout a week. Choose not based on preference, but on what you can stick to with 100 percent consistency, even when life gets messy (revisit pages 455 to 457 for more on the importance of training frequency). From there, the rest is mapped out for you.

Each frequency option—three, four, or five days per week—includes a dynamic warm-up, priming strategy, KPI lift, accessories and prehab, conditioning, and cool-down. What's more, each frequency has a slightly different workout structure, or split based on the time available. The fewer sessions you have, the more you need to accomplish in a single session. The more sessions you commit to, the more focus and variety you can build into the week.

▶ **3 days per week:** Full-body training each session

▶ **4 days per week:** Upper/lower body split with a movement pattern emphasis

▶ **5 days per week:** Upper/lower body split for four days and one full-body day with a movement pattern emphasis that includes a dedicated squat, hinge, lunge, push, and pull day

No matter which frequency you choose, each program in this section follows a three-phase progressive structure:

RECLAIM is your base. You'll establish clean movement patterns, address chronic weak links, and create a pain-free foundation.

REBUILD strengthens that base. You'll add more load, more variation, and more volume to the reclaimed movements.

REGAIN is the performance block. You'll layer in more complexity, and more challenge—earning the right to push harder with better movement and output. This is your bridge to lifelong performance training.

Together, these three phases form a 12-week cycle, and you'll see them directly reflected in the programs that follow.

Each phase includes one week of training, designed to be repeated for four weeks.

Each program also includes a built-in warm-up and cool-down that matches the day's training demands.

Each phase includes one week of training, designed to be repeated for four weeks. That means you'll do the same session structure across the entire phase, progressing from week to week by adjusting reps, load, rest, and strain—as outlined in the Training Tenets chapter (pages 458 to 459). The purpose of repeating a week is threefold: reinforce the pattern, build strength in the right positions, and create space for real, noticeable adaptation.

When a phase feels solid at the end of four weeks, move onto the next phase. If something still feels off, there's no shame in staying put. Repeating a phase isn't a setback—it's a commitment to doing it right. Let your assessments guide you. Use the screens to choose appropriate variations from the movement pattern pyramid. If something hurts, regress it. If you're thriving, stick with it.

Each program also includes a built-in warm-ups and cool-downs that matches the day's training demands—developed to align with the KPI and target the linchpins most commonly stressed by that day's movement pattern.

In this section, you'll also find three distinct program templates based on equipment access:

A **Bodyweight/Bands/Dumbbell Program** designed for training at home or on the go. Most people abandon their routine when they don't have access to a full gym—whether they're traveling, short on time, or working with limited equipment. This program eliminates that excuse. It's built to keep you consistent anywhere, using just your body, resistance bands, and a pair of dumbbells. It follows a three-day, full-body format that includes all three phases: Reclaim, Rebuild, and Regain.

Because external load is limited with minimal equipment, this track creatively blends physical characteristics within each session. You'll notice unique pairings—primers with strength, strength movements integrated with hypertrophy, and hypertrophy exercises combined with conditioning. The goal remains clear: effectively train all six foundational movement patterns while addressing power, strength, hypertrophy, conditioning, athleticism, and mobility.

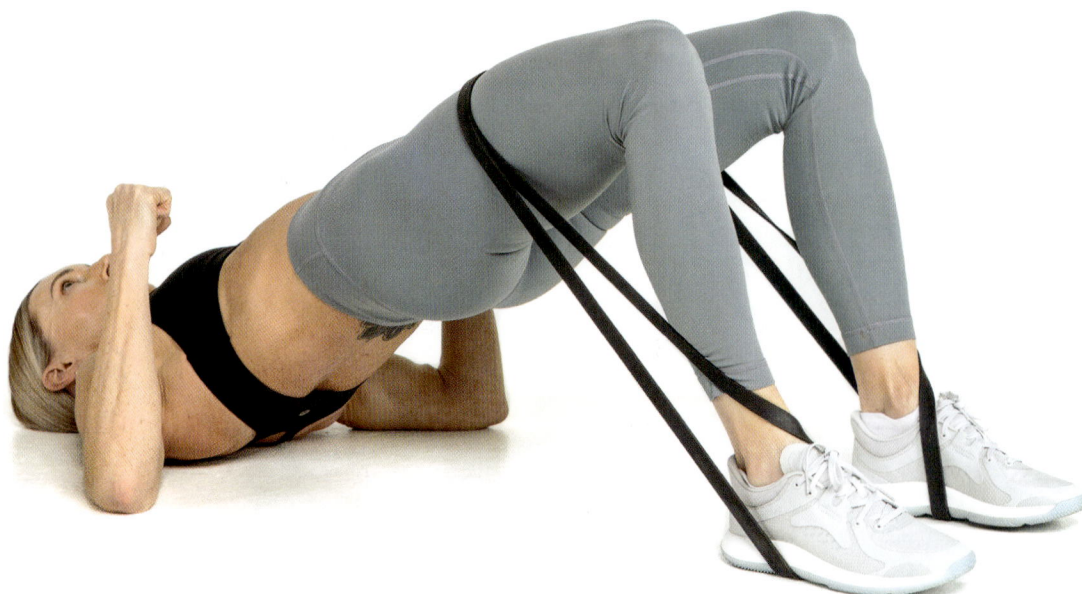

You can follow this as a complete standalone program—or simply pull from it when life throws off your routine. For example, if you're following one of the standard gym programs and find yourself away from your normal setup, you can drop in a session from this track, maintain your momentum, and then seamlessly resume your gym plan when you return. It's an ideal program for minimalist gyms, an approachable starting point if you're new to training, and a practical, flexible solution to ensure you stay consistent when you're on the move.

The **Standard Gym Programs** are built around traditional gym equipment. Whether you're already training in a gym or ready to take that next step, this program gives you access to the tools that make training more effective.

Equipment like dumbbells, kettlebells, barbells, bands, and cables allows for greater variation and better loading options, making it easier to personalize exercises to match your body.

As you advance through the phases (Reclaim, Rebuild, and Regain), you'll be able to challenge patterns in smarter ways, increase intensity without compromising technique, and build each physical characteristic with more precision.

As a special bonus, I've also included the **Ultimate Pain-Free Performance Program**—a hybrid model built around the foundational patterns and most common linchpins.

When I'm taking on new clients, many will say, "Just tell me what to do." No details about linchpins. No movement assessments. No long list of goals. Just a request for a smart, effective program that delivers. This is that program. If I had to design one program to serve 350 million people—built to get them stronger, leaner, healthier, and more resilient—this would be it.

No matter where you start—whether you're new to strength training or just need a smarter plan—there is a program for you.

Pick your frequency. Commit to the process. And let pain-free performance guide the way.

HOW TO APPROACH AND MODIFY THESE PROGRAMS

When I design programs, my goal is to effectively serve 80 percent of people 80 percent of the time. But to truly optimize your results, the remaining 20 percent must be customized specifically for you—your unique body structure, your individual capabilities, and your specific movement needs.

For many people, the best way to approach these programs is to simply follow them exactly as written. However, the smartest way to ensure long-term progress is to **tailor exercises based on your individual results from the screens and assessments**. These assessments clearly identify your strengths, limitations, and ideal movement ranges—guiding you toward safer, more effective setups and executions.

For example, if the program calls for a barbell deadlift and your hinge-back test reveals you can't comfortably reach the bar on the ground without compensating, modify the exercise by elevating the bar onto pins or stacked plates. This small adjustment places you in your ideal, accessible range of motion, removing unnecessary joint stress. Similarly, if overhead movements like vertical presses or pull-downs cause shoulder discomfort or compromise your form, adjust the angle slightly away from vertical—using a landmine press rather than a strict overhead press, for example—to maintain healthy shoulder positions and movement quality.

This guideline specifically applies to key performance indicators (KPIs) and accessory movements. **If an exercise listed is currently too advanced based on your assessment results, choose a regression lower down on the movement pattern pyramid.** Conversely, as you become stronger and your movement improves, you may find you need to progress an exercise to continue challenging your body. The simplest and most effective way to increase difficulty is by gradually adding load while maintaining impeccable form. For instance, if a dumbbell goblet squat becomes comfortable within the recommended rep range, progress by increasing the dumbbell's weight or by using a barbell front squat variation. Always prioritize form and control—progress happens when you're able to handle heavier weights safely and consistently within your optimal ranges.

If you don't have access to a certain piece of equipment, you can substitute a similar variation using the equipment you have available. For example, cable exercises can be effectively performed with resistance bands. The key is to never skip an exercise just because you lack the exact listed equipment; instead, choose a variation that replicates the same movement pattern and action.

Warm-ups also follow a deliberate sequence designed to prime your body for the main workout, improve mobility, and reinforce smooth movement. Although it's encouraged to individualize warm-up exercises according to your specific needs, always select movements that closely match the intended muscle groups and patterns of the original warm-up structure.

The simplest and most effective way to increase difficulty is by gradually adding load while maintaining impeccable form.

This ensures that the purpose behind the warm-up—movement mastery and effective priming—is maintained. This principle of closely matching the intended purpose applies to every exercise throughout all phases of the program.

When choosing loads or resistance in the main workout phases—especially mechanical primers, KPIs, accessory exercises, and conditioning finishers—aim for a level of effort that takes you near, but not to, total muscular failure. This means finishing each set feeling as though you could perform only 2 or 3 more reps with good form if you absolutely had to. It's challenging, but not to the point of compromising your technique. If your form starts breaking down, you've gone too far. For example, during a KPI like a front squat programmed for sets of 6 to 8 reps, select a weight heavy enough that by the end of the sixth rep you feel strong fatigue, yet confident you could have squeezed out just 2 or 3 additional reps with good form. Similarly, accessory exercises performed for higher reps, like a banded push-up done for sets of 15, should become challenging by rep 12 or 13 but not at the expense of good alignment or joint positioning.

Achieving the right balance between effort and form takes practice and experimentation—which is precisely why each phase (Reclaim, Rebuild, Regain) follows a consistent structure for four-week blocks. Sticking with the same exercises over this period allows you to fine-tune loading strategies, understand your body's response, and maximize progress from your training volume.

Ultimately, these programs were created to adapt and evolve with you. Personalizing movements and loads based on your body's unique requirements isn't just recommended—it's essential. This strategic individualization is at the heart of achieving true pain-free performance.

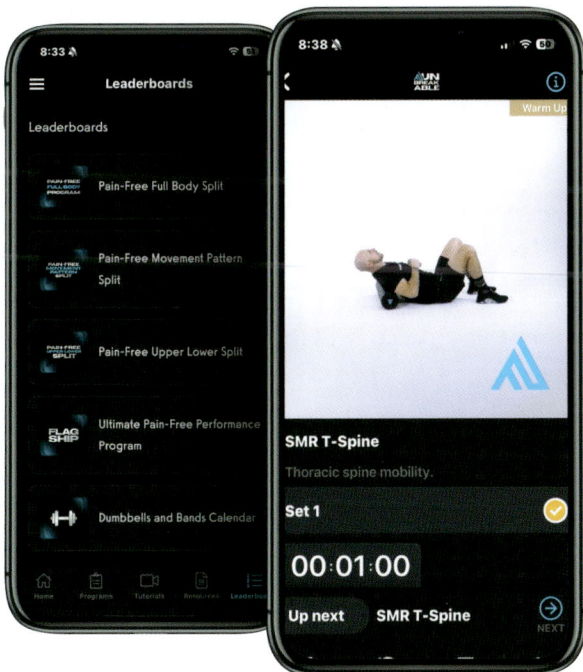

WANT STEP-BY-STEP EXPERT GUIDANCE ON EVERY EXERCISE IN THE PROGRAMS?

Check out the Unbreakable Training App! Get instant access to professionally coached tutorials, personalized guidance, and interactive support for each of the programs you're about to explore. Simply scan the QR code to get started.

HOW TO READ THE PROGRAMS

Each program is structured in clear sections, guiding you from preparation through training to recovery. Here's how to interpret the details.

SETS AND REPS

- **Sets:** The first number listed represents how many times you'll do the given number of repetitions.
- **Reps:** The second number (after the "x") shows how many repetitions you'll perform per set.

For example:

- **4 x 10** *means you'll perform 4 sets, doing 10 repetitions each set.*
- **3 x 15 each side** *means you'll perform 3 sets, with 15 reps per side, per set.*

DURATION (S, M)

- **s:** Indicates seconds.

  Example: 30s *means to hold or perform the movement for 30 seconds.*

- **m:** Indicates minutes.

  Example: 1m *means to perform for 1 minute. Often used in warm-up and cool-down phases.*

AMRAP

- **AMRAP** stands for **"As Many Rounds (or Reps) as Possible."**

  Example: 2m AMRAP *means continuously cycle through the listed exercises, completing as many rounds or reps as you can in 2 minutes, taking minimal rest.*

  If one exercise is listed: *Perform the exercise to near failure, rest for about 15 seconds, and then repeat this process continuously for the entire duration listed.*

  If two exercises are listed: *Alternate between the exercises, performing each to near failure back-to-back with minimal rest (superset) and completing as many rounds as you can within the specified time frame.*

SUPERSET GROUPINGS (A, B, C)

Exercises labeled A, B, or C indicate supersets or grouped exercises, meaning you'll alternate these exercises in sequence before resting.

- **A/B Superset Example:**

  A: Band-Resisted Stretch Push-Up

  B: Half-Kneeling Single-Arm Cable Row

  Complete one set of exercise A, then immediately perform one set of exercise B before resting. Repeat until all listed sets are completed.

- **Tri-Set (three exercises: A, B, C) Example:**

  Phase 4 Rusin Tri-Set

  A: Band Over and Back

  B: Band Face Pull

  C: Band Pull-Apart

  Perform one set of exercise A, immediately followed by one set of B, then one set of C, before resting. Repeat until all listed sets are completed.

ADDITIONAL ABBREVIATIONS/ CLARIFICATIONS

- **Each side:** *Complete the listed repetitions for both the right and left sides separately.*
- **Alternating:** *Switch sides with each repetition, alternating continuously until the total reps are completed.*

By clearly understanding and following this key, you'll confidently execute each session exactly as intended. For a deeper dive into how the programs are structured, guidance on what each training phase should feel like in terms of loading and effort, and specific recommendations for rest periods between sets, refer to the Training Tenets chapter.

BODYWEIGHT, BANDS, AND DUMBBELLS PROGRAM

TRAINING PHASE	FOCUS	EXERCISE	EQUIPMENT/TOOL	SETS/REPS/DURATION/REST
PRE-TRAINING PREPARATION	PHASE 1	Quadriceps & Thoracic Spine	Foam roller	1m each exercise/side (30s oscillation / 30s neurological trigger point)
	PHASE 2	Half-Kneeling Hip Flexor Stretch	None	1m each side (30s oscillation / 30s end-range hold)
	PHASE 3	Bird Dog (Single Arm)	None	30s each side
	PHASE 4	A: Banded Glute Bridge B: Band Pull-Apart	Long resistance band (light)	2–3 x 8–10 each exercise
	PHASE 5	A: Bodyweight Squat B: Standing Band-Under-Feet Bent-Over Row	A: None B: Long resistance band (light)	3 x 5 each exercise
	PHASE 6	A: Vertical Jacks B: Snap-Down	None	A: 3 x 5 B: 3 x 1
PRIMING & POTENTIATION	POWER	A: Jump Squat	None	4 x 5
	STRENGTH	B: Banded Front Squat with Pause	Long resistance band (heavy)	4 x 10
KEY PERFORMANCE INDICATOR (KPI)	LOWER	A: Banded 1.5-Rep Split Squat	Long resistance band (medium/heavy)	3 x 12 each side
	UPPER	B: Self-Supported Single-Arm Dumbbell Row with Rotation	Dumbbell	3 x 15 each side
PUMP ACCESSORIES & PREHAB	SHOULDERS	Supine Banded Pulsing Rear Delt Hold	Long resistance band	3 x 1m
CONDITIONING FINISHER	CARRY	Bodyweight Inchworm Walkout	None	3 x 10
POST-TRAINING COOL-DOWN	BREATHE	Supine 90/90 Breathing	None	1m
	FOAM ROLL	Quadriceps	Foam roller	1m each side
	STRETCH	Prone Quad Stretch with Strap	Stretch strap or long resistance band	1m each side

BODYWEIGHT, BANDS, AND DUMBBELLS PROGRAM

TRAINING PHASE	FOCUS	EXERCISE	EQUIPMENT/TOOL	SETS/REPS/DURATION/REST
PRE-TRAINING PREPARATION	PHASE 1	Adductor Group & Thoracic Spine	Foam roller	1m each exercise/side (30s oscillation / 30s neurological trigger point)
	PHASE 2	Adductor Rock-Back	None	1m each side (30s oscillation / 30s end-range hold)
	PHASE 3	Quadruped T-Spine Rotation	None	30s each side
	PHASE 4	A: Banded Glute Bridge B: Single-Arm Archer Band Row	Long resistance band (light)	2–3 x 8–10 each exercise
	PHASE 5	A: Dumbbell Anterior Good Morning B: Push-Up	A: Dumbbell B: None	3 x 5 each exercise
	PHASE 6	A: Seal Jacks B: Band-Behind-Back Press	A: None B: Long resistance band (light)	3 x 5 each exercise
PRIMING & POTENTIATION	POWER	A: Band-Under-Feet Explosive Glute Bridge	Long resistance band (light)	4 x 15
	STRENGTH	B: Banded Romanian Deadlift (RDL)	Long resistance band (medium) & dumbbell	4 x 10
KEY PERFORMANCE INDICATOR (KPI)	LOWER	A: Goblet Reverse Lunge	Dumbbell	3 x 12 each side
	UPPER	B: Band-Resisted Push-Up	Long resistance band (medium)	3 x 10
PUMP ACCESSORIES & PREHAB	SHOULDERS	Band-Under-Foot Single-Arm Lateral Raise	Long resistance band (light/medium)	3 x 15 each side
CONDITIONING FINISHER	CORE	High Plank Shoulder Taps	None	3 x 30s
POST-TRAINING COOL-DOWN	BREATHE	Prone Breathing	None	1m
	FOAM ROLL	Hamstrings	Foam roller	1m each side
	STRETCH	Supine Hamstring Stretch	Long resistance band	1m each side

486   04. PROGRAMS AND TEMPLATES

BODYWEIGHT, BANDS, AND DUMBBELLS PROGRAM

TRAINING PHASE	FOCUS	EXERCISE	EQUIPMENT/TOOL	SETS/REPS/DURATION/REST
PRE-TRAINING PREPARATION	PHASE 1	Lateral Hip & Posterior Shoulder	Foam roller	1m each exercise/side (30s oscillation / 30s neurological trigger point)
	PHASE 2	90/90 Glute Stretch & Child's Pose (10 & 2)	None	1m each side (30s oscillation / 30s end-range hold)
	PHASE 3	Dead Bug (Opposite Arm & Leg)	None	1m
	PHASE 4	A: Side Plank Hip Drop B: Band Face Pull	A: None B: Long resistance band (light)	2–3 x 8–10 each exercise
	PHASE 5	A: Dumbbell Anterior Good Morning B: Push-Up	A: Dumbbell B: None	3 x 5 each exercise
	PHASE 6	A: Skip B: ¼ Speed Skaters	None	3 x 5 each exercise
PRIMING & POTENTIATION	POWER	A: Explosive Band-Behind-Back Single-Arm Press	Long resistance band (light)	4 x 5 each side
	STRENGTH	B: Banded Bent-Over Row	Long resistance band (medium)	4 x 10
KEY PERFORMANCE INDICATOR (KPI)	LOWER	A: Single-Arm Dumbbell Lateral Lunge	Dumbbell	3 x 10–12 each side
	UPPER	B: Seated Band Around Feet Row	Long resistance band (medium)	3 x 15
PUMP ACCESSORIES & PREHAB	BICEPS	Standing on Band Hammer Curl	Long resistance band (medium)	3 x 15
CONDITIONING FINISHER	CARRY	Single-Arm Dumbbell Overhead March	Dumbbell	3 x 30s each side
POST-TRAINING COOL-DOWN	BREATHE	Supine Butterfly Breathing	None	1m
	FOAM ROLL	Glutes	Foam roller	1m each side
	STRETCH	Supine Figure 4	None	1m each side

BODYWEIGHT, BANDS, AND DUMBBELLS PROGRAM

TRAINING PHASE	FOCUS	EXERCISE	EQUIPMENT/TOOL	SETS/REPS/DURATION/REST
PRE-TRAINING PREPARATION	PHASE 1	Quadriceps & Thoracic Spine	Foam roller	1m each exercise/side (30s oscillation / 30s neurological trigger point)
	PHASE 2	Half-Kneeling Hip Flexor Stretch with Overhead Reach	None	1m each side (30s oscillation / 30s end-range hold)
	PHASE 3	Bird Dog (Single Leg)	None	30s each side
	PHASE 4	A: Banded Glute Bridge B: Band Pull-Apart	Long resistance band (light)	2–3 x 8–10 each exercise
	PHASE 5	A: Bodyweight Squat B: Standing Band-Under-Feet Bent-Over Row	A: None B: Long resistance band (light)	3 x 5 each exercise
	PHASE 6	A: Vertical Jacks B: Triple Extension to Jump	None	A: 3 x 5 B: 3 x 1
PRIMING & POTENTIATION	MECHANICAL PRIMER	A: Foam Roller Hamstring Curl	Foam roller	4 x 5
	STRENGTH	B: Banded Goblet Squat	Long resistance band (medium)	4 x 10
KEY PERFORMANCE INDICATOR (KPI)	LOWER	A: Banded Goblet Split Squat	Long resistance band (heavy)	3 x 12–15 each side
	UPPER	B: High-Angle Band Pull-Apart	None	3 x 15 each side
PUMP ACCESSORIES & PREHAB	GLUTES	Banded Thruster	Long resistance band (heavy)	3 x 12
CONDITIONING FINISHER	CARRY/ARMS	3-Way Plank	None	3 x 45s
POST-TRAINING COOL-DOWN	BREATHE	Supine 90/90 Breathing	None	1m
	FOAM ROLL	Quadriceps & Adductor Group	Foam roller	1m each exercise/side
	STRETCH	Prone Quad Stretch & Frog Stretch	Long resistance band	1m each exercise/side

BODYWEIGHT, BANDS, AND DUMBBELLS PROGRAM

TRAINING PHASE	FOCUS	EXERCISE	EQUIPMENT/TOOL	SETS/REPS/DURATION/REST
PRE-TRAINING PREPARATION	PHASE 1	Adductor Group & Thoracic Spine	Foam roller	1m each exercise/side (30s oscillation / 30s neurological trigger point)
	PHASE 2	Adductor Rock-Back	None	1m each side (30s oscillation / 30s end-range hold)
	PHASE 3	Quadruped T-Spine Rotation	None	30s each side
	PHASE 4	A: Banded Glute Bridge B: Single-Arm Archer Band Row	Long resistance band (light)	2–3 x 8–10 each exercise
	PHASE 5	A: Dumbbell Anterior Good Morning B: Push-Up	A: Dumbbell B: None	3 x 5 each exercise
	PHASE 6	A: Seal Jacks B: Band-Behind-Back Press	A: None B: Long resistance band (light)	3 x 5 each exercise
PRIMING & POTENTIATION	MECHANICAL PRIMER	A: Double-Banded Glute Bridge	Long & short resistance bands (light)	4 x 20
	STRENGTH	B: Banded Hybrid Stance Deadlift	Long resistance band (medium)	4 x 8
KEY PERFORMANCE INDICATOR (KPI)	LOWER	A: Kickstand Band-Under-Foot Romanian Deadlift (RDL)	Long resistance band (medium) & dumbbell	3 x 15 each side
	UPPER	B: Single-Arm Split-Stance Band-Under-Foot Vertical Press	Long resistance band (medium)	3 x 15 each side
PUMP ACCESSORIES & PREHAB	SHOULDERS	Supine Blackburn	None	3 x 15
CONDITIONING FINISHER	CARRY/ARMS	Kneeling Band Under Shins Overhead Triceps Extension	Long resistance band (light)	3 x 15
POST-TRAINING COOL-DOWN	BREATHE	Prone Breathing	None	1m
	FOAM ROLL	Hamstrings & Pecs	Foam roller	1m each exercise/side
	STRETCH	Supine Hamstring Stretch	Long resistance band	1m each side

BODYWEIGHT, BANDS, AND DUMBBELLS PROGRAM

REBUILD **DAY 03**

TRAINING PHASE	FOCUS	EXERCISE	EQUIPMENT/TOOL	SETS/REPS/DURATION/REST
PRE-TRAINING PREPARATION	PHASE 1	Lateral Hip & Lats	Foam roller	1m each exercise/side (30s oscillation / 30s neurological trigger point)
	PHASE 2	90/90 Glute Stretch & Child's Pose (10 & 2)	None	1m each side (30s oscillation / 30s end-range hold)
	PHASE 3	Dead Bug (Opposite Arm & Leg)	None	1m
	PHASE 4	A: Side Plank Hip Drop B: Band Face Pull	A: None B: Long resistance band (light)	2–3 x 8–10 each exercise
	PHASE 5	A: Reverse Lunge B: Seated Band Around Feet Row	A: None B: Long resistance band (light)	3 x 5 each exercise
	PHASE 6	A: Skip B: ¼ Speed Skaters	None	3 x 5 each exercise
PRIMING & POTENTIATION	MECHANICAL PRIMER	A: Band Pull-Apart	Long resistance band (light)	4 x 20 each side
	STRENGTH	B: Banded Hinge Single-Arm Row	Long resistance band (light)	4 x 8 each side
KEY PERFORMANCE INDICATOR (KPI)	LOWER	A: Dumbbell Goblet Curtsy Lunge	Dumbbell	3 x 12 each side
	UPPER	B: Side Plank Banded Powell Raise	Long resistance band (light)	3 x 15
PUMP ACCESSORIES & PREHAB	ACCESSORY	Side-Lying Banded Clam	Short resistance band (medium)	3 x 15 each side
CONDITIONING FINISHER	CARRY/ARMS	Inchworm Walkout with Push-Up	None	3 x 10
POST-TRAINING COOL-DOWN	BREATHE	Supine Butterfly Breathing	None	1m
	FOAM ROLL	Glutes & Lats	Foam roller	1m each exercise/side
	STRETCH	Supine Figure 4 & Child's Pose (10 & 2)	None	1m each exercise/side

BODYWEIGHT, BANDS, AND DUMBBELLS PROGRAM

TRAINING PHASE	FOCUS	EXERCISE	EQUIPMENT/TOOL	SETS/REPS/DURATION/REST
PRE-TRAINING PREPARATION	PHASE 1	Quadriceps & Thoracic Spine	Foam roller	1m each exercise/side (30s oscillation / 30s neurological trigger point)
	PHASE 2	Half-Kneeling Hip Flexor Stretch with Overhead Reach	None	1m each side (30s oscillation / 30s end-range hold)
	PHASE 3	Bird Dog (Arm & Leg Opposites)	None	30s
	PHASE 4	A: Banded Glute Bridge B: Band Pull-Apart	Long resistance band (light)	2–3 x 8–10 each exercise
	PHASE 5	A: Goblet Squat B: Standing Band-Under-Feet Bent-Over Row	A: Dumbbell B: Long resistance band (light)	3 x 5 each exercise
	PHASE 6	A: Vertical Jacks B: Countermovement Jump	None	A: 3 x 5 B: 3 x 1
PRIMING & POTENTIATION	SKILL/ PLYOMETRIC	A: Dumbbell Snatch	Dumbbell	4 x 8
	STRENGTH	B: Banded Zercher Squat	Long resistance band (medium/heavy)	4 x 8–10
KEY PERFORMANCE INDICATOR (KPI)	LOWER	A: Dumbbell Goblet Split Squat with Rotation	Dumbbell	3 x 12 each side
	UPPER	B: Seated Band Around Feet Alternating Row	Long resistance band (medium)	3 x 15 each side
PUMP ACCESSORIES & PREHAB	CORE	Banded Crunch (Lying on Band)	Long resistance band (medium)	2 x AMRAP
CONDITIONING FINISHER	CARRY	Hand Behind Head Alternating Lunge	None	2 x 1m
POST-TRAINING COOL-DOWN	BREATHE	Supine 90/90 Breathing	None	1m
	FOAM ROLL	Quadriceps & Adductor Group	Foam roller	1m each exercise/side
	STRETCH	Prone Quad Stretch & Frog Stretch	Long resistance band	1m each exercise/side

BODYWEIGHT, BANDS, AND DUMBBELLS PROGRAM

REGAIN DAY 02

TRAINING PHASE	FOCUS	EXERCISE	EQUIPMENT/TOOL	SETS/REPS/DURATION/REST
PRE-TRAINING PREPARATION	PHASE 1	Adductor Group & Thoracic Spine	Foam roller	1m each exercise/side (30s oscillation / 30s neurological trigger point)
	PHASE 2	Adductor Rock-Back	None	1m each side (30s oscillation / 30s end-range hold)
	PHASE 3	Quadruped T-Spine Rotation	None	30s each side
	PHASE 4	A: Banded Glute Bridge B: Single-Arm Archer Band Row	Long resistance band (light)	2–3 x 8–10 each exercise
	PHASE 5	A: Dumbbell Anterior Good Morning B: Push-Up	A: Dumbbell B: None	3 x 5 each exercise
	PHASE 6	A: Seal Jacks B: Plyo Push-Up	None	3 x 5 each exercise
PRIMING & POTENTIATION	SKILL/PLYOMETRIC	A: Dumbbell Clean to Rotating Press	Dumbbell	4 x 8
	STRENGTH	B: Sumo Stance Banded Deadlift	Long resistance band (medium/heavy)	4 x 8–10
KEY PERFORMANCE INDICATOR (KPI)	LOWER	A: Foam Roller Supported Banded Single-Leg RDL	Long resistance band (light) & dumbbell	3 x 15 each side
	UPPER	B: Banded Upright Row	Long resistance band (light/medium)	3 x 15
PUMP ACCESSORIES & PREHAB	CORE	Foam Roller Plank Pull Knees In	Foam roller	2 x AMRAP
CONDITIONING FINISHER	CARRY	Quadruped Dumbbell Alternating Lateral Drag	Dumbbell	2 x 1m
POST-TRAINING COOL-DOWN	BREATHE	Prone Breathing	None	1m
	FOAM ROLL	Hamstrings & Pecs	Foam roller	1m each exercise/side
	STRETCH	Supine Hamstring Stretch & Prone Chest Stretch	Long resistance band	1m each exercise/side

492   04. PROGRAMS AND TEMPLATES

BODYWEIGHT, BANDS, AND DUMBBELLS PROGRAM

TRAINING PHASE	FOCUS	EXERCISE	EQUIPMENT/TOOL	SETS/REPS/DURATION/REST
PRE-TRAINING PREPARATION	PHASE 1	Lateral Hip & Lats	Foam roller	1m each exercise/side (30s oscillation / 30s neurological trigger point)
	PHASE 2	90/90 Glute Stretch & Foam Roller Child's Pose (10 & 2)	None	1m each side (30s oscillation / 30s end-range hold)
	PHASE 3	Dead Bug (Opposite Arm & Leg)	None	1m
	PHASE 4	A: Side Plank Hip Drop B: Single-Arm Band Face Pull	A: None B: Long resistance band (light)	2–3 x 8–10 each exercise
	PHASE 5	A: Reverse Lunge with Overhead Reach B: Seated Band-Around-Feet Row	A: None B: Long resistance band (light)	3 x 5 each exercise
	PHASE 6	A: Split Squat Plyo Jump B: ¼ Speed Skaters	None	3 x 5 each exercise
PRIMING & POTENTIATION	SKILL/PLYOMETRIC	A: Dumbbell Lift & Chop	Dumbbell	4 x 8 each side
	STRENGTH	B: Band-Resisted Partial-Rep Wide Push-Up	Long resistance band (light/medium)	4 x 8–10 each side
KEY PERFORMANCE INDICATOR (KPI)	LOWER	A: Dumbbell Hand Switch Alternating Lunge	Dumbbell	3 x 30 each side
	UPPER	B: Half-Kneeling Band Pull-Apart	Long resistance band (light)	3 x 15–20
PUMP ACCESSORIES & PREHAB	CORE	Star Crunch	None	2 x 30s each side
CONDITIONING FINISHER	CARRY	Side-to-Side Lateral Crawl	None	2 x 1m
POST-TRAINING COOL-DOWN	BREATHE	Supine Butterfly Breathing	None	1m
	FOAM ROLL	Glutes & Lats	Foam roller	1m each exercise/side
	STRETCH	Supine Figure 4 & Child's Pose (10 & 2)	None	1m each exercise/side

3-DAY FULL-BODY PROGRAM

RECLAIM DAY 01

TRAINING PHASE	FOCUS	EXERCISE	EQUIPMENT/TOOL	SETS/REPS/DURATION/REST
PRE-TRAINING PREPARATION	PHASE 1	Quadriceps & Thoracic Spine	Foam roller	1m each exercise/side (30s oscillation / 30s neurological trigger point)
	PHASE 2	Half-Kneeling Hip Flexor Stretch & Hinged T-Spine Extension / Bilateral Stretch	Suspension trainer	1m each exercise/side (30s oscillation / 30s end-range hold)
	PHASE 3	Bird Dog (Single Arm)	None	30s each side
	PHASE 4	A: Banded Glute Bridge B: Hinged Straight-Arm Pulldown	A: Long resistance band (medium) B: Long resistance band (light)	2–3 x 8–10 each exercise
	PHASE 5	A: Bodyweight Squat B: Inverted Row	A: None B: Suspension trainer	3 x 5 each exercise
	PHASE 6	A: Vertical Jacks B: Snap-Down	None	A: 3 x 5 B: 3 x 1
PRIMING & POTENTIATION	NEUROLOGICAL PRIMER	A: Med Ball Slam	Med ball	3 x 3
	MECHANICAL PRIMER	B: Prone Band Hamstring Curl	Long resistance band	3 x 15–20 each side
KEY PERFORMANCE INDICATOR (KPI)	LOWER	A: Goblet Box Squat	Dumbbell or kettlebell	3–4 x 10–12
	UPPER	B: Close-Grip Supinated Lat Pulldown	Cable	3 x 15 each side
PUMP ACCESSORIES & PREHAB	HINGE	Romanian Deadlift (RDL)	Dumbbell	3 x 12
	PUSH	Push-Up	None	3 x 12
CONDITIONING FINISHER	CARRY	Farmer's Carry (Bilateral)	Dumbbells	3–4 x 20s
POST-TRAINING COOL-DOWN	BREATHE	Supine 90/90 Breathing	None	1m
	FOAM ROLL	Hamstrings	Foam roller	1m each side
	STRETCH	Supine Hamstring Stretch	Long resistance band / stretch strap	1m each side

3-DAY FULL-BODY PROGRAM

TRAINING PHASE	FOCUS	EXERCISE	EQUIPMENT/TOOL	SETS/REPS/DURATION/REST
PRE-TRAINING PREPARATION	PHASE 1	Adductor Group & Pectoralis Group	Foam roller	1m each exercise/side (30s oscillation / 30s neurological trigger point)
	PHASE 2	Adductor Rock-Back & 90/90 Chest Stretch	None	1m each exercise/side (30s oscillation / 30s end-range hold)
	PHASE 3	Dead Bug (Single Arm)	None	30s
	PHASE 4	A: Banded Glute Bridge B: Band Pull-Apart	A: Long resistance band (medium) B: Long resistance band (light)	2–3 x 8–10 each exercise
	PHASE 5	A: Romanian Deadlift (RDL) B: Push-Up	A: Dumbbell B: None	3 x 5 each exercise
	PHASE 6	A: Seal Jacks B: Bent-Over Med Ball Press (single rep variation)	A: None B: Med ball	3 x 5 each exercise
PRIMING & POTENTIATION	NEUROLOGICAL PRIMER	A: Bilateral Band Press (Explosive)	Long resistance band (light)	3 x 5
	MECHANICAL PRIMER	B: Prone Band Hamstring Curl	Long resistance band (light)	3 x 15–20 each side
KEY PERFORMANCE INDICATOR (KPI)	LOWER	A: Romanian Deadlift (RDL)	Dumbbell	3–4 x 10–12
	UPPER	B: Deficit Push-Up (optional: loaded)	Weight plate (optional)	3–4 x 8–10
PUMP ACCESSORIES & PREHAB	LUNGE	Dumbbell Split Squat	Dumbbells	3 x 10–12
	PULL	Inverted Row	Suspension trainer	3 x 10–12
CONDITIONING FINISHER	GLUTE BURNOUT	Double-Banded Glute Bridge	Long & short resistance bands (medium)	2m AMRAP: do reps to near-failure, rest 15s, repeat for 2m
POST-TRAINING COOL-DOWN	BREATHE	Supine 90/90 Breathing	None	1m
	FOAM ROLL	Glutes	Foam roller	1m each side
	STRETCH	90/90 Glute Stretch	None	1m each side

3-DAY FULL-BODY PROGRAM

TRAINING PHASE	FOCUS	EXERCISE	EQUIPMENT/TOOL	SETS/REPS/DURATION/REST
PRE-TRAINING PREPARATION	PHASE 1	Lateral Hip & Posterior Shoulder	Foam roller	1m each exercise/side (30s oscillation / 30s neurological trigger point)
	PHASE 2	90/90 Glute Stretch & Posterior Shoulder Stretch	Suspension trainer	1m each exercise/side (30s oscillation / 30s end-range hold)
	PHASE 3	Side Plank	None	30s each side
	PHASE 4	A: Single-Leg Glute Bridge B: Band Over & Back	A: None B: Long resistance band (light)	2–3 x 8–10 each exercise
	PHASE 5	A: Bodyweight Reverse Lunge B: Inverted Row	A: None B: Suspension trainer	3 x 5 each exercise
	PHASE 6	A: Triple Extension to Snap-Down B: Seal Jack	None	3 x 5 each exercise
PRIMING & POTENTIATION	NEUROLOGICAL PRIMER	A: Supported Skip (Alternating)	None	3 x 10
	MECHANICAL PRIMER	B: Banded Glute Bridge	Long resistance band (medium)	3 x 20
KEY PERFORMANCE INDICATOR (KPI)	LOWER	A: Dumbbell Goblet Reverse Lunge	Dumbbell or kettlebell	3–4 x 10 each side
	UPPER	B: Single-Arm Row	Dumbbell	3–4 x 10–12 each side
PUMP ACCESSORIES & PREHAB	SQUAT	Landmine Goblet Squat	Landmine	3 x 12
	PUSH	Half-Kneeling Landmine Single-Arm Press	Landmine	3 x 12 each side
CONDITIONING FINISHER	SHOULDER BURNOUT	Double-Banded Rear Delt Fly	Long resistance bands (light)	2m AMRAP: do reps to near-failure, rest 15s, repeat for 2m
POST-TRAINING COOL-DOWN	BREATHE	Supine 90/90 Breathing	None	1m
	FOAM ROLL	Lats	Foam roller	1m each side
	STRETCH	Child's Pose (10 & 2)	None	1m each side

3-DAY FULL-BODY PROGRAM

TRAINING PHASE	FOCUS	EXERCISE	EQUIPMENT/TOOL	SETS/REPS/DURATION/REST
PRE-TRAINING PREPARATION	PHASE 1	Quadriceps & Thoracic Spine	Foam roller	1m each exercise/side (30s oscillation / 30s neurological trigger point)
	PHASE 2	Half-Kneeling Hip Flexor Stretch & Hinged T-Spine Extension / Bilateral Stretch	Suspension trainer	1m each exercise/side (30s oscillation / 30s end-range hold)
	PHASE 3	Bird Dog (Single Leg)	None	30s each side
	PHASE 4	A: Banded Glute Bridge B: Hinged Straight-Arm Pulldown	A: Long resistance band (medium) B: Long resistance band (light)	2–3 x 8–10 each exercise
	PHASE 5	A: Goblet Squat B: Inverted Row	A: Dumbbell or kettlebell B: Suspension trainer	3 x 5 each exercise
	PHASE 6	A: Vertical Jacks B: Vertical Jump	None	A: 3 x 5 B: 3 x 1
PRIMING & POTENTIATION	NEUROLOGICAL PRIMER	A: Anti-Flexion Med Ball Slam	Med ball	3 x 3
	MECHANICAL PRIMER	B: Ball Hamstring Curl	Physio ball	3 x 15 each side
KEY PERFORMANCE INDICATOR (KPI)	LOWER	A: Goblet Squat	Dumbbell or kettlebell	3–4 x 12–15
	UPPER	B: Medium Grip Lat Pulldown	Cable	3–4 x 10–12
PUMP ACCESSORIES & PREHAB	HINGE	Landmine Romanian Deadlift (RDL)	Landmine	3 x 15
	PUSH	Suspension Push-Up	Suspension trainer	3 x 12–15
CONDITIONING FINISHER	CARRY	Front Rack Carry (Bilateral)	Dumbbells	4 x 30s
POST-TRAINING COOL-DOWN	BREATHE	Supine 90/90 Breathing	None	1m
	FOAM ROLL	Hamstrings	Foam roller	1m each side
	STRETCH	Supine Hamstring Stretch	Long resistance band / stretch strap	1m each side

3-DAY FULL-BODY PROGRAM

TRAINING PHASE	FOCUS	EXERCISE	EQUIPMENT/TOOL	SETS/REPS/DURATION/REST
PRE-TRAINING PREPARATION	PHASE 1	Adductor Group & Pectoralis Group	Foam roller	1m each exercise/side (30s oscillation / 30s neurological trigger point)
	PHASE 2	Adductor Rock-Back & 90/90 Chest Stretch	None	1m each exercise/side (30s oscillation / 30s end-range hold)
	PHASE 3	Dead Bug (Single Leg)	None	30s each side
	PHASE 4	A: Banded Glute Bridge B: Band Pull-Apart	A: Long resistance band (medium) B: Long resistance band (light)	2–3 x 8–10 each exercise
	PHASE 5	A: Romanian Deadlift (RDL) B: Push-Up	A: Dumbbell B: Suspension trainer	3 x 5 each exercise
	PHASE 6	A: Seal Jacks B: Bent-Over Med Ball Press (Repeater Variation)	A: None B: Med ball	3 x 5 each exercise
PRIMING & POTENTIATION	NEUROLOGICAL PRIMER	A: Broad Jump	Long resistance band (light)	3 x 1
	MECHANICAL PRIMER	B: Hands-Free Double-Band Face Pull	Long resistance band (light)	3 x 20
KEY PERFORMANCE INDICATOR (KPI)	LOWER	A: Trap Bar Deadlift	Dumbbell or kettlebell	3–4 x 12–15
	UPPER	B: Dumbbell Bench Press	Dumbbells	3–4 x 12–15
PUMP ACCESSORIES & PREHAB	LUNGE	Dumbbell Contralateral Split Squat	Dumbbell	3 x 10–15
	PULL	Half-Kneeling Cable Row	Cable	3 x 15
CONDITIONING FINISHER	GLUTE BURNOUT	A: Banded Hip Thrust B: Banded Side-Lying Hip Abduction	A: Long resistance band (medium) B: Short resistance band (medium)	5m AMRAP: do exercises to near-failure, alternating continuously with minimal rest
POST-TRAINING COOL-DOWN	BREATHE	Supine 90/90 Breathing	None	1m
	FOAM ROLL	Glutes	Foam roller	1m each side
	STRETCH	90/90 Glute Stretch	None	1m each side

3-DAY FULL-BODY PROGRAM

REBUILD DAY 03

TRAINING PHASE	FOCUS	EXERCISE	EQUIPMENT/TOOL	SETS/REPS/DURATION/REST
PRE-TRAINING PREPARATION	PHASE 1	Lateral Hip & Posterior Shoulder	Foam roller	1m each exercise/side (30s oscillation / 30s neurological trigger point)
	PHASE 2	90/90 Glute Stretch & Posterior Shoulder Stretch	Suspension trainer	1m each exercise/side (30s oscillation / 30s end-range hold)
	PHASE 3	Side Plank	None	30s each side
	PHASE 4	A: Single-Leg Glute Bridge B: Band Over & Back	A: None B: Long resistance band (light)	2–3 x 8–10 each exercise
	PHASE 5	A: Bodyweight Reverse Lunge B: Inverted Row	A: None B: Suspension trainer	3 x 5 each exercise
	PHASE 6	A: Counter Movement Jump B: Explosive Band Press	A: None B: Long resistance band	3 x 3 each exercise/side
PRIMING & POTENTIATION	NEUROLOGICAL PRIMER	A: Skip in Place	None	3 x 10 alternating
	MECHANICAL PRIMER	B: Dumbbell Glute Bridge	Dumbbell	3 x 20
KEY PERFORMANCE INDICATOR (KPI)	LOWER	A: Dumbbell Contralateral Reverse Lunge	Dumbbell	3–4 x 12–15 each side
	UPPER	B: Dumbbell Bent-Over Row	Dumbbell	3–4 x 10–15 each side
PUMP ACCESSORIES & PREHAB	SQUAT	Heels Goblet Squat	Dumbbell	3 x 15
	LUNGE	Split Stance Single-Arm Landmine Press	Landmine	3 x 12–15 each side
CONDITIONING FINISHER	SHOULDER/TRICEPS BURNOUT	A: Dumbbell Alternating Lateral Raise B: Half-Kneeling Cable (or Band) Overhead Triceps Extension	A: Dumbbell B: Cable or band	5m AMRAP: do exercises to near-failure, alternating continuously with minimal rest
POST-TRAINING COOL-DOWN	BREATHE	Supine 90/90 Breathing	None	1m
	FOAM ROLL	Lats	Foam roller	1m each side
	STRETCH	Child's Pose (10 & 2)	None	1m each side

3-DAY FULL-BODY PROGRAM

REGAIN DAY 01

TRAINING PHASE	FOCUS	EXERCISE	EQUIPMENT/TOOL	SETS/REPS/DURATION/REST
PRE-TRAINING PREPARATION	PHASE 1	Quadriceps & Thoracic Spine	Foam roller	1m each exercise/side (30s oscillation / 30s neurological trigger point)
	PHASE 2	Half-Kneeling Hip Flexor Stretch & Hinged T-Spine Extension/Stretch	Suspension trainer	1m each exercise/side (30s oscillation / 30s end-range hold)
	PHASE 3	Bird Dog (Single Leg)	None	30s each side
	PHASE 4	A: Banded Glute Bridge B: Hinged Straight-Arm Pulldown	A: Long resistance band (medium) B: Long resistance band (light)	2–3 x 8–10 each exercise
	PHASE 5	A: Goblet Squat B: Inverted Row	A: Dumbbell or kettlebell B: Suspension trainer	3 x 5 each exercise
	PHASE 6	A: Vertical Jacks B: Vertical Jump	None	A: 3 x 5 B: 3 x 1
PRIMING & POTENTIATION	NEUROLOGICAL PRIMER	A: Rotating Med Ball Slam	Med ball	3 x 3
	MECHANICAL PRIMER	B: Glider Hamstring Curl	Gliders	3 x 15 each side
KEY PERFORMANCE INDICATOR (KPI)	LOWER	A: Front Squat	Barbell	3–4 x 12–15
	UPPER	B: Pull-Up	Rack	3–4 x 10–12
PUMP ACCESSORIES & PREHAB	HINGE	Romanian Deadlift (RDL)	Dumbbell	3 x 15
	PUSH	Slight Incline Dumbbell Bench Press	Dumbbells	3 x 12–15
	LUNGE	Dumbbell Lateral Lunge	Dumbbell	3 x 12–15 each side
	SHOULDERS	Seated Dumbbell Halo	Dumbbell	3 x 10 each direction
CONDITIONING FINISHER	CARRY	Overhead Carry	Dumbbells	4 x 30s
POST-TRAINING COOL-DOWN	BREATHE	Supine 90/90 Breathing	None	1m
	FOAM ROLL	Hamstrings	Foam roller	1m each side
	STRETCH	Supine Hamstring Stretch	Long resistance band / stretch strap	1m each side

3-DAY FULL-BODY PROGRAM

TRAINING PHASE	FOCUS	EXERCISE	EQUIPMENT/TOOL	SETS/REPS/DURATION/REST
PRE-TRAINING PREPARATION	PHASE 1	Adductor Group & Pectoralis Group	Foam roller	1m each exercise/side (30s oscillation / 30s neurological trigger point)
	PHASE 2	Adductor Rock-Back & 90/90 Chest Stretch	None	1m each exercise/side (30s oscillation / 30s end-range hold)
	PHASE 3	Dead Bug (Opposite Arm & Leg)	None	30s
	PHASE 4	A: Banded Glute Bridge B: Band Pull-Apart	A: Long resistance band (medium) B: Long resistance band (light)	2–3 x 8–10 each exercise
	PHASE 5	A: Romanian Deadlift (RDL) B: Push-Up	A: Dumbbell B: Suspension trainer	3 x 5 each exercise
	PHASE 6	A: Seal Jacks B: Bent-Over Med Ball Press (Repeater Variation)	A: None B: Med ball	3 x 5 each exercise
PRIMING & POTENTIATION	NEUROLOGICAL PRIMER	A: Explosive Band Press	Long resistance band (light)	3 x 5 each side
	MECHANICAL PRIMER	B: High-Angle Band Face Pull	Long resistance band (light)	3 x 20
KEY PERFORMANCE INDICATOR (KPI)	LOWER	A: Conventional Deadlift (Elevated)	Barbell	4 x 6–8
	UPPER	B: Bench Press	Barbell	4 x 6–8
PUMP ACCESSORIES & PREHAB	LUNGE	Front-Foot-Elevated Dumbbell Split Squat	Dumbbell	3 x 12
	PULL	Inverted Row	Suspension trainer	3 x 10–15
	PULL	Lat Pulldown	Cable	3 x 15
	CALVES	Deficit Calf Raise	Wedge or box	3 x 15
CONDITIONING FINISHER	LOWER BURNOUT	A: Alternating Curtsy Lunge B: Side Plank Hip Thrust C: 90/90 Squat Iso with Band Hip Abduction	A–B: None C: Short resistance band (medium)	3 rounds: A: 20 alternating (10 each side) B: Max reps each side (near failure) C: Max reps (near failure)
POST-TRAINING COOL-DOWN	BREATHE	Supine 90/90 Breathing	None	1m
	FOAM ROLL	Glutes	Foam roller	1m each side
	STRETCH	90/90 Glute Stretch	None	1m each side

3-DAY FULL-BODY PROGRAM

TRAINING PHASE	FOCUS	EXERCISE	EQUIPMENT/TOOL	SETS/REPS/DURATION/REST
PRE-TRAINING PREPARATION	PHASE 1	Lateral Hip & Posterior Shoulder	Foam roller	1m each exercise/side (30s oscillation / 30s neurological trigger point)
	PHASE 2	90/90 Glute Stretch & Posterior Shoulder Stretch	Suspension trainer	1m each exercise/side (30s oscillation / 30s end-range hold)
	PHASE 3	Side Plank Starfish	None	30s each side
	PHASE 4	A: Single-Leg Glute Bridge B: Band Over & Back	A: None B: Long resistance band (light)	2–3 x 8–10 each exercise
	PHASE 5	A: Bodyweight Reverse Lunge B: Inverted Row	A: None B: Suspension trainer	3 x 5 each exercise/side
	PHASE 6	A: Counter Movement Jump B: Explosive Band Press	A: None B: Long resistance band (light)	3 x 3 each exercise/side
PRIMING & POTENTIATION	NEUROLOGICAL PRIMER	A: Forward Skip	None	3 x 10 alternating
	MECHANICAL PRIMER	B: Banded Hip Thrust	Long resistance band (light)	3 x 20
KEY PERFORMANCE INDICATOR (KPI)	LOWER	A: Dumbbells at Sides Reverse Lunge	Dumbbells	4 x 6–8 each side
	UPPER	B: Half-Kneeling Cable Row	Cable	4 x 8–12 each side
PUMP ACCESSORIES & PREHAB	SQUAT	Dumbbell Goblet Squat	Dumbbell	3 x 15
	PUSH	Half-Kneeling Single-Arm Overhead Press	Dumbbell	3 x 12–15 each side
CONDITIONING FINISHER	ARM BURNOUT	A: Band Biceps Curl B: Band Triceps Push Down C: Dumbbell Lateral Raise	A–B: Long resistance band C: Dumbbells	2 x 20 each exercise
POST-TRAINING COOL-DOWN	BREATHE	Supine 90/90 Breathing	None	1m
	FOAM ROLL	Lats	Foam roller	1m each side
	STRETCH	Child's Pose (10 & 2)	None	1m each side

4-DAY UPPER/LOWER PROGRAM
LOWER/HINGE

RECLAIM
DAY 01

TRAINING PHASE	FOCUS	EXERCISE	EQUIPMENT/TOOL	SETS/REPS/DURATION/REST
PRE-TRAINING PREPARATION	PHASE 1	Adductor Group	Foam roller	1m each exercise/side (30s oscillation / 30s neurological trigger point)
	PHASE 2	Adductor Rock-Back	None	1m each exercise/side (30s oscillation / 30s end-range hold)
	PHASE 3	Bird Dog (Single Arm)	None	30s each side
	PHASE 4	Side-Lying Banded Clam	Short resistance band (medium)	2–3 x 8–10 each side
	PHASE 5	A: Romanian Deadlift (RDL) B: Bodyweight Squat	A: Dumbbell B: None	3 x 5 each exercise
	PHASE 6	A: Vertical Jacks B: Broad Jump	None	A: 3 x 5 B: 3 x 3
PRIMING & POTENTIATION	NEUROLOGICAL PRIMER	A: Supported Skip (Alternating)	None	3 x 5
	MECHANICAL PRIMER	B: Banded Glute Bridge	Long resistance band (medium)	3 x 20
KEY PERFORMANCE INDICATOR (KPI)	LOWER/HINGE	Kettlebell Romanian Deadlift (RDL)	Kettlebell	3–4 x 10–12
PUMP ACCESSORIES & PREHAB	SQUAT	A: Heels-Elevated Goblet Squat	Dumbbell	3 x 12
	LUNGE	B: Dumbbell Alternating Reverse Lunge	Dumbbell	3 x 10 each side
	CALVES	C: Calf Raises	None	3 x 15
CONDITIONING FINISHER	GLUTE BURNOUT	Banded Hip Thrust	Long resistance band (heavy)	2m AMRAP: do reps to near-failure, rest 15s, repeat for 2m
POST-TRAINING COOL-DOWN	BREATHE	Supine 90/90 Breathing	None	1m
	FOAM ROLL	Glutes	Foam roller	1m each side
	STRETCH	Supine Figure 4	None	1m each side

4-DAY UPPER/LOWER PROGRAM

UPPER/PUSH

RECLAIM **DAY 02**

TRAINING PHASE	FOCUS	EXERCISE	EQUIPMENT/TOOL	SETS/REPS/DURATION/REST
PRE-TRAINING PREPARATION	PHASE 1	Pectoralis Group	Foam roller	1m each side (30s oscillation / 30s neurological trigger point)
	PHASE 2	90/90 Chest Stretch	None	1m each side (30s oscillation / 30s end-range hold)
	PHASE 3	Quadruped T-Spine Rotation	None	30s
	PHASE 4	Rusin Tri-Set A: Band Over & Back B: Band Face Pull C: Band Pull-Apart	Long resistance band (light)	2–3 x 8–10 each exercise
	PHASE 5	Pause Push-Up	None	3 x 5
	PHASE 6	A: Seal Jacks B: Bent-Over Med Ball Press	A: None B: Med ball	A: 3 x 5 B: 3 x 3
PRIMING & POTENTIATION	NEUROLOGICAL PRIMER	A: Explosive Band Press (Bilateral)	Long resistance band (light)	3 x 5 each side
	MECHANICAL PRIMER	B: Band Face Pull	Long resistance band (light)	3 x 15–20
KEY PERFORMANCE INDICATOR (KPI)	UPPER/PUSH	Deficit Loaded Push-Up	Weight plate	3–4 x 8–10
PUMP ACCESSORIES & PREHAB	PUSH	A: Landmine Single-Arm Press	Landmine	3 x 10–12 each side
	PULL	B: Three-Point Bench Row	Dumbbell	3 x 10–12 each side
	CHEST	C: Dumbbell Floor Pec Fly	Dumbbells	3 x 12–15
CONDITIONING FINISHER	SHOULDER BURNOUT	Double-Banded Rear Delt Fly to Overhead	Long resistance bands (light)	2m AMRAP: do reps to near-failure, rest 15s, repeat for 2m
POST-TRAINING COOL-DOWN	BREATHE	Supine 90/90 Breathing	None	1m
	FOAM ROLL	Pectoralis Group	Foam roller	1m each side
	STRETCH	Prone Pec Stretch	None	1m each side

4-DAY UPPER/LOWER PROGRAM
LOWER/SQUAT

TRAINING PHASE	FOCUS	EXERCISE	EQUIPMENT/TOOL	SETS/REPS/DURATION/REST
PRE-TRAINING PREPARATION	PHASE 1	Quadriceps	Foam roller	1m each side (30s oscillation / 30s neurological trigger point)
	PHASE 2	Half-Kneeling Hip Flexor Stretch	None	1m each side (30s oscillation / 30s end-range hold)
	PHASE 3	Knee-Bend Side Plank	None	30s each side
	PHASE 4	Banded Single-Leg Glute Bridge	Short resistance band (light)	2–3 x 8–10 each side
	PHASE 5	Bodyweight Squat	None	3 x 5
	PHASE 6	A: Vertical Jacks B: Vertical Jump	None	A: 3 x 5 B: 3 x 3
PRIMING & POTENTIATION	NEUROLOGICAL PRIMER	A: Snap-Down	None	3 x 3
	MECHANICAL PRIMER	B: Prone Banded Hamstring Curl	Long resistance band (light)	3 x 20
KEY PERFORMANCE INDICATOR (KPI)	LOWER/SQUAT	Goblet Squat	Dumbbell	3–4 x 10–12
PUMP ACCESSORIES & PREHAB	HINGE	A: Romanian Deadlift (RDL)	Dumbbell	3 x 12
	LUNGE	B: Contralateral Dumbbell Split Squat	Dumbbell	3 x 10–12 each side
	CORE	C: Side Plank	None	3 x 30s each side
CONDITIONING FINISHER	CARRY	Farmer's Carry (Bilateral)	Dumbbells	3–4 x 20s
POST-TRAINING COOL-DOWN	BREATHE	Supine 90/90 Breathing	None	1m
	FOAM ROLL	Adductor Group	Foam roller	1m each side
	STRETCH	Frog Stretch	None	1m each side

4-DAY UPPER/LOWER PROGRAM
UPPER/PULL

TRAINING PHASE	FOCUS	EXERCISE	EQUIPMENT/TOOL	SETS/REPS/DURATION/REST
PRE-TRAINING PREPARATION	PHASE 1	Thoracic Spine	Foam roller	1m (30s oscillation / 30s neurological trigger point)
	PHASE 2	Hinged T-Spine Extension / Bilateral Lat Stretch	Suspension trainer	1m (30s oscillation / 30s end-range hold)
	PHASE 3	Quadruped T-Spine Rotation	None	30s
	PHASE 4	Rusin Tri-Set A: Band Over & Back B: Band Face Pull C: Band Pull-Apart	Long resistance band (light)	2–3 x 8–10 each exercise
	PHASE 5	Inverted Row	Suspension trainer	3 x 5
	PHASE 6	A: Vertical Jacks B: Med Ball Slam	A: None B: Med ball	A: 3 x 5 B: 3 x 3
PRIMING & POTENTIATION	NEUROLOGICAL PRIMER	A: High Kneeling Med Ball Slam	Med ball	3 x 5
	MECHANICAL PRIMER	B: High Kneeling Straight-Arm Pulldown	Long resistance band (light)	3 x 15
KEY PERFORMANCE INDICATOR (KPI)	UPPER/PULL	High-Angle Pulldown	Long resistance band (light)	3–4 x 10
PUMP ACCESSORIES & PREHAB	PUSH	A: Push-Up (optional: loaded)	Weight plate (optional)	3 x 12
	PULL	B: Half-Kneeling High-Angle Face Pull	Long resistance band (light) or cable	3 x 10–15
	CHEST	C: Chest-Supported Dumbbell T	Dumbbells	3 x 12–15
CONDITIONING FINISHER	CORE BURNOUT	Half-Kneeling Cable or Band Chop	Long resistance band (light) or cable	2m AMRAP: do reps to near-failure, rest 15s, repeat for 2m
POST-TRAINING COOL-DOWN	BREATHE	Supine 90/90 Breathing	None	1m
	FOAM ROLL	Lats	Foam roller	1m each side
	STRETCH	Child's Pose (10 & 2)	None	1m each side

4-DAY UPPER/LOWER PROGRAM
LOWER/HINGE

TRAINING PHASE	FOCUS	EXERCISE	EQUIPMENT/TOOL	SETS/REPS/DURATION/REST
PRE-TRAINING PREPARATION	PHASE 1	Adductor Group	Foam roller	1m each side (30s oscillation / 30s neurological trigger point)
	PHASE 2	Adductor Rock-Back	None	1m each side (30s oscillation / 30s end-range hold)
	PHASE 3	Bird Dog (Single Leg)	None	30s each side
	PHASE 4	Side Plank Hip Thrust (Feet Together)	None	30s each side
	PHASE 5	A: Romanian Deadlift (RDL) B: Bodyweight Squat	A: Dumbbell B: None	3 x 5 each exercise
	PHASE 6	A: Vertical Jacks B: Broad Jump	None	A: 3 x 5 B: 3 x 3
PRIMING & POTENTIATION	NEUROLOGICAL PRIMER	A: Forward Skip	None	3 x 5
	MECHANICAL PRIMER	B: Banded Hip Thrust	Long resistance band (medium)	3 x 20
KEY PERFORMANCE INDICATOR (KPI)	LOWER/HINGE	Trap Bar Deadlift	Trap bar	3–4 x 12–15
PUMP ACCESSORIES & PREHAB	SQUAT	A: Landmine Goblet Squat	Landmine	3 x 15
	LUNGE	B: Dumbbell Front-Foot-Elevated Alternating Reverse Lunge	Dumbbell	3 x 12–15 alternating each side
	CALVES	C: Deficit Calf Raise	Wedge or box	3 x 15
CONDITIONING FINISHER	GLUTE BURNOUT	A: Dumbbell Hip Thrust B: Banded Side-Lying Hip Abduction	A: Dumbbell B: Short resistance band (medium)	2m AMRAP: do reps to near-failure, rest 15s, repeat for 2m
POST-TRAINING COOL-DOWN	BREATHE	Supine 90/90 Breathing	None	1m
	FOAM ROLL	Glutes	Foam roller	1m each side
	STRETCH	Supine Figure 4	None	1m each side

4-DAY UPPER/LOWER PROGRAM
UPPER/PUSH

REBUILD **DAY 02**

TRAINING PHASE	FOCUS	EXERCISE	EQUIPMENT/TOOL	SETS/REPS/DURATION/REST
PRE-TRAINING PREPARATION	PHASE 1	Pectoralis Group	Foam roller	1m each side (30s oscillation / 30s neurological trigger point)
	PHASE 2	90/90 Chest Stretch	None	1m each side (30s oscillation / 30s end-range hold)
	PHASE 3	Quadruped T-Spine Rotation	None	30s
	PHASE 4	Rusin Tri-Set A: Band Over & Back B: Band Face Pull C: Band Pull-Apart	Long resistance band (light)	2–3 x 8–10 each exercise
	PHASE 5	Pause Push-Up	None	3 x 5
	PHASE 6	A: Seal Jacks B: Explosive Band Press	A: None B: Long resistance band (light)	A: 3 x 5 B: 3 x 3 each side
PRIMING & POTENTIATION	NEUROLOGICAL PRIMER	A: Bent-Over Med Ball Chest Press (Singles)	Med ball	3 x 5
	MECHANICAL PRIMER	B: Hands-Free Double-Band Face Pull	Long resistance bands (light)	3 x 20
KEY PERFORMANCE INDICATOR (KPI)	UPPER/PUSH	Dumbbell Bench Press	Dumbbells	3–4 x 12–15
PUMP ACCESSORIES & PREHAB	PUSH	A: Half-Kneeling Single-Arm Overhead Press	Dumbbell	3 x 12–15 each side
	PULL	B: Three-Point Bench Row	Dumbbell	3 x 10–12 each side
	CHEST	C: Bench Dumbbell Pec Fly	Dumbbells	3 x 15
CONDITIONING FINISHER	SHOULDER/ BICEPS BURNOUT	A: High-Angle Face Pull B: Alternating Dumbbell Curl	A: Long resistance band (light) B: Dumbbells	5m AMRAP: do exercises to near-failure, alternating continuously with minimal rest
POST-TRAINING COOL-DOWN	BREATHE	Supine 90/90 Breathing	None	1m
	FOAM ROLL	Pectoralis Group	Foam roller	1m each side
	STRETCH	Prone Pec Stretch	None	1m each side

4-DAY UPPER/LOWER PROGRAM
LOWER/SQUAT

TRAINING PHASE	FOCUS	EXERCISE	EQUIPMENT/TOOL	SETS/REPS/DURATION/REST
PRE-TRAINING PREPARATION	PHASE 1	Quadriceps	Foam roller	1m each side (30s oscillation / 30s neurological trigger point)
	PHASE 2	Half-Kneeling Hip Flexor Stretch	None	1m each side (30s oscillation / 30s end-range hold)
	PHASE 3	Side Plank	None	30s each side
	PHASE 4	Banded Single-Leg Glute Bridge	Short resistance band (light)	2–3 x 8–10 each side
	PHASE 5	Bodyweight Squat	None	3 x 5
	PHASE 6	A: Vertical Jacks B: Vertical Jump	None	A: 3 x 5 B: 3 x 3
PRIMING & POTENTIATION	NEUROLOGICAL PRIMER	A: Snap-Down	None	3 x 3
	MECHANICAL PRIMER	B: Prone Banded Hamstring Curl	Long resistance band (light)	3 x 20
KEY PERFORMANCE INDICATOR (KPI)	LOWER/SQUAT	Landmine Goblet Squat	Landmine	3–4 x 10–12
PUMP ACCESSORIES & PREHAB	HINGE	A: Landmine Romanian Deadlift (RDL)	Landmine	3 x 15
	LUNGE	B: Rear-Foot-Elevated Split Squat (Bulgarian)	Dumbbells (optional)	3 x 10–15 each side
	CORE	C: Hip Drop Side Plank	None	3 x 30s each side
CONDITIONING FINISHER	CARRY	Front Rack Carry (Bilateral)	Dumbbells	4 x 30s
POST-TRAINING COOL-DOWN	BREATHE	Supine 90/90 Breathing	None	1m
	FOAM ROLL	Adductor Group	Foam roller	1m each side
	STRETCH	Frog Stretch	None	1m each side

4-DAY UPPER/LOWER PROGRAM
UPPER/PULL

TRAINING PHASE	FOCUS	EXERCISE	EQUIPMENT/TOOL	SETS/REPS/DURATION/REST
PRE-TRAINING PREPARATION	PHASE 1	Thoracic Spine	Foam roller	1m (30s oscillation / 30s neurological trigger point)
	PHASE 2	Hinged T-Spine Extension / Bilateral Lat Stretch	Suspension trainer	1m (30s oscillation / 30s end-range hold)
	PHASE 3	Quadruped T-Spine Rotation	None	30s
	PHASE 4	Rusin Tri-Set A: Band Over & Back B: Band Face Pull C: Band Pull-Apart	Long resistance band (light)	2–3 x 8–10 each exercise
	PHASE 5	Inverted Row	Suspension trainer	3 x 5
	PHASE 6	A: Vertical Jacks B: Med Ball Slam	A: None B: Med ball	A: 3 x 5 B: 3 x 3
PRIMING & POTENTIATION	NEUROLOGICAL PRIMER	A: Anti-Flexion Med Ball Slam	Med ball	3 x 3
	MECHANICAL PRIMER	B: Bent-Over Straight-Arm Pulldown	Long resistance band (light)	3 x 15
KEY PERFORMANCE INDICATOR (KPI)	UPPER/PULL	Lat Pulldown	Cable or long resistance band	3–4 x 10–12
PUMP ACCESSORIES & PREHAB	PUSH	A: Hand-Release Push-Up (optional: loaded)	Weight plate (optional)	3 x 12
	PULL	B: Half-Kneeling High-Angle Single-Arm Row	Cable or long resistance band	3 x 12–15 each side
	SHOULDERS	C: Chest-Supported Dumbbell Y	Dumbbells	3 x 12–15
CONDITIONING FINISHER	SHOULDER/ ARM BURNOUT	A: Seated Dumbbell Lateral Raise B: Lying Neutral Grip Dumbbell Skull Crusher	Dumbbells	5m AMRAP: do exercises to near-failure, alternating continuously with minimal rest
POST-TRAINING COOL-DOWN	BREATHE	Supine 90/90 Breathing	None	1m
	FOAM ROLL	Pectoralis Group	Foam roller	1m each side
	STRETCH	Prone Pec Stretch	None	1m each side

4-DAY UPPER/LOWER PROGRAM
LOWER/HINGE

REGAIN DAY 01

TRAINING PHASE	FOCUS	EXERCISE	EQUIPMENT/TOOL	SETS/REPS/DURATION/REST
PRE-TRAINING PREPARATION	PHASE 1	Adductor Group	Foam roller	1m each side (30s oscillation / 30s neurological trigger point)
	PHASE 2	Adductor Rock-Back	None	1m each side (30s oscillation / 30s end-range hold)
	PHASE 3	Bird Dog (Arm & Leg Opposites)	None	30s
	PHASE 4	Side Plank Hip Thrust	None	30s each side
	PHASE 5	A: Romanian Deadlift (RDL) B: Bodyweight Squat	A: Dumbbell B: None	3 x 5 each exercise
	PHASE 6	A: Vertical Jacks B: Broad Jump	None	A: 3 x 5 B: 3 x 3
PRIMING & POTENTIATION	NEUROLOGICAL PRIMER	A: Band-Resisted Broad Jump	None	3 x 3
	MECHANICAL PRIMER	B: Banded Glute Bridge March	Short resistance band (medium)	3 x 20 alternating
KEY PERFORMANCE INDICATOR (KPI)	LOWER/HINGE	Conventional Deadlift (Elevated to Match Hinge Assessment)	Barbell	4 x 6–8
PUMP ACCESSORIES & PREHAB	SQUAT	1A: Heels-Elevated Dumbbell Goblet Squat	Dumbbell	3 x 15
	LUNGE	1B: Dumbbell Forward Lunge	Dumbbell	3 x 10–15 alternating each side
	CALVES	1C: Single-Leg Deficit Calf Raise	Wedge or box	3 x 10–15 each side
	HINGE	2A: Cable Pull-Through	Cable	2–3 x 15
	CORE	2B: Side Plank Starfish Iso	None	2–3 x 20–30s each side
CONDITIONING FINISHER	LOWER BURNOUT	A: Dumbbell Alternating Curtsy Lunge B: Side Plank Hip Thrust w/ Pause C: 90/90 Squat Iso with Band Hip Abduction	A: Dumbbell B: None C: Short resistance band (medium)	3 rounds: A: 20 alternating (10 each side) B: Max reps (near failure) C: Max reps (near failure)
POST-TRAINING COOL-DOWN	BREATHE	Supine 90/90 Breathing	None	1m
	FOAM ROLL	Glutes	Foam roller	1m each side
	STRETCH	Supine Figure 4	None	1m each side

4-DAY UPPER/LOWER PROGRAM
UPPER/PUSH

TRAINING PHASE	FOCUS	EXERCISE	EQUIPMENT/TOOL	SETS/REPS/DURATION/REST
PRE-TRAINING PREPARATION	PHASE 1	Pectoralis Group	Foam roller	1m each side (30s oscillation / 30s neurological trigger point)
	PHASE 2	90/90 Chest Stretch	None	1m each side (30s oscillation / 30s end-range hold)
	PHASE 3	Quadruped T-Spine Rotation	None	30s
	PHASE 4	Rusin Tri-Set A: Band Over & Back B: Band Face Pull C: Band Pull-Apart	Long resistance band (light)	2–3 x 8–10 each exercise
	PHASE 5	Pause Push-Up	None	3 x 5
	PHASE 6	A: Seal Jacks B: Explosive Band Press	A: None B: Long resistance band (light)	A: 3 x 5 B: 3 x 3 each side
PRIMING & POTENTIATION	NEUROLOGICAL PRIMER	A: Bent-Over Med Ball Chest Press (Repeaters)	Med ball	3 x 5
	MECHANICAL PRIMER	B: High-Angle Band Face Pull	Long resistance band (light)	3 x 20
KEY PERFORMANCE INDICATOR (KPI)	UPPER/PUSH	Bench Press	Barbell	4 x 6–8
PUMP ACCESSORIES & PREHAB	PULL	1A: Lat Pulldown	Cable	3 x 15
	SHOULDERS	1B: Half-Kneeling Dumbbell Halo	Dumbbell	3 x 15 alternating
	PUSH	2A: Single-Arm Dumbbell Overhead Press Split Stance 2B: Single-Arm Landmine Row 2C: Slight Incline Dumbbell Pec Fly	2A: Dumbbell 2B: Landmine 2C: Dumbbells	2A: 3 x 12–15 each side 2B: 3 x 12–15 each side 2C: 3 x 15
CONDITIONING FINISHER	SHOULDER/ BICEPS BURNOUT	A: Dumbbell Hammer Curl B: Dumbbell Tate Press C: Alternating Front/Lateral Raise	Dumbbells	2–3 x 20 each exercise
POST-TRAINING COOL-DOWN	BREATHE	Supine 90/90 Breathing	None	1m
	FOAM ROLL	Pectoralis Group	Foam roller	1m each side
	STRETCH	Prone Pec Stretch	None	1m each side

4-DAY UPPER/LOWER PROGRAM
LOWER/SQUAT

TRAINING PHASE	FOCUS	EXERCISE	EQUIPMENT/TOOL	SETS/REPS/DURATION/REST
PRE-TRAINING PREPARATION	PHASE 1	Quadriceps	Foam roller	1m each side (30s oscillation / 30s neurological trigger point)
	PHASE 2	Half-Kneeling Hip Flexor Stretch	None	1m each side (30s oscillation / 30s end-range hold)
	PHASE 3	Starfish	None	30s each side
	PHASE 4	Banded Single-Leg Glute Bridge	Short resistance band (light)	2–3 x 8–10 each side
	PHASE 5	Bodyweight Squat	None	3 x 5
	PHASE 6	A: Vertical Jacks B: Vertical Jump	None	A: 3 x 5 B: 3 x 3
PRIMING & POTENTIATION	NEUROLOGICAL PRIMER	A: Countermovement Jump	None	3 x 3
	MECHANICAL PRIMER	B: Suspension Hamstring Curl to Hip Thrust	Suspension trainer	3 x 10–15
KEY PERFORMANCE INDICATOR (KPI)	LOWER/SQUAT	Front Squat	Barbell	4 x 6–8
PUMP ACCESSORIES & PREHAB	HINGE	1A: Barbell Romanian Deadlift (RDL)	Barbell	3 x 15
	LUNGE	1B: Contralateral Rear-Foot-Elevated Split Squat (Bulgarian)	Dumbbell	3 x 12 each side
	CORE	1C: Side Plank March	None	3 x 20–30s each side
	LUNGE	2A: Dumbbell Lateral Lunge	Dumbbell	3 x 10–15 alternating each side
	GLUTES	2B: Standing Banded Hip Flexor March	Short resistance band (medium)	3 x 15 each side
CONDITIONING FINISHER	CARRY	Mixed-Grip Carry (Bilateral)	Dumbbells	4 x 30s
POST-TRAINING COOL-DOWN	BREATHE	Supine 90/90 Breathing	None	1m
	FOAM ROLL	Adductor Group	Foam roller	1m each side
	STRETCH	Frog Stretch	None	1m each side

4-DAY UPPER/LOWER PROGRAM
UPPER/PULL

TRAINING PHASE	FOCUS	EXERCISE	EQUIPMENT/TOOL	SETS/REPS/DURATION/REST
PRE-TRAINING PREPARATION	PHASE 1	Thoracic Spine	Foam roller	1m (30s oscillation / 30s neurological trigger point)
	PHASE 2	Hinged T-Spine Extension / Bilateral Lat Stretch	Suspension trainer	1m (30s oscillation / 30s end-range hold)
	PHASE 3	Quadruped T-Spine Rotation	None	30s
	PHASE 4	Rusin Tri-Set A: Band Over & Back B: Band Face Pull C: Band Pull-Apart	Long resistance band (light)	2–3 x 8–10 each exercise
	PHASE 5	Inverted Row	Suspension trainer	3 x 5
	PHASE 6	A: Vertical Jacks B: Med Ball Slam	A: None B: Med ball	A: 3 x 5 B: 3 x 3
PRIMING & POTENTIATION	NEUROLOGICAL PRIMER	A: Anti-Flexion Med Ball Slam	Med ball	3 x 5
	MECHANICAL PRIMER	B: Band Pull Down and Apart	Long resistance band (light)	3 x 15–20
KEY PERFORMANCE INDICATOR (KPI)	UPPER/PULL	Neutral Grip Pull-Up	Rack	4 x 6–8
PUMP ACCESSORIES & PREHAB	PUSH	1A: Deficit Push-Up (optional: loaded)	Weight plate (optional)	3 x 8–12
	PULL	1B: Cable Split Stance High-Angle Row	Cable or long resistance band	3 x 10–15 each side
	SHOULDERS	1C: Chest-Supported Dumbbell Face Pull to External Rotation	Dumbbells	3 x 12–15
	SHOULDERS	2A: Banded Single-Arm Rear Delt Fly	Long resistance band (light)	2–3 x 15 each side
	BICEPS	2B: Suspension Trainer Biceps Curl	Suspension trainer	2–3 x 15
CONDITIONING FINISHER	CORE/HINGE BURNOUT	A: Standing Band Crunch B: Oblique Crunch C: Sumo Stance Banded Good Morning	A: Long resistance band B: None C: Long resistance band	2–3 rounds: A: 15 reps B: 10 reps each side C: 15 reps
POST-TRAINING COOL-DOWN	BREATHE	Supine 90/90 Breathing	None	1m
	FOAM ROLL	Lats	Foam roller	1m each side
	STRETCH	Child's Pose (10 & 2)	None	1m each side

5-DAY MOVEMENT PATTERN SPLIT PROGRAM

RECLAIM DAY 01

LOWER/HINGE

TRAINING PHASE	FOCUS	EXERCISE	EQUIPMENT/TOOL	SETS/REPS/DURATION/REST
PRE-TRAINING PREPARATION	PHASE 1	Adductor Group	Foam roller	1m each side (30s oscillation / 30s neurological trigger point)
	PHASE 2	Adductor Rock-Back	None	1m each side (30s oscillation / 30s end-range hold)
	PHASE 3	Bird Dog (Single Arm)	None	30s each side
	PHASE 4	Side-Lying Banded Clam	Short resistance band (medium)	2–3 x 8–10 each exercise
	PHASE 5	Romanian Deadlift (RDL)	Dumbbell	3 x 5
	PHASE 6	A: Vertical Jacks B: Broad Jump	None	A: 3 x 5 B: 3 x 3
PRIMING & POTENTIATION	NEUROLOGICAL PRIMER	A: Supported Skip (Alternating)	None	3 x 5
	MECHANICAL PRIMER	B: Banded Glute Bridge	Long resistance band (medium)	3 x 20
KEY PERFORMANCE INDICATOR (KPI)	LOWER/HINGE	Kettlebell Romanian Deadlift (RDL)	Kettlebell	3–4 x 10–12
PUMP ACCESSORIES & PREHAB	SQUAT	1A: Goblet Squat	Dumbbell	3 x 12
	LUNGE	1B: Dumbbell Curtsy Lunge	Dumbbell	3 x 16–20 each side
	CALVES	1C: Calf Raise	None	3 x 15
	HAMSTRINGS	2A: Ball Hamstring Curl	Physio ball	2–3 x 12 each side
	CORE	2B: Plank to Pike	None	2–3 x 15
CONDITIONING FINISHER	GLUTE BURNOUT	Banded Hip Thrust	Long resistance band (heavy)	2m AMRAP: do reps to near-failure, rest 15s, repeat for 2m
POST-TRAINING COOL-DOWN	BREATHE	Supine 90/90 Breathing	None	1m
	FOAM ROLL	Glutes	Foam roller	1m each side
	STRETCH	Supine Figure 4	None	1m each side

5-DAY MOVEMENT PATTERN SPLIT PROGRAM
UPPER/PUSH

TRAINING PHASE	FOCUS	EXERCISE	EQUIPMENT/TOOL	SETS/REPS/DURATION/REST
PRE-TRAINING PREPARATION	PHASE 1	Pectoralis Group	Foam roller	1m each side (30s oscillation / 30s neurological trigger point)
	PHASE 2	90/90 Chest Stretch	None	1m each side (30s oscillation / 30s end-range hold)
	PHASE 3	Quadruped T-Spine Rotation	None	30s
	PHASE 4	Rusin Tri-Set A: Band Over & Back B: Band Face Pull C: Band Pull-Apart	Long resistance band (light)	2–3 x 8–10 each exercise
	PHASE 5	Pause Push-Up	None	3 x 5
	PHASE 6	A: Seal Jacks B: Bent-Over Med Ball Press	A: None B: Med ball	A: 3 x 5 B: 3 x 3
PRIMING & POTENTIATION	NEUROLOGICAL PRIMER	A: Band Assisted Plyo Push-Up	Long resistance band (medium)	3 x 5
	MECHANICAL PRIMER	B: Half-Kneeling Band Pull-Apart	Long resistance band (light)	3 x 20
KEY PERFORMANCE INDICATOR (KPI)	UPPER/PUSH	Deficit Push-Up (optional: loaded)	Weight plate (optional)	3–4 x 10–12
PUMP ACCESSORIES & PREHAB	PUSH	1A: Half-Kneeling Single-Arm Cable Press	Cable or long resistance band	3 x 10–12
	PULL (HORIZONTAL)	1B: Inverted Row	Suspension trainer	3 x 12
	PULL (VERTICAL)	1C: Tall Kneeling High-Angle Row	Cable or long resistance band	3 x 12–15 each side
	TRICEPS	2A: Dumbbell Lying Triceps Extension	Dumbbell	2 x 12–15
	FOREARMS/ GRIP	2B: Bench-Supported Dumbbell Wrist Extension	Dumbbells	2 x 12–15 each side
CONDITIONING FINISHER	SHOULDER BURNOUT	Half-Kneeling Band Face Pull to Y Press	Long resistance band (light)	2m AMRAP: do reps to near-failure, rest 15s, repeat for 2m
POST-TRAINING COOL-DOWN	BREATHE	Supine 90/90 Breathing	None	1m
	FOAM ROLL	Pectoralis Group	Foam roller	1m each side
	STRETCH	Prone Pec Stretch	None	1m each side

5-DAY MOVEMENT PATTERN SPLIT PROGRAM

LOWER/SQUAT

TRAINING PHASE	FOCUS	EXERCISE	EQUIPMENT/TOOL	SETS/REPS/DURATION/REST
PRE-TRAINING PREPARATION	PHASE 1	Quadriceps	Foam roller	1m each side (30s oscillation / 30s neurological trigger point)
	PHASE 2	Half-Kneeling Hip Flexor Stretch	None	1m each side (30s oscillation / 30s end-range hold)
	PHASE 3	Side Plank	None	30s each side
	PHASE 4	Banded Single-Leg Glute Bridge	Short resistance band (light)	2–3 x 8–10 each side
	PHASE 5	Bodyweight Squat	None	3 x 5
	PHASE 6	A: Vertical Jacks B: Depth Drop	None	A: 3 x 5 B: 3 x 3
PRIMING & POTENTIATION	NEUROLOGICAL PRIMER	A: Snap-Down	None	3 x 3
	MECHANICAL PRIMER	B: Prone Banded Hamstring Curl	Long resistance band (light)	3 x 20
KEY PERFORMANCE INDICATOR (KPI)	LOWER/SQUAT	Goblet Squat	Dumbbell	3–4 x 10–12
PUMP ACCESSORIES & PREHAB	HINGE	1A: Landmine Romanian Deadlift (RDL)	Landmine	3 x 12
	LUNGE	1B: Dumbbell Contralateral Split Squat	Dumbbell	3 x 10–12
	HIP ER/IR	1C: Shin Box with Rotation (Alternating)	None	3 x 20 alternating between sides
	CORE/GLUTES	2A: Quadruped Banded Leg Extension	Long resistance band (medium)	2–3 x 15
	CORE	2B: Dead Bug Banded Pullover Iso w/ Alternating Leg Extension	Long resistance band (medium)	2–3 x 30s
CONDITIONING FINISHER	CARRY	Farmer's Carry (Bilateral)	Dumbbells	4 x 30s
POST-TRAINING COOL-DOWN	BREATHE	Supine 90/90 Breathing	None	1m
	FOAM ROLL	Adductor Group	Foam roller	1m each side
	STRETCH	Frog Stretch	None	1m each side

5-DAY MOVEMENT PATTERN SPLIT PROGRAM
UPPER/PULL

RECLAIM **DAY 04**

TRAINING PHASE	FOCUS	EXERCISE	EQUIPMENT/TOOL	SETS/REPS/DURATION/REST
PRE-TRAINING PREPARATION	PHASE 1	Thoracic Spine	Foam roller	1m (30s oscillation / 30s neurological trigger point)
	PHASE 2	Hinged T-Spine Extension / Bilateral Lat Stretch	Suspension trainer	1m (30s oscillation / 30s end-range hold)
	PHASE 3	Quadruped T-Spine Rotation	None	30s
	PHASE 4	Rusin Tri-Set A: Band Over & Back B: Band Face Pull C: Band Pull-Apart	Long resistance band (light)	2–3 x 8–10 each exercise
	PHASE 5	Inverted Row	Suspension trainer	3 x 5
	PHASE 6	A: Vertical Jacks B: Med Ball Slam	A: None B: Med ball	A: 3 x 5 B: 3 x 3
PRIMING & POTENTIATION	NEUROLOGICAL PRIMER	A: Dumbbell Ballistic Row	Dumbbell	3 x 5 each side
	MECHANICAL PRIMER	B: Tall Kneeling Straight-Arm Pulldown	Long resistance band (light)	3 x 15
KEY PERFORMANCE INDICATOR (KPI)	UPPER/PULL	Bilateral Half-Kneeling High-Angle Row	Cable or long resistance band	3–4 x 8–10
PUMP ACCESSORIES & PREHAB	PUSH	1A: Single-Arm Dumbbell Bench Press	Dumbbell	3 x 10–12 each side
	PULL	1B: Three-Point Bench Row	Dumbbell	3 x 10–12 each side
	CORE	1C: Side Plank Iso	None	3 x 30s each side
	BICEPS	2A: Hammer Curl	Dumbbells	2–3 x 10
	CORE	2B: Plank	None	2–3 x 30s
CONDITIONING FINISHER	SHOULDER BURNOUT	Band Pull-Apart	Long resistance band (light)	2m AMRAP: do reps to near-failure, rest 15s, repeat for 2m
POST-TRAINING COOL-DOWN	BREATHE	Supine 90/90 Breathing	None	1m
	FOAM ROLL	Lats	Foam roller	1m each side
	STRETCH	Child's Pose (10 & 2)	None	1m each side

5-DAY MOVEMENT PATTERN SPLIT PROGRAM
FULL BODY/LUNGE

RECLAIM DAY **05**

TRAINING PHASE	FOCUS	EXERCISE	EQUIPMENT/TOOL	SETS/REPS/DURATION/REST
PRE-TRAINING PREPARATION	PHASE 1	Lateral Hip	Foam roller	1m each side (30s oscillation / 30s neurological trigger point)
	PHASE 2	Half-Kneeling Hip Flexor Stretch	None	1m each side (30s oscillation / 30s end-range hold)
	PHASE 3	Dead Bug (Single Arm)	None	30s
	PHASE 4	A: Banded Glute Bridge B: Band Pull-Apart	A: Long resistance band (medium) B: Long resistance band (light)	2–3 x 8–10 each exercise
	PHASE 5	Split Squat	None	3 x 5
	PHASE 6	A: Seal Jacks B: Supported Skip (Alternating)	None	A: 3 x 5 B: 3 x 5
PRIMING & POTENTIATION	NEUROLOGICAL PRIMER	A: Landmine Power Thruster	Landmine	3 x 5
	MECHANICAL PRIMER	B: Hip-Banded Bodyweight Good Morning	Long resistance band (medium)	3 x 15
KEY PERFORMANCE INDICATOR (KPI)	LOWER/LUNGE	Dumbbell Reverse Lunge Ipsilateral Load	Dumbbell or kettlebell	3–4 x 10–12
PUMP ACCESSORIES & PREHAB	SQUAT	1A: Hand-Release Push-Up	None	3 x 12
	LUNGE	1B: Suspension-Assisted Lateral Split Squat (Cossack)	Suspension trainer	3 x 20 alternating
	CARRY/CORE	1C: Crawl Hover	None	3 x 30s
	PULL	2A: Inverted Row	Suspension trainer	2–3 x 10–15
	SHOULDERS	2B: Powell Raise	Dumbbells	2–3 x 10–15 each side
CONDITIONING FINISHER	CORE BURNOUT	A: Kneeling Banded Ab Crunch B: Pallof Press from Full Kneeling	A: Long resistance band (medium) B: Cable or long resistance band	5m AMRAP A: 15 reps B: 10 reps each side
POST-TRAINING COOL-DOWN	BREATHE	Supine 90/90 Breathing	None	1m
	FOAM ROLL	T-Spine & Quadriceps	Foam roller	1m each exercise/side
	STRETCH	Prone Quad Stretch & Child's Pose (10 & 2)	None	1m each exercise/side

5-DAY MOVEMENT PATTERN SPLIT PROGRAM
LOWER/HINGE

TRAINING PHASE	FOCUS	EXERCISE	EQUIPMENT/TOOL	SETS/REPS/DURATION/REST
PRE-TRAINING PREPARATION	PHASE 1	Adductor Group	Foam roller	1m each side (30s oscillation / 30s neurological trigger point)
	PHASE 2	Adductor Rock-Back	None	1m each side (30s oscillation / 30s end-range hold)
	PHASE 3	Bird Dog (Single Leg)	None	30s each side
	PHASE 4	Side Plank Hip Thrust (Feet Together)	Short resistance band (medium)	30s each side
	PHASE 5	Romanian Deadlift (RDL)	Dumbbell	3 x 5
	PHASE 6	A: Vertical Jacks B: Broad Jump	None	A: 3 x 5 B: 3 x 3
PRIMING & POTENTIATION	NEUROLOGICAL PRIMER	A: Skip	None	3 x 5
	MECHANICAL PRIMER	B: Banded Hip Thrust	Long resistance band (medium)	3 x 20
KEY PERFORMANCE INDICATOR (KPI)	LOWER/HINGE	Trap Bar Deadlift	Trap bar	3–4 x 12–15
PUMP ACCESSORIES & PREHAB	SQUAT	1A: Heels-Elevated Goblet Squat (Narrow Stance)	Dumbbell	3 x 15
	LUNGE	1B: Dumbbell Curtsy Lunge (Alternating)	Dumbbell	3 x 16–20 alternating
	CALVES	1C: Deficit Calf Raise	None	3 x 15
	HAMSTRINGS	2A: Landmine Single-Leg Romanian Deadlift (RDL)	Landmine	2–3 x 15 each side
	CORE/UPPER	2B: Plank to Pike with Push-Up	None	2–3 x 10–12
CONDITIONING FINISHER	GLUTE BURNOUT	A: Dumbbell Hip Thrust B: Banded Side-Lying Hip Abduction	A: Dumbbell B: Short resistance band (medium)	5m AMRAP A: 15 reps B: 15 reps each side
POST-TRAINING COOL-DOWN	BREATHE	Supine 90/90 Breathing	None	1m
	FOAM ROLL	Glutes	Foam roller	1m each side
	STRETCH	Supine Figure 4	None	1m each side

5-DAY MOVEMENT PATTERN SPLIT PROGRAM
UPPER/PUSH

TRAINING PHASE	FOCUS	EXERCISE	EQUIPMENT/TOOL	SETS/REPS/DURATION/REST
PRE-TRAINING PREPARATION	PHASE 1	Pectoralis Group	Foam roller	1m each side (30s oscillation / 30s neurological trigger point)
	PHASE 2	90/90 Chest Stretch	None	1m each side (30s oscillation / 30s end-range hold)
	PHASE 3	Quadruped T-Spine Rotation	None	30s
	PHASE 4	Rusin Tri-Set A: Band Over & Back B: Band Face Pull C: Band Pull-Apart	Long resistance band (light)	2–3 x 8–10 each exercise
	PHASE 5	Pause Push-Up	None	3 x 5
	PHASE 6	A: Seal Jacks B: Bent-Over Med Ball Chest Press	A: None B: Med ball	A: 3 x 5 B: 3 x 3
PRIMING & POTENTIATION	NEUROLOGICAL PRIMER	A: Band-Assisted Plyo Push-Up	Long resistance band (light)	3 x 5
	MECHANICAL PRIMER	B: Half-Kneeling Face Pull	Long resistance band (light)	3 x 20
KEY PERFORMANCE INDICATOR (KPI)	UPPER/PUSH	Dumbbell Bench Press	Dumbbells	3–4 x 12–15
PUMP ACCESSORIES & PREHAB	PUSH	1A: Half-Kneeling Single-Arm Landmine Press	Landmine	3 x 12–15 each side
	PULL (HORIZONTAL)	1B: Inverted Row	Suspension trainer	3 x 15
	PULL (VERTICAL)	1C: Half-Kneeling High-Angle Row	Cable or long resistance band	3 x 15 each side
	TRICEPS	2A: Half-Kneeling Overhead Triceps Extension	Cable or long resistance band	2–3 x 12–15
	FOREARMS/GRIP	2B: Bench-Supported Hammer Grip Dumbbell Wrist Extension	Dumbbell	2–3 x 10–15 each side
CONDITIONING FINISHER	SHOULDER BURNOUT	A: Chest-Supported Rear Delt Raise B: Supinated Dumbbell Curl	Dumbbells	5m AMRAP A: 15 reps B: 15 reps
POST-TRAINING COOL-DOWN	BREATHE	Supine 90/90 Breathing	None	1m
	FOAM ROLL	Pectoralis Group	Foam roller	1m each side
	STRETCH	Prone Pec Stretch	None	1m each side

5-DAY MOVEMENT PATTERN SPLIT PROGRAM
LOWER/SQUAT

TRAINING PHASE	FOCUS	EXERCISE	EQUIPMENT/TOOL	SETS/REPS/DURATION/REST
PRE-TRAINING PREPARATION	PHASE 1	Quadriceps	Foam roller	1m each side (30s oscillation / 30s neurological trigger point)
	PHASE 2	Half-Kneeling Hip Flexor Stretch	None	1m each side (30s oscillation / 30s end-range hold)
	PHASE 3	Hip Drop Side Plank	None	30s each side
	PHASE 4	Banded Single-Leg Glute Bridge	Short resistance band (light)	2–3 x 8–10 each side
	PHASE 5	Bodyweight Squat	None	3 x 5
	PHASE 6	A: Vertical Jacks B: Depth Drop	None	A: 3 x 5 B: 3 x 3
PRIMING & POTENTIATION	NEUROLOGICAL PRIMER	A: Triple Extension to Snap-Down	None	3 x 3
	MECHANICAL PRIMER	B: Ball Hamstring Curl	Physio ball	3 x 20
KEY PERFORMANCE INDICATOR (KPI)	LOWER/SQUAT	Front Squat	Barbell	3–4 x 10–12
PUMP ACCESSORIES & PREHAB	HINGE	1A: Romanian Deadlift (RDL)	Dumbbell	3 x 15
	LUNGE	1B: Front-Foot-Elevated Dumbbell Split Squat	Dumbbells	3 x 10–15
	HIP ER/IR	1C: Shin Box Lift with Rotation (Alternating)	None	3 x 10 each side
	QUADS	2A: Band-Assisted Reverse Nordic	Long resistance band (medium)	2–3 x 10–12
	CORE	2B: Banded Pullover Iso Double Leg Drop	Long resistance band (medium)	2–3 x 30s
CONDITIONING FINISHER	CARRY	Front Rack Carry (Bilateral)	Dumbbells	4 x 30s
POST-TRAINING COOL-DOWN	BREATHE	Supine 90/90 Breathing	None	1m
	FOAM ROLL	Adductor Group	Foam roller	1m each side
	STRETCH	Frog Stretch	None	1m each side

5-DAY MOVEMENT PATTERN SPLIT PROGRAM
UPPER/PULL

TRAINING PHASE	FOCUS	EXERCISE	EQUIPMENT/TOOL	SETS/REPS/DURATION/REST
PRE-TRAINING PREPARATION	PHASE 1	Thoracic Spine	Foam roller	1m (30s oscillation / 30s neurological trigger point)
	PHASE 2	Hinged T-Spine Extension / Bilateral Lat Stretch	Suspension trainer	1m (30s oscillation / 30s end-range hold)
	PHASE 3	Quadruped T-Spine Rotation	None	30s
	PHASE 4	Rusin Tri-Set A: Band Over & Back B: Band Face Pull C: Band Pull-Apart	Long resistance band (light)	2–3 x 8–10 each exercise
	PHASE 5	Inverted Row	Suspension trainer	3 x 5
	PHASE 6	A: Vertical Jacks B: Med Ball Slam	A: None B: Med ball	A: 3 x 5 B: 3 x 3
PRIMING & POTENTIATION	NEUROLOGICAL PRIMER	A: Explosive Split Stance Cable or Band Row	Cable or long resistance band	3 x 5 each side
	MECHANICAL PRIMER	B: Tall Kneeling Straight-Arm Pulldown	Long resistance band (light)	3 x 15
KEY PERFORMANCE INDICATOR (KPI)	UPPER/PULL	Lat Pulldown	Cable or long resistance band	3–4 x 10–12
PUMP ACCESSORIES & PREHAB	PUSH	1A: Dumbbell Alternating Chest Press	Dumbbells	3 x 12–15 each side
	PULL	1B: Hinged-Supported Row	Dumbbell	3 x 12–15 each side
	CORE	1C: Side Plank March	None	3 x 30s each side
	SHOULDERS	2A: Supine Band Face Pull	Long resistance band (light)	2–3 x 12–15
	T-SPINE MOBILITY	2B: Banded T-Spine Rotations	Long resistance band (light)	2–3 x 30s each side
CONDITIONING FINISHER	BICEPS/ TRICEPS BURNOUT	A: Alternating Dumbbell Curl B: Cable Triceps Push Down	A: Dumbbells B: Cable or long resistance band	5m AMRAP A: 15 reps B: 15 reps
POST-TRAINING COOL-DOWN	BREATHE	Supine 90/90 Breathing	None	1m
	FOAM ROLL	Pectoralis Group	Foam roller	1m each side
	STRETCH	Prone Pec Stretch	None	1m each side

5-DAY MOVEMENT PATTERN SPLIT PROGRAM
FULL BODY/LUNGE

TRAINING PHASE	FOCUS	EXERCISE	EQUIPMENT/TOOL	SETS/REPS/DURATION/REST
PRE-TRAINING PREPARATION	PHASE 1	Lateral Hip	Foam roller	1m each side (30s oscillation / 30s neurological trigger point)
	PHASE 2	Half-Kneeling Hip Flexor Stretch	None	1m each side (30s oscillation / 30s end-range hold)
	PHASE 3	Dead Bug (Single Leg)	None	30s
	PHASE 4	A: Banded Glute Bridge B: Band Pull-Apart	A: Long resistance band (medium) B: Long resistance band (light)	2–3 x 8–10 each exercise
	PHASE 5	Split Squat	None	3 x 5
	PHASE 6	A: Seal Jacks B: Forward Skip	None	A: 3 x 5 B: 3 x 5
PRIMING & POTENTIATION	NEUROLOGICAL PRIMER	A: Landmine Clean & Press	Landmine	4 x 4 each side
	MECHANICAL PRIMER	B: Kickstand Dumbbell Good Morning	Dumbbell or kettlebell	4 x 12 each side
KEY PERFORMANCE INDICATOR (KPI)	LOWER/LUNGE	Dumbbell Reverse Lunge Contralateral Load	Dumbbell or kettlebell	3–4 x 10–12
PUMP ACCESSORIES & PREHAB	SQUAT	1A: Loaded Push-Up	Weight plate	3 x 12–15
	LUNGE	1B: Bodyweight Cossack	None	3 x 20 alternating
	CARRY/CORE	1C: Forward Crawl	None	3 x 30s
	PULL	2A: Feet-Elevated Inverted Row	Suspension trainer	2–3 x 12–15
	SHOULDERS	2B: Dumbbell Rear Delt Fly	Dumbbells	2–3 x 12–15 each side
CONDITIONING FINISHER	CORE BURNOUT	A: Legs-Elevated Crunch B: Pallof Press from Standing	A: None B: Cable or long resistance band	5m AMRAP A: 15 reps B: 10 reps each side
POST-TRAINING COOL-DOWN	BREATHE	Supine 90/90 Breathing	None	1m
	FOAM ROLL	T-Spine & Quadriceps	Foam roller	1m each exercise/side
	STRETCH	Prone Quad Stretch & Child's Pose (10 & 2)	None	1m each exercise/side

5-DAY MOVEMENT PATTERN SPLIT PROGRAM
LOWER/HINGE

TRAINING PHASE	FOCUS	EXERCISE	EQUIPMENT/TOOL	SETS/REPS/DURATION/REST
PRE-TRAINING PREPARATION	PHASE 1	Adductor Group	Foam roller	1m each side (30s oscillation / 30s neurological trigger point)
	PHASE 2	Adductor Rock-Back	None	1m each side (30s oscillation / 30s end-range hold)
	PHASE 3	Bird Dog (Single Leg)	None	30s each side
	PHASE 4	Side Plank Hip Thrust (Feet Together)	Short resistance band (medium)	30s each side
	PHASE 5	Romanian Deadlift (RDL)	Dumbbell	3 x 5
	PHASE 6	A: Vertical Jacks B: Broad Jump	None	A: 3 x 5 B: 3 x 3
PRIMING & POTENTIATION	NEUROLOGICAL PRIMER	A: Band-Resisted Broad Jump	Long resistance band (medium)	3 x 3
	MECHANICAL PRIMER	B: Tall Kneeling Banded Hip Thrust	Long resistance band (medium)	3 x 20
KEY PERFORMANCE INDICATOR (KPI)	LOWER/HINGE	Conventional Deadlift (Elevated)	Barbell	4 x 6–8
PUMP ACCESSORIES & PREHAB	SQUAT	1A: Landmine Goblet Squat	Landmine	3 x 15
	LUNGE	1B: Dumbbell Curtsy Lunge	Dumbbell	3 x 16–20 each side
	CALVES	1C: Single-Leg Deficit Calf Raise	None	3 x 15
	HAMSTRINGS	2A: Kickstand Dumbbell RDL	Dumbbell	2–3 x 12–15 each side
	CORE/UPPER	2B: Pike Push-Up	None	2–3 x 10–12
CONDITIONING FINISHER	GLUTE BURNOUT	A: Lateral Lunge B: Side Plank Hip Thrust w/ Pause C: 90/90 Squat Iso with Band Hip Abduction	A: None B–C: Short resistance band (medium)	5m AMRAP A: 10 reps each side B: 15 reps C: 25 reps
POST-TRAINING COOL-DOWN	BREATHE	Supine 90/90 Breathing	None	1m
	FOAM ROLL	Glutes	Foam roller	1m each side
	STRETCH	Supine Figure 4	None	1m each side

5-DAY MOVEMENT PATTERN SPLIT PROGRAM
UPPER/PUSH

TRAINING PHASE	FOCUS	EXERCISE	EQUIPMENT/TOOL	SETS/REPS/DURATION/REST
PRE-TRAINING PREPARATION	PHASE 1	Pectoralis Group	Foam roller	1m each side (30s oscillation / 30s neurological trigger point)
	PHASE 2	90/90 Chest Stretch	None	1m each side (30s oscillation / 30s end-range hold)
	PHASE 3	Quadruped T-Spine Rotation	None	30s
	PHASE 4	Rusin Tri-Set A: Band Over & Back B: Band Face Pull C: Band Pull-Apart	Long resistance band (light)	2–3 x 8–10 each exercise
	PHASE 5	Pause Push-Up	None	3 x 5
	PHASE 6	A: Seal Jacks B: Bent-Over Med Ball Chest Press	A: None B: Med ball	A: 3 x 5 B: 3 x 3
PRIMING & POTENTIATION	NEUROLOGICAL PRIMER	A: Explosive Band Press	Long resistance band (light)	3 x 5 each side
	MECHANICAL PRIMER	B: Band Pull-Apart	Long resistance band (light)	3 x 10
KEY PERFORMANCE INDICATOR (KPI)	UPPER/PUSH	Barbell Bench Press	Barbell	3–4 x 12–15
PUMP ACCESSORIES & PREHAB	PUSH	1A: Landmine Split Stance Press	Landmine	3 x 12–15 each side
	PULL (HORIZONTAL)	1B: Feet-Elevated Inverted Row	Suspension trainer	3 x 10–15
	PULL (VERTICAL)	1C: Split Stance High-Angle Row	Cable or long resistance band	3 x 12–15 each side
	TRICEPS	2A: Suspension Trainer Triceps Extension	Suspension trainer	2–3 x 12–15
	FOREARMS/ GRIP	2B: Bench-Supported Dumbbell Pronation/Supination	Dumbbell	2–3 x 10–15 each side
CONDITIONING FINISHER	SHOULDER BURNOUT	A: Seated Lateral Raise B: Hammer Curl	Dumbbells	5m AMRAP A: 5 reps B: 10 reps
POST-TRAINING COOL-DOWN	BREATHE	Supine 90/90 Breathing	None	1m
	FOAM ROLL	Pectoralis Group	Foam roller	1m each side
	STRETCH	Prone Pec Stretch	None	1m each side

5-DAY MOVEMENT PATTERN SPLIT PROGRAM
LOWER/SQUAT

TRAINING PHASE	FOCUS	EXERCISE	EQUIPMENT/TOOL	SETS/REPS/DURATION/REST
PRE-TRAINING PREPARATION	PHASE 1	Quadriceps	Foam roller	1m each side (30s oscillation / 30s neurological trigger point)
	PHASE 2	Half-Kneeling Hip Flexor Stretch	None	1m each side (30s oscillation / 30s end-range hold)
	PHASE 3	Hip Drop Side Plank	None	30s each side
	PHASE 4	Banded Single-Leg Glute Bridge	Short resistance band (light)	2–3 x 8–10 each side
	PHASE 5	Bodyweight Squat	None	3 x 5
	PHASE 6	A: Vertical Jacks B: Depth Drop	None	A: 3 x 5 B: 3 x 3
PRIMING & POTENTIATION	NEUROLOGICAL PRIMER	A: Countermovement Jump	None	3 x 3
	MECHANICAL PRIMER	B: Suspension Trainer Ball Hamstring Curl	Suspension trainer	3 x 15–20
KEY PERFORMANCE INDICATOR (KPI)	LOWER/ SQUAT	Back Squat	Barbell	4 x 6–8
PUMP ACCESSORIES & PREHAB	HINGE	1A: Barbell Romanian Deadlift (RDL)	Barbell	3 x 15
	LUNGE	1B: Goblet Bulgarian Split Squat	Dumbbell	3 x 15 each side
	HIP ER/IR	1C: Loaded Shin Box Lift with Rotation (Alternating)	Dumbbell	3 x 10 each side
	QUADS	2A: Reverse Nordic	None	2–3 x 8–10
	CORE	2B: Hollow Body Hold	None	2–3 x 30s
CONDITIONING FINISHER	CARRY	Cross-Body Carry (Bilateral)	Dumbbells	4 x 30s
POST-TRAINING COOL-DOWN	BREATHE	Supine 90/90 Breathing	None	1m
	FOAM ROLL	Adductor Group	Foam roller	1m each side
	STRETCH	Frog Stretch	None	1m each side

5-DAY MOVEMENT PATTERN SPLIT PROGRAM

UPPER/PULL

REGAIN DAY **04**

TRAINING PHASE	FOCUS	EXERCISE	EQUIPMENT/TOOL	SETS/REPS/DURATION/REST
PRE-TRAINING PREPARATION	PHASE 1	Thoracic Spine	Foam roller	1m (30s oscillation / 30s neurological trigger point)
	PHASE 2	Hinged T-Spine Extension / Bilateral Lat Stretch	Suspension trainer	1m (30s oscillation / 30s end-range hold)
	PHASE 3	Quadruped T-Spine Rotation	None	30sv
	PHASE 4	Rusin Tri-Set A: Band Over & Back B: Band Face Pull C: Band Pull-Apart	Long resistance band (light)	2–3 x 8–10 each exercise
	PHASE 5	Inverted Row	Suspension trainer	3 x 5
	PHASE 6	A: Vertical Jacks B: Med Ball Slam	A: None B: Med ball	A: 3 x 5 B: 3 x 3
PRIMING & POTENTIATION	NEUROLOGICAL PRIMER	A: Alternating Lateral Split Squat with Hand Switch Row	Dumbbell	3 x 5 each side
	MECHANICAL PRIMER	B: Band Pull Down and Apart	Long resistance band (light)	3 x 15–20
KEY PERFORMANCE INDICATOR (KPI)	UPPER/PULL	Neutral Grip Pull-Up	Rack	4 x 6–8
PUMP ACCESSORIES & PREHAB	PUSH	1A: Banded Deficit Push-Up	Long resistance band (medium)	3 x 8–12
	PULL	1B: Bent-Over Row	Dumbbells	3 x 12–15 each side
	CORE	1C: Dumbbell Floor Chest Fly	Dumbbells	3 x 12–15
	SHOULDERS	2A: Band Face Pull to Overhead	Long resistance band (light)	2–3 x 12–15
	T-SPINE MOBILITY	2B: Reach and Rotate	Long resistance band (light)	2–3 x 30s each side
CONDITIONING FINISHER	CORE BURNOUT	A: Standing Band Crunch B: Oblique Crunch C: Quadruped Shoulder Tap	A–B: Cable or long resistance band C: None	5m AMRAP A: 15 reps B: 10 reps each side C: 15 reps
POST-TRAINING COOL-DOWN	BREATHE	Supine 90/90 Breathing	None	1m
	FOAM ROLL	Lats	Foam roller	1m each side
	STRETCH	Child's Pose (10 & 2)	None	1m each side

5-DAY MOVEMENT PATTERN SPLIT PROGRAM
FULL BODY/LUNGE

TRAINING PHASE	FOCUS	EXERCISE	EQUIPMENT/TOOL	SETS/REPS/DURATION/REST
PRE-TRAINING PREPARATION	PHASE 1	Lateral Hip	Foam roller	1m each side (30s oscillation / 30s neurological trigger point)
	PHASE 2	Half-Kneeling Hip Flexor Stretch	None	1m each side (30s oscillation / 30s end-range hold)
	PHASE 3	Dead Bug (Single Leg)	None	30s
	PHASE 4	A: Banded Glute Bridge B: Band Pull-Apart	A: Long resistance band (medium) B: Long resistance band (light)	2–3 x 8–10 each exercise
	PHASE 5	Split Squat	None	3 x 5 each side
	PHASE 6	A: Seal Jacks B: Forward Skip	None	A: 3 x 5 B: 3 x 5
PRIMING & POTENTIATION	NEUROLOGICAL PRIMER	A: Landmine Rotating Pull to Press	Landmine	4 x 3 each side
	MECHANICAL PRIMER	B: Sumo Stance Banded Good Morning	Long resistance band (medium)	4 x 15
KEY PERFORMANCE INDICATOR (KPI)	LOWER/ LUNGE	Dumbbell Reverse Lunge (Double Dumbbell at Sides / Farmer's Carry)	Dumbbells	4 x 6–8 each side
PUMP ACCESSORIES & PREHAB	SQUAT	1A: Deficit Loaded Push-Up	Weight plate	3 x 8–12
	LUNGE	1B: Landmine Cossack	Landmine	3 x 20 alternating
	CARRY/CORE	1C: Backward Crawl	None	3 x 30s
	PULL	2A: Single-Arm Landmine Row	Landmine	2–3 x 12–15 each side
	SHOULDERS	2B: Knee Support Shoulder External Rotation	Cable or long resistance band	2–3 x 12–15 each side
CONDITIONING FINISHER	CORE BURNOUT	A: Standing Cable Crunch B: Pallof Press from Split Stance	Cable or long resistance band	5m AMRAP A: 8–15 reps B: 10 reps each side
POST-TRAINING COOL-DOWN	BREATHE	Supine 90/90 Breathing	None	1m
	FOAM ROLL	T-Spine & Quadriceps	Foam roller	1m each exercise/side
	STRETCH	Prone Quad Stretch & Child's Pose (10 & 2)	None	1m each exercise/side

ULTIMATE PAIN-FREE PERFORMANCE PROGRAM
LOWER/HINGE

RECLAIM **DAY 01**

TRAINING PHASE	FOCUS	EXERCISE	EQUIPMENT/TOOL	SETS/REPS/DURATION/REST
PRE-TRAINING PREPARATION	PHASE 1	Adductor Group	Foam roller	1m each side (30s oscillation / 30s neurological trigger point)
	PHASE 2	Adductor Rock-Back	None	1m each side (30s oscillation / 30s end-range hold)
	PHASE 3	Bird Dog (Single Arm)	None	30s each side
	PHASE 4	Side-Lying Banded Clam	Short resistance band (medium)	30s each side
	PHASE 5	A: Romanian Deadlift (RDL) B: Bodyweight Squat	A: Dumbbell B: None	3 x 5 each exercise
	PHASE 6	A: Vertical Jacks B: Broad Jump	None	A: 3 x 5 B: 3 x 3
PRIMING & POTENTIATION	NEUROLOGICAL PRIMER	A: Kneeling Banded Hip Thrust	Long resistance band (medium)	4 x 5
	MECHANICAL PRIMER	B: Banded Glute Bridge	Long resistance band (medium)	4 x 20
KEY PERFORMANCE INDICATOR (KPI)	LOWER/HINGE	Kettlebell Romanian Deadlift (RDL)	Kettlebell	3–4 x 10–12
PUMP ACCESSORIES & PREHAB	SQUAT	A: Heels-Elevated Goblet Squat	Dumbbell & wedge	3 x 12
	LUNGE	B: Dumbbell Single-Arm Contralateral Reverse Lunge	Dumbbell	3 x 10–12 each side
	ADDUCTORS	C: Open Half-Kneeling Dumbbell Adductor Mobilizer	Dumbbell	3 x 30s each side
CONDITIONING FINISHER	GLUTE BURNOUT	Barbell Hip Thrust (Rest-Pause)	Barbell (light load)	2m AMRAP: do reps to near-failure, rest 15s, repeat 2m
POST-TRAINING COOL-DOWN	BREATHE	Supine 90/90 Breathing	None	1m
	FOAM ROLL	Glutes	Foam roller	1m each side
	STRETCH	Supine Figure 4	None	1m each side

ULTIMATE PAIN-FREE PERFORMANCE PROGRAM
UPPER/PUSH

RECLAIM
DAY
02

TRAINING PHASE	FOCUS	EXERCISE	EQUIPMENT/TOOL	SETS/REPS/DURATION/REST
PRE-TRAINING PREPARATION	PHASE 1	Pectoralis Group	Foam roller	1m each side (30s oscillation / 30s neurological trigger point)
	PHASE 2	90/90 Chest Stretch	None	1m each side (30s oscillation / 30s end-range hold)
	PHASE 3	Quadruped T-Spine Rotation	None	30s
	PHASE 4	Rusin Tri-Set A: Band Over & Back B: Band Face Pull C: Band Pull-Apart	Long resistance band (light)	2–3 x 8–10 each exercise
	PHASE 5	Pause Push-Up	None	3 x 5
	PHASE 6	A: Seal Jacks B: Bent-Over Med Ball Press	A: None B: Med ball	A: 3 x 5 B: 3 x 3
PRIMING & POTENTIATION	NEUROLOGICAL PRIMER	A: Bent-Over Med Ball Press	Med ball	4 x 5
	MECHANICAL PRIMER	B: Kneeling Band Pull-Apart	Long resistance band (light)	4 x 15–20
KEY PERFORMANCE INDICATOR (KPI)	UPPER/PUSH	Deficit Loaded Push-Up	Weight plate	3–4 x 8–10
PUMP ACCESSORIES & PREHAB	PUSH	A: Half-Kneeling Landmine Single-Arm Press	Landmine	3 x 10–12 each side
	PULL	B: Inverted Row	Suspension trainer	3 x 10–12
	SHOULDERS	C: Chest-Supported Rear Delt Fly	Dumbbells	3 x 15
CONDITIONING FINISHER	TRICEPS BURNOUT	Dumbbell Skull Crusher	Dumbbell	2m AMRAP
POST-TRAINING COOL-DOWN	BREATHE	Supine 90/90 Breathing	None	1m
	FOAM ROLL	Pectoralis Group	Foam roller	1m each side
	STRETCH	Prone Pec Stretch	None	1m each side

ULTIMATE PAIN-FREE PERFORMANCE PROGRAM
LOWER/SQUAT

RECLAIM **DAY 03**

TRAINING PHASE	FOCUS	EXERCISE	EQUIPMENT/TOOL	SETS/REPS/DURATION/REST
PRE-TRAINING PREPARATION	PHASE 1	Quadriceps	Foam roller	1m each side (30s oscillation / 30s neurological trigger point)
	PHASE 2	Half-Kneeling Hip Flexor Stretch	None	1m each side (30s oscillation / 30s end-range hold)
	PHASE 3	Knee-Bend Side Plank	None	30s each side
	PHASE 4	Banded Single-Leg Glute Bridge	Short resistance band (light)	2–3 x 8–10 each side
	PHASE 5	Bodyweight Squat	None	3 x 5
	PHASE 6	A: Vertical Jacks B: Vertical Jump	None	A: 3 x 5 B: 3 x 3
PRIMING & POTENTIATION	NEUROLOGICAL PRIMER	A: Triple Extension to Snap-Down	None	4 x 3
	MECHANICAL PRIMER	B: Heels-Elevated Alternating Bridge	Long resistance band (light)	4 x 20
KEY PERFORMANCE INDICATOR (KPI)	LOWER/SQUAT	Goblet Squat	Dumbbell	3–4 x 10–12
PUMP ACCESSORIES & PREHAB	HINGE	A: Romanian Deadlift (RDL)	Dumbbell	3 x 12–15
	LUNGE	B: Contralateral Dumbbell Split Squat	Dumbbell	3 x 10–12 each side
	GLUTES	C: Seated Banded Abduction	Short resistance band (medium)	3 x 15
CONDITIONING FINISHER	CARRY	Farmer's Carry (Bilateral)	Dumbbells	4 x 20s
POST-TRAINING COOL-DOWN	BREATHE	Supine 90/90 Breathing	None	1m
	FOAM ROLL	Adductor Group	Foam roller	1m each side
	STRETCH	Frog Stretch	None	1m each side

ULTIMATE PAIN-FREE PERFORMANCE PROGRAM

UPPER/PULL

RECLAIM DAY 04

TRAINING PHASE	FOCUS	EXERCISE	EQUIPMENT/TOOL	SETS/REPS/DURATION/REST
PRE-TRAINING PREPARATION	PHASE 1	Thoracic Spine	Foam roller	1m (30s oscillation / 30s neurological trigger point)
	PHASE 2	Hinged T-Spine Extension / Bilateral Lat Stretch	Suspension trainer	1m (30s oscillation / 30s end-range hold)
	PHASE 3	Quadruped T-Spine Rotation	None	30s
	PHASE 4	Rusin Tri-Set A: Band Over & Back B: Band Face Pull C: Band Pull-Apart	Long resistance band (light)	2–3 x 8–10 each exercise
	PHASE 5	Inverted Row	Suspension trainer	3 x 5
	PHASE 6	A: Vertical Jacks B: Med Ball Slam	A: None B: Med ball	A: 3 x 5 B: 3 x 3
PRIMING & POTENTIATION	NEUROLOGICAL PRIMER	A: High Kneeling Med Ball Slam	Med ball	4 x 5
	MECHANICAL PRIMER	B: High Kneeling Straight-Arm Pulldown	Long resistance band (light)	4 x 15
KEY PERFORMANCE INDICATOR (KPI)	UPPER/PULL	High-Angle Pulldown	Long resistance band (light)	3–4 x 10
PUMP ACCESSORIES & PREHAB	PUSH	A: Push-Up (optional: loaded)	Weight plate (optional)	3 x 12
	PULL	B: Seated Low Cable Row	Cable or long resistance band	3 x 10–15
	CHEST	C: Quadruped Hover	None	3 x 30s
CONDITIONING FINISHER	BICEPS/CORE BURNOUT	A: Alternating Hammer Curl B: Legs-Elevated Crunch	A Dumbbells B: None	2m AMRAP A: 10 reps each side B: 15 reps
POST-TRAINING COOL-DOWN	BREATHE	Supine 90/90 Breathing	None	1m
	FOAM ROLL	Lats	Foam roller	1m each side
	STRETCH	Child's Pose (10 & 2)	None	1m each side

ULTIMATE PAIN-FREE PERFORMANCE PROGRAM
LOWER/HINGE

TRAINING PHASE	FOCUS	EXERCISE	EQUIPMENT/TOOL	SETS/REPS/DURATION/REST
PRE-TRAINING PREPARATION	PHASE 1	Adductor Group	Foam roller	1m each side (30s oscillation / 30s neurological trigger point)
	PHASE 2	Adductor Rock-Back	None	1m each side (30s oscillation / 30s end-range hold)
	PHASE 3	Bird Dog (Single Arm)	None	30s each side
	PHASE 4	Side-Lying Banded Clam	Short resistance band (medium)	30s each side
	PHASE 5	A: Romanian Deadlift (RDL) B: Bodyweight Squat	A: Dumbbell B: None	3 x 5 each exercise
	PHASE 6	A: Vertical Jacks B: Broad Jump	None	A: 3 x 5 B: 3 x 3
PRIMING & POTENTIATION	NEUROLOGICAL PRIMER	A: Kettlebell Swing	Kettlebell	4 x 5
	MECHANICAL PRIMER	B: Elevated Banded Hip Thrust	Long resistance band (medium)	4 x 15–20
KEY PERFORMANCE INDICATOR (KPI)	LOWER/HINGE	Trap Bar Deadlift	Trap bar	3–4 x 12–15
PUMP ACCESSORIES & PREHAB	SQUAT	A: Landmine Goblet Squat	Landmine	3 x 15
	LUNGE	B: Reverse Lunge (Dumbbells at Sides / Farmer's Carry)	Dumbbells	3 x 10–15 each side
CONDITIONING FINISHER	GLUTE BURNOUT	A: Dumbbell Hip Thrust w/ Pause B: Band Around Knees Alternating Side Step	A: Dumbbell B: Short resistance band (medium)	2m AMRAP A: 10 reps B: 15 each direction
POST-TRAINING COOL-DOWN	BREATHE	Supine 90/90 Breathing	None	1m
	FOAM ROLL	Glutes	Foam roller	1m each side
	STRETCH	Supine Figure 4	None	1m each side

ULTIMATE PAIN-FREE
PERFORMANCE PROGRAM

REBUILD DAY 02

UPPER/PUSH

TRAINING PHASE	FOCUS	EXERCISE	EQUIPMENT/TOOL	SETS/REPS/DURATION/REST
PRE-TRAINING PREPARATION	PHASE 1	Pectoralis Group	Foam roller	1m each side (30s oscillation / 30s neurological trigger point)
	PHASE 2	90/90 Chest Stretch	None	1m each side (30s oscillation / 30s end-range hold)
	PHASE 3	Quadruped T-Spine Rotation	None	30s
	PHASE 4	Rusin Tri-Set A: Band Over & Back B: Band Face Pull C: Band Pull-Apart	Long resistance band (light)	2–3 x 8–10 each exercise
	PHASE 5	Pause Push-Up	None	3 x 5
	PHASE 6	A: Seal Jacks B: Bent-Over Med Ball Press	A: None B: Med ball	A: 3 x 5 B: 3 x 3
PRIMING & POTENTIATION	NEUROLOGICAL PRIMER	A: Split Stance Single-Arm Band Press with Rotation	Long resistance band (light)	4 x 5 each side
	MECHANICAL PRIMER	B: Split Stance Hands-Free Double-Band Face Pull	Long resistance bands (light)	4 x 15–20
KEY PERFORMANCE INDICATOR (KPI)	UPPER/PUSH	Dumbbell Bench Press	Dumbbells	3–4 x 12–15
PUMP ACCESSORIES & PREHAB	PUSH	A: Split Stance Landmine Single-Arm Press	Landmine	3 x 12–15 each side
	PULL	B: Feet-Elevated Inverted Row	Suspension trainer	3 x 12–15
	SHOULDERS	C: Bent-Over Rear Delt Fly	Dumbbells	3 x 12–15
CONDITIONING FINISHER	UPPER BURNOUT	A: Tall Kneeling Cable or Band Triceps Press-Down B: Tall Kneeling Lateral Raise	A: Cable or long resistance band (light) B: Dumbbells	5m AMRAP A: 15 reps B: 15 reps
POST-TRAINING COOL-DOWN	BREATHE	Supine 90/90 Breathing	None	1m
	FOAM ROLL	Pectoralis Group	Foam roller	1m each side
	STRETCH	Prone Pec Stretch	None	1m each side

ULTIMATE PAIN-FREE PERFORMANCE PROGRAM
LOWER/SQUAT

TRAINING PHASE	FOCUS	EXERCISE	EQUIPMENT/TOOL	SETS/REPS/DURATION/REST
PRE-TRAINING PREPARATION	PHASE 1	Quadriceps	Foam roller	1m each side (30s oscillation / 30s neurological trigger point)
	PHASE 2	Half-Kneeling Hip Flexor Stretch	None	1m each side (30s oscillation / 30s end-range hold)
	PHASE 3	Side Plank	None	30s each side
	PHASE 4	Banded Single-Leg Glute Bridge	Short resistance band (light)	2–3 x 8–10 each side
	PHASE 5	Bodyweight Squat	None	3 x 5
	PHASE 6	A: Vertical Jacks B: Vertical Jump	None	A: 3 x 5 B: 3 x 3
PRIMING & POTENTIATION	NEUROLOGICAL PRIMER	A: Paused Jump	None	4 x 1
	MECHANICAL PRIMER	B: Stability Ball Hamstring Curl	Physio/Stability ball	4 x 15–20
KEY PERFORMANCE INDICATOR (KPI)	LOWER/SQUAT	Front Squat	Barbell	3–4 x 10–12
PUMP ACCESSORIES & PREHAB	HINGE	A: Landmine Romanian Deadlift (RDL)	Landmine	3 x 15
	LUNGE	B: Double Dumbbell at Sides Split Squat (Farmer's Carry)	Dumbbells	3 x 10–15 each side
	GLUTES	C: Quadruped Banded Fire Hydrant	Short resistance band (light)	3 x 15 each side
CONDITIONING FINISHER	CARRY	Front Rack Carry (Bilateral)	Dumbbells	4 x 20s
POST-TRAINING COOL-DOWN	BREATHE	Supine 90/90 Breathing	None	1m
	FOAM ROLL	Adductor Group	Foam roller	1m each side
	STRETCH	Frog Stretch	None	1m each side

ULTIMATE PAIN-FREE
PERFORMANCE PROGRAM
UPPER/PULL

REBUILD **DAY 04**

TRAINING PHASE	FOCUS	EXERCISE	EQUIPMENT/TOOL	SETS/REPS/DURATION/REST
PRE-TRAINING PREPARATION	PHASE 1	Thoracic Spine	Foam roller	1m (30s oscillation / 30s neurological trigger point)
	PHASE 2	Hinged T-Spine Extension / Bilateral Lat Stretch	Suspension trainer	1m (30s oscillation / 30s end-range hold)
	PHASE 3	Quadruped T-Spine Rotation	None	30s
	PHASE 4	Rusin Tri-Set A: Band Over & Back B: Band Face Pull C: Band Pull-Apart	Long resistance band (light)	2–3 x 8–10 each exercise
	PHASE 5	Inverted Row	Suspension trainer	3 x 5
	PHASE 6	A: Vertical Jacks B: Med Ball Slam	A: None B: Med ball	A: 3 x 5 B: 3 x 3
PRIMING & POTENTIATION	NEUROLOGICAL PRIMER	A: Anti-Flexion Med Ball Slam	Med ball	4 x 3
	MECHANICAL PRIMER	B: Half-Kneeling Single-Arm High-Angle Row	Cable or long resistance band (light)	4 x 15 each side
KEY PERFORMANCE INDICATOR (KPI)	UPPER/PULL	Medium Grip Lat Pulldown	Cable	3–4 x 10–12
PUMP ACCESSORIES & PREHAB	PUSH	A: Deficit Push-Up (optional: loaded)	Weight plate (optional)	3 x 12–15
	PULL	B: Seated Single-Arm Cable Row	Cable or long resistance band	3 x 15 each side
	CHEST	C: Forward Crawl	None	3 x 30s
CONDITIONING FINISHER	BICEPS/CORE BURNOUT	A: Hammer Curl B: Crunch to Extend	A: Dumbbells B: None	2m AMRAP A: 10 reps B: 10 reps each leg
POST-TRAINING COOL-DOWN	BREATHE	Supine 90/90 Breathing	None	1m
	FOAM ROLL	Lats	Foam roller	1m each side
	STRETCH	Child's Pose (10 & 2)	None	1m each side

ULTIMATE PAIN-FREE PERFORMANCE PROGRAM

LOWER/HINGE

TRAINING PHASE	FOCUS	EXERCISE	EQUIPMENT/TOOL	SETS/REPS/DURATION/REST
PRE-TRAINING PREPARATION	PHASE 1	Adductor Group	Foam roller	1m each side (30s oscillation / 30s neurological trigger point)
	PHASE 2	Adductor Rock-Back	None	1m each side (30s oscillation / 30s end-range hold)
	PHASE 3	Bird Dog (Single Arm)	None	30s each side
	PHASE 4	Side-Lying Banded Clam	Short resistance band (medium)	30s each side
	PHASE 5	A: Romanian Deadlift (RDL) B: Bodyweight Squat	A: Dumbbell B: None	3 x 5 each exercise
	PHASE 6	A: Vertical Jacks B: Broad Jump	None	A: 3 x 5 B: 3 x 3
PRIMING & POTENTIATION	NEUROLOGICAL PRIMER	A: Band-Resisted Broad Jump	Long resistance band (medium)	4 x 3
	MECHANICAL PRIMER	B: Barbell Hip Thrust	Barbell (light load)	4 x 15–20
KEY PERFORMANCE INDICATOR (KPI)	LOWER/HINGE	Conventional Deadlift (Elevated)	Barbell	4 x 6–8
PUMP ACCESSORIES & PREHAB	SQUAT	1A: Heels-Elevated Landmine Goblet Squat	Landmine & wedge	3 x 10–15
	LUNGE	1B: Front-Foot-Elevated Reverse Lunge (Dumbbells at Sides / Farmer's Carry)	Dumbbells	3 x 10–15
	LUNGE	2A: Rear-Foot-Elevated Split Squat (Dumbbells at Sides / Farmer's Carry)	Dumbbells	3 x 10–15
	CALVES	2B: Deficit Calf Raise	Wedge or box	3 x 20
CONDITIONING FINISHER	LOWER/GLUTE BURNOUT	A: Bodyweight Curtsy Lunge B: Side Plank Hip Thrust C: Side-Lying Banded Leg Abduction	A: None B: None C: Short resistance band (medium)	5m AMRAP A: 10 reps B: 10 reps C: 15 reps
POST-TRAINING COOL-DOWN	BREATHE	Supine 90/90 Breathing	None	1m
	FOAM ROLL	Glutes	Foam roller	1m each side
	STRETCH	Supine Figure 4	None	1m each side

ULTIMATE PAIN-FREE PERFORMANCE PROGRAM
UPPER/PUSH

TRAINING PHASE	FOCUS	EXERCISE	EQUIPMENT/TOOL	SETS/REPS/DURATION/REST
PRE-TRAINING PREPARATION	PHASE 1	Pectoralis Group	Foam roller	1m each side (30s oscillation / 30s neurological trigger point)
	PHASE 2	90/90 Chest Stretch	None	1m each side (30s oscillation / 30s end-range hold)
	PHASE 3	Quadruped T-Spine Rotation	None	30s
	PHASE 4	Rusin Tri-Set A: Band Over & Back B: Band Face Pull C: Band Pull-Apart	Long resistance band (light)	2–3 x 8–10 each exercise
	PHASE 5	Pause Push-Up	None	3 x 5
	PHASE 6	A: Seal Jacks B: Bent-Over Med Ball Press	A: None B: Med ball	A: 3 x 5 B: 3 x 3
PRIMING & POTENTIATION	NEUROLOGICAL PRIMER	A: Band-Assisted Plyo Push-Up	Long resistance band (light)	4 x 5
	MECHANICAL PRIMER	B: Half-Kneeling Double-Band Face Pull	Long resistance bands (light)	4 x 15–20
KEY PERFORMANCE INDICATOR (KPI)	UPPER/PUSH	Bench Press	Barbell	4 x 6–8
PUMP ACCESSORIES & PREHAB	PUSH	1A: Standing Alternating Dumbbell Press	Dumbbell	3 x 12–15 each side
	PULL	1B: Chest-Supported Alternating Dumbbell Row	Incline bench & dumbbell	3 x 15 each side
	SHOULDERS	1C: Suspension Face Pull	Suspension trainer	3 x 12–15
	PULL	2A: Lat Pulldown	Cable or long resistance band	2–3 x 12–15
	CORE	2B: Plank Shoulder Taps	None	2–3 x 20 alternating
CONDITIONING FINISHER	UPPER BURNOUT	A: Cable Push-Down B: Seated Band Lateral Raise C: Alternating Biceps Curl	A: Cable or long resistance band (light) B: Long resistance band (light) C: Dumbbells	5m AMRAP A: 25 reps B: 10 reps C: 10 reps each side
POST-TRAINING COOL-DOWN	BREATHE	Supine 90/90 Breathing	None	1m
	FOAM ROLL	Pectoralis Group	Foam roller	1m each side
	STRETCH	Prone Pec Stretch	None	1m each side

ULTIMATE PAIN-FREE PERFORMANCE PROGRAM
LOWER/SQUAT

TRAINING PHASE	FOCUS	EXERCISE	EQUIPMENT/TOOL	SETS/REPS/DURATION/REST
PRE-TRAINING PREPARATION	PHASE 1	Quadriceps	Foam roller	1m each side (30s oscillation / 30s neurological trigger point)
	PHASE 2	Half-Kneeling Hip Flexor Stretch	None	1m each side (30s oscillation / 30s end-range hold)
	PHASE 3	Side Plank Starfish	None	30s each side
	PHASE 4	Banded Single-Leg Glute Bridge	Short resistance band (light)	2–3 x 8–10 each side
	PHASE 5	Bodyweight Squat	None	3 x 5
	PHASE 6	A: Vertical Jacks B: Vertical Jump	None	A: 3 x 5 B: 3 x 3
PRIMING & POTENTIATION	NEUROLOGICAL PRIMER	A: Countermovement Jump	None	4 x 1
	MECHANICAL PRIMER	B: Suspension Trainer Hamstring Curl to Hip Thrust	Suspension trainer	4 x 12–20
KEY PERFORMANCE INDICATOR (KPI)	LOWER/SQUAT	Back Squat	Barbell	4 x 6–8
PUMP ACCESSORIES & PREHAB	HINGE	1A: Barbell Romanian Deadlift (RDL)	Barbell	3 x 15
	LUNGE	1B: Double Dumbbell at Sides Rear-Foot-Elevated Split Squat (Bulgarian)	Dumbbells	3 x 12 each side
	GLUTES	1C: Banded Single-Leg Fire Hydrant	Short resistance band (light)	3 x 10–15 each side
	LUNGE	2A: Low Dumbbell Hand Switch Alternating Lateral Lunge	Dumbbell	2–3 x 10–15 each side
	GLUTES	2B: Side-Lying Adductor Raise	None	2–3 x 15 each side
CONDITIONING FINISHER	CARRY	Cross-Body Carry (Bilateral)	Dumbbells	4 x 30s
POST-TRAINING COOL-DOWN	BREATHE	Supine 90/90 Breathing	None	1m
	FOAM ROLL	Adductor Group	Foam roller	1m each side
	STRETCH	Frog Stretch	None	1m each side

ULTIMATE PAIN-FREE PERFORMANCE PROGRAM
UPPER/PULL

REGAIN **DAY 04**

TRAINING PHASE	FOCUS	EXERCISE	EQUIPMENT/TOOL	SETS/REPS/DURATION/REST
PRE-TRAINING PREPARATION	PHASE 1	Thoracic Spine	Foam roller	1m (30s oscillation / 30s neurological trigger point)
	PHASE 2	Hinged T-Spine Extension / Bilateral Lat Stretch	Suspension trainer	1m (30s oscillation / 30s end-range hold)
	PHASE 3	Quadruped T-Spine Rotation	None	30s
	PHASE 4	Rusin Tri-Set A: Band Over & Back B: Band Face Pull C: Band Pull-Apart	Long resistance band (light)	2–3 x 8–10 each exercise
	PHASE 5	Inverted Row	Suspension trainer	3 x 5
	PHASE 6	A: Vertical Jacks B: Med Ball Slam	A: None B: Med ball	A: 3 x 5 B: 3 x 3
PRIMING & POTENTIATION	NEUROLOGICAL PRIMER	A: Rainbow Med Ball Slam	Med ball	4 x 10 alternating
	MECHANICAL PRIMER	B: Hinged Straight-Arm Band Pulldown	Cable or long resistance band (light)	4 x 20
KEY PERFORMANCE INDICATOR (KPI)	UPPER/PULL	Neutral Grip Pull-Up	Rack	4 x 6–8
PUMP ACCESSORIES & PREHAB	PUSH	1A: Band-Resisted Stretch Push-Up	Long resistance band	3 x 8–10
	PULL	1B: Half-Kneeling Single-Arm Cable Row	Cable or long resistance band	3 x 15 each side
	CHEST	1C: Backward Crawl	None	3 x 30s
	SHOULDERS	2A: Powell Raise	Dumbbells	2–3 x 10–15 each side
	SHOULDERS	2B: Suspension Trainer Y Fly	Suspension trainer	2–3 x 10–15
CONDITIONING FINISHER	BICEPS/CORE BURNOUT	A: Dumbbell Supinated Curl B: Kneeling Band/Cable Crunch	A: Dumbbells B: Cable or long resistance band	5m AMRAP A: 15 reps B: 15 reps
POST-TRAINING COOL-DOWN	BREATHE	Supine 90/90 Breathing	None	1m
	FOAM ROLL	Lats	Foam roller	1m each side
	STRETCH	Child's Pose (10 & 2)	None	1m each side

PAIN-FREE PERFORMANCE PRODUCTS

DR. JOHN RUSIN'S
UNBREAKABLE TRAINING APP

**⋀⋀UN
BREAKABLE**

STRONG. LEAN. RESILIENT.

UNBREAKABLE TRAINING APP

Continue your Pain-Free Performance training inside the Unbreakable App.

**PAIN-FREE PERFORMANCE
SPECIALIST CERTIFICATION**
Train Smarter. Train Harder. Stay Healthier

PAIN-FREE PERFORMANCE SPECIALIST CERTIFICATION

Earn your Pain-Free Performance Specialist Certification (PPSC) credential.

**DR. JOHN RUSIN'S
COACHING**

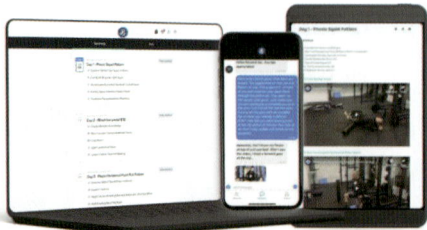

DR. JOHN RUSIN PERSONALIZED ONLINE COACHING

Work directly with Dr. John Rusin as your personal online coach.

PPSC OFFICIAL RESISTANCE BAND SET (8 TOTAL)

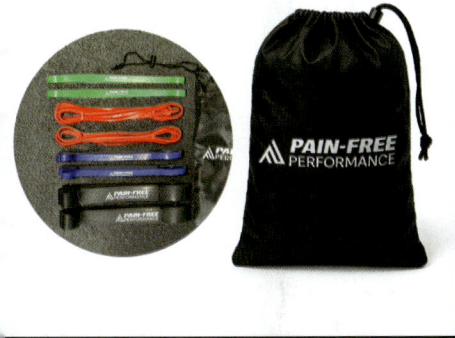

Train with the official Pain-Free Performance 8-Pack Band Set featuring 4 different resistance profiles perfect for every type of exercise, strength level & skill set.

SQUAT WEDGIEZ

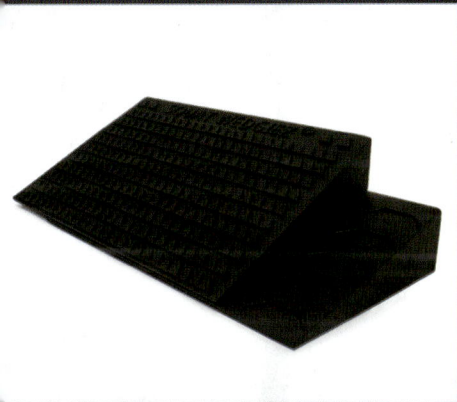

Optimize your biomechanics and unlock more complete ranges of motion for a smarter, more customized pain-free training approach.

PAIN-FREE PERFORMANCE APPAREL

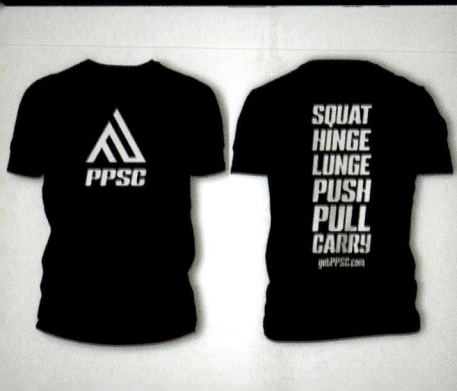

Rep the foundations of Pain-Free Performance with our official apparel line featuring the iconic pyramid on the front and 6 foundational movement patterns on the back.

REFERENCES

PART 1: PRINCIPLES OF PAIN-FREE PERFORMANCE

THE MOVEMENT MASTERY MINDSET

1. Ericsson, K. Anders, Ralf Th. Krampe, and Clemens Tesch-Römer. "The Role of Deliberate Practice in the Acquisition of Expert Performance." *Psychological Review* 100, no. 3 (1993): 363–406.

2. Fitts, Paul M., and Michael I. Posner. *Human Performance*. Belmont, CA: Brooks/Cole Publishing Company, 1967.

Deliberate Practice and Skill Acquisition

Schmidt, Richard A., and Timothy D. Lee. *Motor Control and Learning: A Behavioral Emphasis*. 6th ed. Champaign, IL: Human Kinetics, 2019.

Explains the core principles behind motor learning, helping you understand the progression through cognitive, associative, and autonomous stages. Supports efforts to systematically build and refine movement quality through deliberate practice.

Magill, Richard A., and David I. Anderson. *Motor Learning and Control: Concepts and Applications*. 11th ed. New York: McGraw-Hill Education, 2016.

Offers practical strategies for improving motor control and skill development. Their insights will help you effectively apply deliberate practice, enabling you to enhance your movement proficiency and achieve greater performance mastery.

THE PILLAR

1. McGill, Stuart M., and Leigh Marshall. "Kettlebell Swing, Snatch, and Bottoms-up Carry: Back and Hip Muscle Activation, Motion, and Low Back Loads." *Journal of Strength and Conditioning Research* 26, no. 1 (2012): 16–27.

Bracing and Core Stability

Vera-Garcia, Francisco J., Stuart M. McGill, and Joan S. Brown. "Effects of Abdominal Hollowing and Bracing Maneuvers on the Control of Spine Motion and Stability Against Sudden Trunk Perturbations." *Journal of Electromyography and Kinesiology* 17, no. 5 (2007): 556–567.

Supports the understanding of core bracing by illustrating how specific bracing techniques can significantly improve spine stability, reducing unwanted movement and protecting against injury.

Joint Centration and Neutral Zone

Sahrmann, Shirley A. *Diagnosis and Treatment of Movement Impairment Syndromes*. St. Louis, MO: Mosby, 2002.

Highlights the importance of joint centration (aligning joints for optimal stability and muscle activation), reinforcing strategies for maintaining neutral joint positions.

Biomechanics of the Shoulder and Hip

Neumann, Donald A. *Kinesiology of the Musculoskeletal System: Foundations for Rehabilitation*. 3rd ed. St. Louis, MO: Elsevier, 2016.

Provides clear explanations of shoulder and hip biomechanics, emphasizing the importance of proper alignment for effective and pain-free movement, which underpins pillar stability principles.

Neutral Spine and Movement Variability

Panjabi, Manohar M. "The Stabilizing System of the Spine. Part I. Function, Dysfunction, Adaptation, and Enhancement." *Journal of Spinal Disorders* 5, no. 4 (1992): 383–389.

Details the role of spinal stabilization and explains why maintaining movement within your individual neutral zone is crucial for preventing injuries and enhancing overall stability.

BREATHING STRATEGIES

Diaphragmatic Breathing and Parasympathetic Response

Ma, Xue-Qiang, Yue-Jie Yue, Zi-Ying Gong, Hua-Xin Zhang, Na Duan, Yong-Tai Shi, Wei Wei, and Ying Li. "The Effect of Diaphragmatic Breathing on Attention, Negative Affect, and Stress in Healthy Adults." *Frontiers in Psychology* 8 (2017): 874.

Underscores how diaphragmatic breathing can enhance focus, reduce stress, and positively affect mood.

Laborde, Sylvain, Emma Mosley, and Julian F. Thayer. "Heart Rate Variability and Cardiac Vagal Tone in Psychophysiological Research—Recommendations for Experiment Planning, Data Analysis, and Data Reporting." *Frontiers in Psychology* 8 (2017): 213.

Highlights the role of slow, controlled breathing in enhancing heart rate variability and cardiac vagal tone—crucial markers for recovery and stress management.

Grudzińska, Ewa, et al. "Benefits from one session of deep and slow breathing on vagal tone and state anxiety." *Scientific Reports* 11 (2021): 98736.

Demonstrates how brief deep-breathing sessions can immediately boost vagal tone and reduce anxiety, validating breathing exercises to quickly facilitate recovery.

Box Breathing (Tactical Breathing) and Performance

Divine, Mark. *Unbeatable Mind: Forge Resiliency and Mental Toughness to Succeed at an Elite Level.* Carlsbad, CA: CreateSpace Independent Publishing Platform, 2015.

Provides insight into "box breathing" and its role in building mental resilience, optimizing recovery, and enhancing performance under pressure.

Breathing Techniques for CNS and Stress Management

Russo, Marc A., Danielle M. Santarelli, and Dean O'Rourke. "The Physiological Effects of Slow Breathing in the Healthy Human." *Breathe* 13, no. 4 (2017): 298–309.

Illustrates the physiological impacts of controlled breathing on stress and CNS regulation, reinforcing use of breathing strategies for enhancing calmness and recovery.

Breathing, Core Stability, and Athletic Performance

Janssens, Lotte, Annick Brumagne, Bertine Feys, Maarten Pijnenburg, Barbara Claeys, and Alice Troosters. "The Effect of Inspiratory Muscles Fatigue on Postural Control in People with and without Recurrent Low Back Pain." *Spine* 35, no. 10 (2010): 1088–1094.

Supports breathing as integral to maintaining core stability and posture, especially under conditions of fatigue, to reduce injury risk and enhance performance.

PART 2: THE 6-PHASE DYNAMIC WARM-UP

PREPARATION TENETS

Physical, Mental, and Emotional Readiness

Davies, Michael J., Jonathan K. Sinclair, Paul J. Taylor, and Lindsay Bottoms. "Revisiting the 'Whys' and 'Hows' of the Warm-Up: Are We Asking the Right Questions?" *Frontiers in Physiology* 14 (2023): 1196247.

Provides clarity on the physiological and psychological reasons behind an effective warm-up, reinforcing its role in optimizing physical, mental, and emotional preparedness for training.

van Raalte, Judy L., et al. "Effects of a Mental Warmup on Workout Readiness and Stress of College Student Exercisers." *Journal of Functional Morphology and Kinesiology* 4, no. 2 (2019): 42–52.

Supports the use of mental preparation strategies, highlighting their impact on enhancing readiness, reducing stress, and elevating overall workout quality.

Central Nervous System Regulation and Performance

Bishop, David. "Warm Up I: Potential Mechanisms and the Effects of Passive Warm Up on Exercise Performance." *Sports Medicine* 33, no. 6 (2003): 439–454.

Outlines the underlying mechanisms behind warming up, providing scientific support for the strategies that optimize CNS regulation for better exercise performance.

Bishop, David. "Warm Up II: Performance Changes Following Active Warm Up and How to Structure the Warm Up." *Sports Medicine* 33, no. 7 (2003): 483–498.

Complements structuring warm-ups strategically to gradually elevate CNS activity, reinforcing the step-by-step sequence of preparation.

Sympathetic and Parasympathetic Balance for Training and Recovery

Stanley, Jamie, Brad Peake, and Jonathan M. Buchheit. "Cardiac Parasympathetic Reactivation Following Exercise: Implications for Training Prescription." *Sports Medicine* 43, no. 12 (2013): 1259–1277.

Highlights the importance of quickly shifting from a sympathetic to a parasympathetic state post-exercise, aligning with CNS balance for optimized recovery.

Laborde, Sylvain, Emma Mosley, and Julian F. Thayer. "Heart Rate Variability and Cardiac Vagal Tone in Psychophysiological Research—Recommendations for Experiment Planning, Data Analysis, and Data Reporting." *Frontiers in Psychology* 8 (2017): 213.

Validates the effectiveness of breathing strategies to manage stress and enhance recovery through improved heart rate variability.

Effectiveness of Dynamic Warm-ups in Reducing Injury and Enhancing Performance

Fradkin, Andrea J., Bronwyn J. Gabbe, and Paul A. Cameron. "Does Warming Up Prevent Injury in Sport? The Evidence from Randomised Controlled Trials." *Journal of Science and Medicine in Sport* 9, no. 3 (2006): 214–220.

Provides robust evidence supporting the rationale for dynamic warm-ups as effective tools in reducing injury risk.

McCrary, J. Matt, Sheila L. Ackermann, and Barbara A. Halaki. "A Systematic Review of the Effects of Upper Body Warm-up on Performance and Injury." *British Journal of Sports Medicine* 49, no. 14 (2015): 935–942.

Reinforces the impact of dynamic warm-ups on enhancing upper body performance and minimizing the risk of injury.

Mindfulness, Breathing, and Parasympathetic Activation

Russo, Marc A., Danielle M. Santarelli, and Dean O'Rourke. "The Physiological Effects of Slow Breathing in the Healthy Human." *Breathe* 13, no. 4 (2017): 298–309.

Highlights how intentional slow breathing positively affects the nervous system, supporting strategies for using mindful breathing techniques to manage stress and facilitate recovery.

Hopper, Sarah I., Daniel J. Murray, Timothy Ferrara, and Maryam Singleton. "Effectiveness of Diaphragmatic Breathing for Reducing Physiological and Psychological Stress: A Review." *Journal of Evidence-Based Integrative Medicine* 24 (2019): 2515690X19842803.

Strengthens advocacy of diaphragmatic breathing for reducing physiological and psychological stress.

PHASE 1: SOFT TISSUE TECHNIQUES

1. Cheatham, Scott W., Morey J. Kolber, Matt Cain, and Matt Lee. "The Effects of Self-Myofascial Release Using a Foam Roll or Roller Massager on Joint Range of Motion, Muscle Recovery, and Performance: A Systematic Review." *International Journal of Sports Physical Therapy* 10, no. 6 (2015): 827–838.

Foam Rolling, Parasympathetic Activation, and Central Nervous System Regulation

Behm, David G., Duane C. Button, Eric J. Drinkwater, and Mike M. Behm. "Foam Rolling as a Recovery Tool after an Intense Bout of Physical Activity." *Medicine & Science in Sports & Exercise* 52, no. 8 (2020): 1804–1812.

Highlights foam rolling's effectiveness in promoting recovery post-exercise by activating the parasympathetic nervous system, directly supporting how foam rolling calms the CNS and reduces muscle tension.

Wilke, Jan, Lukas Müller, Andreas L. Giesche, Paul Ackermann, and David Behm. "Acute Effects of Foam Rolling on Range of Motion in Healthy Adults: A Systematic Review with Multilevel Meta-analysis." *Sports Medicine* 50, no. 2 (2020): 387–402.

Provides evidence that foam rolling temporarily enhances joint range of motion, reinforcing its role in preparing the body for effective movement during warm-ups.

Foam Rolling, Pain Perception, and Reduction of Muscle Tone

Aboodarda, Saied Jalal, Duane C. Button, Jordan Andersen, and David G. Behm. "Acute Effects of Foam Rolling on Quadriceps Pain, Muscle Function, and Performance." *International Journal of Sports Physiology and Performance* 10, no. 8 (2015): 1147–1153.

Underscores foam rolling's immediate impact on reducing pain perception and muscle soreness, validating its inclusion in pre-training warm-up to improve movement comfort and quality.

Pearcey, Gregory E. P., David J. Bradbury-Squires, Jon-Erik Kawamoto, Eric J. Drinkwater, Duane G. Behm, and David G. Behm. "Foam Rolling for Delayed-Onset Muscle Soreness and Recovery of Dynamic Performance Measures." *Journal of Athletic Training* 50, no. 1 (2015): 5–13.

Demonstrates foam rolling's ability to alleviate delayed-onset muscle soreness (DOMS), reduce muscle tone, and manage discomfort to enhance performance.

Psychological Benefits and Mental Readiness through Foam Rolling

Monteiro, Estêvão Rios, Bianca Škarabot, and Anthony J. Blazevich. "Foam Rolling Improves Mental Readiness for Subsequent Physical Activity." *International Journal of Sports Physiology and Performance* 12, no. 6 (2017): 833–839.

Confirms that foam rolling enhances mental preparedness, directly reinforcing the psychological benefits of soft tissue techniques for improved focus and performance.

PHASE 2: BIPHASIC POSITIONAL STRETCHING

1. Pinto, Matheus D., Fabio L. Wilhelm, Cesar A. Radaelli, Thiago Bottaro, Gabriel N. Blazevich, Marco Aurélio Vaz, and Martim Bottaro. "Differential Effects of 30- Vs. 60-Second Static Muscle Stretching on Vertical Jump Performance." *Journal of Strength and Conditioning Research* 28, no. 12 (2014): 3440–3446.

2. Ayala, Francisco, Antonio Sainz de Baranda, David De Ste Croix, and Alejandro Santonja. "Acute Effects of Two Different Stretching Techniques on Passive Torque and Range of Motion in Healthy Adults." *Journal of Sports Science & Medicine* 11, no. 1 (2012): 190–197.

Effect of Stretching on Parasympathetic Activation and CNS Downregulation

Behm, David G., Anthony J. Blazevich, Anthony D. Kay, and Malachy McHugh. "Acute Effects of Muscle Stretching on Physical Performance, Range of Motion, and Injury Incidence in Healthy Active Individuals: A Systematic Review." *Applied Physiology, Nutrition, and Metabolism* 41, no. 1 (2016): 1–11.

Summarizes the benefits of stretching in modulating muscle tone, reducing injury risk, and activating a parasympathetic response, clearly aligning with phase 2 objectives of reducing tension and stress before training.

Weerapong, Pornratshanee, Patria A. Hume, and Gregory S. Kolt. "Stretching: Mechanisms and Benefits for Sport Performance and Injury Prevention." *Physical Therapy Reviews* 9, no. 4 (2004): 189–206.

Explains how stretching can support injury prevention and enhance overall sports performance.

Mobility, Stability, and Stretching Techniques

Page, Phil. "Current Concepts in Muscle Stretching for Exercise and Rehabilitation." *International Journal of Sports Physical Therapy* 7, no. 1 (2012): 109–119.

Outlines the role of stretching in improving mobility and rehabilitation, supporting controlled stretching techniques to restore functional range of motion and stability.

Blazevich, Anthony J., Gillian S. Gill, and David G. Behm. "Stretching and Flexibility: A Critical Review of the Literature." *Applied Physiology, Nutrition, and Metabolism* 44, no. 2 (2019): 179–188.

Provides a comprehensive review, validating strategic approaches to stretching for enhancing mobility, improving biomechanics, and minimizing compensation in training.

Neuromuscular Responses to Stretching

Lima, Carlos D., Lucas D. Ruas, Frederico T. Behm, et al. "Acute Effects of Static vs. Ballistic Stretching on Strength, Power, and Neuromuscular Performance." *Journal of Strength and Conditioning Research* 33, no. 2 (2019): 333–341.

Demonstrates the differential effects of stretching types, aligning with the biphasic approach that combines oscillatory (dynamic) and static end-range stretching to optimize neuromuscular readiness.

Trajano, Gabriel S., Anthony J. Blazevich, and Glen Lichtwark. "Neural Mechanisms of Muscle Stretching and Flexibility." *Scandinavian Journal of Medicine & Science in Sports* 27, no. 7 (2017): 781–791.

Offers insights into the neurological mechanisms involved in stretching, emphasizing the effectiveness of stretching to improve movement quality by targeting neuromuscular control and flexibility.

PHASE 3: CORRECTIVE EXERCISE

1. Uehara, Luiz, Keith Davids, and Duarte Araújo. "Constraints on Exploration of Perceptual-Motor Workspace and Creativity in Soccer." *Brazilian Journal of Motor Behavior* 15, no. 5 (2021): 315–338.

2. Casazza, Brian A. "Diagnosis and Treatment of Acute Low Back Pain." *American Family Physician* 61, no. 6 (2000): 1779–1786.

Corrective Exercises and Movement Quality Enhancement

Cook, Gray, Lee Burton, and Barb Hoogenboom. "Pre-Participation Screening: The Use of Fundamental Movements as an Assessment of Function – Part 1." *North American Journal of Sports Physical Therapy* 1, no. 2 (2006): 62–72.

Supports the idea of using fundamental movement screens to pinpoint functional limitations, reinforcing corrective exercises to enhance movement quality.

Kiesel, Kyle, Phillip Plisky, and Michael L. Voight. "Can Serious Injury in Professional Football Be Predicted by a Preseason Functional Movement Screen?" *North American Journal of Sports Physical Therapy* 2, no. 3 (2007): 147–158.

Validates the principle of proactively addressing weak links through corrective exercises, highlighting their effectiveness in preventing injuries by improving fundamental movement patterns.

Neuromuscular Activation and Corrective Exercise Efficacy

Clark, Micheal, Scott Lucett, and Brian Sutton. *NASM Essentials of Corrective Exercise Training*. Burlington, MA: Jones & Bartlett Learning, 2021.

Provides practical insights into corrective exercise strategies, offering readers clear guidelines on effectively activating muscles and improving motor control to enhance their training sessions.

Page, Phil, Clare C. Frank, and Robert Lardner. *Assessment and Treatment of Muscle Imbalance: The Janda Approach*. Champaign, IL: Human Kinetics, 2010.

Clarifies the importance of addressing muscle imbalances, directly reinforcing the use of corrective exercises to improve symmetry, stability, and functional strength.

Motor Control, Stability, and Injury Prevention

Huxel Bliven, Kellie C., and Barton Anderson. "Core Stability Training for Injury Prevention." *Sports Health* 5, no. 6 (2013): 514–522.

Demonstrates how effective core stability training is in reducing injury risk, clearly supporting pillar and corrective exercises designed to maintain stable, pain-free movements.

McGill, Stuart. *Ultimate Back Fitness and Performance*. Waterloo, ON: Backfitpro Inc., 2009.

Underscores recommendations on bracing and core stabilization, supporting functional movement and preventing injury through corrective exercise.

PHASE 4: ACTIVATION DRILLS

1. Schoenfeld, Brad J., Bret Contreras, Jeffrey M. Vigotsky, and Andrew Alto. "Mind-Muscle Connection: A Review of Mechanisms and Practical Applications." *Strength and Conditioning Journal* 40, no. 5 (2018): 27–33.

Neuromuscular Activation and Injury Prevention

Lehecka, B. Jeffrey, et al. "Gluteal Muscle Activation during Common Therapeutic Exercises." *Journal of Orthopaedic & Sports Physical Therapy* 51, no. 7 (2021): 340–347.

Validates the use of glute activation exercises like glute bridges and single-leg variations, emphasizing their effectiveness for stabilizing the hips and preventing lower body injuries.

Reiman, Michael P., John Bolgla, and Christopher Lorenzetti. "Hip Function's Influence on Lower Extremity Kinematics and Kinetics." *Journal of Orthopaedic & Sports Physical Therapy* 39, no. 2 (2009): 90–104.

Highlights the crucial role hip stability plays in controlling lower body movements, with an emphasis on targeted hip activation drills to enhance movement quality and reduce injury risk.

Posterior Chain Emphasis and Pillar Stability

Kibler, W. Ben, Aaron Sciascia, and Timothy L. Uhl. "Prevention and Rehabilitation of Upper Extremity Injuries in Sports: Integration of the Kinetic Chain into Practice." *North American Journal of Sports Physical Therapy* 3, no. 2 (2008): 98–105.

Aligns directly with pillar stability and posterior chain activation, highlighting how activation drills improve kinetic chain integration and safeguard against upper body injuries.

Pearcey, Gregory E. P., David J. Bradbury-Squires, Jon-Erik Kawamoto, Eric J. Drinkwater, Duane G. Behm, and David G. Behm. "Foam Rolling for Delayed-Onset Muscle Soreness and Recovery of Dynamic Performance Measures." *Journal of Athletic Training* 50, no. 1 (2015): 5–13.

Reinforces the rationale for integrating activation exercises to prime muscles, reduce soreness, and prepare the body for dynamic performance.

Activation and Performance Optimization

Monteiro, Estêvão Rios, Bianca Škarabot, and Anthony J. Blazevich. "Foam Rolling Improves Mental Readiness for Subsequent Physical Activity." *International Journal of Sports Physiology and Performance* 12, no. 6 (2017): 833–839.

Validates the approach of activation drills not only for physical preparation but also for enhancing mental readiness and focus prior to engaging in demanding movements.

PHASE 5: MOVEMENT PATTERN DEVELOPMENT

1. Moore, Aaron, and Jared W. Coburn. "Attentional Focus Cueing: How and When to Use Internal and External Focus Cues to Optimize Exercise Performance." *ACSM's Health & Fitness Journal* 25, no. 6 (2021): 20–26.

Internal Cueing, Attentional Focus, and Motor Learning

Wulf, Gabriele. "Attentional Focus and Motor Learning: A Review of 15 Years." *International Review of Sport and Exercise Psychology* 6, no. 1 (2013): 77–104.

Clarifies how attentional focus influences skill learning and performance, directly supporting the use of internal cues to develop precise, controlled movements in practice.

Becker, Katrina A., and David E. Smith. "Effects of Attentional Focus on Performance and Learning of a Motor Skill." *Journal of Exercise Science & Fitness* 13, no. 2 (2015): 34–41.

Emphasizes the effectiveness of internal focus cues for skill acquisition, aligning with the chapter's approach of breaking down movements to refine technique.

Slow, Deliberate Movement and Neuromuscular Control

Suchomel, Timothy J., Sophia Nimphius, and Michael H. Stone. "The Importance of Muscular Strength in Athletic Performance." *Sports Medicine* 46, no. 10 (2016): 1419–1449.

Underscores the value of developing muscular strength through deliberate, controlled movements—reinforcing strategies of slow movement and intentional muscle engagement for better neuromuscular control.

Schoenfeld, Brad J., Jozo Grgic, Dan Ogborn, and James W. Krieger. "Strength and Hypertrophy Adaptations between Low- vs. High-Load Resistance Training: A Systematic Review and Meta-analysis." *Journal of Strength and Conditioning Research* 31, no. 12 (2017): 3508–3523.

Supports the principle that slow, deliberate movement at lighter loads can effectively stimulate muscular adaptation, confirming the approach to movement pattern development without heavy weights.

Motor Control and Skill Refinement

Schmidt, Richard A., and Timothy D. Lee. *Motor Control and Learning: A Behavioral Emphasis*. 6th ed. Champaign, IL: Human Kinetics, 2019.

Offers foundational insights into motor learning, helping you apply deliberate practice techniques in phase 5 to refine and master complex movement patterns.

Magill, Richard A., and David I. Anderson. *Motor Learning and Control: Concepts and Applications*. 11th ed. New York: McGraw-Hill Education, 2016.

Provides practical guidance for skill refinement and motor control, supporting the methodology of gradual, controlled progression toward movement mastery.

PHASE 6: CENTRAL NERVOUS SYSTEM STIMULATION

1. Seitz, Laurent B., Gabriel J. Trajano, and G. Gregory Haff. "The Acute Effects of Postactivation Potentiation on Explosive Strength Performance: A Systematic Review and Meta-Analysis." *Sports Medicine* 46, no. 2 (2016): 231–240.

2. Carvalho, Arthur, Irineu Loturco, Lucas A. Pereira, João Pedro Lopes-Silva, Felipe Romano Medeiros, Rodrigo Ramirez-Campillo, and Tomás T. Freitas. "Optimal Rest Interval to Maximize Post-Activation Performance Enhancement in Vertical Jumps: A Systematic Review and Meta-Analysis." *Scientific Reports* 14, no. 1 (2024): 5899.

Dynamic Movement, CNS Stimulation, and Injury Prevention

Haff, G. Gregory, and Sophia Nimphius. "Training Principles for Power." *Strength and Conditioning Journal* 34, no. 6 (2012): 2–12.

Outlines the foundational principles of training for power, supporting the dynamic, explosive movements in phase 6 to enhance neuromuscular coordination and athletic performance.

Ebben, William P. "Complex Training: A Brief Review." *Journal of Sports Science & Medicine* 1, no. 2 (2002): 42–46.

Supports the use of explosive movements to activate the central nervous system, reinforcing strategies for injury prevention and enhancing performance by priming the body with high-intensity, fast-twitch activities.

External Cueing and Enhanced Athletic Performance

Wulf, Gabriele, and Rebecca Lewthwaite. "Optimizing Performance through Intrinsic Motivation and Attention for Learning: The OPTIMAL Theory of Motor Learning." *Psychonomic Bulletin & Review* 23, no. 5 (2016): 1382–1414.

Validates the effectiveness of external cues to optimize performance, aligning precisely with phase 6 to transition from internal cues during practice to external cues during performance.

Halperin, Israel, David B. Pyne, and Dale W. Chapman. "Using Attentional Focus Instructions to Improve Explosive Performance." *Journal of Strength and Conditioning Research* 30, no. 5 (2016): 1215–1221.

Directly reinforces external cueing to enhance explosive power and athletic performance, and why specific, goal-oriented cues are critical during high-intensity movements.

Athletic Movement and Neuromuscular Coordination

Myer, Gregory D., Kevin R. Ford, Joseph M. Palumbo, and Timothy E. Hewett. "Neuromuscular Training Improves Performance and Lower-Extremity Biomechanics in Female Athletes." *Journal of Strength and Conditioning Research* 19, no. 1 (2005): 51–60.

Underscores the importance of neuromuscular coordination training for improving biomechanics and performance, clearly supporting fast, coordinated exercises in phase 6 to enhance athletic attributes and reduce injury risk.

Faigenbaum, Avery D., Gregory D. Myer, Ivan P. Paterno, and Timothy E. Hewett. "Neuromuscular Training to Reduce Sports-Related Injuries in Youth: Effectiveness of Integrative Neuromuscular Training." *Exercise and Sport Sciences Reviews* 41, no. 3 (2013): 161–166.

Demonstrates how neuromuscular training reduces injury risk and enhances athletic performance, highlighting the critical role of dynamic exercises in developing resilient, responsive movement patterns.

PART 3: THE 6 FOUNDATIONAL MOVEMENT PATTERNS

MOVEMENT TENETS

Foundational Movement Patterns and Functional Training

Cook, Gray, Lee Burton, and Barb Hoogenboom. "Pre-Participation Screening: The Use of Fundamental Movements as an Assessment of Function—Part 1." *North American Journal of Sports Physical Therapy* 1, no. 2 (2006): 62–72.

Provides foundational insights into movement screening, emphasizing its importance in identifying functional limitations and guiding exercise selection.

Kiesel, Kyle, Phillip Plisky, and Michael L. Voight. "Can Serious Injury in Professional Football Be Predicted by a Preseason Functional Movement Screen?" *North American Journal of Sports Physical Therapy* 2, no. 3 (2007): 147–158.

Validates the effectiveness of functional movement screening to predict injury risk, reinforcing the importance of assessing and addressing weak links in foundational movements.

Biomechanics and Individualized Training

McGill, Stuart. *Ultimate Back Fitness and Performance.* Waterloo, ON: Backfitpro Inc., 2009.

McGill's comprehensive guide to spinal biomechanics supports individualized movement adaptations, helping you understand how a personalized setup and execution can minimize injury risk and enhance performance.

Sahrmann, Shirley A. *Diagnosis and Treatment of Movement Impairment Syndromes.* St. Louis, MO: Mosby, 2002.

Emphasizes individualized training based on movement impairments, which supports customizing exercises to match each person's unique biomechanics and functional needs.

Screens, Assessments, and Injury Prevention

Frost, David M., Tyson A. Beach, Callaghan P. Jack, and Stuart M. McGill. "An Appraisal of the Functional Movement Screen™ Grading Criteria: Is the Composite Score Sensitive to Functional Changes?" *Journal of Strength and Conditioning Research* 26, no. 6 (2012): 1620–1626.

Provides evidence supporting the sensitivity of movement screens in tracking functional improvements, aligning closely with the idea of continuous reassessment and optimization of foundational patterns.

Huxel Bliven, Kellie C., and Barton Anderson. "Core Stability Training for Injury Prevention." *Sports Health* 5, no. 6 (2013): 514–522.

Emphasizes core stability as critical for injury prevention, directly reinforcing the tenets of using foundational movements to build a stable, resilient body.

SQUAT

1. Tiwari, Vivek, Sandeep Kumar, Pradeep Kumar, Mukesh Kumar, and Sameer Aggarwal. "Is Femoral Anteversion Different in Various Ethnic Groups? A Retrospective Computed Tomography Study." *Journal of Clinical Orthopaedics and Trauma* 11, no. 1 (2020): 101–105.

Squat Biomechanics and Anthropometry

Escamilla, Rafael F. "Knee Biomechanics of the Dynamic Squat Exercise." *Medicine & Science in Sports & Exercise* 33, no. 1 (2001): 127–141.

Provides essential insights into knee mechanics during squatting, reinforcing the discussion on maintaining proper alignment and minimizing joint stress.

Individualized Squat Technique and Anatomical Variability

Horsak, Brian, Arnold Baca, Stefan Pobatschnig, and Mario Greber-Platzer. "Individual Variation in Hip Anatomy and Its Implications for Movement: A Systematic Review." *Journal of Sports Sciences* 33, no. 15 (2015): 1587–1598.

Emphasizes the importance of recognizing individual anatomical differences, directly supporting a personalized squat stance and depth for comfort, safety, and performance.

Vigotsky, Andrew D., Bret Contreras, Chris Beardsley, and Brad J. Schoenfeld. "Biomechanical Implications of Squat Depth: A Review." *Journal of Strength and Conditioning Research* 33, no. 7 (2019): 1974–1986.

Reinforces the recommendation to tailor squat depth based on individual biomechanics, highlighting why deeper isn't always better and how individual anatomy influences safe squat depth.

Movement Screens, Assessments, and Squat Optimization

Kritz, Matthew, John Cronin, and Patria Hume. "The Bodyweight Squat: A Movement Screen for the Squat Pattern." *Strength and Conditioning Journal* 31, no. 1 (2009): 76–85.

Validates the approach of using the bodyweight squat as a foundational movement screen, helping readers understand how to identify and address limitations before loading the squat.

Frost, David M., Tyson A. Beach, Callaghan P. Jack, and Stuart M. McGill. "An Appraisal of the Functional Movement Screen™ Grading Criteria: Is the Composite Score Sensitive to Functional Changes?" *Journal of Strength and Conditioning Research* 26, no. 6 (2012): 1620–1626.

Underscores the value of regular movement screening and assessment, supporting the methodology for continuously refining squat mechanics.

Addressing Common Squat Compensations and Injuries

Kang, Min-Hyeok, et al. "Comparison of Ankle and Knee Kinetics between Normal and Valgus Squats." *Journal of Physical Therapy Science* 27, no. 7 (2015): 2091–2093.

Reinforces guidance on correcting knee valgus collapse, clearly demonstrating why proper ankle and knee alignment are essential for preventing injuries during squats.

Bell, David R., Michael J. Padua, and Michael A. Clark. "Muscle Strength and Flexibility Characteristics of People Displaying Excessive Medial Knee Displacement." *Archives of Physical Medicine and Rehabilitation* 89, no. 7 (2008): 1323–1328.

Provides evidence supporting strategies for addressing medial knee displacement (valgus collapse), emphasizing the importance of targeted muscle strengthening and flexibility to correct and prevent this common squat compensation.

HINGE

Hinge Pattern Biomechanics and Individualized Hip Hinge Mechanics

Escamilla, Rafael F., et al. "Biomechanical Analysis of the Deadlift During the 1999 Special Olympics World Games." *Medicine & Science in Sports & Exercise* 33, no. 8 (2001): 1345–1353.

Reinforces the emphasis on hinge mechanics by detailing how deadlift biomechanics impact lower body joint stresses, underscoring the importance of individualized form.

Addressing Compensations and Optimizing the Hinge

Hales, Michael E., Brendan D. Johnson, and Jeffery W. Johnson. "Kinematic Analysis of the Powerlifting Style Squat and the Conventional Deadlift During Competition: Is There a Cross-Over Effect Between Lifts?" *Journal of Strength and Conditioning Research* 23, no. 9 (2009): 2574–2580.

Clarifies distinctions between hinge and squat mechanics, validating strategies for correcting compensations such as excessive knee bend or squat-like patterns during the hinge.

Schoenfeld, Brad J. "Squatting Kinematics and Kinetics and Their Application to Exercise Performance." *Journal of Strength and Conditioning Research* 24, no. 12 (2010): 3497–3506.

Highlights how squat-like compensations can negatively affect hinge performance. This supports maintaining a pure hip hinge pattern to protect the spine and optimize movement.

LUNGE

1. Helliwell, Philip N., John Howell, and Valerie Wright. "Tibiofemoral Ratio and Its Association with Osteoarthritis of the Knee." *Annals of the Rheumatic Diseases* 55, no. 1 (1996): 51–52.

Biomechanics and Importance of Single-Leg and Split-Stance Movements

McCurdy, Kevin W., George A. Langford, Michael Doscher, R. Todd Wiley, and Keith E. Mallard. "The Effects of Short-Term Unilateral and Bilateral Lower-Body Resistance Training on Measures of Strength and Power." *Journal of Strength and Conditioning Research* 19, no. 1 (2005): 9–15.

Highlights the distinct advantages of unilateral training over bilateral exercises in improving lower body strength and power.

Myer, Gregory D., Kevin R. Ford, Joseph M. Palumbo, and Timothy E. Hewett. "Neuromuscular Training Improves Performance and Lower-Extremity Biomechanics in Female Athletes." *Journal of Strength and Conditioning Research* 19, no. 1 (2005): 51–60.

Underscores how neuromuscular training through single-leg movements like lunges can significantly improve biomechanics and athletic performance.

Individualized Anatomical Assessment and Movement Optimization

Horsak, Brian, Arnold Baca, Stefan Pobatschnig, and Mario Greber-Platzer. "Individual Variation in Hip Anatomy and Its Implications for Movement: A Systematic Review." *Journal of Sports Sciences* 33, no. 15 (2015): 1587–1598.

Emphasizes individual anatomical variability in hip structure, supporting the use of the TF Ratio Hip Flexion Test to personalize lunge mechanics and optimize performance while minimizing discomfort.

Vigotsky, Andrew D., Bret Contreras, Chris Beardsley, and Brad J. Schoenfeld. "Biomechanical Implications of Squat Depth: A Review." *Journal of Strength and Conditioning Research* 33, no. 7 (2019): 1974–1986.

Provides biomechanical context for the depth and alignment considerations in split-stance movements, reinforcing guidance on customized range-of-motion adjustments based on individual limb proportions.

Assessments and Injury Prevention

Bell, David R., Michael J. Padua, and Michael A. Clark. "Muscle Strength and Flexibility Characteristics of People Displaying Excessive Medial Knee Displacement." *Archives of Physical Medicine and Rehabilitation* 89, no. 7 (2008): 1323–1328.

Supports strategies for correcting excessive knee displacement during lunges, emphasizing the importance of targeted strength and flexibility training to prevent injuries.

PUSH

Overtraining and Muscular Imbalances in Push Patterns

Kolber, Morey J., and Mitchell S. Cheatham. "Shoulder Joint and Muscle Characteristics among Weight-Training Participants with and without Shoulder Pain." *Journal of Strength and Conditioning Research* 31, no. 4 (2017): 1024–1032.

Supports how overtraining the push pattern can lead to shoulder imbalances and pain, highlighting the importance of balanced training for joint health.

Borstad, John D. "Resting Position Variables at the Shoulder: Evidence to Support a Posture-Impairment Association." *Physical Therapy* 86, no. 4 (2006): 549–557.

Demonstrates the direct connection between chronic poor posture from excessive pushing movements and compromised shoulder mechanics.

Poor Mechanics and Shoulder Pain Associated with Barbell Bench Pressing

Green, Chad M., and Paul Comfort. "The Effect of Grip Width on Bench Press Performance and Risk of Injury." *Strength and Conditioning Journal* 29, no. 5 (2007): 10–14.

Highlights how grip width impacts shoulder stress during bench pressing, validating recommendations for optimizing hand position to prevent injury.

Fees, Marcus, Dennis N. Brown, and Andrew Jensen. "Bench Press Modifications to Minimize Shoulder Injury." *Strength and Conditioning Journal* 24, no. 6 (2002): 14–19.

Suggests practical modifications to reduce shoulder injury risk during bench pressing, directly reinforcing the concept of movement mastery (proper form and controlled execution).

Importance of Scapular Movement and Stability

Kibler, W. Ben, Aaron Sciascia, and Timothy L. Uhl. "Prevention and Rehabilitation of Upper Extremity Injuries in Sports: Integration of the Kinetic Chain into Practice." *North American Journal of Sports Physical Therapy* 3, no. 2 (2008): 98–105.

Validates the importance of proper scapular mechanics and kinetic chain integration, strongly supporting scapular stability in pressing movements.

Paine, Russell, and Michael L. Voight. "The Role of the Scapula." *International Journal of Sports Physical Therapy* 8, no. 5 (2013): 617–629.

Emphasizes the critical role scapular positioning plays in safe and effective pressing, aligning precisely with guidance on maintaining optimal shoulder blade mechanics.

Influence of Overhead Mobility Restrictions

Kolber, Morey J., Scott W. Hanney, and Mitchell S. Cheatham. "Shoulder Joint Range of Motion Deficits in Competitive Swimmers." *Journal of Athletic Training* 45, no. 5 (2010): 514–519.

Highlights how overhead mobility restrictions lead to compensatory patterns and shoulder pain, directly reinforcing strategies for improving mobility before loading overhead pressing movements.

Wilk, Kevin E., Michael M. Reinold, and James R. Andrews. "Rehabilitation of the Thrower's Shoulder." *Clinics in Sports Medicine* 21, no. 2 (2002): 271–287.

Supports recommendations for addressing overhead mobility and stability deficits to enhance pressing performance and reduce injury risk.

PULL

Importance of Balanced Push-Pull Training and Posture Improvement

Borstad, John D., and Paula M. Ludewig. "The Effect of Long Versus Short Pectoralis Minor Resting Length on Scapular Kinematics in Healthy Individuals." *Journal of Orthopaedic & Sports Physical Therapy* 35, no. 4 (2005): 227–238.

Highlights how tightness from excessive pushing affects scapular positioning, validating the importance of balancing push-pull exercises for improved posture and shoulder health.

Kang, Ji-Hae, Kyoung-Sim Jung, and Do-Youn Lee. "The Effects of Bodyweight-Based Exercise with Push-Pull Patterns on the Posture of University Students." *Journal of Physical Therapy Science* 30, no. 7 (2018): 935–938.

Provides direct evidence that balanced push-pull training significantly improves postural alignment, supporting recommendations for correcting posture through pull-focused training.

Shoulder Health, Stability, and Injury Prevention Through Pulling Movements

Kibler, W. Ben, Aaron Sciascia, and Timothy L. Uhl. "Prevention and Rehabilitation of Upper Extremity Injuries in Sports: Integration of the Kinetic Chain into Practice." *North American Journal of Sports Physical Therapy* 3, no. 2 (2008): 98–105.

Confirms the critical role of proper scapular mechanics and balanced pulling exercises in preventing upper body injuries.

Reinold, Michael M., Kevin E. Wilk, Leonard C. Macrina, Stephen J. Sheheane, Charles A. Dun, Glenn S. Fleisig, and James R. Andrews. "Changes in Shoulder and Elbow Passive Range of Motion After Pitching in Professional Baseball Players." *American Journal of Sports Medicine* 36, no. 3 (2008): 523–527.

Reinforces the focus on restoring shoulder mobility and stability through targeted pulling patterns, illustrating their importance in maintaining long-term shoulder health.

Importance of Thoracic Mobility and Scapular Mechanics in Pulling Exercises

Kolber, Morey J., Mitchell S. Cheatham, Joseph C. Salamh, and Justin T. Hanney. "Characteristics of Individuals with Chronic Shoulder Pain: A Systematic Review." *Musculoskeletal Science and Practice* 29 (2017): 11–20.

Emphasizes the direct link between restricted thoracic mobility, impaired scapular mechanics, and chronic shoulder pain, supporting strategies for targeted pulling exercises.

Cools, Ann M., and Filip Struyf. "Shoulder Scapular Rehabilitation." *British Journal of Sports Medicine* 48, no. 8 (2014): 692–697.

Supports scapular control and thoracic mobility exercises as fundamental components of effective pulling strategies, crucial for shoulder rehabilitation and injury prevention.

Effects of Modern Sedentary Lifestyle on Shoulder Mechanics and Posture

Szeto, Grace P., Leon M. Straker, and Peter B. O'Sullivan. "The Effects of Sedentary Office Work on Musculoskeletal Health: A Systematic Review." *Journal of Occupational Rehabilitation* 20, no. 1 (2010): 7–22.

Demonstrates how modern sedentary lifestyles negatively impact posture and shoulder mechanics, validating the necessity of targeted pull-based training to offset these effects.

Borstad, John D. "Resting Position Variables at the Shoulder: Evidence to Support a Posture-

Impairment Association." *Physical Therapy* 86, no. 4 (2006): 549–557.

Emphasizes addressing lifestyle-induced postural dysfunction through consistent, corrective pulling exercises.

CARRY

1. Leong, Darryl P., et al. "Prognostic Value of Grip Strength: Findings from the Prospective Urban Rural Epidemiology (PURE) Study." *The Lancet* 386, no. 9990 (2015): 266–273.

2. Huxel Bliven, Kellie C., and Barton Anderson. "Core Stability Training for Injury Prevention." *Sports Health* 5, no. 6 (2013): 514–522.

3. Newman, Anne B., Tamara B. Harris, Rita C. Fallat, et al. "Strength, Not Muscle Mass, Is Associated with Mortality in the Health, Aging, and Body Composition Study Cohort." *Journals of Gerontology Series A: Biological Sciences and Medical Sciences* 71, no. 6 (2016): 678–683.

Functional Strength, Locomotion, and Real-World Carry Patterns

McGill, Stuart, Jordan Andersen, and Edward K. Cannon. "Muscle Activity and Spine Load during the Farmer's Walk Exercise." *Journal of Strength and Conditioning Research* 29, no. 8 (2015): 2196–2201.

Reinforces the emphasis on the farmer's walk, highlighting its unique ability to build core stability, protect spinal integrity, and develop practical strength for daily life.

Winwood, Paul W., et al. "Strongman Implements: A Review of Biomechanical and Physiological Effects." *International Journal of Sports Science & Coaching* 9, no. 5 (2014): 1207–1222.

Supports the effectiveness of loaded carries like farmer's walks for enhancing functional strength, stability, and performance in real-world activities.

Importance of Grip Strength and Longevity

Bohannon, Richard W. "Grip Strength: An Indispensable Biomarker for Older Adults." *Clinical Interventions in Aging* 14 (2019): 1681–1691.

Provides strong evidence supporting grip strength as an essential marker for aging health, emphasizing the critical role loaded carries play in maintaining functional independence.

Pillar Stability, Injury Prevention, and Carry Mechanics

Kibler, W. Ben, Aaron Sciascia, and Timothy L. Uhl. "Prevention and Rehabilitation of Upper Extremity Injuries in Sports: Integration of the Kinetic Chain into Practice." *North American Journal of Sports Physical Therapy* 3, no. 2 (2008): 98–105.

Underscores the critical importance of integrating kinetic chain mechanics into training, reinforcing the chapter's emphasis on loaded carries to enhance pillar stability and prevent injuries.

Shinkle, Justin, Todd W. Nesser, Thomas J. Demchak, and David M. McMannus. "Effect of Core Strength on the Measure of Power in the Extremities." *Journal of Strength and Conditioning Research* 26, no. 2 (2012): 373–380.

Supports the focus on building core (pillar) strength through carries, demonstrating the clear link between improved core stability and enhanced performance in all foundational movements.

The Significance of Loaded Carries for Assessing and Enhancing Movement Quality

McGill, Stuart, Edward K. Cannon, and Jordan T. Andersen. "Analysis of Muscle Activation and Spine Load in Farmer's Walk Exercises." *Clinical Biomechanics* 43 (2017): 110–116.

Highlights the importance of loaded carries for evaluating movement mechanics, spinal loading, and muscle activation.

Rusin, John, and Scotty Butcher. "Loaded Carries: A Missing Link to Strength and Performance." *Strength and Conditioning Journal* 40, no. 2 (2018): 31–38.

Validates claims about the role of loaded carries as critical diagnostic and performance tools.

PART 4: PROGRAMS AND TEMPLATES

TRAINING TENETS

Wave Loading and Structured Programming

Haff, G. Gregory, and Sophia Nimphius. "Training Principles for Power." *Strength and Conditioning Journal* 34, no. 6 (2012): 2–12.

Supports wave loading principles, emphasizing structured intensity and strategic fluctuations in an effort to optimize performance and recovery.

Conditioning and Cardiovascular Training

Gorzelitz, Jessica, Britton Trabert, Hormuzd A. Katki, Steven C. Moore, Eleanor L. Watts, and Charles E. Matthews. "Independent and Joint Associations of Weightlifting and Aerobic Activity with All-Cause, Cardiovascular Disease and Cancer Mortality in the Prostate, Lung, Colorectal and Ovarian Cancer Screening Trial." *British Journal of Sports Medicine* 56, no. 22 (2022): 1277–1283.

Highlights that while weightlifting independently reduces mortality risk, the combination of aerobic and strength training significantly enhances longevity benefits. Reinforces why aerobic conditioning must complement weightlifting in a balanced training program for optimal cardiovascular health and lifespan.

Buchheit, Martin, and Paul B. Laursen. "High-Intensity Interval Training, Solutions to the Programming Puzzle: Part I: Cardiopulmonary Emphasis." *Sports Medicine* 43, no. 5 (2013): 313–338.

Validates the use of heart rate–based conditioning and interval training, outlining why high-intensity intervals are effective for enhancing cardiovascular performance.

Accessory Work, Prehab, and Movement Optimization

Cook, Gray, Lee Burton, and Barb Hoogenboom. "Pre-Participation Screening: The Use of Fundamental Movements as an Assessment of Function—Part 1." *North American Journal of Sports Physical Therapy* 1, no. 2 (2006): 62–72.

Provides strong support for integrating accessory and prehab exercises, highlighting their essential role in identifying and correcting movement limitations to optimize function.

Kiesel, Kyle, Phillip Plisky, and Michael L. Voight. "Can Serious Injury in Professional Football Be Predicted by a Preseason Functional Movement Screen?" *North American Journal of Sports Physical Therapy* 2, no. 3 (2007): 147–158.

Emphasizes targeted accessory work to address compensations and prevent injuries by proactively managing weak links identified through screening.

Importance of Balanced Programming and Ratios

Contreras, Bret, and Brad J. Schoenfeld. "Latissimus Dorsi and Teres Major: Functional Anatomy and Application." *Strength and Conditioning Journal* 35, no. 1 (2013): 15–20.

Supports this book's recommended push-to-pull training ratio, highlighting the importance of horizontal pulling movements for improved scapular control and shoulder balance.

McGill, Stuart, Jordan Andersen, and Edward K. Cannon. "Muscle Activity and Spine Load during the Farmer's Walk Exercise." *Journal of Strength and Conditioning Research* 29, no. 8 (2015): 2196–2201.

Underscores the strategic use of carry patterns, validating their role in balanced training to enhance core stability, spine health, and functional performance.

Movement Frequency and Exercise Selection

Schoenfeld, Brad J., Dan Ogborn, and James W. Krieger. "Effects of Resistance Training Frequency on Measures of Muscle Hypertrophy: A Systematic Review and Meta-analysis." *Sports Medicine* 46, no. 11 (2016): 1689–1697.

Confirms the effectiveness of training frequencies, providing scientific backing for the optimal weekly exposure to maximize hypertrophy and strength gains.

Intelligent Progression and Technical Limits

Zourdos, Michael C., Andrew W. Dolan, Eric R. Helms, et al. "Novel Resistance Training-Specific Rating of Perceived Exertion Scale Measuring Repetitions in Reserve." *Journal of Strength and Conditioning Research* 30, no. 1 (2016): 267–275.

Supports recommendations for using repetitions-in-reserve (RIR) as an intelligent strategy to gauge effort, manage fatigue, and maintain optimal technique while progressively increasing load.

Suchomel, Timothy J., Sophia Nimphius, and Michael H. Stone. "The Importance of Muscular Strength in Athletic Performance." *Sports Medicine* 46, no. 10 (2016): 1419–1449.

Reinforces the approach of prioritizing quality movement and technical precision during strength training, emphasizing the long-term benefits of intelligent progression over maximal intensity.

INDEX

authentic hinge stance, 275–277

authentic positioning, compensation vs., 113

authentic squat stance, 240

autonomous stage, of motor control, 18–19

autopilot movement, 16–17

B

back emphasis, activation drills for, 167

back squat, 260, 266–267

backward crawl, 152

balance, for squat, 237

ball-and-socket joints, 26

band face pull

    about, 158

    for shoulders, 169–170

band over and back, for shoulders, 168–169

band pull-apart, for shoulders, 170–171

band-assisted pull-up, 411

banded distraction variation

    for dynamic pigeon stretch, 122

    for half-kneeling hip flexor stretch, 119

banded glute bridge, for hips, 162–163

banded single-leg glute bridge variation, 164–165

barbell back squat, 260

barbell bench press, 353, 354, 360–361

barbell bent-over row, 402

barbell front squat, 260

barbell overhead press, 353, 354, 368–369

bent-over lat pulldown, for back, 167

bent-over med ball press, 204–205

bent-over row progression, 392–394

bent-over row, 399–402

bilateral high-angle row, 403

bilateral lat stretch, for upper body, 123

bilateral stance dumbbell overhead press, 364–365

biomechanical efficiency, improving with Rhythmic Breathing, 59–61

biphasic positional stretching

    about, 106–107

central nervous system (CNS) and, 197

    exercises, 118–129

    goals of, 108–111

    for lower body, 118–122

    recommendations and guidelines, 112–115

    in 6-phase dynamic warm-up, 66–67, 75, 76, 81

    supplemental options, 124–129

    for upper body, 122–124

bird dog, 135, 149–151

blood flow, activation drills and, 156

body composition, relationship to relative strength, 424

body position

    for hinge, 271–272

    for pulling, 375

    for reverse lunge, 299

    for single-leg RDL, 300

    for split squat, 297–298

    for squat, 236

Bodyweight, Bands, and Dumbbells Program

    about, 480–481

    Rebuild, 488–490

    Reclaim, 485–487

    Regain, 491–493

bodyweight hinge, 285, 286

bodyweight pull-up, 411

bodyweight split squat, 315, 316–317

bodyweight squat, 260, 261, 314

Box Breathing. *See* Tactical Breath

box jumps, 210

box pistol squat, 328–329

bracing

    about, 24–25

    in cueing sequence, 34, 35

    Double Breath Technique and, 49–53

    for hinge, 272

    preplanned strategy for, 36

    reactive strategy for, 36

    for reverse lunge, 299